Foundations of Clinical Nurse Specialist Practice

Janet S. Fulton, PhD, RN, ACNS-BC, FAAN, is professor and program coordinator of the Adult Clinical Nurse Specialist (CNS) program at Indiana University School of Nursing, Science of Nursing Care Department, where she teaches CNS and other graduate courses. She has been teaching CNSs since 1995, having previously worked as a CNS and also having served as clinical preceptor for CNS students. She is most recently known for designing an innovative distance-accessible CNS program called *Learn Where You Live*. She currently is editor in chief of Lippincott Williams Wilkins's *Clinical Nurse Specialist: The International Journal of Advanced Nursing Practice*, the official journal of the National Association of Clinical Nurse Specialists (NACNS), having previously served as president (2002) and treasurer (2000–2001). Dr. Fulton holds memberships in the American Nurses Association, the Oncology Nursing Society, the Multinational Association for Supportive Care in Cancer, and the International Society of Oral Oncology, where she is currently serving as treasurer. She is an ANCC-certified Adult CNS. Her work has been recognized by her peers with awards from Sigma Theta Tau and the NACNS for leadership and from Indiana University School of Nursing for public service; she also was awarded an Indiana University Trustee Teaching Award three different years. She is a fellow in the American Academy of Nursing.

Brenda L. Lyon, PhD, RN, CNS, FAAN, is professor emerita at Indiana University School of Nursing Department of Adult Health. She has taught master of science in nursing (MSN) courses such as the Scientific Basis of CNS Practice, Advanced Practice Roles—Adult Health CNS, Dynamics of Stress and Coping; and PhD courses in Stress and Coping, Self-Care Science, and Health Promotion Science at the School of Nursing. She conducted a private practice as a CNS in Stress-Related Physical Illness from 1975 to 2013. She is a founder of the NACNS and served as president of that organization from 1996 to 1997 and was chair of its Legislative/Regulation Committee from 1997 to 2004. She is a past president of the Indiana State Nurses Association and past chair of that organization's Legislative Committee. As chair, she led the state's effort to change the Nurse Practice Act to incorporate nursing's autonomous scope of practice in 1975 and to establish mandatory licensure for nursing in 1981 as well as title protection for CNSs in 1991. Dr. Lyon served as a consultant to numerous hospitals and corporations in helping to make organizational climates less conducive to stress and consulted with many hospital nursing service departments in advancing the practice of nursing through clinical reasoning and focusing on nursing's autonomous scope of practice. She has conducted hundreds of workshops on conquering stress through learning skills to manage thoughts, thereby eliminating or preventing stress emotions. She is the recipient of the Midwest Nursing Research Society's Advancement in Stress and Coping Research Award and is a fellow in the American Academy of Nursing as well as a fellow in the National Academies of Practice. She is executive vice president, Aircom Manufacturing, Inc., and Medivative Technologies, LLC, and president of Health Potentials Unlimited, LLC (since 1975).

Kelly A. Goudreau, PhD, RN, ACNS-BC, FAAN, is associate director Patient Care Services and nurse executive at the VA Southern Oregon Rehabilitation Center and Clinics (VA SORCC), White City, oregon, and associate editor for *Clinical Nurse Specialist: The International Journal of Advanced Nursing Practice*, Lippincott Williams and Wilkins, from 2008 to present, and is past president, past secretary, and past board member of the NACNS. She has worked clinically as a CNS in a wide variety of specialties and has held a variety of positions including consultant, director of nursing, and nurse administrator. She is licensed as a CNS in Oregon and is certified by the ANCC as a CNS in Adult Health. Among other honors and awards, Dr. Goudreau has received honors from the Oregon Nurses Association for nursing education for 4 years of service as chair of the Oregon Council of CNS, is an NACNS Brenda L. Lyon Leadership award recipient, and is an invited fellow of the American Academy of Nursing. She received the first President's Award from the NACNS in 2013 in recognition of long-term, outstanding contributions to the organization and CNSs everywhere. She has published more than 30 journal articles.

Foundations of Clinical Nurse Specialist Practice

Second Edition

Janet S. Fulton, PhD, RN, ACNS-BC, FAAN
Brenda L. Lyon, PhD, RN, CNS, FAAN
Kelly A. Goudreau, PhD, RN, ACNS-BC, FAAN

Editors

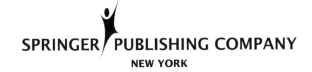

SPRINGER PUBLISHING COMPANY
NEW YORK

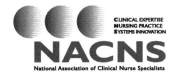

NACNS
National Association of Clinical Nurse Specialists

Springer Publishing Company, LLC
11 West 42nd Street
New York, NY 10036
www.springerpub.com

Acquisitions Editor: Margaret Zuccarini
Composition: Newgen Knowledge Works

ISBN: 978-0-8261-2966-6
e-book ISBN: 978-0-8261-2967-3

17 18 19/ 6 5 4

The author and the publisher of this Work have made every effort to use sources believed to be reliable to provide information that is accurate and compatible with the standards generally accepted at the time of publication. Because medical science is continually advancing, our knowledge base continues to expand. Therefore, as new information becomes available, changes in procedures become necessary. We recommend that the reader always consult current research and specific institutional policies before performing any clinical procedure. The author and publisher shall not be liable for any special, consequential, or exemplary damages resulting, in whole or in part, from the readers' use of, or reliance on, the information contained in this book. The publisher has no responsibility for the persistence or accuracy of URLs for external or third-party Internet websites referred to in this publication and does not guarantee that any content on such websites is, or will remain, accurate or appropriate.

Library of Congress Cataloging-in-Publication Data
Foundations of clinical nurse specialist practice / [edited by] Janet S. Fulton, Brenda L. Lyon, Kelly A. Goudreau. – Second edition.
    p. ; cm.
Includes bibliographical references and index.
ISBN 978-0-8261-2966-6 – ISBN 978-0-8261-2967-3 (e-book)
I. Fulton, Janet S., editor. II. Lyon, Brenda L., editor. III. Goudreau, Kelly A., editor.
[DNLM: 1. Nurse Clinicians—organization & administration. 2. Nursing Process–organization & administration. WY 128]
RT82.8
610.7306'92–dc23
                                                                                                    2014009247

Special discounts on bulk quantities of our books are available to corporations, professional associations, pharmaceutical companies, health care organizations, and other qualifying groups. If you are interested in a custom book, including chapters from more than one of our titles, we can provide that service as well.

For details, please contact:
Special Sales Department, Springer Publishing Company, LLC
11 West 42nd Street, 15th Floor, New York, NY 10036–8002
Phone: 877-687-7476 or 212-431-4370; Fax: 212-941-7842
E-mail: sales@springerpub.com

Printed in the United States of America by McNaughton & Gunn.

Like the first edition, this second edition is dedicated to CNSs everywhere. We know you share our enthusiasm for the role because of your response to the first edition. We salute you! To those who preceded this work, thank you for showing us the way. For our contemporary colleagues, we again thank you and celebrate your dedication to creativity, leadership, and innovation. To future generations, your success is assured with great leaders such as the authors of these chapters guiding your footsteps. May you continue to grow in wisdom while carrying on a proud tradition of advancing the practice of nursing.

Contents

Contributors

Taletha M. Askew, MS, RN, CNS, CCRN
Clinical Nurse Specialist
The Ohio State University Comprehensive Cancer
  Center
Arthur G. James Cancer Hospital and
  Richard J. Solove Research Institute
Columbus, Ohio

Carol L. Baird, PhD, RN, GCNS-BC
Associate Professor Emerita
Indiana University
Indianapolis, Indiana

Nancy Benton, PhD, RN, CNS
Associate Director/Patient Care Services
  Mann-Grandstaff VA Medical Center
Spokane, Washington

Diane Billay, RN, BN, MN, PhD
Nurse Educator–Professional Development
Health Canada
First Nations & Inuit Health Branch
Alberta Region, Edmonton, Alberta, Canada

Janet M. Bingle, RN, MS
Clinical Nurse Specialist, Nursing Care of
  the Adult
Retired, CNO, Community Health Network
Indianapolis, Indiana

Leeann Blue, MSN, RN
Chief Nursing Officer and Executive Vice
  President
Eskenazi Health
Indianapolis, Indiana

Jane L. Bromund, MSN, RN
Clinical Research Scientist
Eli Lilly and Company
Indianapolis, Indiana

**Garrett K. Chan, PhD, APRN, FAEN,
  FPCN, FNAP, FAAN**
Director of Advanced Practice Stanford Hospital
  and Clinics
Stanford, California
Associate Adjunct Professor University of
  California San Francisco
San Francisco, California

**Kathleen Chapman, MSN, RN, NEA-BC,
  FACHE**
Deputy Director-Patient Care Services, CNO
Portland VA Medical Center
Portland, Oregon

Victoria Church, MS, RN, CNS-BC
Associate Director Portland Informatics
  Center
Clinical Nurse Specialist Cardiac Telemetry
Portland VA Medical Center
Portland, Oregon

**Cheryl L. Crisp, PhD, RN, PCNS-BC,
  CRRN**
Assistant Professor
Indiana University-Purdue University at
  Columbus
Columbus, Indiana

Ann L. Cupp Curley, PhD, RN
Nurse Research Specialist
Capital Health
Trenton, New Jersey

Sue B. Davidson, PhD, RN, CNS
Independent Nursing Practice Consultant
Portland, Oregon

Tammie DiPietro, MN, RN
Lawrence S. Bloomberg Faculty of Nursing
University of Toronto
Toronto, Ontario, Canada

Diane M. Doran, RN, PhD, FCAHS
Professor Emerita
Lawrence S. Bloomberg Faculty of Nursing
University of Toronto
Toronto, Ontario, Canada

Kathleen L. Dunn, MS, RN, CRRN,
  CNS-BC
Clinical Nurse Specialist and Rehab Case
  Manager
Spinal Cord Injury/Disease Center (128)
VA San Diego Healthcare System
San Diego, California

Patricia R. Ebright, PhD, RN, FAAN
Associate Professor and Associate Dean for
  Graduate Programs
Indiana University School of Nursing
Indianapolis, Indiana

Naomi E. Ervin, PhD, RN, PHCNS-BC,
  FAAN
Nursing and Health Consultant
Shelby, Michigan

Courtney Federspiel, MBA, MHA
Director, Value-Based Programming
Franciscan Alliance Accountable Care
  Organization
Franciscan St. Francis Health
Indianapolis, Indiana

Ginette G. Ferszt, PhD, RN, PMHCNS-BC
Professor
College of Nursing
University of Rhode Island
Kingston, Rhode Island

Mary L. Fisher, PhD, RN
Associate Vice Chancellor for Academic
  Affairs
Professor of Nursing
Indiana University School of Nursing
Indianapolis, Indiana

Janet S. Fulton, PhD, RN, ACNS-BC, FAAN
Professor
Indiana University School of Nursing
Indianapolis, Indiana

Kelly A. Goudreau, PhD, RN, ACNS-BC,
  FAAN
Associate Director Patient Care Services/
  Nurse Executive
VA Southern Oregon Rehabilitation Center
  and Clinics (VA SORCC)
White City, Oregon

Desiree Hensel, PhD, RN, PCNS-BC, CNE
Assistant Professor
Indiana University School of Nursing
Bloomington, Indiana

Frank D. Hicks, PhD, RN
Professor, Adult Health and Gerontological
  Nursing
Assistant Dean for Generalist Education
Director, Center for Nursing Education
  Innovation and Scholarship
Rush University College of Nursing
Chicago, Illinois

Kimberly S. Hodge, MSN, RN, ACNS-BC,
  CCRN-CMC
Care Coordination Manager
Clinical Nurse Specialist
Franciscan Alliance Accountable Care
  Organization
Franciscan St. Francis Health
Indianapolis, Indiana

Lisa Hopp, PhD, RN FAAN
Professor, College of Nursing
Director, Indiana Center for Evidence-Based
  Nursing Practice
Purdue University Calumet
Hammond, Indiana

Mary Pat Johnston, RN, MS, AOCN®
Oncology Clinical Nurse Specialist
ProHealth Care, Regional Cancer Center
Waukesha Memorial Hospital
Waukesha, Wisconsin

Diana Jones, MSN, RN, ACNS-BC
Medical Clinical Nurse Specialist
St. Vincent Hospital
Indianapolis, Indiana

Jeffrey S. Jones, DNP, PMHCNS-BC, CST, LNC
Pinnacle Mental Health Associates, Inc.
Mansfield, Ohio

Tracey Loudon, MN, RN, CNS, CCNS, CCRN
Critical Care Clinical Nurse Specialist
Portland Veterans Affairs Medical Center
Portland, Oregon

Brenda L. Lyon, PhD, RN, CNS, FAAN
Professor Emerita, Indiana University School
    of Nursing
Executive Vice President, Aircom
    Manufacturing, Inc. and Medivative
    Technologies, LLC
Indianapolis, Indiana
President, Health Potentials Unlimited, LLC
Noblesville, Indiana

Patricia S. Moore, MSN, RN, CDE, CNS
Cofounder and Managing Partner
Clinical Solutions, LLC
Columbus, Indiana

Florence Myrick, PhD, MScN, BN, RN
Professor and Associate Dean, Teaching and
    Learning
Faculty of Nursing
University of Alberta
Edmonton, Alberta, Canada

Barbara S. O'Brien, PhD, CNS
Associate Professor (Retired)
College of Nursing
University of Rhode Island
Kingston, Rhode Island

Colleen O'Leary, MSN, RN, AOCNS
Clinical Nurse Specialist Head and Neck
    Cancer
Coordinator of Nursing Evidence-Based
    Practice
The Ohio State University Comprehensive
    Cancer Center Arthur G. James Cancer
    Hospital and Richard J. Solove Research
    Institute
Columbus, Ohio

Patricia O'Malley, PhD, RN, CNS, CCRN
Nurse Researcher and APRN
Center of Nursing Excellence
Miami Valley Hospital
Dayton, Ohio
Faculty, Indiana University East School of
    Nursing
Richmond, Indiana

Christine M. Pacini, PhD, RN
Dean and Professor
College of Health Professions and McAuley
    School of Nursing
University of Detroit Mercy
Detroit, Michigan

Geraldine S. Pearson, PhD, PMH-CNS, FAAN
Associate Professor
University of Connecticut School of
    Medicine
Farmington, Connecticut

Ginger S. Pierson, MSN, RN, CCRN, CNS
Clinical Nurse Specialist, Emergency
    Department
Hoag Memorial Hospital Presbyterian
Newport Beach, California

Jan M. Powers, PhD, RN, CCRN, CCNS, CNRN, FCCM
Director of Clinical Nurse Specialists and
    Nursing Research
St. Vincent Hospital
Indianapolis, Indiana

Jeannette Richardson, MS, RN, CNS-BC, CCRN
Primary Care Clinical Nurse Specialist
Portland Veterans Affairs Medical Center
Portland, Oregon

Jo Ellen Rust, MSN, RN, CNS
Clinical Nurse Specialist for Children with
 Complex Health Care Needs
Riley Circle of Care Program
Riley Hospital for Children
Indianapolis, Indiana

Maria R. Shirey, PhD, MBA, RN, NEA-BC,
 FACHE FAAN
Assistant Dean, Clinical Affairs and
 Partnerships
Professor, Community Health, Outcomes
 and Systems
The University of Alabama at Birmingham
School of Nursing
Birmingham, Alabama

Mary A. Short, MSN, RN
Clinical Research Scientist
Eli Lilly and Company
Indianapolis, Indiana

Souraya Sidani, PhD
Professor and Canada Research Chair
Ryerson University School of Nursing
Toronto, Ontario, Canada

Kathleen C. Solotkin, MSN, RN
Clinical Research Scientist
Lilly USA, LLC
Indianapolis, Indiana

Lori D. Stark, MSN, RN, ONC
Orthopaedic Clinical Nurse Specialist
St. Vincent Hospital
Indianapolis, Indiana

Michelle L. Treon, MSN, RN, OCN,
 CNS-BC
Oncology Clinical Nurse Specialist
Indiana University Health, University
 Hospital
Indianapolis, Indiana

Kathleen M. Vollman, MSN, RN, CCNS,
 FCCM, FAAN
Clinical Nurse Specialist, Educator,
 Consultant
Advancing Nursing LLC
Northville, Michigan

Jane A. Walker, PhD, RN
Associate Professor and Graduate Program
 Coordinator College of Nursing
Purdue University Calumet
Hammond, Indiana

Stacy Webster-Wharton, PE, VA FAC P/PM
Chief Engineer/Chief of Facilities
 Maintenance
VA Southern Oregon Rehabilitation Center
 and Clinics
White City, Oregon

Kathy D. Wright, MSN, RN, CWOCN-AP,
 ACHRN
Community Education Specialist
Nanticoke Wound Care and Hyperbaric
 Center
Seaford, Delaware

Foreword

The mission of the National Association of Clinical Nurse Specialists (NACNS) is to enhance and promote the unique, high-value contribution of the clinical nurse specialist to the health and well-being of individuals, families, groups, and communities, and to promote and advance the practice of nursing. As health care organizations respond to financial losses and increased expenditures, technology changes at a rapid pace, and frontline staff experience knowledge-acquisition fatigue, the CNS is in a pivotal position to continue to work within all spheres of influence to explore and provide short- and long-term solutions, plan and facilitate change, and positively impact the safety and quality of patient care delivery and patient outcomes. In this era of national health care transformation and reform, the clinical nurse specialist advanced practice nurse is uniquely positioned to lead, guide, and transform care delivery and interprofessional teams in a variety of settings and with a variety of specialty populations. A demand for improved quality and safety, evidence-based practice, and the demonstration of clinical and process outcome measures combined with cost savings is the system and organizational work of the CNS. Thus, the expectation for an increase in demand for CNSs who possess the sophisticated knowledge and skills necessary to successfully accomplish change and improvement at this challenging and complex time is palpable.

This second edition of *Foundations of Clinical Nurse Specialist Practice* is being released at a crucial time. Drs. Fulton, Lyon, and Goudreau have provided a comprehensive textbook for the CNS in practice across the continuum. An excellent resource for students and their faculty, novices, and the most experienced CNSs, the text provides an overview of the essentials of CNS practice including chapters on the professional attributes of the CNS and the framework for clinical practice. The CNS spheres of client and direct care, nurses and nursing practice, and organizations and systems are reflected throughout the various chapters of this book with consultation, education, coaching, mentorship, and leadership addressed. The material presented is certain to provide direction and to strengthen the core competencies of the CNS.

New chapters address program evaluation, accountable care organizations, and CNS practice in primary care. These are timely and will provide direction to those expanding or re-envisioning their roles at this time. The exemplars also provide important information as it relates to establishing a new and unique program, identifying new populations and methods to improve outcomes for unique services.

NACNS is honored to support this all-inclusive work that has targeted essential and key components of CNS practice today.

Carol Manchester, MSN, ACNS-BC,
BC-ADM, CDE
President
National Association of Clinical
Nurse Specialists

Preface

Clinical nurse specialists (CNSs) make unique contributions to the health and safety of the public by working directly and indirectly with patients, families, groups, and communities. These contributions often occur through clinical intervention and leadership at the point of nursing care delivery and are carried out by influencing factors that impact the point of delivery and leading multidisciplinary teams in system-focused practice improvement. CNSs are clinical experts in a specialty area of practice. They provide their clinical expertise while also diffusing expert knowledge about phenomena central to nursing practice, such as pain (symptoms), mobility, nutrition, and skin integrity, which cut across specialties. CNSs help to shape specialty-focused practice innovations by identifying new or changing nursing care needs and by bringing new advanced nursing knowledge to well-established specialty practice areas.

Across diverse specialties, CNSs exhibit core practice competencies that cluster into three domains. The domains, also referred to as spheres of influence, are client, nursing practice/nurses, and system/organization. CNSs bridge the gap between what is known through research and what is practiced. They also collaborate with all system stakeholders in the removal of system barriers that impede the delivery of safe and cost-effective care. A wide range of knowledge is required to practice effectively in all three domains. Today, perhaps more than ever before in the context of health care reform, the contributions of CNSs to quality, cost-effective care are vital.

The second edition of this book is written again as a textbook to be used in the education of CNSs and the continuing development of practicing CNSs, and is consistent with the competencies required to effectively practice in the three spheres of influence. No one book can ever include the expanse of knowledge needed by CNSs. As editors, we included content believed to be core foundational knowledge for CNS practice, knowledge that will help CNS students and practicing CNSs achieve the core competencies. The basic organizational structure of the book has not changed from the first edition. Chapters are updated and new chapters are added. Unit I begins with an overview of the evolution of CNSs from the 1940s to present, setting the stage for understanding contemporary CNS practice. Also included are chapters describing the professional attributes of CNSs, the philosophical underpinnings of CNS practice, and nurse-sensitive outcome measures. Units II, III, and IV include content supporting the *how* of CNS practice. For example, there are chapters devoted to clinical reasoning, designing and evaluating interventions, working in complex systems, influencing quality, and promoting patient safety. Unit V addresses the business of CNS practice such as entrepreneurship, billing and reimbursement, and understanding the regulation of CNS practice. Unit VI includes exemplars demonstrating CNS practice in different settings—hospital, private practice, business and industry, and entrepreneurship ventures. The last unit, Unit VII, offers 10 short vignettes describing CNS practice in various specialties.

It is our fervent belief that the future of CNSs and of CNS practice is brighter than ever and that the need for the unique contributions of CNSs will be increasingly in demand as hospitals and other health care settings are moved to accountable care organizations (ACOs) and performance-based reimbursement. We hope that faculty teaching in programs preparing CNSs, CNS students, and practicing CNSs will find this book to be a helpful resource.

Janet S. Fulton, PhD, RN, ACNS-BC, FAAN
Brenda L. Lyon, PhD, RN, CNS, FAAN
Kelly A. Goudreau, PhD, RN, ACNS-BC, FAAN

Acknowledgments

Many thanks are in order to the individuals who supported development of the second edition of this book. To our contributors, you are the best. And since we know you are supported by family, friends, secretaries, administrators, and others, we are most grateful to this legion of unknown but very important people. Thanks to the staff at Springer Publishing Company, especially Margaret Zuccarini, Publisher, for her guidance, patience, and support. A special thanks to Linda Wright and Barbara Saligoe for the million things they do in support of Dr. Fulton's work.

We also thank our family, friends, and colleagues for their support in our continued efforts to ensure a knowledgeable, well-prepared CNS workforce. To the leadership, past and present, of the NACNS, we salute you for all you have contributed to advancing the CNS role and practice.

J.S.F., B.L.L., K.A.G.

Many thanks to my husband, Morgan, and sons Alexander and David Fulton. Your spirit, humor, and support make a project like this possible. I'm forever grateful to have you in my life.

Janet S. Fulton

Thanks to CNS leaders of the past on whose shoulders we stand! Thanks, again, to my many CNS colleagues/ friends who inspire me every day with your talent and unwavering commitment to the improvement of patient care and outcomes. Because of you and the staff you empower, patients are better off and even saved every day!

Brenda L. Lyon

To my family... especially my husband Serge now that we have entered into the empty-nester phase of our lives. I know that there were many times that you wanted to do something and I simply could not because of one thing or another. To the students whom I have had the great privilege of working with over the years who have said to me "You mean you are THAT Kelly Goudreau?!" Your energy and enthusiasm for the role of the CNS is enduring and will ensure the positive future safety and quality outcomes in health care for years to come. Thank you!

Kelly A. Goudreau

Evolution of the Clinical Nurse Specialist Role and Practice in the United States

Janet S. Fulton

*B*eginning in the 1940s, much has been written about the need for a clinical expert in nursing practice and the clinical nurse specialist (CNS) role. An electronic search of the Cumulative Index to Nursing and Allied Health Literature (CINAHL) database from 1971 (earliest date available for e-search) to 2013 found about 5,000 articles, and a search of OVID Nursing from 1950 to 2013 found over 6,000 articles, both using the search term CNS. With so much literature available, it is possible to look back at the history of the CNS not just as a series of events but also as the development of the profession's thinking about advanced practice, a sort of evolution of thinking where it is possible to see the rationale for the role as shaped by history and the expectations for practice across the decades. This kind of look-back provides a good base for envisioning the opportunities and challenges in the future. To achieve an understanding of the historical development of the CNS role, this chapter explores the rationale for creating the role, educational and social challenges, and past and current conceptualization of practice. From the 1940s to the present, it is possible to trace the CNS role and its legacy of leadership for advancing the practice of nursing.

EARLY HISTORICAL ROOTS

Evidence indicates that the idea for a clinical expert in nursing emerged in the 1940s. In the first textbook written for CNSs, *The Clinical Nurse Specialist: Interpretations* by Riehl and McVay (1973), the editors suggested that the 1923 Winslow-Goldmark Committee report on nursing education, sponsored by the Rockefeller Foundation, set in motion events creating a need for clinical experts in nursing practice. Also called *The Study of Nursing and Nursing Education in the United States*, the report noted inadequacies in hospital nursing education and identified as a central problem the extended hours of service worked by students in apprenticeship hospital training programs. A poor educational option, hospital training was made worse by lack of curricular standards, insufficient pedagogical knowledge among faculty, and inadequate instruction in the application of science and theory to practice (Bullough & Bullough, 1979; Ellis & Hartley, 2004; McHenry, 1983). As a result of these findings, nursing placed great emphasis on roles of teaching and administration in an effort to improve academic curricula, the scientific quality of nursing content, and clinical education experiences. Evidence of this focus on educators and clinical supervisors can be seen in the preface to Wolf's (1947) textbook for nurses:

> The never-ending task of improving the quality of nursing practice falls squarely upon the shoulders of the teaching personnel in schools of nursing and in public health nursing agencies. Those who are responsible for planning and providing the classroom and field practice experiences for nurse students are constantly striving to enrich these learning experiences and keep them in line with newer developments in the broad field of public health and preventative medicine. (p. v)

The 1948 release of Esther Lucile Brown's *The Future of Nursing* (Brown, 1948) further reinforced the need to improve nursing education. Called the *Brown Report*, it also criticized hospital training programs while strongly advocating for collegiate-level nursing education. Less well noted in the report was Brown's observation of an overemphasis on teaching and administration at the expense of patient care—the pendulum had swung too far. She called for increasing efforts to help students develop clinical knowledge and expert skill necessary for supporting direct care of patients; to better prepare nurses for the care of persons both sick and well; and to teach scientific knowledge and create opportunities for students to apply knowledge in the care of patients. Nurses, Brown argued, needed to possess discriminative judgment and be able to exert leadership. In particular, she noted that nurses needed to be able to (a) make a unique contribution to the prevention and treatment of illness; (b) improve nursing skills and develop new nursing skills; (c) teach and supervise other nurses and ancillary workers; and (d) cooperate with other professions in planning for health at community, state, national, and international levels (Allen, Koos, Bradley, & Wolf, 1948).

In 1956, the National League for Nursing (NLN) sponsored the National Working Conference in Williamsburg, Virginia, to discuss the need for a psychiatric clinical expert (NLN, 1958). With the prevailing emphasis on programs to train teachers and administrators, conference participants determined that a new role should be created. The purpose of this new role, labeled *clinical specialist*, was "to bring about advances in the art and science of psychiatric nursing and to promote the application of new knowledge and methods in the care of patients" (NLN, 1958/1973, p. 8). The new specialist role was to be prepared at the graduate degree level. The final conference report included a description of clinical competencies for the new role and basic elements of a graduate-level curriculum.

Concerns about the lack of attention to developing clinical nursing experts continued. Appointed the first dean of the Graduate School of Nursing at New York Medical College, Frances Reiter became a leading voice for developing educational programs to prepare advanced clinical experts in many different specialty areas (Hiestand, 2006). Reiter's 1961 essay *Improvement in Nursing Practice* criticized hospital nursing service departments for devaluing direct patient care provided by the graduate nurses (*graduate nurse* being the term used for what are now called registered nurses). She asserted that hospital nursing services were controlled by nurses who were not clinically skilled but rather were highly influenced by policies of hospital administration (Reiter, 1961). In addressing the American Nurses Association (ANA), she forecast a preferred future:

> I believe that someday an Academy of Nursing will be established. Membership in this academy will be an honorable one. The members will be selected from those practitioners who are clinical nursing specialists. Because of their values in practice, their clinical knowledge and their judgment, this corps of practitioners will give us professional leadership in advancing the excellence of our practice. (Reiter, 1961, p. 18)

As a dean, Reiter's goal was to prepare a new kind of expert clinical nurse. In 1948, she had chaired the second of five studies funded by the W. K. Kellogg Foundation to develop teaching and learning experiences for nurses, the *Study of Advanced Clinical Nursing Education* (Hiestand, 2006). In 1966, she again called for a renewed emphasis on clinical practice and described an expert nurse-clinician. This expert nurse-clinician was to be a master practitioner for all dimensions of nursing practice—able to provide both basic and technical care while using discriminative judgment in "assessing problems" [diagnosis], "determining care priorities," and "selecting nursing measures" [interventions] to achieve "therapeutic objectives" [outcomes]. The expert nurse-clinician would possess sound knowledge of basic sciences and principles underlying care and would use this knowledge to promote quality of care and remove system-level barriers to care delivery. As she expressed it, the expert nurse-clinician would be "committed to 'hacking' her way down through the personnel pyramid so that her professional knowledge and judgment are exerted on behalf of every patient" (Reiter, 1966, p. 9). Further, the expert nurse-clinician's motivation, judgment, and expert skills were envisioned to benefit patients both directly and indirectly because the visible expertise of this clinician was expected to provide leadership for the nursing staff in the delivery of patient care.

In summary, the early history of the CNS was a vision of a clinically expert role in nursing in response to a growing need for knowledgeable and skilled nurses to provide direct care and to lead the delivery of nursing care by others. An expert clinical nurse was expected to be grounded in theory and scientific evidence, possess high-level clinical skill, and be able to advance nursing care techniques, mentor nursing staff, assure excellence and quality, collaborate with other care providers, and remove system barriers to care delivery. This vision of the clinical expert created the CNS role.

THE CNS ROLE TAKES SHAPE

Role is defined as a set of expected functions of a person and is characterized by a pattern of behavior in a given social context. CNS is a functional role in nursing actualized through a set of professional practice competencies. These competencies are learned through formal academic preparation at the graduate level. The commitment to graduate education—education that included a practice component—was championed as the best educational approach. In 1971, Plawecki wrote,

> Through formal, higher education the nurse gains deeper knowledge into theories and principles as they pertain to nursing. Through practice the nurse gains insight into the applicability of the principles in the care of patients. The combination makes the clinical nurse specialist. (p. 49)

Multiple articles, which began to appear in the 1960s, helped to define and establish the core practice competencies of the CNS role. MacPhail (1971), assistant dean for clinical nursing, Case Western Reserve University, and associate to assistant administrator for nursing, University Hospitals of Cleveland, summarized much of the prevailing thinking about the expectation for the role from her combined academic and practice perspective. The competencies of the new clinical expert role were expected to include synthesizing physical, biological, and behavioral sciences for application to practice; serving as role model for staff; assessing the care given by other staff and identifying needs for improvement; providing consultation in an area of specialization; teaching both patients and personnel; understanding group dynamics; demonstrating high-level interpersonal skills; working effectively with the health care team; serving as change agent; fostering inquiry; identifying problems for investigation; participating in research; and fostering initiative, resourcefulness, and creativity in improving patient

outcomes. Table 1.1 summarizes the role description and core competencies identified in the literature of the 1960s and early 1970s. Not until 1998 were the common functional role competencies of CNS practice enunciated (NACNS, 1998). These first-ever CNS core practice competencies, issued by a professional organization, relied heavily on a review of the literature and the job descriptions of practicing CNSs (Baldwin et al., 2007). The common agreed-upon expectations summarized by MacPhail were evident in the job descriptions of contemporary CNSs, and most of the early expectations were incorporated into the first set of competencies. Subsequent iterations of CNS role competencies (NACNS, 2004, 2008) have included these same competencies, making for remarkable consistency in the expectations of the CNS role across the past 50 years.

ADVANCED SPECIALTY PRACTICE

At the same time the CNS role was being conceptualized, specialization in health care was evolving and creeping into nursing practice. In 1949, the idea of specialization was introduced at a conference of graduate program directors convened at the University of Minnesota (Sills, 1983). In 1967, Little (1967) noted that specialization in nursing had moved well beyond the usual fields of public health and hospital nursing and the usual functions of teaching and supervision. Specialization was emerging in clinical areas based on body systems, age, type of illness, and scientific content areas and, with reluctance, Little (1967) conceded that specialization in nursing had indeed arrived.

The idea of specialty-focused practice for nurses was discussed in the first issue of the *American Journal of Nursing* in an article by Katherine DeWitt (1900). DeWitt's comments were prompted by the turn-of-the-century emergence of specialties in medicine and health care practices. Physicians were becoming more focused on medical practice; dentistry and pharmacology were becoming autonomous specialty practices and no longer services provided by the physician. DeWitt stated a belief that all nurses should first be trained as generalists and, while she saw no immediate need for specialists, conceded that a nurse could pursue a specialty out of personal interest. Should a nurse choose a specialty, she (all nurses were referred to using the feminine pronoun in most early nursing literature) should engage in additional and continued studies in the specialty area and likewise should keep abreast of advances in science in the specialty.

The importance of specialization in nursing continued to be debated. In a landmark paper, Peplau

TABLE 1.1

SUMMARY OF SELECTED EARLY PUBLICATIONS ABOUT CNS ROLE AND COMPETENCIES DESCRIPTIONS			
Descriptions of CNS Role	**Descriptions of CNS Competencies**	**Year**	**Reference**
Independent provider for continuity of care; clinical leader for nursing staff	Explore and study (research) ways to improve patient care; understand patient needs; apply theory to practice; observe and report results objectively	1964	Crawford
Independent clinician; model of expertness representing advanced or newly developing practices	Clinical expert; develop innovations in practice based on emerging knowledge; interprofessional collaboration	1965	Peplau
Expert nurse in direct care of patients; working with other nurses to improve performance	Work with difficult patients; analyze needs; problem solve; interpret nursing care principles to nursing personnel	1966	Anderson
Expert professional practitioner; assumes direct and continuing responsibility for nursing care of patients	High levels of knowledge and cognitive ability demonstrated in practice; skilled decision maker; high level of ability in identifying patient problems and selecting intervention	1967	Johnson, Wilcox & Moidel
Professional nurse with advanced knowledge and competence in nursing	Activities include many things: teaching, providing leadership in planning patient care, or exclusively practicing direct nursing care	1968	Towner
A nurse who practices nursing by applying specific, relevant theories and knowledge from nursing and allied disciplines to person requiring specialized nursing services	Deliver expert care; guide allied nursing personnel as teacher and model; innovate or initiate change; contribute to nursing knowledge through research and practice; coordinate activities with persons in allied disciplines; consult with those requiring clinical nursing judgment and knowledge	1969	Berlinger
Expert nurse with definite responsibility for influencing patient care	Uses a theoretical framework for change—one that allows for description and analysis of problems for organizing and interpreting what the nurse perceives; brings about through conscious, deliberate, and collaborative effort the improvement of patient care	1969	Gorden
Nurse with special preparation through education and experience to serve as expert practitioner and consultant	Practitioner providing direct care; consultant directing, guiding, and assisting nursing staff to provide nursing care to patients; educator providing staff development to improve clinical competence; collaborates in initiating and facilitating patient care programs with health team members	1973	Kurihara

(1965) discussed the nature of specialties in clinical nursing practice and noted three social trends that gave rise to specialty practice: (a) increasing knowledge about a phenomenon, (b) new technology emerging from new knowledge, and (c) emerging areas of public need. *Specialization* was defined as a division or partitioning of a more general area of practice along some logical lines. It involves a narrowing and deepening of focus or a combination of aspects of different areas of knowledge and practice

competencies with a simultaneous narrowing and deepening of focus (Peplau, 1965). Specialties were acknowledged as the inevitable result of new knowledge and demands of the public for new services (Smoyak, 1976). As such, specialties are adaptations arising in response to scientific and technological discoveries and continuously evolving to meet health concerns in a society. Specialties evolve and are refined, promoted, and molded, become outdated and are discarded. Most importantly, specialties are determined by society's needs for nursing care. Specialization gives the nursing profession the ability to address the public's need for services by expanding and contracting focus. Areas for specialty practice suggested by Peplau in 1965, summarized in Table 1.2, were intended as examples and expressly considered as neither exhaustive nor static, only suggestions based on observation about nursing practice at the time.

Creating specialties required thoughtful consideration and attention to possible problems. Peplau (1965) offered two cautions where specialty practice was concerned. The first caution addressed the growing complexity of health care delivery, particularly in post–World War II hospitals, which saw the emergence of multiple types of care providers. She noted that "nurses must pinpoint intersecting, overlapping, and identical functions and activities which they share with other professional disciplines. *And nurses must identify their unique nursing functions*" (Peplau, 1965, p. 276). Peplau's caution echoes Brown's (1948) earlier recommendation that nursing identify its unique contribution to patient care anchored in nursing knowledge and skill. Peplau was concerned that nurses not gravitate into practice areas and specialties where they would merely be duplicating the services offered by others. Peplau's second caution addressed keeping specialization efforts focused on developing *clinical experts* in patient care. Experts in the delivery of patient care services, such as care coordinators or others with responsibilities for supervisory or administrative duties, were different from,

and should not be substituted for, clinical experts in specialty patient care.

Specialties ebb and flow, adapting to the availability of knowledge, advances in technology, and public health demands. Today, due to advances in antibiotic therapies, nurses specializing in tuberculosis hospital care are not needed. Similarly, Peplau could not have foreseen a need for clinical specialists in AIDS, a disease that was only described in the 1980s. It has been, and remains, the responsibility of CNSs, grounded in nursing theory, science, and use of evidence in practice, to interpret needs and bring nursing expertise to new and emerging specialties for the public good.

Defining Specialty Practice

Specialization eventually was recognized as a mark of advancement for the profession (ANA, 1980; Snyder, 1990). In 1980, ANA defined specialization in nursing as

> a narrowed focus on a part of the whole field of nursing involving the application of [a]broad range of theories to selected phenomena within the domain of nursing in order to secure depth of understanding as a basis for advances in nursing practice. (p. 21)

At present, *specialty* is defined by the ANA (2010) as a delimited or concentrated area of expert clinical practice with focused knowledge and competencies. The American Board of Nurse Specialties

TABLE 1.2

AREAS OF SPECIALIZATION SUGGESTED BY PEPLAU (1965)	
Areas of Specialization	**Examples**
Areas of practice	General hospitals, psychiatric hospitals, tuberculosis hospitals, mental retardation centers, industry
Organs and body systems	Cardiac, renal, and cardiac surgery
Age of client	Infant, premature infant, child, juvenile, adolescent, adult, and geriatric
Degree of illness	Progressive care, acute illness, convalescent care, and chronic illness services
Length of illness	Short-term (ambulatory), intermediate, and long-term
Fields of knowledge	Knowledge gives rise to new terminology; for example, nuclear nursing, interpersonal nursing, electronics nursing, and space nursing
Subroles of the work role of staff nurse	Mother-surrogate nurse, expert technical nurse, health teacher, nurse counselor
Professional goal	Rehabilitation nursing, prevention nursing, curative nursing, ameliorative nursing
Clinical services	Medical, surgical, maternal, pediatric, psychiatric-mental health

Source: From Peplau (1965).

(ABNS) defined a *specialty* as (a) a distinct and well-defined field of nursing that subscribes to the overall purpose and function of nursing and is national in scope, and (b) possessing a tested body of research or data-based knowledge related to the nursing specialty (Accreditation Board for Specialty Nurse Certification [ABSNC], 2012; Burns & Welk, 1997).

The method for determining specialties in nursing has developed along with the total number of specialties. Styles (1990) advocated for a single, central authority designated to recognize specialties and specialty standards to give nursing a source of authority for its specialties. Without a central authority in nursing, Styles argued, specialties would be self-declared and self-ordained, susceptible to internal fluctuations and disorganization, and vulnerable to outside forces competing for power and resources. In contrast, Snyder (1990) noted that because nursing is continuously developing its body of knowledge and is also part of a dynamic health care system and society, any organizing framework for specialization in nursing would be, of necessity, continuously evolving.

At present, many CNSs practice well-established specialties attached to large professional organizations, several of which have created scope and standards for CNS practice in the specialty, such as the *Scope of Practice and Standards of Professional Performance for Acute and Critical-Care Clinical Nurse Specialist* (American Association of Critical Care Nurses, 2010) and the *Oncology Clinical Nurse Specialist Competencies* (Oncology Nursing Society, 2008). For these established specialties, Styles's vision of a central authority that recognizes and regulates the specialty is a good fit. However, for smaller, emerging specialties, Snyder's arguments are a better fit. ABSNC's (2012) criterion for determining a specialty includes role delineation and job analysis data as evidence of a unique role for providers practicing in the specialty. Small and emerging specialties often lack the number of providers to conduct role delineation studies. Further, role delineation studies may simply codify existing practice and not provide the insights necessary for advancing practice in new directions. The inability to be recognized in a specialty is an ongoing concern for CNSs who, as practice leaders, historically have been, and likely will continue to serve, on the forefront of newly emerging specialties. In 2004, NACNS stated that CNS practice specialties could be identified as population, type of problem, setting, type of care, or disease. The fluidity of specialty practice can be seen by reviewing Table 1.2, where many of the specialties proposed by Peplau in 1965 are no longer relevant, made obsolete by changes in medical treatment, technology, and economics, changes that have in turn given rise to newer and different specialties.

Evolving CNS Specialty Practice

There is a dearth of information describing the process for evolving CNS and other advanced practice nursing roles; only one reference could be located, a three-stage model proposed by Hanson and Hamric (2003). According to their model, in Stage I a specialty emerges from within a practice setting in response to unmet patient needs in a health care system, and often involving activities not valued by physicians yet not really a nursing role. Nurses in this stage attain on-the-job skills and expand practice to encompass the new activity. In Stage II, organized training develops for nurses performing the new, special activity. Training is institution- or agency-specific and uses an apprentice model with emphasis on skill development. Anesthesia, midwifery, and nurse practitioner are offered as examples of specialties that began with apprentice-based training programs (Hanson & Hamric, 2003). In Stage III, graduate nursing education with a standardized curriculum emerges for the specialty. The model was modified and a Stage IV proposed by Salyer and Hamric (2008). Stage IV encompasses the period when the specialty role is clearly articulated within the profession, is recognized by other providers, and has corresponding certification available for nurses in the specialty.

While descriptive of some advanced practice roles, this model fails to describe the evolution of CNS practice. CNS role was conceived by nursing leaders to address a void in clinical practice expertise in nursing and, from the beginning, was intended to be an advanced nursing role—not a role to fill gaps for hospital tasks or chores viewed as undesirable by physicians. CNS education did not begin as an institutional apprenticeship; it was designed to be graduate education from the very beginning. Apprentice-type training programs never existed for preparing the CNS for practice. Standardized educational expectations for CNSs were not developed, however, resulting in an array of consequences to be discussed later in this chapter. Certification programs were developed to validate expertise and were limited to those with at least 3 years of CNS practice experience, and certification options were created for some but not all CNS specialties.

Uncoupling *role* from *specialty* is critical to understanding the evolution of the CNS. The role, which is a set of functions, is different from specialty knowledge and skills and the context in which the role is practiced. Making a distinction between role and specialty facilitates development of core role competencies that can apply to all practitioners in the role while also facilitating implementation of the same role in different specialties. The NACNS (1998, 2004, 2008) core CNS practice competencies identify CNS role competencies regardless of specialty. Also, distinguishing role from specialty allows CNSs to expand practice into emerging and narrow specialties and thus fulfill the original intent of the role: to lead the advancement of nursing in meeting the public need. An appropriate model describing the evolution for CNS role and practice, based on historical development of the role, is as follows:

- Stage I: Scientific discovery, knowledge, and technology create a public need for nursing services in a new area. CNSs practicing in related specialties begin to interpret needs for nursing services in the new area.
- Stage II: CNSs combine new and existing scientific knowledge with existing clinical expertise and begin defining and providing nursing services in the area of need.
- Stage III: CNSs provide leadership for other nurses in providing services in the emerging specialty area by disseminating knowledge, role modeling, and mentoring to improve clinical outcomes. CNSs lead the development of norms and standards of care for nursing practice in the newly emerging specialty.
- Stage IV: CNSs engage in developing and promoting competency validation for nurses providing care to the specialty. Practice competencies are validated by professional certification or other mechanisms.

With the roots of advanced practice nursing firmly grounded in clinical practice, it was easy to confuse professional role with employer job description. In 1989, Hamric wrote that the CNS title was, unfortunately, being seen by some nurses as a professional attribute based on education and not a discrete work role. Boyle (1996) noted that the use of the CNS title by master's-prepared nurses not functioning in the job role contributed to confusion about the role. Such statements represent confusion within the profession about the difference between professional role preparation and an employer-based job description. For a more in-depth discussion about CNS title use and protection, see Chapter 28.

CNS EDUCATION

In 1943, the NLN appointed a committee to identify guiding assumptions and basic principles for developing clinically grounded postgraduate nursing courses (Mayo, 1944). The third guiding assumption stated,

The fundamental purpose of all advanced clinical nursing courses is the further preparation of qualified graduate nurses as clinical nursing specialists in order to ensure a constantly improving quality of nursing practice. (Mayo, 1944, p. 581)

This guiding assumption used the term *clinical nursing specialist* and linked the role to improved nursing practice. Written prior to the release of the 1948 Brown report, it is evidence of the nursing profession's self-awareness of the need to promote and advance quality clinical care, and a clinical nursing specialist was the vision for achieving this goal. It was also noted that advanced clinical courses would provide a path for professional advancement and dispel the prevailing myth that career advancement meant leaving nursing for another profession. Between 1944 and 1946, a Subcommittee of Nurse Specialists under the direction of the NLN Education Committee on Postgraduate Clinical Nursing Courses used the guiding assumptions and basic principles to develop four advanced specialty nursing practice curricula: maternity, pediatrics, psychiatry, and tuberculosis.

Graduate education slowly became available, yet very few nurses held bachelor's degrees and it was difficult to establish cohorts of baccalaureate-prepared nurses for master's-level classes. Throughout the 1940s and 1950s, diploma- and bachelor-prepared nurses often enrolled in the same courses; the only determinant of the degree granted was the degree held upon enrollment. Course content varied widely and classes did not always contain theory and science. During this same time, specialty education was largely controlled by hospitals and used by administrators to recruit nurses and manipulate the nursing workforce for hospital goals (Smoyak, 1976). Not until theory, science, and specialty practice knowledge were embedded in academic curricula did the reality of a graduate-prepared specialist as expert clinician emerge. The first graduate specialty program to prepare only CNSs as expert clinicians was the graduate program in advanced psychiatric nursing at Rutgers University in New Jersey. The design and delivery of the program as a specialty-focused graduate program was important because up to that point graduate courses included students seeking options in administration or teaching and were not necessarily always taught by faculty in the specialty or with an advanced degree (Smoyak, 1976).

Curriculum recommendations were developed for CNS educational programs but not formally organized as a curricular standard. The 1969 NLN report, *Extending the Boundaries of Nursing Education* (NLN, 1969), failed to reach a single definition of the clinical specialist and called for the role to be flexible. However, a cluster of role components were identified: therapist/practitioner, teacher, consultant, researcher, and change agent. The therapist/practitioner component was a direct care provider in a specialty area of expertise and included assessment, interpreting cues, and intervention. The teacher component included one-on-one bedside work with staff nurses, formal (classes) and informal (in-service) staff development programs, assessment of staff competencies, interpretation of the nursing literature, and building of staff nurses' skills. The consultant component was linked to the ability to move about in the system—"unit to unit"—offering expertise and knowledge as needed and responding to calls by staff nurses for assistance in solving problems. Change agent was described as ability to effect changes in the health care delivery system. No description of research was included. The report emphasized placing a CNS in the clinical setting so she would be able to move about without interference while being an integral part of the staff because she would be able to identify staff needs and help them develop professionally. To prepare a graduate student to perform competently in the role components, four educational requirements were recommended. These requirements are listed in Table 1.3.

The 1969 NLN report advocated four educational strands for all CNS education: the process of nursing, the process of clinical nursing specialization, the process of scientific investigation, and the process of communication (Berlinger, 1969). In addition, each student was expected to evolve a philosophy of nursing practice congruent with her philosophy of nursing and adopt or develop a conceptual framework

TABLE 1.3

EARLY CNS EDUCATIONAL REQUIREMENTS
1. A broad base in the psychopathology and pathophysiology related to the clinical specialty. Even though the nurse planned to specialize in the nursing care of patient with neurological conditions, for example, her preparation should include a sound foundation in the whole medical-surgical nursing area
2. Knowledge and skills in the clinical practice of the specialty and in teaching and research
3. The behavioral sciences essential to the leadership role and to prepare the person to be a change agent
4. Knowledge and understanding of the social framework in which health care is given. Some participants felt that public health nursing concepts would be sufficient; others suggested a breadth of knowledge of social agencies and societal influences

Source: From NLN (1969).

for nursing practice. Clinical experiences in the specialty area were recommended for the purpose of knowledge of scientific investigation, critical analysis of current research, the conduct of independent research, and the care of patients in the specific specialty.

Subsequent descriptions of CNS curricula were published with similarities but not agreement. McIntyre (1970) listed five essential content areas underpinning the CNS program at the University of California, San Francisco: (a) intense study and experience with complex, specialized health problems; (b) opportunity to use advanced technology; (c) deliberative and continuous exchange with members of other health professions; (d) participation with members of the community in the improvement of nursing care; and (e) opportunity to identify the unknowns in care, including participation in research. Rhein (1973) outlined the curriculum at University of California Los Angeles, noting a strong emphasis on the care of patients and families with one academic quarter of introduction to clinical practice and two quarters of actual clinical practice. The focus of clinical practice was assessment, diagnosis, and planning interventions for patients within a philosophy-conceptual framework. Rubin (1969) reported implementing a specialty-focused PhD degree for maternity and pediatric nursing at the University of Pittsburgh.

The number of CNS programs began to expand after the Nurse Training Act of 1964 (PL 88–581), Title II of the 1968 Health Manpower Act (PL 92–158), and the Nurse Training Act of 1975 (PL 94–63; Hawkins & Thibodeau, 1993). From 1974 to 1975, the NLN reported 65 universities offering master's programs in nursing; of these, 90% offered some type of clinical focus. Program titles varied, making it difficult to distinguish the specialty focus and depth of clinical experiences (Smoyak, 1976). By 1984, the NLN reported 129 accredited programs preparing CNSs (NLN, 1984). In 2003, Walker and colleagues identified 157 separate CNS programs/majors offered by 139 different schools (Walker et al., 2003). In a national survey conducted several years later, Spross and colleagues reported a total of 215 schools self-reporting CNS programs/majors (Spross, Gerard, & France, 2006). In 2013, the American Association of Colleges of Nursing (AACN) reported a total of 250 CNS programs/majors in the United States (Fang, Li, & Bednash, 2013).

The CNS title was rarely protected by statute or regulation. Nurses not prepared in CNS graduate programs assumed the title or were given the title *clinical specialist* by employers. In 1980, the ANA published the first edition of its *Social Policy Statement*, recognizing the CNS as an expert clinician with a specialty focus and a graduate degree. This document helped further to entrench the expectation for CNS graduate education with a specialty focus.

> The specialist in nursing practice is a nurse who, through study and supervised practice at the graduate level (master's or doctorate) has become an expert in a defined area of knowledge and practice in a selected clinical area of nursing. (ANA, 1980, p. 23)

Although CNS educational programs were becoming widely available, CNS curricula varied by school and specialty. Throughout the 1980s and most of the 1990s, publications discussing CNS education appeared in the literature, but no organized effort came together to create national standards for CNS education. Schools continued to rely on the NLN recommendations to guide curricula. CNS graduate programs varied in length from 9 to 28 months, with most programs taking 2 full academic years to complete (Sills, 1983). Some programs were not designated CNS but were labeled the "clinical" option to distinguish them from administration and teaching-focused programs. Other CNS programs were linked to a specialty with separate curricular tracks for each specialty. For example, between mid-1970 and mid-1990, the University of Cincinnati College of Nursing offered distinct CNS specialty tracks for pulmonary, medical-surgical, burn-trauma, occupational health, gerontology, oncology, adult mental health, and child/adolescent mental health.

In 1996, the AACN published *The Essentials of Master's Education for Advanced Practice Nursing* (AACN, 1996). The *Essentials* recommended content for advanced practice nursing curricula preparing clinical specialists, nurse midwives, nurse anesthetists, and nurse practitioners. In 1999, the National Advisory Council on Nurse Education and Practice (NACNEP), established by Title VIII of the Public Health Service Act to advise the secretary on nursing workforce issues, completed a comprehensive report addressing federal support for the preparation of the CNS workforce (NACNEP, 1999). Among the recommendations, the report called for the federal government to support and encourage the profession's efforts to standardize requirements for educational preparation for core competencies of the CNS role. In 1998, NACNS published the first edition of *The Statement on Clinical Nurse Specialist Practice and Education*, which included both core practice competencies for the CNS role and recommendations for educational preparation of the CNS. In 2003, Walker and colleagues found that 56% of schools preparing CNSs used the NACNS recommendations to guide curricula. The second edition of the NACNS *Statement* was published in 2004 and again

included core practice competencies and curricular recommendations.

The Advanced Practice Registered Nurse (APRN) Consensus Model (2008) included educational recommendations for core content and clinical experience. Consistent with all APRN education programs, CNS programs were to include course work in physiology/ pathophysiology, physical assessment, and pharmacology and a minimum of 500 supervised clinical practice hours in the CNS role. In 2011, NACNS released the *Criteria for the Evaluation of Clinical Nurse Specialist Master's, Practice Doctorate, and Post-Graduate Certificate Educational Programs* (NACNS, 2011). These criteria reflected the requirements necessary to ensure quality CNS education at the master's, postgraduate, and practice doctorate levels and provided guidance to CNS programs for curricula design and delivery.

MODELS OF CNS PRACTICE

The CNS role components identified in earlier works and summarized in the 1969 NLN report—therapist/practitioner, teacher, consultant, researcher, and change agent—became unifying descriptions of the CNS. Beginning in the 1980s, a number of models and frameworks were developed to further explain CNS practice, with the identified role components serving as central concepts. Some models described the structure of CNS where others showed CNS practice as a process linked to clinical outcomes. Few were developed using theory-development and testing methods. Table 1.4 briefly summarizes models describing the CNS role and/or CNS practice.

The Subroles Model of CNS Practice

Throughout the 1980s, the "Subroles" model was dominant, though it was more a description—a listing of expected practice activities—than it was a model demonstrating the relationships between and among the activities. Hamric (1983) was an early contributor to describing the CNS role as a constellation of subroles, including expert practitioner, role model, and patient advocate, identified as direct care functions; and change agent, consultant/resource person, clinical teacher, supervisor, researcher, liaison, and innovator, identified as indirect care functions. In 1986, the ANA Council of Clinical Nurse Specialists published *The Role of the Clinical Nurse Specialist*, which listed the dimensions of the CNS role as specialist in clinical practice, educator, consultant, researcher, and administrator (ANA, 1986). The administrator dimension

TABLE 1.4

SUMMARY OF MODELS AND FRAMEWORKS FOR CNS PRACTICE	
Reference	**Summary**
Roy and Martinez (1983)	A systems framework for CNS practice. Concepts include input, process, output, and feedback. A circular process where input influences processes, which in turn influence output, which generates feedback, which serves as continuing input. Outcomes described as "effects on nursing practice and nursing profession"
Girouard (1983)	The linkage model. Composed of two major systems—expert knowledge application system and internal problem solving system. Each system has internal circular steps that lead to problem solving. The systems interact through feedback loops. Outcome is "the nurse implements the planned change"
Hamric (1983)	Subroles of the CNS. Lists the direct care functions as expert practitioner, role model, and patient advocate. Indirect care functions are identified as change agent, consultant/resource person, clinical teacher, supervisor, researcher, liaison, and innovator. Relationships between/among subroles not defined or linked to outcomes
Calkin (1984)	Developed for nurse administrators to use in distinguishing novice, expert-by-experience, and advanced nurses' performance. Used a series of normal distribution curves to illustrate levels of knowledge, skill, and patient population response (outcome). The model links practice to patient outcomes, but was never tested
Holt (1984)	Anatomy of a clinical nurse specialist. Provides a structural description of the role, including nature of the unit; goal of the unit; growth and development of the unit; deviations from expected developmental pattern; other units in the universe; and relationships and interventions
Fenton (1985)	An ethnographic study confirmed CNS practice in Benner's seven domains of nursing practice—helping role; administrating and monitoring therapeutic interventions and regimes; effective management of rapidly changing situations; diagnostic and monitoring function; teaching-coaching function; monitoring and ensuring quality of health care practices; and organizational and work–role competencies—and suggested an additional domain: Consulting role
Brown (1998)	Framework proposed to consolidate and integrate concepts from multiple sources to create a comprehensive model of advanced practice nursing. Consists of four domains—role legitimacy, advanced practice nursing, outcomes and environment—and proposed relationships among the domains
National Association of Clinical Nurse Specialists (1998)	Describes core CNS competencies and relationships among competencies, skills, attributes, and outcomes in environmental context that includes organizational structure, culture and processes, public policy, social factors, and human and fiscal resources

was controversial, with arguments against including administrative functions related to negating the clinical focus of the role. Arguments for including an administrative component were building an important option for situations where the CNS assumed responsibility for direct care programs in the area of specialization and maintains direct client-based practice (ANA, 1986).

Multiple articles appeared through the 1980s and early 1990s using a Subroles model to describe, explain, and measure CNS practice in many different specialties. Hamric (1989) expanded her initial description to include three foundational elements,

called primary criteria, and to distinguish skills/competencies from subroles. Primary criteria were those conditions required for beginning practice in the role: earned graduate degree in nursing with a focus on clinical practice, certification by a professional nursing organization, and a practice focus on patient/client/family. Skills and competencies included in the model were change agent, collaborator, clinical leader, role model, and patient advocate. Subroles were expert practice, consultation, education, and research. The rationale for categorizing an item as a competency or a subrole was not stated, appeared arbitrary, and did little to clarify the role within nursing or to the public.

Nonetheless, by the end of the 1980s, the subroles of expert clinician, educator, and researcher were solidified as the structural description of the CNS role. Other subroles frequently associated with the CNS role were consultant, collaborator, role model, and change agent.

The subroles description became a de facto organizing framework for describing the structural components of the CNS role. Textbooks began emphasizing the subroles. Hamric and Spross's 1989 book included chapters on the subroles, one each discussing direct patient care provider, consultant, educator, researcher, collaborator, and clinical leader (Hamric & Spross, 1989). Sparacino, Cooper, and Minarik's (1990) book included a chapter on each subrole—clinician, consultant, educator, researcher, administrator, and clinical leader. Gawlinski and Kern's (1994) text for critical care CNSs was organized according to subroles and included sections on practitioner, educator, consultant, researcher, and leader/manager. Multiple additional publications, articles, and books used the subroles framework.

At the same time, research about the CNS role was appearing in the literature using subroles as the organizing framework for the studies. This body of work helped codify the subroles by designing data collection instruments for identifying activities associated with each subrole. It was typical for researchers to use questionnaires that asked CNSs to identify a percentage of time spent in each of the subroles and/or to identify activities in the subroles.

Critique of the Subroles Model

Despite its familiarity, or perhaps because of it, the Subroles model has not been subject to sufficient critique as a model for describing CNS practice. A description of the CNS role as the additive sum of subroles is inadequate. Each of the subroles can be a unique role in its own right, raising even more questions about the difference between a CNS, for example, acting in the "educator subrole" and a nurse educator acting in the educator role, especially where the nurse educator is in a clinical setting working directly with clients or staff. The subroles' description of a CNS became the equivalent of painting a "white dog in a snowstorm."

Three shortcomings of the Subroles model were as follows:

1. Conceptualizing the CNS role as an assemblage of discrete activities. In practice, the CNS role is highly integrated with the CNSs' bringing a unique perspective to identifying clinical questions and seeking alternative solutions. CNS practice is a way of thinking that incorporates complex, interdependent actions. This way of thinking is not easily captured in discrete units of time or activities.

2. Using subroles as proxy indicators for professional competencies. The lack of core practice competencies, coupled with no consensus on curricular standards for the CNS education, allowed the subroles, being broad and nonspecific, to serve as the only guide for education and contributed to inconsistency in role preparation and implementation. In addition, the lack of clear distinction between subrole, skills, and competencies in some models contributed to confusion between CNS role definition and CNS practice competencies.

3. Failing to level CNS practice relative to other levels of nursing practice. The subrole, skill, and competency descriptors for CNSs—practitioner, educator, researcher, consultant, collaborator, change agent, patient advocate, and leader—are expected professional nursing performance requirements for all nurses. The level of performance varies by type of nursing educational preparation. For example, bachelor-prepared nurses engage in research activities, as do master's and doctorally prepared nurses, albeit not at the same level. The subroles framework did little to distinguish the CNS level of performance from other nursing roles.

As a description of the CNS role, the Subroles model emerged as an outgrowth of many of the early writings outlining the need for an advanced clinical expert, but it was never empirically tested for its own validity. It was, however, codified by a body of research work that accepted it prima facia, never questioning underlying assumptions.

AN INTEGRATED MODEL OF CNS PRACTICE

Core CNS Practice Competencies

After far too many years of waiting, core competencies for CNS practice were identified in the 1998 publication of the NACNS *Statement on Clinical Nurse Specialist Practice and Education*. The core practice competencies were created through a rigorous content analysis process, including an extensive review of the literature and interviews of practicing CNSs and administrators. A national external review panel was used to validate the final list of competencies (Baldwin et al., 2007). The final list of core competencies reflected CNS practice regardless of specialty. The core competencies were updated in 2004 (NACNS, 2004), and were subsequently validated through research (Baldwin, Clark, Fulton, & Mayo, 2009). The content analysis process used to define the core competencies also identified an organizing framework with three distinct domains.

Domains of Practice

The organizing framework for the core competencies was an integrated representation of CNS practice. The domains were patient/client, nurses and nursing practice, and organizations and systems (NACNS, 1998). The domains were labeled *spheres of influence* to denote the scope or breadth of practice activities and the target outcomes associated with a particular sphere. The patient/client sphere was considered central, reinforcing the longstanding view of CNSs as clinical experts. The nurses and nursing practice sphere recognized that the CNS practice included influencing the clinical practice by working one-on-one with nurses to deliver care and improving norms and standards of care for directing the actions of nurses and nursing personnel. The organizations/system sphere reflected the practice of CNSs in articulating the value of nursing care at the organizational level and influencing decision making at the system level to remove barriers and facilitate quality care and improved patient outcomes (NACNS, 2004). CNSs are advanced practice nurses with a specialty focus; thus, the role core competencies were seen as actualized in specialty knowledge, standards, and skills, as demonstrated in Figure 1.1. Outcomes of CNS practice were also identified for each domain, demonstrating the link between CNS practice consistent with the core competencies and anticipated clinical outcomes.

This integrated model of CNS practice, commonly referred to as the *Spheres of Influence* model, is more descriptive of CNS practice than the previous additive Subroles model. The creation of core competencies brought greater clarity to curriculum content because educators could identify performance expectations for graduates. Identifying core competencies and expected outcomes also informed employers, the public, and other providers what to expect from CNS practice.

Continuing Challenges in Describing CNS Practice

Competencies should reflect contemporary practice and therefore must be updated. The 2008 update of the core competencies created a furor among groups with vested political and economic interests. Among the competing forces were the National Council of State Boards of Nursing's model for clarifying regulatory standards (known as the APRN Consensus Model), the AACN introduction of the doctor of nursing practice (DNP) degree, and the new role of clinical nurse leader (CNL), and organizations like the ANA, American Association of Critical Care Nurses, and Oncology Nursing Society, with affiliated advanced practice certifying bodies. The outcome of this clash was, sadly, a return to a list of competencies disconnected from associated outcomes. In attempting to accommodate competing political agendas, the revised standards incorporated the Subroles, the synergy model (American Association of Critical Care Nurses), and the NACNS spheres of influence model. The resulting document was logically inconsistent for the purpose of directing practice. Valid, research-driven frameworks for explaining CNS practice and outcomes are needed. Efforts to create such frameworks should adhere to methods for theory development and theory testing.

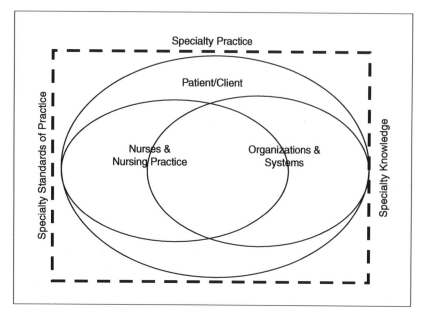

FIGURE 1.1 Clinical nurse specialist practice conceptualized as core competencies in three interacting spheres actualized in specialty practice and guided by specialty knowledge and specialty standards.

Source: ©J. S. Fulton (2004). Used with permission.

OPPORTUNITIES FOR THE FUTURE

The CNS is an expanded nursing role prepared at the graduate level, either master's or doctorate. CNSs acquire and apply scientific knowledge and skills for the purpose of meeting the public need for clinically expert nursing services with both newly emerging and established specialty populations. CNSs are leaders in providing innovative nurse-initiated interventions, resulting in improved health outcomes for specialty populations. The federal Accountable Care Act is opening up opportunities for CNSs to embrace new responsibilities and identify emerging needs for nursing care. Technology and informatics are shaping the future. CNSs should embrace opportunities and be prepared to shape new legislative initiatives and technologies for practice. Affordable care organizations, telehealth, health/medical homes, genetically optimal pharmaceuticals, expanded end-of-life care, and other emerging health care innovations provide endless opportunity for CNSs to lead nursing into the future.

The hundreds of existing articles about the CNS present a consistent core representation of the CNS role and practice. It is curious, however, that so many publications include commentary noting CNS role ambiguity and a poor understanding by nurses, administrators, and other health care providers. Continued assertion about CNS role ambiguity is a curiosity, given the many CNSs successfully practicing in the role and the many administrators supporting the role. With the focus of the CNS role on interpreting and advancing nursing practice, ambiguity about the CNS role is further reflection of a lack of clarity about nursing, nursing practice, and the unique contributions nursing makes to the public good. Understanding the CNS role and practice is inextricably tied to the ability to articulate the value of nursing. As a profession, nursing too frequently lacks the ability to express its contributions and value and, thus, it becomes even more challenging to describe nursing practiced at an advanced level.

This is the dual challenge for CNSs in the future to continue moving forward with the advice offered by Brown (1948): to clearly articulate the unique contributions of nursing to patient care while describing, implementing, and evaluating nursing practice at an advanced level. It's difficult to manage what is not measured. The next decade should be dedicated to intense efforts to measure the outcomes of CNS practice, which, in turn, demonstrates the value of nursing practiced at the advanced level and the inherent value of nursing in general. To do this, models and frameworks that link CNS practice to clinical outcomes need to be developed—models with theoretical and empirical support. As CNSs successfully address practice model development and outcomes measurement,

much will be achieved for the benefit of our patients, their families, and general public welfare.

■ DISCUSSION QUESTIONS

- Discuss the significance of collegiate education on the emergence of the CNS role. What social and/or professional influences surrounded moving nursing education from the hospital training program to university academic programs? How have these influences changed over time, and are they similar or nonexistent today?
- Discuss the development of a framework for the CNS role and practice. Identify themes in early descriptions of the CNS role. How are those same themes found in today's CNS practice?

■ ANALYSIS AND SYNTHESIS EXERCISES

- Clinical expertise in nursing practice is central to the CNS role and practice. Trace the development of a selected specialty practice. Explore the relationships among the specialty and scientific knowledge development, technological influences, and public need for nursing services.
- Analyze trends in nursing that influenced development of nursing and the CNS role. The *American Journal of Nursing* is electronically archived in JSTOR and available through Google Scholar; explore this historical literature for influences on today's CNS role.

■ CLINICAL APPLICATION

Identify methods for measuring outcomes related to CNS practice. Compare and contrast variations in methods and data needed to measure the same outcome in different specialties.

REFERENCES

Accreditation Board for Specialty Nurse Certification (ABSNC). (2012). *The American Board of Nursing Specialties accreditation standards.* Aurora, OH: Author.

Allen, R. B., Koos, E. L., Bradley, F. R., & Wolf, L. K. (1948). The Brown report. *American Journal of Nursing, 48*(12), 736–742.

American Association of Colleges of Nursing (AACN). (1996). *The essentials of master's education for advanced practice nursing.* Washington, DC: Author.

American Association of Critical Care Nurses. (2010). *Scope of practice and standards of professional performance for the acute and critical care clinical nurse specialist.* Aliso Viejo, CA: Author.

American Nurses Association (ANA), Council of Clinical Nurse Specialists. (1986). *The role of the clinical nurse specialist.* Kansas City, MO: Author.

American Nurses Association (ANA). (1980). *Social policy statement.* Kansas City, MO: Author.

American Nurses Association (ANA). (2010). *Nursing scope and standards of practice.* Washington, DC: Author.

Anderson, L. C. (1966). The clinical nursing expert. *Nursing Outlook, 14,* 62–64.

Baldwin, K. M., Clark, A. P., Fulton, J. S., & Mayo, A. (2009). Validation of the NACNS clinical nurse specialist core competencies through a national survey. *The Journal of Nursing Scholarship, 41*(2), 193–201.

Baldwin, K. M., Lyon, B. L., Clark, A. P., Fulton, J., Davidson, S., & Dayhoff, N. (2007). Developing clinical nurse specialist practice competencies. *Clinical Nurse Specialist, 21*(6), 297–302.

Berlinger, M. R. (1969). The preparation and roles of the clinical specialist at the master's level. In *Extending the boundaries of nursing education* (pp. 15–21). New York, NY: National League for Nursing.

Boyle, D. M. (1996). The clinical nurse specialist. In A. B. Hamric, J. A. Spross, & C. M. Hanson (Eds.), *Advanced nursing practice: An integrative approach* (pp. 299–336). Philadelphia, PA: W.B. Saunders.

Brown, E. L. (1948). *Nursing for the future.* New York, NY: Russell Sage Foundation.

Brown, S. J. (1998). A framework for advanced practice nursing. *Journal of Professional Nursing, 14*(3), 157–164.

Bullough, V. L., & Bullough, B. (1979). *Care of the sick: The emergence of modern nursing.* London, UK: C. Helm.

Burns, K., & Welk, D. (1997). American Board of Nursing Specialties: Past, present and future. *Nursing Outlook, 45,* 114–117.

Calkin, J. D. (1984). A model for advanced nursing practice. *Journal of Nursing Administration, 14*(1), 24–30.

Consensus Model for Advanced Practice Registered Nursing: Licensure, Accreditation, Certification and Education (2008, July 7). Retrieved September 30, 2013, from https://www.ncsbn.org/4213.htm

Crawford, M. I. (1964). Use of the clinical specialist. In *Blueprint for action in hospital nursing* (pp. 87–90). New York, NY: National League for Nursing.

DeWitt, K. (1900). Specialties in nursing. *American Journal of Nursing, 1*(1), 14–17.

Ellis, J. R., & Hartley, C. L. (2004). *Nursing in today's world: Trends, issues and management* (8th ed.). Philadelphia, PA: Lippincott Williams Wilkins.

Fang, D., Li, Y., & Bednash, G. D. (2013). *2012–2013 enrollment and graduations in baccalaureate and graduate programs in nursing.* Washington, DC: American Association of Colleges of Nursing.

Fenton, M. V. (1985). Identifying competencies of clinical nurse specialists. *Journal of Nursing Administration, 15*(2), 31–37.

Gawlinski, A., & Kern, L. S. (1994). *The clinical nurse specialist role in critical care.* Philadelphia, PA: W. B. Saunders.

Girouard, S. (1983). Theory-based practice: Functions, obstacles and solutions. In A. B. Hamric & J. Spross (Eds.), *The clinical nurse specialist in theory and practice* (pp. 21–36). New York, NY: Grune & Stratton.

Gorden, M. (1969). The clinical nurse specialist as change agent. *Nursing Outlook, 17,* 37–39.

Hamric, A. B., (1983). Role development and functions. In A. B. Hamric & J. Spross (Eds.), *The clinical nurse specialist in theory and practice* (pp. 39–56). New York, NY: Grune & Stratton.

Hamric, A. B., (1989). History and overview of CNS role. In A. B. Hamric & J. A. Spross (Eds.), *The clinical nurse specialist in theory and practice* (pp. 1–18). Philadelphia, PA: Saunders.

Hamric, A. B., & Spross, J. A. (1989). *The clinical nurse specialist in theory and practice.* Philadelphia, PA: Saunders.

Hanson, C. M., & Hamric, A. B. (2003). Reflections on the continuing evolution of advanced practice nursing. *Nursing Outlook, 51*(5), 203–211.

Hawkins, J. W., & Thibodeau, J. A. (1993). *The advanced practitioner: Current practice issues.* New York, NY: Tiresias Press.

Hiestand, W. C. (2006). Frances U. Reiter and the Graduate School of Nursing at the New York Medical College, 1960–1973. *Nursing History Review, 14,* 213–226.

Holt, F. M. (1984). A theoretical model for clinical nurse specialist practice. *Nursing and Healthcare, 5*(8), 445–449.

Johnson, D. E., Wilcox, J. A., & Moidel, H. C. (1967). The clinical specialist as a practitioner. *American Journal of Nursing, 67*(11), 2298–2303.

Kurihara, M. (1973). A nursing care specialist in cardiopulmonary disease and medical intensive care unit. In J. P. Riehl & J. W. McVay (Eds.), *The clinical nurse specialist: Interpretations* (pp. 258–267). New York, NY: Appleton-Century-Crofts.

Little, D. (1967). The nurse specialist. *American Journal of Nursing, 67,* 552–556.

MacPhail, J. (1971). Reasonable expectations for the nurse clinician. *Journal of Nursing Administration, 1,* 16–18.

Mayo, A. A. (1944). Advanced courses in clinical nursing: A discussion of basic assumptions and guiding principles. *American Journal of Nursing, 44*(6), 579–585.

McHenry, R. (1983). *Famous American women: A biographical dictionary from colonial times to present.* New York, NY: Dover Publications.

McIntyre, H. M. (1970). The nurse-clinician—One point of view. *Nursing Outlook, 18*(9), 26–29.

National Advisory Council on Nurse Education and Practice (NACNEP). (1999). *Federal support for the preparation of the clinical nurse specialist workforce through Title VIII.* Department of Health and Human Services, Health Resources and Services Administration, Bureau of Health Professions, Division of Nursing. HRSA 99–40. Retrieved March 25, 2009, from http://www.eric.ed.gov/ERICDocs/data/ericdocs2sql/content_storage_01/0000019b/80/16/36/30.pdf

National Association of Clinical Nurse Specialists (NACNS). (1998). *Statement on clinical nurse specialist practice and education.* Harrisburg, PA: Author.

National Association of Clinical Nurse Specialists (NACNS). (2004). *Statement on clinical nurse specialist practice and education* (2nd ed.). Harrisburg, PA: Author.

National Association of Clinical Nurse Specialists (NACNS). (2008). *Clinical nurse specialist core competencies.* Retrieved September 30, 2013, from http://www.nacns.org/html/competencies.php

National Association of Clinical Nurse Specialists (NACNS). (2011). *Criteria for the evaluation of clinical nurse specialist master's, practice doctorate, and post-graduate certificate educational programs.* Philadelphia, PA: Author.

National League for Nursing (NLN). (1958). *Report of the National Working Conference: Education of the clinical specialist in psychiatric nursing.* New York, NY: Author.

National League for Nursing (NLN). (1958/1973). Report of the National Working Conference: Education of the clinical specialist in psychiatric nursing. In J. P. Riehl & J. W. McVay (Eds.), *The clinical nurse specialist: Interpretations* (p. 8). New York, NY: Appleton-Century-Crofts.

National League for Nursing (NLN). (1969). *Extending the boundaries of nursing education.* New York, NY: Author.

National League for Nursing (NLN). (1984). *Master's education in nursing: Route to opportunities in contemporary nursing.* New York, NY: Author.

Oncology Nursing Society. (2008). *Oncology clinical nurse specialists competencies.* Pittsburgh, PA: Author.

Peplau, H. (1965). Specialization in professional nursing. *Nursing Science, 3,* 268–287.

Plawecki, J. A. (1971). A viewpoint on the preparation of the clinical nurse specialist. *Supervisor Nurse, 2*(1), 49–63.

Reiter, F. (1961/1973). Improvement in nursing practice. In J. P. Riehl & J. W. McVay (Eds.), *The clinical nurse specialist: Interpretations* (pp. 9–18). New York, NY: Appleton-Century-Crofts.

Reiter, F. (1966). The nurse-clinician. *American Journal of Nursing, 66,* 274–280.

Rhein, M. (1973). The education of the clinical specialist. In J. P. Riehl & J. W. McVay (Eds.), *The clinical nurse specialist: Interpretations* (pp. 131–144). New York, NY: Appleton-Century-Crofts.

Riehl, J. P., & McVay, J. W. (1973). *The clinical nurse specialist: Interpretations.* New York, NY: Appleton-Century-Crofts.

Roy, C., & Martinez, C. (1983). A conceptual framework for CNS practice. In A. B. Hamric & J. Spross (Eds.), *The clinical nurse specialist in theory and practice* (pp. 3–20). New York, NY: Grune & Stratton.

Rubin, R. (1969). Graduate programs in maternity and pediatric nursing leading to the degree of doctor of philosophy at the University of Pittsburgh. In *Extending the boundaries of nursing education* (pp. 22–27). New York, NY: National League for Nursing.

Salyer, J., & Hamric, A. B. (2008). Evolving and innovative opportunities for advanced practice nursing. In A. B. Hamric, J. A. Spross, & C. M. Hanson (Eds.), *Advanced practice nursing: An integrative approach* (pp. 520–540). St. Louis, MO: Saunders.

Sills, G. M. (1983). The role and function of the clinical nurse specialist. In N. L. Chaska (Ed.), *The nursing profession: A time to speak* (pp. 563–579). New York, NY: McGraw-Hill.

Smoyak, S. A. (1976). Specialization in nursing: From then to now. *Nursing Outlook, 24*(11), 565–681.

Snyder, M. (1990). Specialization in nursing: Logic or chaos. In N. L. Chaska (Ed.), *The nursing profession: Turning points.* St. Louis, MO: C. V. Mosby.

Sparacino, P. A. S., Cooper, D. M., & Minark, P. A. (1990). *The clinical nurse specialist: Implementation and impact.* Norwalk, CT: Appleton & Lange.

Spross, J. A., Gerard, P. S., & France, N. (2006). Directory of clinical nurse specialist programs in the United States, 2005. *Clinical Nurse Specialist, 20*(1), 34–48.

Styles, M. M. (1990). Clinical nurse specialists and the future of nursing. In P. S. A. Sparacino, D. M. Cooper, & P. A. Minarik (Eds.), *The clinical nurse specialist: Implementation and impact* (pp. 279–298). Norwalk, CT: Appleton-Century-Crofts.

Towner, A. M. (1968). No more supervisors? *Nursing Outlook, 16,* 56–58.

Walker, J., Gerard, P. S., Bayley, E. W., Coeling, H., Clark, A. P., Dayhoff, N., & Goudreau, K. (2003). A description of clinical nurse specialist programs in the United States. *Clinical Nurse Specialist, 17*(1), 50–57.

Wolf, L. K. (1947). *Nursing.* New York, NY: Appleton-Century-Crofts.

Professional Attributes in the Context of Emotional Intelligence, Ethical Conduct, and Citizenship of the Clinical Nurse Specialist

Janet M. Bingle and Sue B. Davidson

Note to reader. The content of this chapter has provided the professional opportunity for reflection on our rich and extensive careers over a 45-year period in a continually changing context of nursing, health care, and society. In this reflection, we realize that there are different ways that the professional attributes discussed in this chapter have been acquired/developed or enhanced. A good part of this development did not occur in our various academic and professional practice experiences as CNSs; rather, the development has occurred through interactions in life experiences that we regard as our personhood. There were times in this reflection that we were joyful and other times that we became sad or angry. This reflection has, however, made conscious our thoughts for your consideration, and our hope is that learning and growth will occur.

In the context of the current health care system in the United States, there is a level of conflict, a need for positive influence, and the requirement to deliver cost-effective care. Given the context of health care

reform, the student clinical nurse specialist (CNS) or practicing CNS stands at the intersection of practice and outcomes. This is true not only in acute care but also in every place in which health care and nursing care are provided. The recipients of CNS practice are patients, families, groups, organizations, and communities where primary and specialty care populations receive care from direct care nurses and other health care providers. The essential characteristics of the student or practicing CNS, which are described in the second CNS scope statement (National Association of Clinical Nurse Specialists [NACNS], 2004), are as follows: (a) clinical expertise in the specialty; (b) collaboration skills; (c) leadership skills; (d) consultation skills; (e) *professional attributes*, including but not limited to honesty, integrity, emotional competence, a willingness for self-review, and a value for diversity; (f) *ethical conduct*; and (g) *professional citizenship*. These seven essential characteristics are critical to the CNS's ability to influence in the absence of position or line authority. *Influence* is the power to produce desired effects or outcomes by moving others to action (*Webster's Dictionary of the American Language,*

1962; see also Chapter 11). For a CNS to be effective in today's health care system, development of these essential characteristics is not a luxury but a requisite. The characteristics taken together reflect a gestalt that is partly innate, partly developed, and continuously refined in the practice so that the CNS is growing and expanding his or her practice in these areas.

This chapter begins with an overview of the development of essential characteristics of the CNS. Then the professional attributes of the CNS are discussed in the context of emotional intelligence (EI), followed by an overview of ethical conduct, including ethical principles and dealing with ethical dilemmas. The chapter concludes with an overview of professional citizenship, including organizational citizenship. The three characteristics discussed in this chapter form the basis for other essential characteristics of the CNS, such as clinical expertise, leadership, consultation, and collaboration, which are addressed in other chapters.

DEVELOPMENT OF THE ESSENTIAL CHARACTERISTICS OF A CNS

The professional attributes, ethical conduct, and citizenship attributes are critical elements of CNS practice. Knowing where you stand with reference to them is critical in choosing to become a CNS, in learning to be a CNS, and in practicing as a CNS (Table 2.1).

The curriculum in a CNS program hones the intellectual abilities in mastery of the discipline of nursing and within a nursing specialty and assumes that these attributes are present. These attributes, however, require attention and development across the career because they are significant predictors of the success of the CNS in practice.

Undergraduate nursing education is designed to ensure that the graduate has competency and skill in the *caring* delivery of safe patient care as a generalist. Clinical practice experiences following completion of the program are assumed to enable the nurse to become competent in the delivery of specialized nursing care in a variety of settings to a specific population of patients, for example, oncology, critical care, mother/baby, and so on.

There is an assumption that intellectual development in courses combined with clinical experiences in the nursing program and the student's *intention to care for others* will be sufficient. Several factors suggest that this assumption is questionable. First, research has shown that emotional competency is critical to provision of caring assessment and intervention—the basis for nursing practice (Codier, 2012; Porter O'Grady & Malloch, 2002). Second, the presence of high turnover, burnout, lower overall effectiveness of teams/units, reduced patient satisfaction, ineffective communication resulting in error and/or workplace injury, as well as nurse-to-nurse horizontal violence in the workplace are problems that plague the nursing component in the health

TABLE 2.1

DEFINITIONS OF SELECTED ESSENTIAL CHARACTERISTICS AND PROFESSIONAL ATTRIBUTES OF A CNS	
Essential Characteristics of CNS	**Definition**
Professional attributes	Personal characteristics such as honesty, integrity, mastery in managing thoughts and emotions, positive self-regard and confidence, willingness to take risks, knowledge of one's own strengths and weaknesses coupled with openness to continued learning and development, self-review, willingness to solicit and accept peer review, ability to value and support diversity
	Self-awareness
	Self-management
	Social awareness
	Relationship management (communication, negotiation, and team building)
Ethical conduct	Application of ethical principles to the identification and analysis of ethical dilemmas, and demonstration of decision making characterized by thoughtful consideration of multiple competing values in an ethical dilemma
Professional citizenship	Awareness and action that is based on membership in the community of all CNSs, with rights and obligations to shape and influence the destiny of all CNSs

care system (Bartholomew, 2005, 2006; Walrefen, Brewer, & Mulvernon, 2012). Many of these situations are directly or indirectly linked to emotional/social intelligence, effective communication, and positive workplaces.

These persistent troublesome characteristics of nurses' work environment suggest that preparation in content related to EI is needed. Research studies are emerging that focus on EI in nursing. These studies demonstrate that nursing students can learn EI competencies (Benson, Martin, Ploeg, & Wessel, 2012). Among practicing nurses, where it has been predicted that knowledge of EI can enhance clinical practice, clinical rounds and other nursing processes were improved (Cosby & Croskerry, 2004; Kerfoot, 1999, 2005; Lynch & Cole, 2006). It has also been found that where hospital restructuring has occurred, nursing leadership with EI competencies have had a mitigating effect on the restructuring in terms of nurses' emotional health and patient outcomes (Cummings, Hayduk, & Estabrooks, 2005).

If there is not an equivalent focus in the undergraduate and graduate nursing programs on the development of emotional competency as well as intellectual competency, the nurse may lack self-awareness, have self-doubt, and be unskilled or undeveloped in controlling his or her emotions, understanding patterns of behavior, and having organizational and political savvy (Arena & Page, 1992). A lack of emotional competency can have a significant impact on the nurse's ability to thrive and grow in the clinical practice of nursing. As an example, practice competencies of an experienced registered nurse (RN) and those of an experienced CNS with full role development are depicted in Table 2.2.

The preparation of the CNS must include content, experience, and self-assessment of EI/competency, including understanding and dealing with stress emotions, relationship building, and citizenship in organizations and external entities. The CNS role includes expectations of EI and emotional competency because the role is built on role modeling and persuasion and not line authority.

TABLE 2.2

DESCRIPTION OF THE DEVELOPMENTAL DIFFERENCES BETWEEN AN EXPERIENCED RN AND A CNS		
Developmental Difference	**Registered Nurse**	**CNS**
Focus	Within a specialty unit	Within specialty populations and organization/system
Clinical expertise	Competency and excellence with patients and families	Excellence with patient, families, and related system-level initiatives
System skills	Some	Role models skills to other nurses; coaches development of skills; collaborates with and provides consultation to other members of the health care team
Emotional competence	Varies from novice to expert given the variability in expectations for emotional competence in the practice	Expectation is for expert competence in self-awareness, resilience, handling of difficult information, openness in thinking and feeling, openness to differing viewpoints, active coaching and mentoring, well-developed impulse control (Goleman, 1998; Goleman & Boyatzis, 2008; Porter O'Grady & Malloch, 2002, p. 210)
Ethical conduct	Uses Code of Ethics for nurses to guide practice; delivers care that preserves and protects patient autonomy, dignity, and rights; maintains patient confidentiality within legal/regulatory parameters; maintains therapeutic/professional patient–nurse relationship; contributes to resolution of ethical issues of patients, colleagues, and unit of work. *Source:* ANA, 2008	Involved in bioethics (patient, family) as well as organizational and business ethical dilemmas; educates others and has knowledge competency within the organization around ethical issues; informs patient of risks, benefits, and outcomes of health care regimens; participates in interprofessional teams addressing ethical risks and outcomes; leads ethics consultation and completes causal analysis of ethical dilemmas
Professional citizenship	Varies from novice to expert, given the organization and the practice	Meets expectations for strong stewardship/citizen of professional practice in an organization, within the specialty, and at the state and national levels

PROFESSIONAL ATTRIBUTES IN THE CONTEXT OF EI

Why is there a need to describe professional attributes of the CNS? First, because these professional attributes link to competencies for effectiveness of the CNS in organizations (Goleman, 1998; NACNS, 2004). Individuals who provide leadership in health care are judged by a different yardstick, not just by clinical expertise but also by how well they manage themselves and others. New leaders are not predicted based solely on academic learning but also on the attributes and personal qualities of initiative, empathy, adaptability, and persuasiveness (Skinner & Spurgeon, 2005; see Chapter 11). For example, in a national survey of employers, the skills, competencies, and attributes that were highly valued were not technical skills but competence in reading and writing, communication, interpersonal skills, initiative, and team building (Goleman & Boyatzis, 2008). Additionally, the general and specialty-based scope and standards of nursing practice presuppose these professional attributes (American Association of Critical Care Nurses [AACN], 2008a; American Nurses Association [ANA], 2010a, 2012; ANA Council of Clinical Nurse Specialists, 1986).

Professional attributes, as described by NACNS (2004), include

> honesty and integrity, personal mastery in managing thoughts and emotions; positive self regard and confidence; willingness to take risks and be wrong, knowledge of one's own strengths and weaknesses coupled with openness to continued learning goals for development; self review and willingness to solicit and accept peer review, and ability to value and support diversity. (p. 16)

These attributes collectively have been described in the literature in relation to emotional competence and EI of the leader and, in particular, the transformational leader (Beauman, 2006; IOM, 2004). EI is measured as EI quotient (EQ). The emotional competency of the CNS is critical to personal and professional success and fulfillment. Although traditionalists in health care have often looked at this competency and EQ as the soft side of work, research evidence has emerged over the past decade to demonstrate the interdependence between IQ and EQ (McKinnon, 2005). In fact, the attributes most coveted in many types of professionals and businesses are those of emotional and social intelligence (Goleman, 2008). Porter-O'Grady points out that EI is like other intelligences in that it provides the potential to learn, in this case, how to be emotionally competent.

Social intelligence, in which EI has its roots, was first described in the 1920s (McQueen, 2004). In the 1990s, this intelligence was further elucidated to include *intra*- and *inter*personal intelligence, with *intra*personal intelligence being the knowledge of self and *inter*personal intelligence being the knowledge of self and others. Building on that work, the research and work of Goleman (1995, 1998) gave substance and definition to EQ so that its requisite skills and competencies could be elucidated and studied (Goleman & Boyatzis, 2008; Goleman, Boyatzis, & McKee, 2002). Goleman outlined four leadership competencies associated with EQ: self-awareness, self-management, social awareness, and relationship management. Each competency has subcompetencies that resonate with the professional attributes identified in the NACNS's *Statement on CNS Practice and Education* (2004).

Self-Awareness

CNSs must recognize their moods, emotions, and drives. They need to understand how these emotions affect their own performance and that of others. This self-awareness requires disciplined inquiry into their personal thoughts and experiences. It requires deliberate analysis of their feelings and how these emotions drive thoughts and behaviors. Humans often have automatic reactions to certain interpersonal stimuli. These reactions may result from deep-seated assumptions that have taken root over time. Probably the best example of an automatic reaction can be seen when watching a group of cows head out to pasture. For whatever reasons, the cows always follow the same path. Day in and day out, they create the "cow path" for their route. Humans also create symbolic "cow paths" in their responses to certain situations (e.g., responses to failure or interpersonal conflict), thoughts, and emotions. The CNS needs to understand his or her "cow paths" in order to raise his or her self-knowledge and to have confidence in situations fraught with the various emotional triggers found in health care.

Self-Management

Self-management or self-control is critical to a professional who is immersed in daily conflict. The CNS, regardless of what sphere of influence he or she is functioning within, must remain clearheaded, exhibit composure, and find ways to steer the emotions to positive outcomes. Professionals with a high degree of self-regulation are transparent to others. Through personal disclosure, humor, and optimism, they are open to discussing their feelings and behaviors, receiving feedback, and experiencing personal learning. This transparency allows the individual to suspend judgment, assume accountability, and take the initiative to be solution oriented. Self-management is critical to the CNS who is expected to be the expert in situations that are loaded with intense emotions, a steep authority gradient, and unclearly defined outcomes. The self-confidence that comes with personal awareness and control gives the CNS the courage to navigate critical situations and create a model for managing them (Arena & Page, 1992; LaSala & Bjornson, 2010; Murray, 2010; Patterson, Grenny, McMillan, & Switzler, 2002).

Social Awareness

The CNS is the role model for emotional competence. His or her EQ provides for social awareness, organizational savvy, and agility. Given high levels of empathy, CNSs are sensitive to a wide range of emotions from individuals, groups, and the organization as a whole. As CNSs move through their setting, they cultivate relationships with diverse groups of professionals and clients. They can astutely read the political climate at the time and accurately describe the emotional reality of the situation (Goleman et al., 2002). Social awareness implies engagement, availability, and service competence. In this competence, there's a level of approachability that keeps the communication lines open, relationships intact, and social networks functioning.

Relationship Management

Relationship management is the fourth leadership competency associated with EI, and it builds on the previous three competencies (Goleman et al., 2002). As Goleman describes the leader with relationship competency, he draws a clear picture of the transformational leader, in general, and the CNS, in particular (Institute of Medicine [IOM], 2011; see also Chapter 11). This leader is inspirational, has power derived from his or her ability to influence, and is committed to the development of others. Because of these attributes, the leader is a trusted change agent skilled in conflict management and collaboration. Being able to effectively manage relationships to ensure desired outcomes is fundamental to the core competencies outlined in the *Statement on CNS Practice and Education* (NACNS, 2004). The CNS is expected to serve as a leader, consultant, mentor, and change agent among nurses and across systems. The role is also required to lead multidisciplinary groups and to establish and enhance collaboration with other disciplines to attain mutually agreed-upon outcomes. These core competencies are essential for establishing and maintaining a highly reliable care delivery system

and healthy work environment. Fundamental to these functions and outcomes, however, are effective communication and team building skills.

The communication skills of the CNS must be as proficient as the clinical skills. One's ability to communicate effectively creates the pathway to successful organizational change through influence and inspiration. The ability to articulate ideas, opportunities for improvement, and the mission, vision, and values inherent in those concepts and improvements requires a command of the language, knowledge of the power of linguistics, the ability to find the right appeal to a diverse audience, and the knowledge of how to build buy-in from key stakeholders. To be able to communicate a controversial, conflict-laden issue so that all participants can hear and become engaged in solution building is critical to CNS credibility and organizational success. As CNSs today become immersed in error management, root cause analysis, and sentinel event disclosure to professional as well as public audiences, skilled communication will be a required competency (Frankel, Leonard, & Denham, 2006). Through active listening, respectful interaction, and compassionate dialogue, trust is built so that crucial conversations can be had that result in learning and a safe, high-quality health care environment (Patterson, Grenny, McMillan, & Switzler, 2002). Conflicts and confrontations need to be managed effectively, keeping them as part of a solution and not the focus of the problem or an issue to be avoided. Knowing how to "language" one's way through the confrontation is essential and often needs to be role played or rehearsed so that all individuals emerge from the conversation intact and are able to grow from the experience (Patterson, Grenny, McMillan, & Switzler, 2002).

Another critical skill in managing relationships is the art of negotiation. As the CNS brings together multiple disciplines to weigh in on a system issue or care improvement opportunity, many lines may be drawn in the sand, none of which connects or leads to a solution. These lines may be discipline-specific and compartmentalized, not system-focused and in alignment. Don Berwick, chief executive officer for the Institute for Health Care Improvement, stated, "System-mindedness means cooperation. It means skills such as conflict resolution. It means asking yourself... not what are the parts of me, not what do I do, but what am I part of?" (IOM, 2003).

Berwick is talking about high levels of cooperation, coordination, and collaboration. The CNS, in leading multidisciplinary teams, is the catalyst for collaboration by helping members negotiate their differences and establish concessions without damaging relationships. The CNS needs to establish rapport and know how to find a common ground or platform on which all can agree. Storytelling, humor, self-disclosure, and a patient focus often allow the members to become grounded in the overall system and venture out of their specific paradigms. Successful negotiation can be thrilling for a CNS as long as he or she remains open to all possibilities and to the influence from others. EI and the competencies of self-awareness, self-management, and social awareness are critical to this process because the success of negotiating is more about the relationships than management of the deal itself. Many can relate to situations in which one has much time, energy, and emotional investment in an idea, policy and procedure, or plan for improvement. There is often fear and trepidation when bringing them forward for external or team review. One's emotional competency can wane as the critique becomes negative, and the desire to defend one's position inhibits the ability to listen, understand, and learn from the input. This is when the CNS needs to be at the top of his or her game in relationship management.

The ability to self-correct and take in the collective wisdom of the team is essential. To stop oneself from personalizing the feedback and focus on maintaining friendly collegiality is necessary for strong team building and collaboration. Keeping in mind there is no "I" in the word "TEAM," the CNS uses the words "we," "us," and "the team" when referring to results and outcomes of a particular initiative. Creating a collective identity drives cohesion in the group, which, in turn, facilitates high performance. Other characteristics of high-performing teams are that they have a common vision, the members trust each other and will cover for each other, the members collectively have the talent to get the work done, and the team has the group skills to work effectively and efficiently. The CNS can create a spirit of innovation and experimentation in the team by communicating a learning attitude toward mistakes or failures. This type of team culture has fun while being highly productive. An atmosphere of learning, trust, and fun helps members develop into leaders. It also allows the CNS leader to coach and mentor through timely and effective feedback, because the members feel safe and genuinely cared about.

The emotional competency of the CNS is critical to his or her success in the role. Both as a student and a practitioner, the CNS must conduct periodic self-reflection and seek structured feedback regarding his or her emotional competence. Role playing, improvisational theater, or simulation can provide great insight into one's self-awareness, social awareness, and self-management. Soliciting feedback from peers, coaches, mentors, and customers can facilitate this personal inquiry into how others perceive these competencies. Conducting a 360° feedback (Nowack & Mashihi, 2012) and similar approaches may give

the CNS a well-rounded view from multiple, varied customers and lenses. Working on transparency through storytelling can help others to see the attributes that the CNS is working on and brings to each situation.

ETHICAL CONDUCT

Ethical conduct, an essential characteristic of the CNS, is embedded in beliefs and values. It involves application of knowledge related to ethical principles, analysis of situations that contain ethical dilemmas, and decision making in responding to these situations. Ethical conduct is based on the presence of emotional competency (self-awareness, self-management, social awareness, relationship competency) and knowledge of health care ethics and moral reasoning. It is also based on the foundational principles that the profession has articulated in two documents: the *Code of Ethics with Interpretive Statements* (ANA, 2008) and the *Scope and Standards of Nursing Practice* (ANA, 2010a).

Code of Ethics

Nursing's ethical conduct is derived from universal principles of ethics (Table 2.3). These principles include autonomy, truth telling, beneficence, nonmaleficence, confidentiality, justice, and role fidelity. The universal principles were the source for, and are woven into, the Code of Ethics for nursing.

Of the nine provisions of the Code of Ethics for Nursing, three provisions address basic values and commitments of the nurse, three address duty and loyalty, and three address the health care environment, the nursing profession, and its relationships with other health care professionals. For example, the Code of Ethics establishes the expectation that the nurse will practice with compassion and respect for the dignity and worth of every individual, unrestricted by status and personal attributes. This provision is linked to the ethical principles of dignity of all, respect for persons, and primacy of the interests of the patient. In the Code of Ethics provisions having to do with the boundaries of duty and loyalty, the nurse is expected to be responsible for his or her individual nursing practice and appropriately delegate consistent with the provision of optimum patient care. The associated ethical principles for these provisions are accountability and responsibility for nursing judgment, professional growth and maintenance of competency, and exercise of moral virtue and values. Finally, the Code of Ethics provisions having to do with duties beyond patient

TABLE 2.3

	UNIVERSAL PRINCIPLES OF ETHICS AND THE LINKAGE TO THE COMPONENTS OF THE CODE OF ETHICS FOR NURSES	
	Universal Ethical Principles	**Code of Ethics for Nurses (ANA, 2008)**
Autonomy	Individual is free to choose and implement his or her own decisions. Includes the ability to decide, the power to act on the decision, and respect for the autonomy of others	Respect for human dignity. Delivery of nursing with respect for human needs and value and without prejudice and irrespective of disease, disability, functional status, or proximity to death. Right of self-determination. Respect for all persons with whom nurse interacts
Veracity (truth telling)	Applies to both patient and health care giver; patient must tell the truth so that appropriate care is given; provider discloses information so that patient can exercise personal autonomy	Nurse's primary commitment is to promote, advocate for, and protect individual, family, group, community health and safety Maintain professional boundaries Act on questionable practices
Beneficence	Action that benefits another, obligation to help, to promote health and welfare above other considerations. Means one ought to prevent harm or evil, ought to remove evil or harm, out to do or promote good	Act on questionable practice(s) Accept accountability/responsibility Be accountable in nursing judgments Be responsible for nursing actions Delegate nursing activities
Nonmaleficence	Ought not to inflict evil or harm	Address impaired practice
Confidentiality	Patient has the right to privacy regarding his own care program, treatments are conducted discreetly and confidentially, those not involved in the care must have permission to be present	Privacy Confidentiality Protection of those in research projects Standards and review mechanisms
Justice	Equal distribution of scarce resources	
Role fidelity	Individual must practice within the constraints of the role	Act on questionable practice(s) Assert values Exhibit moral self-respect Professional growth and maintenance of competency Advance the profession through research Wholeness of character Preservation of integrity Advance the profession through assertion of values, intra- and interprofessional integrity, social reform

encounters are associated with advancement of the profession of nursing, responsibility to the public, conduct consistent with the profession, and intraprofessional integrity. Conduct consistent with the Code is part of what it means to be a nurse, and such conduct is expected of all nurses regardless of level, role, or setting. The nurse commits to being reflective about his or her ethical conduct in practice situations. The Code of Ethics for Nursing is prescriptive and should be predictive of a nurse's ethical conduct.

The *Scope and Standards of Nursing Practice* "reflect the values of the nursing profession" (ANA, 2010a, p. 1). One of the standards of professional performance of a nurse is to provide ethically sensitive care as described in this document.

These foundational documents of the profession of nursing lay the groundwork for ethical professional practice. Integration of these statements into practice behavior ensures ethical conduct at the level of the RN, an RN practicing in a specialty, and the CNS.

The setting of a CNS's practice may be an office in which the CNS provides care independently or with other health care providers, in a business or the health care industry, within a health care organization, on a unit, a group of units, or all units where a particular population of patients exists, or less commonly, in a nonprofit organization related to health care or nursing. Regardless of setting, the CNS may recognize conflicts in care delivery that give rise to moral distress in nurses and present ethical dilemmas that may have implications for ethical conduct.

Issues

Here are some examples of ethical issues and dilemmas that may arise within components of the health care delivery and its associated management processes:

1. Conflicts over ownership and/or authorship of intellectual property and/or new products, or patient care process innovations; *Potential ethical issue/dilemma*: Justice, conflict of interest.
2. Preeminence of personal versus institutional self-interest (Swidler, Seastrum, & Shelton, 2007); *Potential ethical issue/dilemma*: Justice, autonomy.
3. Insufficient or underestimated resources to support care delivery that results in limitation or no access to care; *Potential ethical issue/dilemma*: Justice.
4. Emergence of unintended consequences from redesign efforts (Rie & Kofke, 2007); *Potential ethical issue/dilemma*: Beneficence, nonmaleficence.
5. Practice outside of scope of practice; *Potential ethical issue/dilemma*: Role fidelity.
6. Dishonest or deceptive interactions with patients, families, nurses, or others (Mohr & Mahon, 1996); *Potential ethical issue/dilemma*: Role fidelity, truth telling, autonomy.
7. Inability or unwillingness to provide the best-practice standard of care even though national guidelines for its use have been disseminated (Golomb, McGraw, Evans, & Dimsdale, 2007); *Potential ethical issue/dilemma*: Justice, beneficence/nonmaleficence, fidelity, autonomy.
8. Presence of policies that deliberatively use the least experienced rather than appropriately experienced staff for nursing care delivery (Mohr & Mahon, 1996; Robert, 1983); *Potential ethical issue/dilemma*: Beneficence/nonmaleficence.
9. Work environments where patients and the nurse are not treated with dignity and respect (Bartholomew, 2005); *Potential ethical issue/ dilemma*: Respect, autonomy.
10. Insufficient safeguards in clinical research projects with some patient populations (psychiatry, trauma) and in some clinical situations such as end of life (Curtin, 2007; Mohr & Mahon, 1996); *Potential ethical issue/dilemma*: Confidentiality, truth telling, beneficence/nonmaleficence.
11. Conflicts in care management, such as futility of care, refusal of treatment, issue of second opinions; *Potential ethical issue/dilemma*: Justice, autonomy, truth telling, fidelity.
12. Patient/provider issues in chronic disease self-management (Redman, 2013).

Some researchers suggest that agreement over ethical issues and dilemmas varies between nurses who lead and nurses who deliver nursing care. A survey of nurse executives identified the failure to provide service of the highest quality in the eyes of the consumer, health care providers not employed by the organization, and by the purchasers of care (insurance companies) as being the most significant ethical issue they face, whereas staff nurses identified economic constraints and quality as the top issues (Cooper, Frank, Hansen, & Gouty, 2004).

DeWolf (1989) found, in a study of medical surgical nurses, that five precipitating factors were present before ethical issues arose to the unit-level discourse: (a) nurses experienced an emotional reaction and felt uncomfortable with a patient situation; (b) there was a sense of urgency with little time available to address the issue; (c) nurses personalized the situation and wondered how they would want to be treated if they were the patient, thus using the personal to act on the professional domain; (d) nurses recognized that a communication failure had occurred and information with which to make a decision was lacking; and (e) there was disagreement among the health care team regarding what should happen. These studies suggest that there was a gap between awareness of ethical dilemmas and action related to these dilemmas among staff nurses, or that there are varying skills/abilities to articulate ethical dilemmas (Moland, 2006). Alternatively, others suggest that, due to the demands of today's care environment, "fully capable health care professionals feel powerless and voiceless," even though they have awareness of ethical dilemmas and concerns (Austin, 2007).

Ethical problems, dilemmas, and issues arise when an individual perceives there is a conflict regarding the right thing to do (Bozek & Savage, 2007). The CNS may be among the first to recognize an ethical dilemma that is causing moral distress to the CNS, to staff nurses, and/or to other health care providers. Early recognition by the CNS of moral distress requires sensitivity, the ability to listen without judgment or premature closure, and maintenance of confidentiality of parties. Ethical conduct, demonstrated in any and all of the domains of CNS practice, includes direct and indirect actions based on the presence of "power, trust, inclusion, role flexibility, and inquiry" (Wlody, 2007, p. S30). It means that the CNS thinks and acts, rather than retreats, in situations where there is moral distress and an ethical dilemma.

Examples illustrative of direct and indirect CNS ethical conduct include fostering truth telling in nursing staff in clinical situations with patients, families, and others; advocating for the rights of patients, families, and others, directly or indirectly; and participating in development and creation of protocols, policies, and/or practice guidelines that are consistent with ethical principles. It means the CNS supports identification, analysis, and response to ethical dilemmas that arise in the practice, rather than avoiding the issue. The CNS skilled in ethics and values clarification will demonstrate adherence to an appropriate and effective set of core values and beliefs during good and bad times, will act in accord with those values, will provide constructive guidance to others in values clarification, and will seek alignment between ethical practices and the organization/setting and practice (Lombardo & Eichinger, 2006).

Role of the CNS in Ethical Analysis and Reasoning

The CNS may be a catalyst for early identification of ethical problems through assisting nursing staff to address issues in rounds, report, care conferences, and dialogue with each other and other disciplines. The CNS may also act as an educator by ensuring that staff and patients and/or their families understand the issues, the language, and the options being discussed; this may be achieved by the CNS's leading or participating in an ethics consultation or conference. The CNS may lead or assist in clarifying assumptions that are affecting the ethical decision making of staff nurses and others. For example, the nursing staff may assume that there is limited time in which to consider the ethical dilemma, that ethical reasoning is relatively easy, that exploration of the ethical problem is unnecessary, and lastly, that the business of health care "trumps" the ethics of health care. The role the CNS plays in ethical analysis and reasoning will also depend on whether the ethical issue relates to the CNS's professional values, the patient's values, or the organization's values (Bozek & Savage, 2007).

Ethical dilemmas are one type of conflict in care management. Conflicts in care management can arise from many sources, and confusion may exist about the root cause(s). For issues arising from questionable medical management, gaps in communication, legal issues, perceived harassment, and other conflicts, the resolution of conflict takes different paths, depending on the cause(s). If an issue is confirmed to be an ethical dilemma, it may be resolved through bedside consultation with members of the Ethics Committee, or, if the ethical dilemma is an issue of sufficient complexity and scope, resolution may take place in the Ethics Committee. The point is that conflicts in practice may have different root causes, some of which are ethical in nature. The CNS can be a valuable resource in clarifying the root causes in care management, thus enabling the organization to direct its resources toward the appropriate resolution of the dilemma (Community Hospitals Indianapolis, 1995).

There are two frameworks for ethical reasoning. It is important that the CNS understand these ethical frameworks, because the individuals with whom he or she is practicing may see the dilemma and its solution from a unique, individual framework. One framework for ethical reasoning, based on adult males, holds that decision making about abstract concepts such as justice, respect for the rights and dignity of others, equality, or listening to one's own conscience is the framework by which ethical dilemmas are analyzed and resolved. The focus is on rights and has been referred to a justice-based ethical framework. This model, however, has come under criticism for several reasons: (a) rules apply, no matter who is involved; (b) this approach focuses on some aspects of an ethical dilemma and ignores others; (c) the individual using this approach to an ethical dilemma is stepping outside of the situation, and the unintended outcome may be to objectify the person/patient; and (d) some ethical principles (for example, autonomy) may lead to ethical uncertainty because they are not universally applicable and because they apply in one situation but not in another situation. Others have criticized the justice-based approach because it is markedly different from the ethical reasoning of women.

A second model, inductive in style, focuses on "concern for individual cases" and is called care-based reasoning. This approach has been associated with ethical reasoning in women (Gilligan, 1982) and is characterized by full knowledge of the particularities of the case through knowledge of the relationships between the principals in the situation. It is called the "ethics of attachment" because it focuses on the responsibility to give care to the patient and less on people as carriers of rights. Care-based approaches are criticized because (a) the ethical dilemma/situation is "ruleless" but contains the possibility of the good, the moral thing to do; (b) this approach damages the patient–provider relationship, which, although unequal, is not necessarily bad; (c) this approach does not result in generalizable knowledge to be used in the other/all patient–provider relationships.

Despite differing frameworks, ethical issues for nurses and nursing continued to be reported and include situations where rules or policies are used for decision making versus identifying ethical issues and/or moral distress related to various clinical practices. Other conditions that contribute to moral distress include compromised standards, unsafe nurse staffing, caring for patients for whom the nurse is not prepared, nurses caring for patients whose needs are beyond their competency, and issues related to difficult discharge such as the patient being unwilling to leave or a patient/family who requests an unsafe discharge (Cooper, Frank, Hansen, & Gouty, 2004; Swidler, Seastrum, & Shelton, 2007). More recently, issues related to ethical reasoning with individuals self-managing chronic illness have arisen (Redman, 2013). Depending on clinical specialty and/or practice setting, the CNS will need to consider ways to address these ethical issues using a variety of strategies such as recognition of moral distress (LaSala & Bjornson, 2010; Murray, 2010), support of moral courage (Gallagher, 2010), assessment of ethical competency of staff nurses in clinical areas (Cooper, Frank, Hansen, & Gouty, 2004), clinical development of care-based reasoning, and development or participation in nursing ethics rounds (Cohen & Erickson, 2006).

The patient, family, CNS, relevant nursing staff, ethics team, and other providers such as physicians, chaplains, and social workers need to be part of ethical decision making, depending on the situation and the issues (Clark, 2010). A multidisciplinary team approach avoids biased or unilateral decision making and fosters/sustains an environment of open discussion around ethical dilemmas. The common processes used, regardless of ethical framework, include identification of the ethical problem, identification and consideration of alternatives, implementation of a choice and the associated ethical rationale, and evaluation of the decision-making process and its outcome (Bozek & Savage, 2007). Other approaches include intentional creation of ethical environments, accessible ethics rounds, and access to ethics consultation (Shirey, 2005). Ethical decision making can occur in a context that involves significant distress. To assist in such situations, a variety of other process approaches to ethical decision making have been suggested, such as concerned argumentation, consensus formation, clarification, ranking, reassurances, review of cases, and rehearsal of arguments, as ways to uncover the various layers and nuances that may exist in ethical dilemmas (Häyry, 2005).

CITIZENSHIP

Citizenship is defined as "membership in a community with rights to political participation," for example, political rights of an individual within a society. This citizenship is similar to the *polis citizenship* of ancient Greece, when citizenship was not seen as a public matter separate from a person's life. The obligations of citizenship were deeply connected to everyone's life in the *polis* (Leydet, 2006). A core concept of the *polis citizenship* was that the destiny of an individual was strongly linked to the destiny of the community. Applied to nursing, this would suggest that the destiny of an individual nurse or CNS is tied to the destiny of the community of all nurses and all CNSs. This viewpoint suggests that being a good citizen or steward of the profession enables the CNS to influence an organization as well as to influence the profession at the local, state, and national levels. Professional citizenship is presented in the context of the CNS as an employee in an organization and, as a member of the nursing profession, a professional citizen in nursing.

Organizational Citizenship

An organizational citizen is someone who exhibits behaviors that exceed formal job requirements but that contribute indirectly to the organization's effectiveness. These behaviors include helping behaviors (helping others, volunteering, orienting others), keeping up with matters that affect the organization (civic virtue), sportsmanship (not complaining about trivial matters), organizational loyalty, organizational compliance, individual initiative, and self-development (Joireman, Kamdar, Daniels, & Duell, 2006). These behaviors are different from tasks; rather, they are directed at supporting the organizational environment in which tasks take place. Other facets of organizational citizenship are demonstrating concern for the well-being of others, concern with future consequences of one's actions, expectations that individual work will be identified as well as linked to groups, and the belief that contributions have a meaningful impact on the group outcome. These behaviors have been studied and, after meta-analysis across many studies, are now considered to be reflective of organizational citizenship (LePine, Erez, & Johnson, 2002).

The CNS moves through and across many layers of an organization as he or she conducts his or her clinical practice. Clinical expertise in a specialty serves as one kind of "passport" to traverse the organization; organizational citizenship is another kind of passport that creates visible fidelity of the CNS with the organization and its mission, vision, and goals. For example, the CNS who is tremendously gifted in the clinical practice but is at odds with his or her organization will be hampered until this dissonance is resolved.

Organizational citizenship behaviors are similar, overlap, and, potentially, have synergy with emotional competency within an organization. Thus, both as an advanced practice nurse and as an employee in an organization, the CNS who demonstrates competency in self- and social awareness, self-management, and relationships is also likely to demonstrate behaviors associated with organizational citizenship.

Organizational citizenship behaviors can create dilemmas or, as these theorists call it, a social delayed fence. This refers to a situation that requires immediate effort ("hurdling the fence") to obtain a long-term collective goal (Joireman, Kamdar, Daniels, & Duell, 2006). For example, a CNS is working on nursing care with staff and the family of a very complex patient; the CNS is asked to leave that work and refocus on participation in a failure mode effect analysis (FMEA) or another complicated project with equal or higher priority over the current work. The new priority moves the CNS from direct care with a patient family situation to another issue of importance to the organization. This scenario is an accurate description of the practice of the CNS who is interacting with multiple "customers" who have differing priorities.

The CNS can resolve such conflicts between equally meaningful projects and activities by considering the short-term and long-term outcomes of the priorities, and through alignment of the new priority with other projects, so that one project advances the other, and, finally, by assessing the resources needed to respond to both priorities. These responses to competing priorities require the CNS to step around the either/or dilemma and use the both/and response. It may be that to accomplish this, the CNS will ask the organization to bring its resources to temporarily bear on his or her work so that his or her expertise can be given to both priorities. This discussion highlights the dilemmas and the solutions that can be used by the CNS as an organizational citizen while fulfilling the unique characteristics of his or her clinical practice.

Organizational citizenship can be influenced by organizational politics. For example, when the organizational environment supports high levels of informal leader and coworker feedback, the perceptions of organizational politics (in this research defined as intrusive and negative) will be low, and higher morale is present. Research has shown that when there is a high-quality feedback environment, employees are more likely to know the standards of good modulate performance, to believe that performing well leads to desired rewards, and to use the feedback to improve their performance, resulting in low perceptions of organizational politics (Rosen, Levy, & Hall, 2006). This means that when issues arise in the organization, the CNS predicts the organizational response to that issue, identifies how he or she can contribute, and makes adjustments in the practice to be responsive.

Professional Citizenship

If a person's choices and activities indicate his or her values, needs, and beliefs, then it would be predicted that future behavior in conceptually similar situations would be consistent with those values, needs, and beliefs. Thus, if a CNS valued and demonstrated organizational citizenship, it could be predicted that the CNS would also value and demonstrate professional citizenship. Professional citizenship behaviors are conceptually similar to those of organizational citizenship; the difference is that organizational citizenship occurs within the context of an organization, and professional citizenship behavior occurs beyond the CNS's organization and in the nursing profession, the community, and in the legislative or political area.

Professional citizenship may be reflected in many differing ways. For example, a CNS may be a member or a leader/officer of a state nursing association and the ANA, a nursing specialty organization such as the Oncology Nurses Society, or a national organization related to his or her role, such as the NACNS. Professional citizenship may also be reflected by the CNS's use and integration of various products and services from national organizations into his or her practice, for example, the use of national standards in the CNS's specialty or of the ANA, or through use of the Code of Ethics (ANA, 2008).

A CNS may demonstrate professional citizenship through leadership or participating in a project in his or her community. For example, recently, scholarship awardees of the national association for CNSs were selected because of their involvement in issues facing a particular patient population in their community (e.g., institutionalized teens, high-risk mothers, etc.; see www.nacns.org).

CNSs may determine that an issue affecting their practice requires resolution in the state legislature or with a regulatory board. An example of this occurred when CNSs in the state of Oregon sought changes in the statutes and participated in writing the language of administrative rules related to CNS practice and CNS prescriptive privileges (Davidson et al., 2001; Klein, 2013). Other examples of professional citizenship include writing for publication about CNS practice on topics such as validation of CNS competencies (Baldwin, Clark, Fulton, & Mayo, 2009) and CNS practice patterns (Mayo et al., 2010).

It may be that the CNS, through his or her professional organization(s), joins others at the national level in addressing issues such as health care reform, tobacco control, or end-of-life care (Long, 2005). Each and all of these levels of involvement add dimension and give meaning to professional citizenship of the CNS.

There are indications that nurses in particular have been reluctant to engage in professional citizenship. The reasons are complex and include the following factors: (a) perception of ethical conflict between professional values and political involvement (Gordon & Nelson, 2006), (b) lack of awareness or comfort with the political process (Buresh & Gordon, 2000; Stone, 2000), (c) sense of powerlessness and apathy (Des Jardin, 2001a, 2001b), (d) inability to frame and defend issues and present them so the public can understand (Mason, 2006), and (e) fear of retribution from peers and others.

The impact of these factors and the reluctance that nurses may have at the national level has limited, but not extinguished, the efforts of nursing to extend its reach beyond the clinical setting. Through professional citizenship, nursing has achieved many of its goals in national nursing organizations as well as seeing an increase in the numbers of nurses elected to political office. These elected nurses have helped secure intermittent increases in federal budgets that support nursing education and practice, have secured funds supporting recruitment into nursing, and have obtained the passage of some laws addressing health care reform (ANA, 2012; Twedell & Webb, 2007).

Many baccalaureate programs now include curriculum content related to professional citizenship, so that as graduates enter practice and then seek to become CNSs they have received preparation in professional citizenship (Byrd, Costello, Shelton, Thomas, & Petrarca, 2004; Des Jardin, 2001a, 2001b; Rains & Barton-Kriese, 2001). Most, if not all, graduate programs include course work on health policy in the graduate core courses.

Professional citizenship by the CNS may take many forms. It is, however, dependent on the voice of CNSs in various arenas outside of the CNS's primary practice site, unit, and organization. Full development of professional citizenship competency is not only an expectation of the CNS but also a requisite for the role.

SUMMARY

This chapter has presented three of the essential characteristics of CNSs, including the professional attributes of a CNS with an emphasis on EI, ethical conduct, and professional citizenship, incorporating theoretical tenets and relevant research. The ability of CNSs to understand emotions as drivers of thoughts and behaviors, including how these emotions affect relationships, allows CNSs to interact ethically and as good citizens in the communities in which they live and work.

CNSs are often evaluated on their intellectual capacity, knowledge competence, and clinical acumen. While these are essential characteristics, the abilities of the CNS within an organization will be incompletely realized should the professional characteristics, including emotional competence, ethical conduct, and professional citizenship, be underdeveloped. Conversely, when emotional competence, ethical conduct, and professional citizenship are highly tuned, the effectiveness of the CNS is ensured and will be recognized by staff, peers, the organization, and by society. It is essential that curricula, work experiences, and lifelong learning be dedicated, in part, to the continual refinement of these attributes and characteristics. As a recognized clinical leader, the role modeling of these behaviors creates understanding and potential cultural transformation within the organization. This transformation supports the growth and development of all members of the team and, subsequently, results in more effective teamwork, reduced conflict, and better outcomes.

■ DISCUSSION QUESTIONS

Self-Awareness/Self-Management

Scenario: With your class, identify a professional situation in which you experienced the emotion of anger or frustration.

a. *Discussion, analysis, synthesis*: Describe the incident and disclose your responses to the incident, both behavioral as well as your thoughts. Does a symbolic "cow path" emerge? What would you do differently next time as you experience these emotions to realize a healthier outcome for you and others in this scenario?
   Caution: Honesty and transparency in this exercise are essential to one's growth.
b. *Clinical application*: Establish a journal in which you narrate your emotional responses to professional situations, focusing on self-awareness and self-management. Has the self-management of your emotions over time reflected a change?

Social Awareness

Scenario: A multidisciplinary group is assigned to refine and implement a clinical practice guideline. This guideline impacts pharmacy, medicine, social work, nursing, and the dietitian. Members of the class assume the roles of the different disciplines.

a. *Discussion, analysis, synthesis*: From the lens of the discipline to which you have been assigned, discuss barriers and facilitators to implementation. Reflect on your thoughts and emotions as you view this situation from a totally different perspective. Discuss how that experience increases your organizational savvy and political acumen.

   Caution: Reverse role playing can uncover deep-seated mental models regarding other disciplines or individuals with whom you have previously worked.

b. *Clinical application*: The next time a conflict arises between yourself and another discipline, practice reverse role playing, step into the shoes of the other discipline, and now look at the situation. Is your response to the conflict different? Make journal entries as to whether your view of the situation has been enhanced to result in a win/win for both parties.

Relationships

Scenario: An accrediting agency is at the doorstep. You need to implement a policy rapidly in order to fulfill the requirements of the standards. The policy will require a substantive change in practice (e.g., national patient safety goals). You have been assigned to outline the implementation process for the policy. You bring together a group of stakeholders. Everybody is grumbling; "It's the other person's work" and "I'm not changing my practice" are the mantras.

a. *Discussion, analysis, synthesis*: How would you move the group to a win/win situation for all, moving from "you/they" to "I/we"? A collective identity for the group is essential to negotiating this conflict.

   Caution: This exercise focuses on accelerated group process, appropriate linguistics, and effective communication. Avoid getting stuck in silos.

b. *Clinical application*: In a group in which you currently participate, reflect on how your interaction patterns and style either accelerate or inhibit group productivity. Reflect on whether the group productivity is different when you are absent as compared to when you are present. Make journal entries related to this.

Ethical Conduct

Scenario: You have been approached by three staff nurses who tell you that there is a serious ethical dilemma in one of the units. The nurses express extreme frustration over the physician's lack of

engagement, the family's veiled threats of suit, and the lack of agreement among the caregivers as to what is appropriate care for this patient. The patient wants to refuse treatment for a very treatable condition.

a. *Discussion, analysis, synthesis*: Discuss the root causes involved in this care conflict; for example, is this a legal matter, or poor communication and understanding, or truly an ethical dilemma? How would you, as a CNS, proceed to analyze which of the root causes is driving the conflict? Talk this through with your group, focusing on the values that are in conflict for you personally, the members of the team involved, the patient, and the family.

   Caution: Be clear with the members involved in the conflict as to what their expectations are of you and the process that you will use to clarify the drivers involved in the conflict.

b. *Clinical application*: Have conversations with nurses in your work unit regarding their perception of conflicts in care management. Is moral distress among the nurses evident? Think about your role in working through these conflicts. How would you know if moral distress was reduced?

Professional Citizenship

Scenario: You are the CNS within a specific specialty. This specialty has a national professional organization and a national certification examination. You work on a unit where only two of the nurses belong to the professional organization, and no one is certified. It is the organization's intent to receive magnet status within the next 3 years. The unit leadership wants you to get the majority of the RNs on the unit certified and actively engaged in their professional organization. There is a local chapter of the national specialty organization in the city in which you work. In fact, you are the vice president of that local chapter and an author of questions that are in the certification examination.

a. *Discussion, analysis, synthesis*: Discuss how to move the nurses from employee to organizational citizen to reach the goals established by the system.

   Caution: Are the nurses with whom you are working connected to the magnet vision? Do they see themselves as professionals within an organization, or employees to do a job?

b. *Clinical application*: Assess the level of professional citizenship in the work unit in which you currently are employed. What variables would you use to assess professional citizenship?

REFERENCES

American Association of Critical Care Nurses (AACN). (2008a). *AACN standards for establishing and sustaining healthy work environments: A journey to excellence.* Aliso Viejo, CA: Author.

American Association of Critical Care Nurses (AACN). (2008b). *Scope and standards for acute and critical care nursing practice.* Alisa Viejo, CA: Author.

American Nurses Association (ANA). (2008). *Code of ethics for nurses with interpretive statements.* Washington, DC: Author.

American Nurses Association (ANA). (2010a). *Nursing: Scope and standards of practice.* Washington, DC: Author.

American Nurses Association (ANA). (2010b). *Nursing's social policy statement.* Washington, DC: Author.

American Nurses Association (ANA). (2012). *The essential guide to nursing practice.* Washington, DC: Author.

American Nurses Association (ANA), Council of Clinical Nurse Specialists. (1986). *The role of the clinical nurse specialist.* Washington, DC: Author.

Arena, D. M., & Page, N. E. (1992). The imposter phenomenon in the clinical nurse specialist role. *Image: Journal of Nursing Scholarship, 24,* 121–125.

Austin, W. (2007). The ethics of everyday practice: Health care environments as moral communities. *Advances in Nursing Sciences, 30,* 81–88.

Baldwin, K. M., Clark, A. P., Fulton, J., & Mayo, A. (2009). National validation of the NACNS clinical nurse specialist core competencies. *Journal of Nursing Scholarship, 41,* 193–201.

Bartholomew, K. (2005). *Speak your truth: Proven strategies for effective nurse-physician communication.* Marblehead, MA: HCPro, Inc.

Bartholomew, K. (2006). *Ending nurse to nurse hostility: Why nurses eat their young and each other.* Marblehead, MA: HCPro, Inc.

Beauman, S. S. (2006). Leadership and the clinical nurse specialist: From traditional to contemporary. *Newborn and Infant Nursing Reviews, 6,* 22–24.

Benson, G., Martin, L., Ploeg, J., & Wessel, J. (2012). Longitudinal study of emotional intelligence, leadership and caring in undergraduate nursing students. *Journal of Nursing Education, 51*(2), 95–101.

Bozek, M. S., & Savage, T. A. (2007). *The ethical component of nursing education: Integrating ethics into clinical experience.* Philadelphia, PA: Lippincott, Williams & Wilkins.

Buresh, B., & Gordon S. (2000). *From silence to voice: What nurses know and must communicate to the public.* Ottawa, Ontario: Canadian Nurses Association.

Byrd, M. E., Costello, J., Shelton, C. R., Thomas, P. A., & Petrarca, D. (2004). An active learning experience in health policy of baccalaureate nursing students. *Public Health Nursing, 21,* 501–506.

Carson, W. Y., & Minarik, P. A. (2007). Advanced practice nurses: A new skirmish in the continuing battle over scope of practice. *Clinical Nurse Specialist, 21,* 52–54.

Clark, A. P. (2010). A model for ethical decision making in cases of patient futility. *CNS Journal, 24*(9), 189–190.

Codier, E. (2012). Emotional intelligence: Why walking the talk transforms nursing care. *American Nurse Today, 7*(4).

Cohen, J. S., & Erickson, J. M. (2006). Ethical dilemmas and moral distress in oncology nursing practice. *Clinical Journal of Oncology Nursing, 10*(6), 775–782.

Community Hospitals Indianapolis. (1995). *Patients rights & responsibilities: The partnership.* Indianapolis, IN: Author.

Cooper, R. W., Frank, G. L., Hansen, M. M., & Gouty, C. A. (2004). Key ethical issues encountered in healthcare organizations: The perceptions of staff nurses and nurse leaders. *Journal of Nursing Administration, 34,* 149–156.

Cosby, K. S., & Croskerry, P. (2004). Profiles in patient safety: Authority gradients in medical error. *Academy of Emergency Medicine, 11,* 1341–1345.

Cummings, G., Hayduk, L., & Estabrooks, C. (2005). Mitigating the impact of hospital restructuring on nurses. *Nursing Research, 54*(1), 2–12.

Curtin, L. L. (2007). Facing up to fallibility: A manager's guide to ethical decision-making. *Nurse Leader, 5,* 23–27.

Davidson, S. B., Beardsley, K., Busch, A. H., Garner, A., Heresa, S., Hodges N. D.,...Rosenfeld, A. (2001). Statutory and regulatory recognition of clinical nurse specialists in Oregon. *Clinical Nurse Specialist, 15,* 276–283.

Des Jardin, K. E. (2001a). Political involvement in nursing—Education and empowerment, Part I. *Association of Perioperative Registered Nurses Journal, 74,* 468–477.

Des Jardin, K. E. (2001b). Political involvement in nursing—Politics, ethics, and strategic action, Part II. *Association of Perioperative Registered Nurses Journal, 74,* 614–622.

DeWolf, M. S. (1989). Clinical ethical decision-making: A grounded theory method. *Dissertation Abstracts International, 50*(11), 4980.

Ennen, K. A. (2001). Shaping the future of practice through political activity. *American Association of Occupational Health Nurses Journal, 49,* 557–569.

Frankel, A. S., Leonard, M. W., & Denham, C. R. (2006). Fair and just culture, team behavior and leadership engagement. *Health Services Research, 41,* 1690–1709.

Gallagher, A. (2010). Moral distress and moral courage in everyday nursing practice. *Online Journal of Nursing, 16*(2).

Gilligan, C. (1982). *In a different voice.* Cambridge, MA: Harvard University Press.

Goleman, D. (1995). *Emotional intelligence: Why it can matter more than IQ* (10th ed.). New York, NY: Bantam Books.

Goleman, D. (1998). *Working with emotional intelligence.* New York, NY: Bantam Books.

Goleman, D., & Boyatzis, L. (2008). Social intelligence and the biology of leadership. *Harvard Business Review, 86*(9), 74–81.

Goleman, D., Boyatzis, L., & McKee, A. (2002). *Primal leadership: Learning to lead with emotional intelligence.* Boston, MA: Harvard Business School Press.

Golomb, B. A., McGaw, J. J., Evans, M. A., & Dimsdale, J. E. (2007). Physician response to patient reports of adverse drug effects: Implications for patient-targeted adverse effect surveillance. *Drug Safety, 30,* 669–675.

Gordon, S., & Nelson, S. (2006). *The complexities of care: Nursing reconsidered.* New York, NY: ILR Press.

Häyry, M. (2005). Can arguments address concerns? *Journal of Medical Ethics, 31,* 598–600.

Institute of Medicine (IOM). (2003). *Health professions education: A bridge to quality.* Washington, DC: National Academies Press.

Institute of Medicine (IOM). (2004). *Keeping patients safe: Transforming the work environment of nurses.* Washington, DC: National Academies Press.

Institute of Medicine (IOM). (2011). *The future of nursing.* Washington, DC: National Academies Press.

Joireman, J., Kamdar, D., Daniels, D., & Duell, B. (2006). Good citizens to the end? Empathy and concern with future consequences moderate the impact of a short-term time horizon on organizational citizenship behaviors. *Journal of Applied Psychology, 91,* 1307–1320.

Kerfoot, K. (1999). The culture of courage. *Pediatric Nursing, 25,* 558–559.

Kerfoot, K. (2005). Healthy work environments: En route to excellence. *Critical Care Nurse, 25,* 71–72.

Klein, T. A. (2013). Implementing automous CNS prescriptive authority. *CNS Journal, 26*(5), 254–262.

LaSala, C., & Bjornson, D. (2010). Creating workplace environments that support moral courage. *Online Journal of Nursing, 15*(3), Manuscript 3.DOI: 10.3912/OJIN.Vol15No03Man04.

LePine, J. A., Erez, A., & Johnson, D. E. (2002). The nature and dimensionality of organizational citizenship behaviors: A critical review and meta-analysis. *Journal of Applied Psychology, 87,* 52–65.

Leydet, D. (2006). *Citizenship.* Retrieved June 21, 2009, from http://plato.stanford.edu/entries/citizenship

Lombardo, M. M., & Eichinger, R. W. (2006). *For your improvement: A guide for development and coaching* (4th ed.). Minneapolis, MN: Lominger International.

Long, R. E. (2005). From revelation to revolution: Critical care nurses' emerging roles in public policy. *Critical Care Nursing Clinics of North America, 17,* 191–199.

Lynch, A. E., & Cole, E. (2006). Human factors in emergency care: The need for team resource management. *Emergency Nurse, 14,* 32–35.

Mason, D. (2006). Pride and prejudice: Nurses' struggle with reasoned debate. In S. Nelson & S. Gordon (Eds.), *The complexities of care: Nursing reconsidered* (pp. 40–49). Ithaca, NY: ILR Press.

Mayo, A., Agocs-Scott, L., Khaghani, F., Meckes, P. G., Moti, N., Redeemer, J.,... Cuenca, E. (2010). Clinical nurse specialist practice patterns. *CNS Journal, 24*(2), 60–68.

McKinnon, J. (2005). Feeling and knowing: Neural scientific perspectives on intuitive practice. *Nursing Standard, 20,* 41–46.

McQueen, A. C. H. (2004). Emotional intelligence in nursing work. *Journal of Advanced Nursing, 47,* 101–108.

Mohr, W. K., & Mahon, M. M. (1996). Dirty hands: The underside of marketplace health care. *Advances in Nursing Science, 19,* 28–37.

Moland, L. L. (2006). Moral integrity and regret in nursing. In S. Nelson & S. Gordon (Eds.), *The complexities of care: Nursing reconsidered* (pp. 50–68). Ithaca, NY: Cornell University Press.

Murray, J. S. (2010). Moral courage in healthcare: Acting ethically even in the presence of risk. *Online Journal of Nursing, 15*(3), Manuscript 2. DOI: 10.3912/OJIN. Vol15No03Man02.

National Association of Clinical Nurse Specialists (NACNS). (2004). *Statement on clinical nurse specialist practice and education* (2nd ed.). Harrisburg, PA: Author.

Nelson, S. (2006). Ethical expertise and the problem of the good nurse. In S. Nelson & S. Gordon (Eds.), *The complexities of care: Nursing reconsidered* (pp. 69–87). Ithaca, NY: ILR Press.

Nowack, K. M., & Mashihi, S. (2012). Evidence-based answers to 15 questions about leveraging 360 degree feedback. *Consulting Psychology Journal: Practice and Research, 64*(3), 157–182.

Patterson, K., Grenny, J., McMillan, R., & Switzler, A. (2002). *Crucial conversations: Tools for talking when stakes are high.* Provo, UT: Vital Smarts.

Porter O'Grady, T. P., & Malloch, K. (2002). *Quantum leadership: A textbook for new leadership.* Gaithersburg, MD: Aspen Publications.

Rains, J. W., & Barton-Kriese, P. (2001). Developing political competence: A comparative study across disciplines. *Public Health Nursing, 18,* 219–224.

Redman, B. K. (2013). *Advanced practice nursing ethics in chronic disease self-management.* New York, NY: Springer.

Rie, M. A., & Kofke, W. A. (2007). Nontherapeutic quality improvement: The conflict of organizational ethics and societal rule of law. *Critical Care Medicine, 35*(Suppl. 2), S66–S84.

Robert, S. J. (1983). Oppressed group behavior: Implication for nursing. *Advances in Nursing Science, 5,* 21–30.

Rosen, C. C., Levy, P. E., & Hall, R. J. (2006). Placing perceptions of politics in the context of feedback environment, employee attitudes, and job performance. *Journal of Applied Psychology, 91,* 211–220.

Shirey, M. R. (2005). Ethical climate of nursing practice: The leaders' role. *JONA's Healthcare Law, Ethics, and Regulation, 7*(2), 59–67.

Skinner, C., & Spurgeon, P. (2005). Empathy: 4 distinct dispositions: Empathetic concern, perspective taking, personal distress and empathetic matching. 3 empathy scales related to transformational behaviors. *Health Services Management Research, 18,* 1–12.

Stone, D., Patton, B., & Heen, S. (2000). *Difficult conversations: How to discuss what matters most.* New York, NY: Penguin Books.

Swidler, R. N., Seastrum, T., & Shelton, W. (2007). Difficult hospital inpatient discharge decisions: Ethical, legal and clinical practice issues. *American Journal of Bioethics, 7,* 23–28.

Twedell, D. M., & Webb, J. A. (2007). The value of the political action committee: Dollars and influence for nurse leaders. *Nursing Administration Quarterly, 31,* 279–283.

Walrefen, N., Brewer, M. K., & Mulvernon, C. (2012). Sadly caught up in the moment: An exploration of horizontal violence. *Nursing Economics, 30*(1), 6–12, 49–50.

Webster's Dictionary of the American Language. (1962). Cleveland, OH: The Word Publishing Company.

Wlody, G. S. (2007). Nursing management and organizational ethics in the intensive care unit. *Critical Care Medicine, 35,* S29–S35.

Philosophical Underpinnings of Advanced Nursing Practice: A Synthesizing Framework for Clinical Nurse Specialist Practice

Frank D. Hicks

Professional nursing has made significant progress since its inception 150 years ago. Moving from a skills-based vocation to a profession and discipline, nursing has produced talented practitioners, scientists, entrepreneurs, and executives. Despite its increasingly recognized contribution to health care, nursing continues to justify its unique place among other health care professions. The need for this justification arose, in my opinion, as a response to two factors. First, as nursing matured and moved into academe, it became increasingly important to establish and justify a unique identity and body of knowledge to be acceptable to the other scholarly and scientific disciplines. Second, as nurses began to take on more sophisticated roles, it became necessary to establish nurses' efficacy and cost effectiveness. At the heart of this justification was, and continues to be, the need to clearly articulate what it is about nursing that is so crucial and necessary to the health and well-being of humankind. Thus, the search to uncover, describe, and categorize nursing's body of knowledge continues.

The generation of nursing science, a body of knowledge unique to nursing with direct applicability to nursing practice, has led to numerous philosophical and theoretical formulations that attempt to give voice to a fundamental and seemingly implicit understanding of the nature of nursing. Importantly, these theoretical formulations have led to philosophical considerations that have helped to elucidate nursing's nature and the structure of its knowledge.

As a clinical nurse specialist (CNS), I have often grappled with questions of the nature of nursing (nursing's ontology) and the structure of its knowledge (nursing's epistemology). I believe that it is important for the CNS to have an understanding of these concepts, for several reasons. First, understanding nursing's ontology and epistemology helps us to understand that our practice emerges from a particular worldview. As nurses, each of us has a view about the nature of health, people, environment, and discipline and practice of nursing. This worldview comes from our education and experience and most certainly influences the way in which we deliver nursing care, and this ultimately influences client outcomes. Second, as CNSs, we are in a remarkable position to influence the generation of theory that is grounded in practice, something that has long been advocated by several theorists and philosophers of science (Ellis, 1969). As championed by Reed (2006), the time has come to end the dichotomy between theory and practice and place the development of theory where it should be, in a practice-oriented discipline such as nursing, with the nurse engaged in the practice of nursing. Given the varied roles and responsibilities of the CNS and the breadth of CNS influence, there is no one better to engage in the generation and application of theory. To that end, this chapter has three goals:

Describe nursing's metatheoretical space as it helps define nursing's autonomous domain of practice.

Discuss nursing's ontological perspective as it informs nursing processes for CNS practice.

Discuss nursing's epistemological perspective related to phenomena of concern for CNS practice and nursing's unique contribution to health care outcomes.

Exploration of these topics addresses concerns generated by the growing emphasis on pathology, pharmacology, and the diagnosis and treatment of disease, readily apparent in current advanced practice nursing (APN) education and practice. This emphasis may be obfuscating the essential core of nursing knowledge (Arslanian-Engorin, Hicks, Whall, & Algase, 2005; Whall & Hicks, 2002). CNSs, and indeed all APNs, need to be able to clearly articulate the unique role of nursing in health care.

METATHEORY AND AUTONOMOUS CNS PRACTICE

Metatheory deals with the broad conceptual issues concerning how theory is situated, discussed, and developed within a particular discipline. As such, metatheory proffers an overarching framework (the metaparadigm) for understanding important concepts within a field of study. The metaparadigm of nursing—considered to be the concepts of person, environment, health, and nursing—has gained acceptance as the essential concept that underlies nursing's view of reality. A majority of scholarly work undertaken in the past four decades can be seen to address, to some degree, the four concepts. Virtually, all theories of nursing deal with these four concepts to one degree or another, though the definitions of these concepts vary greatly, depending upon the theorist's paradigm. The essential message implied by the metaparadigm, however, is that disciplinary focus of nursing is concerned with the person–environment–health interface. The metaparadigm provided the framework for nursing scholars to begin to think about the relationships among the essential concepts of person, environment, health, and nursing. Accordingly, the metaparadigm has given rise to several paradigms.

A *paradigm* is a worldview that frames the assumptions, methods, and theories scientists use to engage in the work of discovery and understanding (Kuhn, 1972). Logical positivism and phenomenology are two such examples of paradigms that have influenced science over the last 100 years, including nurse scientists (Whall & Hicks, 2002). Parse (1981) posited that nursing's scientific endeavors arose from two predominant worldviews: totality and simultaneity. Essential differences in these paradigms arise from how each one defines the nature of person, environment, and health.

In the totality paradigm, the person is viewed as a holistic being comprised of biological, psychological, sociological, and spiritual components that are in constant interaction with the environment. The person and environment are believed to influence one another, as well as to determine health. Health is often seen as well-being or wholeness that results from the human–environment interaction. The simultaneity paradigm, based in the science of unitary human beings (Rogers, 1970), sees person and environment as inseparable energy fields that are in continuous and mutual exchange with one another. Health is viewed as a social construction (Rogers, 1970); thus, it has no inherent value in itself. Newman (1986), who was influenced by Rogers, sees health as a transcendental process resulting in expanding consciousness. Both of these paradigms have assisted nurses in constructing unique ways of viewing nursing and of delineating the focus and work of nursing. From these paradigms arose the grand theories of nursing, such as Orem (1971), King (1971), Roy (1984), Parse (1981), and Newman (1986).

The argument could be made that none of the concepts contained in the metaparadigm are unique to nursing. Certainly, physicians, occupational and physical therapists, social workers, and other health care workers would say they were concerned with aspects of person, environment, and health. The unique view of nursing, however, comes from the belief that these realities are viewed as holistic and inseparable, in mutual process, and ever evolving. The particularities and specifics of each of these concepts, as defined by the various theorists, may differ, but the unifying theme found in these various theories and worldviews is that nurses deal with humans in their totality and unity and are concerned with the continual and mutual interactions and reactions that occur as a result of the human–environment–health interface. The uniqueness of the discipline, science, and practice of nursing lies at the heart of this interaction and emerges from both trying to understand its results and dealing with its consequences.

To summarize, I suggest that the theories of nursing, though diverse, have some strong underlying, unified themes that speak to essential truths and that can be used to help construct a framework for CNS practice:

1. Nursing is relational by nature. Effective nursing cannot occur if the nurse cannot establish a therapeutic relationship with the patient/client.
2. Nursing does not occur in a vacuum. There must always be consideration of the context in which the person, environment, and resulting patterns of health occur.
3. Nursing focuses on health, wholeness, and well-being rather than disease, dysfunction, and disability.
4. Nursing always strives not only to maintain but also to enhance the unique and indivisible wholeness inherent in the human being and his or her environment.

NURSING'S ONTOLOGICAL PERSPECTIVE: NURSING PROCESSES

Ontology is the branch of philosophy that deals with understanding being, existence, or reality. Thus, as applied to nursing (and nursing science), ontology explores the nature of nursing and essential elements defining that nature. For nearly 40 years, nursing scholars attempted to define the nature of nursing, with several unique ontological formulations coming to the fore. As previously noted, Rogers (1970) asserted that humans and their environment could best be understood as energy fields in mutual exchange. The science of nursing, therefore, emerged from the study of patterns generated by the mutual processes of human and environmental energy fields. Roy (1995) posited nursing's purpose as understanding human adaptive processes for attaining or maintaining health, while Orem (1971) focused on understanding self-care needs of nursing's clients. Alternatively, Parse (1981) saw nursing as understanding the process of human becoming (an evolving self-knowledge) and quality of life. Summarizing and unifying these seemingly diverse outlooks on the nature of nursing, Donaldson (2002) asserted that nursing is "the science of personal and familial human health ecology" (p. 61). Hence, we return to the basic elements of nursing's ontology: human–environment–health.

More recently, Reed (1997) offered another ontological view of nursing that has much potential. Reed's unique view of the discipline of nursing is a synthesis of the work of several philosophers and theorists, including Nightingale (1859/1969), Henderson (1964), and Rogers (1970), among others (Kauffman, 1995; Lerner, 1986; von Bertalanffy, 1981; Waldrop, 1992; Werner, 1957). In Reed's

view (1997), nursing's focus of concern is the innate processes of well-being possessed by all human systems, which are manifested by their complexity and integration. The idea that human beings (and their systems) possess innate characteristics that foster well-being is not new in nursing. Similar ideas can be found in the writings of Nightingale (1859/1969), who maintained that the work of nursing was to put the patient in the right state so the body could heal itself. Similarly, Henderson (1964) asserted that nursing was the work of supporting those activities and processes already possessed by the individual, while Watson (1985) referred to self-healing processes. Similarly, Schlotfeldt (1994) believed humans were able and disposed to seek and attain their health. Reed takes these ideas a step further. She asserts that inherent nursing processes are not necessarily an attempt to reverse disease; rather, nursing processes are intent on moving the human system (individual, group, community) forward toward a sense of well-being (Reed, 1997).

Thus, nursing processes are not external mechanistic devices imposed by nurses, but are essentially relational, contextual, and transformational conceptions of the world perceived and employed by human systems. Reed believes that nursing is a participatory process transcending the boundary between patient and nurse and deriving value from the human system's inherent propensity for innovation and change. Human systems emanate and participate in these nursing processes. For example, nursing processes can be seen in an individual experiencing fear and anxiety over a diagnosis of cancer (e.g., the physiological and psychosocial responses that result from the attempt to understand and integrate this event) or in the rituals and activities that emerge from the healing practices of a culture, which attempt to aid the individual as well as the community. The patterns emerging from these processes are potentially limitless, thus providing fodder for research and application to practice. Thus, for Reed (1997), the quest of the nursing discipline is to "understand the nature of and to facilitate nursing processes in diverse contexts of health experiences" (p. 77). The unique characteristic of the discipline of nursing is found in the intersection of three important concepts: complexity, integration, and well-being.

Complexity refers to the number of variables, factors, or events influencing an individual or group. Variables can be psychological, social, cultural, or physiological; the greater the number of variables, the greater the complexity. For example, consider the variables introduced into the life of a patient who sustains a spinal cord injury (SCI). Not only are there functional and physiological limitations for the individual to overcome, but there are also many psychosocial and emotional challenges to meet, which influence not only the patient but the family and health care system as well. Complexity results in quantitative change, not qualitative change of the whole (Reed, 1997).

Integration occurs when variables are synthesized and organized. Synthesis implies a change in form, not simply the number of events (Reed, 1997, p. 78). Change occurs through integration of an event's meaning and symbolism into one's life. Thus, integration is transformative and results in qualitative change (Reed, 1997). Integration is more than adaptation, however. Integration involves constructing meaning of or identifying a pattern (or patterns) among variables experienced and incorporating these new meanings and patterns into a new understanding of the human–health experience. Elaborating on the example of a patient with SCI, integration occurs when the multiple variables confronting the patient and family become understood, interpreted, and incorporated into a new way of being for both the patient and those with whom the patient interacts and relates. Thus, out of this integration comes a new way of being, a synthesized reality that attempts to regain a sense of well-being.

Well-being emerges from the interaction of complexity and integration. As Reed (1997) stated, "Complexity provides life with the diversity, specialization, and depth in experiences, whereas integration provides organization, coherence, and breadth" (p. 78). The rhythm between complexity and integration determines well-being. The inability to achieve harmony between complexity and integration may result in a feeling of dis-harmony or dis-ease.

Reed's ontology provides the CNS with a unique view of nursing that holds great promise for helping to redefine and refine practice. By synthesizing views commonly expressed in nursing's theoretical history, Reed's ontology provides a flexible way of telescoping from the patient to the system. The concepts of complexity, integration, and well-being can be readily applied to a plethora of human experiences and systems. The idea that well-being evolves out of the way in which the system, whether that be the cardiovascular system or a nursing unit, integrates the complexity of its patterns and experiences provides a unique view to understand various phenomena at any level of abstraction.

PHENOMENA OF CONCERN FOR CNS PRACTICE

Having explicated a new ontological view of nursing, let us turn to a discussion of epistemology or the structure of nursing knowledge. Until recently, the only valid form of scientific knowledge was empirical

(Whall & Hicks, 2002), an idea championed by logical positivists who believed that only observable and verifiable knowledge was worthy of consideration for scientists. With the advent of postmodernism, philosophers of science have entertained the possibility that there may be multiple ways of knowing that may arise out of personal experience and knowledge as well as from observables. This view has been embraced in nursing as well.

One of the best-known treatises on the structure of nursing knowledge is Carper's (1978) "Fundamental Patterns of Knowing in Nursing." This work is significant because it went beyond empirical methods of knowledge development. Indeed, Carper argued that the complexities in the nature of nursing and in nursing practice required more than mere observation and confirmation of phenomena. Nurses require knowledge that not only builds their science but that can also inform their art, morality, and self-knowledge.

Carper (1978) identified four patterns by which nursing knowledge can be understood. *Empirical* knowledge is knowledge acquired through the scientific process. *Ethical* knowledge arises out of the moral imperatives related to the right thing to do in patient/client encounters and is grounded in fundamental ethical principles. *Personal* knowledge refers to the understanding of self and how self influences interactions with others. Finally, *aesthetic* knowledge addresses the creative and original interpretation and application of other forms of knowledge. Each of these patterns helps structure observations and experiences encountered on a daily basis by nurses in practice. The complexity of nursing practice requires depth and breadth of empirical knowledge, a sound understanding of knowing the right thing to do (ethics), and understanding of how self-knowledge "promotes wholeness and integrity in the personal encounter" (personal knowledge; Carper, as cited in Reed, Shearer, & Nicoll, 2004, p. 226). These ways of knowing culminate in the application of knowledge in a given context. Repeated application in similar contexts gives rise to knowledge based on experience. Although others have analyzed and expanded upon Carper's initial epistemological conceptualization (Munhall, 1993; Schultz & Meleis, 1988; White, 1995), these fundamental patterns still provide a solid foundation for exploring knowledge generation and categorization, and these ways of knowing can be used in conjunction with Reed's (1997) ontology to develop an organizing framework that helps to delineate the phenomena of concern for CNS practice.

If we accept the assumption that human systems generate patterns of innate nursing processes that compel the system toward integration and well-being, then it is possible to begin to examine nursing situations for these emerging patterns. Further, if we accept that there are four fundamental forms of nursing knowledge (empirical, aesthetic, personal, and ethical), then each pattern emerging from the human system should lend itself to examination within one of these four forms. By relating the patterns of innate processes to patterns of knowing, then a framework develops that assists in the generation and categorization of patterns that arise out of practice. As the CNS has the theoretical and empirical knowledge of a specialist and engages regularly in the advanced practice of nursing, there is no individual better suited to generate and test nursing knowledge.

Knowledge Development: The Practitioner's Imperative

The development of knowledge from CNS practice may seem, at first, a daunting task that should be left to nursing scientists. Interestingly, when substantive work began in nursing to develop its knowledge base, it was felt that this knowledge should come from and be directly applicable to practice (Conant, 1967; Dickoff & James, 1968, Dickoff, James, & Wiedenbach, 1968a, 1968b; Ellis, 1968, 1969; Wald & Leonard, 1964). However, other scholars at the time believed that nursing was a basic science and thus its knowledge should be generated from this science and then applied to practice. Hence, the rise of the nursing theories of the 1970s and 1980s (Risjord, 2010) and the widening of the theory–practice gap.

Of late, as a result of recognizing multiple ways of knowing and acknowledging multiple paradigms with multiple methods, there is a shift toward closing the theory–practice gap: hence the need for practitioners in nursing to be involved in the generation of theory that arises from and is directly applicable to practice. Again, though this may seem daunting to the CNS, there is no other individual better prepared to engage in this endeavor.

We all generate thoughts about the experiences we encounter in life and we analyze them in an attempt to describe and categorize these thoughts and impressions. This description and categorization is the foundation of theory development. Theory is merely a set of hypotheses that create a framework to understand phenomena (Ellis, 1969). The works of Reed (1997) and Carper (1978) provide the CNS with a unique nursing lens through which the observations of phenomena encountered in practice can be described, categorized, and interpreted. As knowledge of these practice-related phenomena accumulates and multiplies, the CNS has a rich and varied resource upon which to design, implement, and evaluate nursing care. Furthermore,

a synthesis of these two works provides a unique way of examining the nursing phenomenon. Given the multiple roles in which most CNSs must engage today, it is increasingly important that they have the ability to see the wide-ranging connections and ramifications that phenomena have for the patient and the system within which they all interact.

A Pragmatic Application

The difficulty in reading a chapter such as this is that it often leaves the reader asking questions such as, "So, what can I do with this?" and "How can I apply this to my practice?" The application of philosophy finds its voice in the way in which it is embraced and the resulting influence it has in shaping how one looks at the world. Philosophy is not directly applicable to practice, but it can profoundly influence the values and beliefs of the practitioner. The beliefs and values of the practitioner, in turn, influence the theories chosen to direct nursing interventions. Thus, if a CNS were to accept the ontological perspective forwarded by Reed (1997), then the resulting worldview of nursing practice may be very different. For example, instead of concerning oneself with a low hemoglobin level, the CNS looking at nursing with a grounding in Reed's ontology would consider the nursing systems that are being influenced by the reduction in oxygen-carrying capacity of the blood and how that ultimately influences the client's well-being.

SUMMARY AND CONCLUSION

In this chapter, I have tried to provide a philosophical basis for CNS practice by positing a new way to look at nursing practice based on Reed's (1997) and Carper's (1978) work. This ontological and epistemological synthesis is not meant to replace ontological and epistemological perspectives from which previous nursing theories have evolved. Rather, it is meant to provide the CNS with another way to examine and understand nursing phenomena. Indeed, there is still disagreement on whether nursing is a basic or an applied science, nor is there any agreement as to what knowledge is appropriate for practice, or who should develop this knowledge.

To recapitulate the beginning of the chapter, I assert that the need to establish nursing as a discipline and profession that brings a unique and clearly articulated perspective to health care cannot be overemphasized. This articulation is important not only to ensure that nursing has a role on the health care team but also to keep this unique perspective before the eyes of educators of advanced practice nurses to ensure that nursing is not lost in APN programs. Finally, nursing scientists need a perspective from which to develop a science that serves the needs of not only nurses but also the patients for whom they care. Though knowledge from other disciplines may be helpful in improving and expanding the practice of nursing, it is crucial that the essence of nursing's role in improving the health and well-being of individuals, families, and communities be preserved and developed.

■ DISCUSSION QUESTIONS

- What beliefs and values most influence your views of nursing and nursing care? Try to develop your own philosophy of nursing.
- Is nursing an applied science or a basic science? Does this distinction help or hinder the practice of nursing?
- Examine the theories you use in your practice. What are the predominant paradigmatic views from which these theories are derived, and how do these views influence the development and implementation of nursing interventions?

■ ANALYSIS AND SYNTHESIS EXERCISES

- Take two nursing theories and analyze them in terms of what the theorist says about each of the metaparadigm concepts (i.e., person, environment, nursing, health). How have the theorist's underlying assumptions (i.e., philosophy) driven the interpretation/definition of these concepts?
- Observe a CNS in his or her practice. In the course of his or her interactions with clients and other health care workers, what philosophical beliefs influence his or her practice?

■ CLINICAL APPLICATION

- Take a recent client/family for whom you cared and evaluate the case from Reed's ontological perspective. Can you identify where and how the complexity and integration in the various nursing systems occurred?
- Take a phenomenon from practice, such as anxiety or treatment adherence, and analyze the phenomenon from the perspective of nursing as a basic science (i.e., a particular nursing theory) and then from nursing as an applied science. Is there a difference in the approach that each of these analyses would suggest?

REFERENCES

Arslanian-Engoren, C., Hicks, F. D., Whall, A. L., & Algase, D. L. (2005). An ontological view of advanced practice nursing. *Research and Theory for Nursing Practice, 19*(4), 315–322.

Carper, B. (1978). Fundamental patterns of knowing in nursing. *ANS; Advances in Nursing Science, 1*(1), 13–23.

Conant, L. H. (1967). Closing the practice-theory gap. *Nursing Outlook, 15*(11), 37–39.

Dickoff, J., & James, P. (1968). A theory of theories: A position paper. *Nursing Research, 17*(3), 197–203.

Dickoff, J., James, P., & Wiedenbach, E. (1968a). Theory in a practice discipline. I. Practice oriented discipline. *Nursing Research, 17*(5), 415–435.

Dickoff, J., James, P., & Wiedenbach, E. (1968b). Theory in a practice discipline. II. Practice oriented research. *Nursing Research, 17*(6), 545–554.

Donaldson, S. K. (2002). Nursing science defined in less than 10 words. *Journal of Professional Nursing, 18*(2), 61–112.

Ellis, R. (1968). Characteristics of significant theories. *Nursing Research, 17*(3), 217–222.

Ellis, R. (1969). The practitioner as theorist. *The American Journal of Nursing, 69*(7), 1434–1438.

Henderson, V. (1964). The nature of nursing. *The American Journal of Nursing, 64*, 62–68.

Kauffman, S. (1995). *At home in the universe: The search for the laws of self-organization and complexity.* New York, NY: Oxford University Press.

King, I. (1971). *Toward a theory of nursing: General concepts of human behavior.* New York, NY: Wiley.

Kuhn, T. S. (1972). *The structure of scientific revolutions* (2nd ed.). Chicago, IL: University of Chicago Press.

Lerner, R. M. (1986). *Concepts and theories of human development* (2nd ed.). New York, NY: Random House.

Munhall, P. L. (1993). "Unknowing": Toward another pattern of knowing in nursing. *Nursing Outlook, 41*(3), 125–128.

Newman, M. (1986). *Health as expanding consciousness.* St. Louis, MO: C. V. Mosby.

Nightingale, F. (1969). *Nursing: What it is and what it is not.* New York, NY: Dover. (Original work published 1859)

Orem, D. E. (1971). *Nursing: Concepts of practice.* New York, NY: McGraw-Hill.

Parse, R. R. (1981). *Man-living-health: A theory of nursing.* New York, NY: Wiley.

Reed, P. G. (1997). Nursing: The ontology of the discipline. *Nursing Science Quarterly, 10*(2), 76–79.

Reed, P. G. (2006). The practice turn in nursing epistemology. *Nursing Science Quarterly, 19*(1), 36–38.

Reed, P. G., Shearer, N. C., & Nicoll, L. H. (2004). *Perspectives on nursing theory* (4th ed.). Philadelphia, PA: Lippincott, Williams & Wilkins.

Risjord, M. (2010). *Nursing knowledge: Science, practice, and philosophy.* Ames, IA: Wiley-Blackwell.

Rogers, M. E. (1970). *Introduction to the theoretical basis of nursing.* Philadelphia, PA: F. A. Davis.

Roy, C. (1984). *Introduction to nursing: An adaptation model* (2nd ed.). Englewood Cliffs, NJ: Prentice Hall.

Roy, C. L. (1995). Developing nursing knowledge: Practice issues raised from four philosophical perspectives. *Nursing Science Quarterly, 8*(2), 79–85.

Schlotfeldt, R. (1994). Resolving opposing viewpoints: Is this desirable? Is it practicable? In J. E. Kikuchi & H.

Simmons (Eds.), *Developing a philosophy of nursing* (pp. 67–74). Thousand Oaks, CA: Sage.

Schultz, P. R., & Meleis, A. I. (1988). Nursing epistemology: Traditions, insights, questions. *Image: Journal of Nursing Scholarship, 20*(4), 217–221.

von Bertalanffy, L. (1981). *A systems view of man* (Ed. P. A. LaViolette). Boulder, CO: Westview Press.

Wald, F. S., & Leonard, R. C. (1964). Towards development of nursing practice theory. *Nursing Research, 13*(4), 309–313.

Waldrop, M. M. (1992). *Complexity: The emerging science at the edge of order and chaos*. New York, NY: Simon and Schuster.

Watson, J. (1985). *Nursing: Human science and human care*. Norwalk, CT: Appleton-Century-Crofts.

Werner, H. (1957). The concept of development from a comparative and organismic point of view. In D. B. Harris (Ed.), *The concept of development* (pp. 125–148). Minneapolis, MN: University of Minnesota Press.

Whall, A. L., & Hicks, F. D. (2002). The unrecognized paradigm shift in nursing: Implications, problems, and possibilities. *Nursing Outlook, 50*(2), 72–76.

White, J. (1995). Patterns of knowing: Review, critique, and update. *ANS; Advances in Nursing Science, 17*(4), 73–86.

Nurse-Sensitive Outcomes

Diane M. Doran, Souraya Sidani, and Tammie DiPietro

Outcomes measurement has become a primary focus as health care organizations tackle the major challenges of today and tomorrow, namely, cost and quality, effectiveness of care, and organizational performance. All practitioners in the health care field are being challenged to find ways to demonstrate that the care they provide leads to improvement in outcomes for patients. To accomplish that, practitioners are attempting to identify the relevant outcomes that can be linked in a meaningful way to their own practices. In this chapter, we review the most recent accumulated evidence related to patient and system outcomes that are associated with the role of the clinical nurse specialist (CNS). We review both the theoretical and empirical literature about patient outcomes that are sensitive to the CNS role, with the goal of providing sound evidence to clinicians, health care leaders, and researchers for evaluating the impact of CNSs in our health care system.

The three objectives of this chapter are the following:

1. To identify the essential characteristics or attributes defining CNS practice. This first objective is critical to developing a clear conceptual definition of their scope of practice, which will lay the foundation for identifying outcomes relevant for measuring the impact of their role. In particular, the framework for CNS practice described in the National Association of Clinical Nurse Specialists (NACNS) Statement on Clinical Nurse Specialist Practice and Education (www.nacns.org) will be reviewed as a foundation for identifying specific outcomes associated with the CNS role

2. To identify outcomes associated with the CNS role
3. To determine the extent to which each outcome has demonstrated sensitivity to the CNS role. This will be accomplished by examining relationships between CNS role variables and patient/team/system outcomes

METHODOLOGY FOR LITERATURE REVIEW ON CNS PRACTICE

Step 1: Literature Search

The first step of the literature review/analysis consisted of identifying conceptual and empirical references that discuss or investigate advanced nursing practice, excluding nurse practitioners (NPs). The search involved three strategies:

1. Generating a comprehensive list of relevant articles, book chapters, books, or other documents that we have accumulated through our involvement in previous work.
2. Completing a computerized literature search to identify relevant literature about the outcomes of the CNS role. The computerized literature bases included in this step were the Cumulative Index to Nursing and Allied Health Literature (CINAHL), Health Planning, MEDLINE, CANCERLIT, SocioFile, and PsychLit. This search strategy used the following key words to identify relevant articles:
   a. Advanced practice nursing/nurses and/or
   b. CNS and

c. Nursing sensitive patient outcomes, role impact, role effectiveness, CNS interventions, quality of nursing care, patient outcomes, nursing organization
d. Patient satisfaction with nursing care, patient satisfaction, patient and quality of care, system outcomes
3. The references reported within the articles, in particular those reporting the results of meta-analytic studies or integrative literature review/synthesis, were traced to identify additional references.

Step 2: Literature Selection

The references identified were included in the literature review if they met the following criteria:

1. For theoretical/conceptual references:
   a. They discussed the definition and the domains/dimensions of advanced nursing practice.
   b. They presented the findings of a concept analysis or literature review performed to identify the essential characteristics, domains, and dimensions as well as the empirical indicators or manifestations of the outcome concepts of interest.
   c. They reported the results of a qualitative study conducted to explore the understanding of role implementation or perception of outcomes related to advanced nursing practice.
2. For empirical references:
   a. They reported the results of studies that examined the relationships among the structure, process, and outcome variables for CNS practice.
   b. Studies with descriptive, experimental, or quasi-experimental designs were included. The inclusion of quasi-experimental studies was important for two reasons:
3. i. It increased the number of references for a comprehensive literature review, particularly if the studies were conducted in the context of actual/everyday practice where randomization may not have been feasible or possible; and
   ii. It provided evidence for determining the extent to which the outcomes are responsive to change.

Differences in research designs across studies were accounted for when synthesizing the findings to address the objectives set for this literature review.

Step 3: Literature Compilation

1. A list of references was generated for each outcome variable.
2. Standardized tables for extracting the relevant data were used to review the literature.

3. Word files were generated for anecdotal observations and synthesis of the literature.
4. Two of the coauthors independently reviewed all of the empirical studies.

CONCEPTUALIZING CNS PRACTICE

In this section, we present a conceptualization of the CNS role, derived from a synthesis of essential characteristics developed by the NACNS (2004) and pertinent theoretical and empirical literature. The literature consisted of:

1. Reviews about the CNS role components done either as independent initiatives (Conger & Craig, 1998; Harrington & Smith, 2005; McAlpine, 1997; Raja-Jones, 2002) or in preparation for a research study (Barnason, Merboth, Pozehl, & Tietjen, 1998; Carroll, Robinson, Buselli, Berry, & Rankin, 2001; Mick & Ackerman, 2000; Wojner & Kite-Powell, 1997); or
2. Quantitative or qualitative studies that investigated the CNS role implementation in various settings (Bousfield, 1997; Dickerson, Wu, & Kennedy, 2006; Froggatt & Hoult, 2002; Linck & Phillips, 2005; McCreaddie, 2001; Scott, 1999)

A clear and sound understanding of the CNS role is required to appreciate its contribution to outcomes. Knowledge of the CNS domains of practice and role functions and activities is critical for delineating the mechanisms underlying the impact of CNSs' care on patient, nurse, and system outcomes (Sidani, Doran, & Mitchell, 2004).

CNSs are "licensed registered professional nurses with graduate preparation" demonstrated in an earned master's or doctorate degree (NACNS, 2004, p. 12). Through graduate preparation, CNSs acquire advanced knowledge and clinical expertise that enable them to function independently and in collaboration with other health care professionals for the purpose of achieving high-quality, cost-effective outcomes. Although CNSs develop expertise in particular specialty areas (Darmody, 2005), they exert their influence in three spheres: patients or clients and patient care; nurse and nursing practice; and organization and system (NACNS, 2004).

Patient and Patient Care

Within this sphere or domain of practice, CNSs follow the nursing process of assessment, diagnosis, intervention, and evaluation in order to maintain or improve health. CNSs focus on identifying the needs of patients, selecting and implementing theory and evidence-based interventions to remedy or alleviate symptoms, enhancing physical and psychosocial functioning, and modifying risk behaviors and promoting healthy lifestyles (NACNS, 2004). In addition, CNSs manage patients' care through consultation and collaboration with health care professionals (Brooten, Youngblut, Deatrick, Naylor, & York, 2003; Harrington & Smith, 2005; Naylor, Bowles, & Brooten, 2000). Consultation and collaboration are directed toward clarifying complex patient problems, finding appropriate solutions to those problems, and providing and coordinating services to achieve the collaboratively identified goals or outcomes (NACNS, 2004).

The role functions and activities comprising the patient and patient care practice domain are specified in the conceptual and empirical literature included in this review. The specific activities are consistent with the NACNS's (2004) statement but are categorized into direct and indirect patient care activities. Direct patient care activities reflect the basic elements of the

nursing process (assessment, diagnosis, intervention, and evaluation) and encompass surveillance, provision of care, and facilitation of support groups for patients and families. Indirect patient care activities include case management and the provision of consultation regarding patient care (Brooten et al., 2003; Conger & Craig, 1998; Fowler Byers & Brunnell, 1998; Linck & Phillips, 2005; Naylor et al., 2000; Scott, 1999; Wojner & Kite-Powell, 1997). Table 4.1 presents a list of specific activities illustrating direct and indirect patient care functions of the CNS role.

Nurse and Nursing Practice

This domain of CNS practice focuses on supporting nursing personnel in the delivery of high-quality, safe, and evidence-based care. CNSs engage in role modeling, consultation, and education to improve nursing practice (NACNS, 2004). The specific activities representing this domain are classified into formal and informal education. Formal education consists of the organization of and

TABLE 4.1

SPECIFIC ACTIVITIES ILLUSTRATING DIRECT AND INDIRECT PATIENT CARE FUNCTIONS	
Direct care	
Surveillance	1. Assessing patients' physical and psychosocial conditions, health behaviors, and environmental situations
	2. Diagnosing patient and family needs
	3. Monitoring patients' condition and progress toward achieving outcomes
Provision of care	1. Planning comprehensive care for patients and family
	2. Providing extended education and counseling
	3. Troubleshooting complex patient care problems
	4. Assessing effectiveness of interventions
Facilitation of support groups for patients and family	1. Planning support groups for patients and family
	2. Organizing logistics of support groups
Indirect care	
Case management	1. Overseeing delivery of patient care
	2. Facilitating interprofessional patient care conference
	3. Coordinating intra-/interprofessional services
	4. Discharge planning, including arrangement for required community services
Provision of consultation regarding patients' care	1. Applying advanced knowledge in crisis intervention
	2. Providing support for frontline problem solving, including equipment problems

participation in staff orientation to the specialty area and the design and provision of programs concerned with the continuous professional development of nurses (Barnason et al., 1998; Carroll et al., 2001; Fowler Byers & Brunnell, 1998; Martin, 1999; McCreaddie, 2001; Phillips, 2005; Scott, 1999). Informal education entails the role modeling and consultation activities mentioned in the NACNS (2004) statement. For a list of specific activities related to formal and informal education provided by CNSs, refer to Table 4.2.

Organization and System

CNSs are leaders who advocate for patient care and professional nursing within the organization and the health care system. They initiate, implement, and coordinate innovative programs that address the needs of patients, nurses, and organizations and aim at achieving high-quality and cost-efficient health care across the full continuum of care (NACNS, 2004). The specific activities pertaining to this organizational domain of CNS practice and mentioned in the literature are grouped into those associated with continuous quality improvement initiatives (Arbour, 2003; Conger & Craig, 1998; Wojner & Kite-Powell, 1997); policies, procedures, and best-practice guidelines development (Froggatt & Hoult, 2002; Harrington & Smith, 2005; McCreaddie, 2001); program development and evaluation (Scott, 1999); evidence-based practice (EBP; Harrington & Smith, 2005; McCreaddie, 2001; Scott, 1999); and committee work. These activities operationalize the CNS role within the organizational domain, as described by the NACNS (2004) and presented in Table 4.3.

Only one study was found that investigated CNSs' implementation of role functions and activities related to the three domains of practice as identified by the NACNS (2004). Darmody (2005) conducted a pilot study to explore CNS ($n = 5$) engagement in patient care, nursing practice, and organization-related activities. CNS performance of these activities was assessed with direct observation and time study. The results provided a useful overview indicating that the CNSs spent 30% of their time in patient care, 44% in activities associated with improvement of nursing practice, 10% in organization activities, and 16% in other activities such as personal time and managing e-mail communication.

CONCEPTUALIZING OUTCOMES OF CNS PRACTICE

In this section, we present a conceptualization of outcomes expected of CNS practice. The conceptualization was derived from a synthesis of the NACNS's (2004) statement, which identified specific outcomes for the three domains of CNS practice, and the available conceptual literature reflecting nursing scholars' propositions of outcomes sensitive to CNS care. We define CNS-sensitive outcomes as those that can be theoretically linked to the activities of CNSs and observed in the three domains of CNS practice: patient and patient care, nurse and nursing practice, and organization and system.

TABLE 4.2

SPECIFIC ACTIVITIES ILLUSTRATING FORMAL AND INFORMAL EDUCATION FUNCTIONS	
Formal	1. Participating in development, organization, and coordination of nursing staff orientation to specialty unit
	2. Participating in initial and continuous assessment of nursing staff competencies
	3. Designing and implementing ongoing educational programs for nursing staff based on identified learning needs/competencies
	4. Providing certification review courses to nursing staff
	5. Participating in and/or providing courses to undergraduate and/or graduate nursing students
	6. Serving as clinical preceptor to nursing staff and students
Informal	1. Providing mentorship to nursing staff at bedside
	2. Serving as role model in problem solving and case management
	3. Serving as information resource to nursing staff (e.g., responding to questions related to unfamiliar policies, procedures, clinical problems; discussing evidence base for nursing interventions)

TABLE 4.3

SPECIFIC ACTIVITIES PERTAINING TO ORGANIZATION-SYSTEM DOMAIN OF PRACTICE	
Continuous quality improvement initiatives	1. Designing methods and tools for continuous collection of data (related to process and outcome of care)
	2. Analyzing and synthesizing data obtained from multiple sources
	3. Identifying care-related issues requiring remediation
	4. Collaborating with members of intra/interprofessional team in formulation of remedial strategies and change of practice
	5. Overseeing implementation of remedial strategies and practice change
	6. Facilitating ongoing outcome monitoring
Policies, procedures, and best-practice guidelines development	1. Developing organization policies and procedures related to care delivery
	2. Developing best-practice guidelines based on available evidence
	3. Providing leadership in dissemination and implementation of policies, procedures, and practice guidelines
Program development and evaluation requiring intervention	1. Collaborating with administrators and professionals (nursing and others) to identify clinical issues
	2. Designing programs to address identified clinical issues
	3. Coordinating implementation of programs and evaluation of their effects
Evidence-based practice	1. Leading or participating in research related to area of specialty
	2. Assisting professionals (nursing and others) in conduct of clinical research
	3. Participating in dissemination of research findings within organization and at conferences
	4. Supporting nursing staff in change of practice or research utilization
Committee work	1. Participating in committees within organization, community, and profession

Patient-Related Outcomes

CNSs have an impact on patient outcomes through the accurate diagnosis of patients' needs and problems and the provision of appropriate interventions to remedy the problems, promote health, and prevent error. CNSs' practice in this domain is expected to achieve four categories of desired patient-focused outcomes: clinical, functional, perception, and cost of care (Fowler Byers & Brunnell, 1998; NACNS, 2004).

The *clinical* outcomes are subdivided into (a) the successful management of disease-specific signs and of physical and psychosocial symptoms experienced as a result of disease, illness, or treatment, manifested by normal test values (e.g., blood glucose level, FEV1) and reduced symptom frequency and severity; and (b) the early identification and prevention of complications (e.g., nosocomial infections and deep vein thrombosis) and side effects of medications (Arbour, 2003; Barnason et al., 1998; Darmody, 2005).

Functional outcomes encompass physical, psychological, and social functioning; ability to participate in activities of daily living and to meet role expectations; overall well-being; quality of life; and self-management knowledge and skills related to current condition and modification of risky health behaviors (Barnason et al., 1998; Carroll et al., 2001; Conger & Graig, 1998; Darmody, 2005).

Perception of care outcomes relates to the patient and family rating of the quality of services and satisfaction with the care received (Harrington & Smith, 2005).

Cost outcomes are associated with utilization of resources across the health care continuum operationalized in indices such as length of hospital stay, readmission, return visit to clinic, and visit to the emergency department (ED; Harrington & Smith, 2005; Linck & Phillips, 2005; McAlpine, 1997; Scott, 1999). CNSs' engagement in indirect patient care activities promotes coordination of patient care, which is reflected in prompt services required for patients (Harrington & Smith, 2005).

Nurse-Related Outcomes

CNSs' involvement in formal and informal education is anticipated to contribute to improving nursing staff's knowledge, skills, and practice that is theory and evidence based, enhancing nurse participation in continuing professional development, increasing nurse job satisfaction, and retaining competent nursing personnel (Arbour, 2003; Barnason et al., 1998; Darmody, 2005; NACNS, 2004).

Organization-Related Outcomes

The implementation of activities within this domain of CNS practice is expected to result in improved organizational performance in terms of innovative evidence-based models of care and cost savings associated with the purchase and use of equipment, supplies, and services (Fowler Byers & Brunnell, 1998; NACNS, 2004).

CNSs' achievement of these specific outcomes will contribute to the attainment of the ultimate goal summarized by the NACNS (2004) as "quality, cost-effective, patient-focused outcomes" (p. 6). The empirical evidence supporting the impact of CNS role on patient, nurse, and organization outcomes is presented next.

CATEGORIZING NURSING-SENSITIVE PATIENT OUTCOMES

In this section, we provide an overview of the historical work in classifying nursing-sensitive patient outcomes as a foundation for situating our discussion of outcomes sensitive to CNS practice. Nursing-sensitive outcomes are outcomes that can be empirically or theoretically linked to the actions of registered nurses (RNs) or registered practical nurses (RPNs; Doran et al., 2003). There have been several attempts to generate a taxonomy of patient outcomes that can be expected to occur from the provision of nursing care (Hegyvary, 1991; Jennings, Staggers, & Brosch, 1999; Lohr, 1985).

Early categorizations of nursing-sensitive outcomes focused on the adverse aspects of treatment and have included mortality, morbidity (iatrogenic complications), unscheduled readmission, unscheduled repeat surgery, and unnecessary hospital procedures (e.g., cesarean section rates). Lohr (1985) proposed a list of six categories based on the continuum of care: mortality, adverse events and complications during hospitalization, inadequate recovery, prolongation of the medical problem, decline in health status, and

decline in quality of life. Using a different approach, Hegyvary (1991) suggested four categories of outcome assessment from the perspectives of patients, providers, and purchasers: (a) clinical (patients' responses to interventions), (b) functional (improvement or decline in physical functioning), (c) financial (cost and length of stay), and (d) perceptual (patient satisfaction with care received and persons providing the care).

Jennings et al. (1999) reviewed the nursing, medical, and health services research literature from 1974 and on to locate all indicators of outcomes. These were classified as patient focused, provider focused, or organization focused. Although not specific to the CNS role, this classification has potential applicability because of its broad conceptualization of outcomes and its recognition that nurses do impact system-level outcomes. Within the patient-focused category, a further subdivision into diagnosis focused and holistically focused was proposed. Examples of the diagnosis-specific outcomes are laboratory values, Apgar scores, and vital signs. The holistically oriented outcomes include health status, health-related quality of life, patient satisfaction ratings, assessments of patient knowledge, and symptom management. Care provider–focused outcomes included complication rates, appropriate use of medications, and, when a family caregiver is involved, a measure of caregiver burden. Adverse events such as falls, deaths, and unplanned readmission were categorized as organization-focused outcomes.

In the Quality Health Outcomes Model developed by the American Academy of Nursing Expert Panel on Quality Health Care, five outcome categories expected to be sensitive to nursing care inputs were delineated: achievement of appropriate self-care, demonstration of health-promoting behaviors, health-related quality of life, perception of being well cared for, and symptom management to criterion (Mitchell, Armstrong, Simpson, & Lentz, 1989; Mitchell & Lang, 2004). In the Nursing Role Effectiveness Model, proposed by Irvine, Sidani, and McGillis Hall (1998), the following patient outcomes were hypothesized as sensitive to nursing: patient satisfaction, functional status, self-care, symptom control, and safety/adverse occurrences.

These different frameworks for categorizing nursing-sensitive outcomes are quite consistent with the conceptualization of outcomes of CNS practice that were derived from the NACNS's (2004) statement on CNS practice and education. Most frameworks recognize that nurses have an impact on a broad set of patient outcomes, reflecting improvement in clinical, functional, and psychosocial outcomes, and that nurses minimize or mitigate the effect of adverse outcomes. The conceptualization of outcomes of CNS practice that was synthesized from the NACNS's statement has been used to organize our discussion of the evidence from the empirical literature presented in the next section.

EVIDENCE CONCERNING OUTCOMES SENSITIVE TO CNS PRACTICE

In identifying outcomes relevant for evaluating the impact of the CNS role within the health care system, we considered both the empirical evidence concerning the influence of CNS practice on patient outcomes and the empirical evidence concerning the influence of CNS practice on unit or system outcomes, recognizing that the processes by which CNSs impact outcomes is often mediated through other system variables, such as changes in the quality of nursing care. The studies that were identified through our search of the literature are summarized in the Table 4.4. Each study was reviewed using the following framework: research design, setting for practice, sample, method of accounting for confounding/control variables that could influence the results, CNS role activities, intervention tested, and research results. This information was helpful in determining the level of consistency in the evidence across studies with regard to outcomes sensitive to CNS practice.

Patient-Related Outcomes

As previously noted, patient-related or patient-focused outcomes include clinical, functional, perception, and cost of care (Fowler Byers & Brunnell, 1998; NACNS, 2004). The *clinical* outcomes have been subdivided into (a) successful management of disease-specific signs and symptoms, and (b) early identification and prevention of complications.

Under subdivision (a), there are a number of *disease/condition-specific outcomes* that were identified from the empirical literature on CNS practice. These include arthritis disease activity for a rheumatoid arthritis population (Ryan, Hassell, Lewis, & Farrell, 2006; Tijhuis, Zwinderman, Hazes, Breedveld, & Vliet, 2003), wound healing (Capasso, 1998), glycemic control for a diabetic population (Vrijhoef, Diederiks, Spreeuwenberg, & Wolffenbuttel, 2001), mobility for patients with Parkinson disease (Hurwitz, Jarman, Cook, & Bajekal, 2005), physiological indicators (Graveley & Littlefield, 1992), and full-term delivery for high-risk women (Brooten et al., 2001). The types of CNS role activities that were investigated in these studies were case management (Ryan et al., 2006; Vrijhoef et al., 2001), patient education

(Brooten et al., 2001; Tijhuis et al., 2003), multidisciplinary collaborative practice (Hurwitz et al., 2005), assessment, patient monitoring, counseling, and referrals (Brooten et al., 2001; Graveley & Littlefield, 1992). With the exception of the research by Vrijhoef et al. (2001) and by Gravely and Littlefield (1992), these studies employed a randomized controlled trial (RCT) design and focused on the expanded role of the CNS in outpatient settings. When this research was reviewed, we found that there was mixed evidence concerning the relationship between CNS practice and disease/condition-specific outcomes. Three studies found a significant positive relationship between CNS practice and the disease/condition-specific outcomes, whereas three studies did not. Two of the studies that did not find a significant relationship might have lacked power to detect significant effects because of small sample size (Graveley & Littlefield, 1992; Tijhuis et al., 2003). However, the third study had a large sample size, included a 2-year follow-up, and utilized objective approaches to outcomes measurement (Hurwitz et al., 2005). Therefore, the empirical evidence suggests that CNSs can have a significant positive influence on patients' disease/condition-specific outcomes, however, this evidence is mixed and requires further validation in future research.

The second type of outcome reviewed under subdivision (a), "successful management of disease-specific signs and symptoms," was *physical and psychosocial symptoms*. Under this grouping, researchers have investigated pain outcomes (Gaston-Johansson et al., 2000; Tranmer & Parry, 2004; White, 1999), perceived stress (Tsay, Lee, & Lee, 2005), depression (Gaston-Johansson et al., 2000; Naylor et al., 1999; Tsay et al., 2005), symptom distress (McCorckle et al., 1989; Tranmer & Parry, 2004), and nausea and fatigue (Gaston-Johansson et al., 2000). These studies have investigated the full scope of CNS practice from case management (McCorckle et al., 1989; Tranmer & Parry, 2004; Tsay et al., 2005) to direct clinical practice (White, 1999) to group intervention (Gaston-Johansson et al., 2000) and to discharge follow-up (Naylor et al., 1999). The empirical evidence suggests that CNSs have a significant positive effect on physical and psychosocial outcomes through practice in inpatient settings (Gaston-Johansson et al., 2000; White, 1999) and outpatient settings (McCorckle et al., 1989; Tsay et al., 2005).

The third category of outcome we consider in the *clinical* category is under subdivision (b), *early identification and prevention of complications*. Two types of outcomes are considered in this category: unanticipated mortality (Brooten et al., 2001) and hospital-acquired complications, such as respiratory infection, foot drop, surgical wound infection, urinary tract

(text continues on pg. 60)

TABLE 4.4

STUDIES INVESTIGATING CLINICAL NURSE SPECIALIST PRACTICE AND PATIENT OUTCOMES

Author(s)	Design	Setting/ Subjects	Control Variables	Outcome	CNS Role Components/ Domains	Intervention	Results
Ahrens et al. (2003)	Quasi-experiment	Medical ICU patients at high risk of dying ($N = 43$ intervention, $N = 108$ control)	Patient demographics (chart review)	Clinical (chart review); Severity of Illness "Apache II scoring system"; resource consumption (ICU and hospital length of stay, mortality and fixed cost per case, hospital variable indirect charge per case, hospital variable direct charge per case)	Physician and CNS collaborative ICU managed care vs. rotating physician managed care. Education, physical functioning, psychosocial functioning, administration, case management	Daily information to families, clarify issues and develop care plan	Patients receiving collaborative physician/CNS care had > improvements in severity of illness (32.1–28.6); length of stay in ICU (6.1–9.5 days); costs ($5,320–$8,484); and mortality (74%–93%) than physician managed care only.
Brooten et al. (2001)	RCT	173 women and 194 infants		Fetal/infant mortality; full-term deliveries; rehospitalization; maternal affect "Multiple Affect Adjective State Form Checklist" (Zuckerman et al., 1983), α 0.73; satisfaction with care "LaMonica-Oberst Patient Satisfaction Scale" (LaMonica-Oberst, 1986), α 0.92	Assessment, monitoring, environmental supports, individual teaching and counseling, referrals	Home visits by APNs	Experimental group had lower fetal/infant mortality (2 vs. 9), fewer preterm infants, more twin pregnancies carried to term (77% vs. 33%), fewer prenatal hospitalizations (41 vs. 49), fewer infant rehospitalizations (18 vs. 24), and lower costs.

Study	Design	Sample	Data source	Measures	Intervention/Comparison	Nursing intervention	Findings
Charles et al. (1999)	Descriptive, comparative, randomly assigned	80 patients from emergency department in Melbourne, Australia		Patient wait times; patient perceptions of wait time; patient satisfaction; wound complications	Low-acuity patients requiring simple suture receiving CNS managed care vs. physician managed care. Physical functioning, administration, psychosocial functioning, role functioning	Nursing educational sessions related to suturing of minor lacerations	More patients were satisfied with CNS than physician care (mean rank 47.65 and 33.35, 2 tailed $P = 0.0016$). No other significant findings
Crimlisk et al. (1997)	Prospective	Adult patients requiring endotracheal intubation in a trauma center during a 3-month period. Phase 1 $N = 862$; Phase 2 $N = 808$		Reintubation rate (the number of reintubations per total hospital intubations) Duration of intubation (# of patient ventilated days)	Reintubation events documented for 3 months. Interventions instituted and evaluated for reintubation (3-month period). Similar data collected at 2 years	Continuous quality screening of high-risk patients. Staff nurses provided with inservices, education, and posted signs	Multiple reintubation events decreased from 45% to 18.8% of all intubations
De Jong (2004)	Descriptive, convenience sampling. Baseline, 8, 12 weeks after initial questionnaire	Community-based COPD screening clinic $N = 243$	Questionnaire: demographics, symptoms, treatments, smoking history	Spirometry "GOLD"; "Stage of Smoking" (author-prepared questionnaire)	CNS-managed COPD clinic to identify at-risk adults. Physical functioning, psychosocial functioning, counseling, self-care	COPD screening questionnaire, spirometry testing, counseling, and follow-up survey.	86% participants identified as current or past smokers. Of these, 23% had evidence of obstruction. 78% had never had spirometry testing. Post screening, 40% stated they were contemplating quitting smoking and 5 had.
Forster et al. (2005)	RCT	General medical in-hospital patients $N = 307$ CNS care; $N = 313$ regular hospital care. Post discharge $N = 175$ CNS care; $N = 186$ regular hospital care	Medical information demographics (chart review, patient interviews)	In-hospital: mortality, length of stay. Post discharge: time to ED visit, readmission or death; patient satisfaction (Cleary et al., 1991); risk of adverse events	Regular hospital care vs. CNS care	CNS arranged in-hospital consultations and investigations, organized follow-up visits and telephone calls post discharge	Addition of CNS to a medical team improved patient satisfaction but did not impact hospital efficiency or patient safety

(continued)

TABLE 4.4

STUDIES INVESTIGATING CLINICAL NURSE SPECIALIST PRACTICE AND PATIENT OUTCOMES (CONTINUED)

Author(s)	Design	Setting/ Subjects	Control Variables	Outcome	CNS Role Components/ Domains	Intervention	Results
Gaston-Johansson et al. (2000)	RCT	Patients with breast cancer with autologous bone marrow/ peripheral blood stem cell transplantation $N = 58$ control; $N = 52$ treatment group	Socio-demographic questionnaire	Pain "(POM)-Gaston-Johansson Painometer" (Gaston-Johansson, 1996); nausea "Nausea VAS" (Gift, 1989); fatigue "Fatigue VAS" (Piper, 1989); anxiety "State Trait Anxiety Inventory" (Spielberger et al., 1971); depression "Beck depression Inventory" (Beck & Steer, 1993)	Treatment group given CCSP vs. regular care. Pain, fatigue, psychological distress, nausea	CNS developed Comprehensive Coping Strategy Program (CCSP); conducted baseline questionnaires (social worker taught CCSP)	CCSP effective in reducing nausea/ fatigue. Treatment group experienced mild anxiety; control group experienced moderate anxiety
Graveley & Littlefield (1992)	Descriptive/cost comparative analysis	3 prenatal clinics: Study period = 3 months; $N = 156$	Demographics	Physiological— "Kessner Index" (Kessner et al., 1973); patient satisfaction tool "PST" (Reed et al., 1978), α 0.83; costs (personal costs/number of kept appointments)	CNS managed prenatal clinic compared to physician/NP managed and physician care. Maternal and infant physical function, psychosocial function, role function, administration, case management, research	CNS delivered total prenatal care & referrals to community agencies	CNS care was significantly lower cost per visit over physician and physician/NP managed care ($7.81, $11.18, and $9.23, respectively). No other differences noted

Hall et al. (1994)	Retrospective 3-, 6-month reviews	N = 70 referrals	Patient compliance (diary cards); mean peak expiratory flow (PEF); nursing consultation time (diary)	Home nebulizer CNS managed care	Patient assessment and nebulizer trial. Referral assessment for appropriateness	19% CNS time spent on patient/nebulizer assessment. 24% CNS time spent on clerical duties. 54% of patients used nebulizer as prescribed. 18% used not at all/very little. 4 referrals inappropriate. PEF not reported
Hurwitz et al. (2004)	RCT over 2 years	Total participants with Parkinson's disease in general practice N = 1859; N = 1028 CNS group; N = 808 control group	Function well-being "PDQ-39" (Jenkinson, Peto, Fitzpatrick, Greenhall, & Hyman, 1995); health-related quality of life "Euroqol" (Williams, 1995); health care costs "Personal Social Services Research Unit" (Netten & Denett, 1996); medicine use "Monthly Index of Medical Specialists 1996 net ingredients costs" (MIMS, 1996); mortality "National Health Services Central Registry"; visuomotor coordination (Gersten-Brand et al., 1973); ability to rise from sitting "Columbian Rating Scale" (Wade, 1994)	Attended by CNS vs. standard care with GP	CNS worked in collaboration with GP providing counseling, education, and monitoring of patients	CNS had little effect on clinical conditions, but did improve patients' sense of well-being. No additional costs to care

(continued)

TABLE 4.4

STUDIES INVESTIGATING CLINICAL NURSE SPECIALIST PRACTICE AND PATIENT OUTCOMES (CONTINUED)

Author(s)	Design	Setting/Subjects	Control Variables	Outcome	CNS Role Components/Domains	Intervention	Results
Jacavone et al. (1999)	Retrospective chart review. Pre/post clinical pathway implement	$N = 602$ preimplement (control), $N = 598$ postimplement (intervention); Cardiac surgery patients		Surgical complications; prolonged ventilation (mechanical vent > 24 hours); pneumonia (+ ve sputum cultures or chest x-ray): complications "Summit Medical Systems Inc database"; length of stay "Information Technology Systems Department"; costs "Information Technology Systems Department"	CNS facilitated cardiac surgery clinical pathway program. Role development, physical function, administration, practice development, health policy	CNS facilitated interdisciplinary development/implementation of a clinical pathway for post cardiac surgery patients	Intervention group had decreased prolonged ventilation (10.3%–9.03%), pneumonia (2.49%–1.67%) and GI (0.66%–0.33%). Intervention group had shorter length of stay (8–7 days) and total cost savings of $201,000
Lacko et al. (2001)	Quasi-experimental	Medical patients aged 65+ in community hospital $N = 34$ experimental; $N = 11$ control	Demographics (chart review)	Mental status "Memory Concentration Test (OMC)"; delirium "Confusion Assessment Method (CAM)" α 0.87, IRR = 1.0. Algorithm for both tests based on guidelines developed by the Task Force on Aging, American College of Physicians, 1995	Experimental group nurses educated to utilize a delirium screening tool vs. control nurses	CNS/NP developed algorithm that identified tools to be used by staff nurses for screening delirium and defining physician vs. nurse responsibilities	Experimental nurses were able to identify all cases of delirium (100%). Control nurses identified none

McCorkle et al. (1989)	Longitudinal, RCT	N = 166 lung cancer patients Nursing home 3 groups: specialized oncology home care (OHC)-APN care; standard home care—interdisciplinary care (SHC); and office care—physician only (OC)	Baseline interview	Symptom distress "The Symptom Distress Scale"; pain "McGill-Melzack Pain Questionnaire"; concern "Inventory of Current Concerns" (Weisman & Worden, 1976); mood state "Profile of Mood States" (Moinpour et al., 1992); functional status "Enforced Social Dependency Scale"; health perceptions "General Health Rating Index"; utilization of services "Medical Record Review"	CNS home care managed personalized care for persons diagnosed with advanced cancer and their family members vs. interdisciplinary home care vs. physician managed care. Pain management, communication, self-care, psychosocial function	5 interviews—1 within 8–10 days of diagnosis 4 at 6-week intervals following. CNS conducted in-depth interviews re: physical and psychosocial health condition, hospitalization	OC experienced symptom distress and social dependency 6 weeks sooner than SHC and OHC. OHC and SHC reported worse health perceptions over time. OHC had fewer hospitalizations, but higher mean LOS in hospital. No difference in post-discharge acute care visits, functional status, depression, or patient satisfaction
Naylor et al.	RCT 2, 6, 12, and 24 weeks follow-up	At-risk elders, 65+ for hospital readmission N = 138 control; N = 124 experimental		Acute/hospital readmission Function "Enforced Social Dependency Scale" (Moinpour et al., 1992); depression "Centre for Epidemiological Studies Depression Scale" (Radloff, 1997); patient satisfaction (author-prepared); costs "Standardized Medicare reimbursements"	CNS transitional care vs. routine acute care discharge planning. Physical function, psychological function	APN visit within 48 hours of hospital admission, comprehensive discharge planning, 2 home follow-up visits and weekly telephone calls	Control group had more hospital readmissions (14.5% and 6.2%, respectively); Greater length of stay (760 vs. 270, $p < 0.001$); and two times greater health care costs ($1,238,928 vs. $642,595, $p < 0.001$)

(continued)

TABLE 4.4

STUDIES INVESTIGATING CLINICAL NURSE SPECIALIST PRACTICE AND PATIENT OUTCOMES (CONTINUED)

Author(s)	Design	Setting/ Subjects	Control Variables	Outcome	CNS Role Components/ Domains	Intervention	Results
Rankin and Butzlaff (2005)	RCT	Unpartnered elders, 65+ post cardiac event, medically stable $N = 40$		Number of contacts with nurse (nursing log); number of minutes spent talking to patients (nursing log); nurse dose "FAMISHED"	Collaborative CNS/peer advisor intervention to improve social networks and enhance social efficacy by promoting social integration	2 CNSs contacted recovering patients 16 times with home visits and telephone calls. CNSs provided social support, emotional-informative-instrumental aid	Nurse dose calculated as amount of time, intensity of nursing time, and percentage of proposed intervention strategies completed = 270 minutes per 12-week period. Most important CNS role identified = emotional support
Ryan et al. (2006)	RCT baseline, 2, 7, 12 months follow-up	Rheumatology clinic (hospital based) $N = 36$ intervention; $N = 35$ control	Demographics (chart review)	Ability to control arthritis "Arthritis Impact Measure Scale" (Meenan et al., 1980); "Rheumatology Attitude Index" (Nicassio et al., 1985); disease activity "Disease Activity Score" (Prevoo et al., 1995); medications (Nursing records/ notes)	Rheumatology clinic vs. outpatient clinic care. Management, role function	CNSs reviewed and monitored patients' conditions once per week for 4 weeks and then once monthly × year for drug reactions, changes in disease	Intervention group: improved scores in perception of ability to control arthritis, control group scores declined at 12 months (1.8 and 0.3, respectively) and had greater improvements in disease activity (0.9 and 0.1, $p = 0.048$, respectively)

Author/Year	Design	Sample	Variables	Measures	Role/Description	Intervention	Implications
Savage & Grap (1999)	Descriptive	Convenience sample of open-heart surgery patients N = 342		Questionnaire related to post surgery recovery: areas investigated—healing of wounds/incisions, physical signs/symptoms, "Appetite Activity" (author-prepared)	Cardiovascular CNS role described in relation to facilitative recovery. Problems patients encounter post hospital discharge defined	CNS conducted telephone interviews 7–14 days post discharge asking patients about certain aspects of care. Provided patients with written material on symptoms of infection, incision care and use of incentive spirometer	Implications noted for CNS postoperative management. Recommended scheduled telephone follow-up interviews post discharge, particularly within first 2 weeks of discharge
Tijhuis et al. (2003)	RCT Study period = 2 years Follow-up at 12, 52, and 104 weeks	Rheumatoid arthritis patients N = 210	Clinical and socio-demographic	Quality of life "RAND 36 Health Survey" (Hays et al., 1993); Rheumatoid Arthritis Quality of Life "RAQoL" (De Jong et al., 1997); function "Health Assessment questionnaire," "HAQ" (Siegert, Vleming, Vandenbroucke, & Cats, 1984); "McMaster Toronto arthritis" "MACT AR" (Tugwell, Bombardier, & Buchanan, 1987); disease activity "DAS" "Disease Activity Scale' (Prevoo et al., 1995); uptake of paramedical services and practical aids and adaptations	CNS provided care in outpatient clinic vs. inpatient care	CNS provided information about RA, medications prescribed, equipment, home adaptations, and additional referrals at 1-hour educational sessions and 9-day clinic treatment days. Patients also received 1.5 hours of bed rest per clinic visit	Care provided by CNS had similar long-term clinical outcomes to inpatient and day patient care in RA patients

(continued)

TABLE 4.4

STUDIES INVESTIGATING CLINICAL NURSE SPECIALIST PRACTICE AND PATIENT OUTCOMES (CONTINUED)

Author(s)	Design	Setting/ Subjects	Control Variables	Outcome	CNS Role Components/ Domains	Intervention	Results
Tranmer et al. (2004)	RCT	Cardiac surgery patients N = 200 Followed during first 5 weeks post hospital discharge		Health-related quality of life "Medical Outcomes Study Short Form 36" (Ware et al., 1994); symptom distress "Memorial Symptom Assessment Scale" (Portenoy et al., 1994); satisfaction with care recovery; rate of unexpected health care contacts (ED/hospital admissions)	APN managed care vs. usual care	APN familiar with patient clinical condition/care needs conducted telephone calls twice in first week and then weekly × 4 weeks	No significant effects on selected outcomes noted
Tsay et al. (2005)	RCT, convenience sampling, pre/post intervention N = 33 control; N = 33 intervention	End-stage renal disease patients from Taiwan		Perceived stress "Hemodialysis Stressor Scale" (Baldree et al., 1982), α 0.85; depression "Beck Depression Scale" (Beck et al., 1961), α 0.89; quality of life "Medical Outcome Short Form 36" (Ware et al., 1994)	CNS managed care vs. usual care (pamphlet and routine treatment), psychosocial function, mental health, self-care management, role function, counseling	Coping and cognitive behavioral group sessions × 8 weeks	Intervention group improved in perception of stress ($t = 3.39$, $p = 0.002$), depression ($t = 3.54$, $p = 0.001$) and quality of life ($t = 4.35$, $p = 0.001$). Control group worsened in perception of stress ($t = 0.05$, $p = 0.96$), depression ($t = 3.69$, $p = 0.001$) and quality of life ($t = 2.68$, $p = 0.01$)

Vrijhoef et al. (2001)	Quasi-experimental, nonequivalent control group, baseline, 2-, 6-, 9-, and 12-month follow-up	Type 2 diabetics from hospital in Netherlands $N = 47$ control $N = 74$ intervention		Clinical status: hemoglobin A1C, fasting total cholesterol triglycerides, BMI, BP, health status "Dutch Version of COOP/WONCA charts" (Nelson et al., 1987); quality of life "Visual Analogue Scale" (Maxwell et al., 1978); self-care "Self care behaviour checklist" (Pennings-van der Eerden, 1992);disease knowledge "Dutch Diabetes Specific Knowledge Instrument" (Ripken et al., 1990) α 0.80; patient satisfaction "Industrial Marketing Management"; number of consults (chart review	CNS substituted diabetes managed care vs. internist led diabetes managed care. Physical function, self-care management, patient satisfaction, education, role function	3 quarterly CNS consultations & annual internist follow-up	Intervention group improved while control declined for: Hemoglobin A1C (8.6–8.3% vs. 8.6–8.8%, respectively); self-care behaviors (3.2–3.5 and 3.6–3.5, respectively); and number of consultations (4–24 and 21–9, respectively). At baseline, 96% intervention group preferred internist care, but at 24 weeks, 89% preferred CNS managed care
Wheeler (2000)	Comparative, correlational, retrospective, random chart review	4 hospital orthopedic units (2 with CNS, 2 without) 32 patients undergoing total knee replacement	Demographics	Quality of care "Acute Pain Process Instrument, APRI" "High Risks for Disuse Syndrome Process Instrument, HRDSPI" (author-prepared). APRI IRR 90.4%, HRDSPI 91%; length of stay (date of discharge—date of admission); number of preventable complications (physician notes, x-rays, laboratory tests)	Orthopedic unit based CNS vs. non-CNS care to delineate CNS processes and patient outcomes. Role function, physical function, role performance	Nursing processes within first 24 hours post surgery	CNS units had fewer complications than non-CNS (6 and 17 respectively), shorter length of stay (4.87 days vs. 6.84 days, $p = 0.001$), and better quality of care (140.44 and 102.16, $p = 0.0001$, respectively)

(continued)

TABLE 4.4

STUDIES INVESTIGATING CLINICAL NURSE SPECIALIST PRACTICE AND PATIENT OUTCOMES (CONTINUED)							
Author(s)	Design	Setting/ Subjects	Control Variables	Outcome	CNS Role Components/ Domains	Intervention	Results
White (1999)	Descriptive, prospective chart audits on nursing documentation at 3 months and 2 years	Acute care patients undergoing spinal surgery N = 35		Present pain "Present Pain Index of McGill Pain Questionnaire" (Melzack et al., 1975); analgesia administration "Agency for home care policy guidelines for acute pain management equivalency table" (Acute Pain Management Guideline Panel, 1992); nursing documentation "Pain Management Audit Tool" (Ferrell et al., 1991); education program	Baseline: 1) Assess patient pain intensity and nursing documentation of pain assessment/analgesia administration; 2) Assess nursing documentation of pain assessment/ management. Evaluate 1 & 2 with chart audit for changes in patient intensity and nursing documentation (with same population). Pain management, physical function, role function, education	4-week pain assessment and management focused educational program & new routes for post-op analgesia	Assessment: PPI = 3.4 mean, 40% charts documented pain assessment, 50% received analgesia as ordered. Evaluation: PPI < 3.0 mean, 3 months 90% charts documented pain assessment and 85% received analgesia as ordered
Willoughby & Burrows (2001)	Descriptive, random selection	N = 48 Outpatient foot care clinic N = 15 Did not attend clinic	Demographics	Questionnaire re: Foot pathology and foot care behaviors (author-prepared)	CNS managed foot care clinic vs. inpatient or outpatient care with no clinic visits	CNS foot assessment, education re: foot care, referrals, lesion treatment	69% attendees reported calluses/corns vs. 40% nonattendees. 8% attendees vs. 0% nonattendees reported ulcers. 60% nonattendees vs. 25% attendees walk barefoot. 20% nonattendees vs. 2% attendees would treat own lesions

York et al. (1997)	RCT, baseline, 2, 4, 8 weeks postpartum	High-risk pregnant woman with diabetes or hypertension (N = 52 control, N = 44 intervention) and their infants (N = 51 control, N = 42 intervention)	Function "Enforced social dependent scale" (Benoliel et al., 1980), α 0.65; patient satisfaction "La Monica Oberst Patient Satisfaction Scale" (LaMonica et al., 1986), α 0.98; maternal/infant length of stay; number of hospital/acute care visits; cost of care	Perinatal CNS care vs. routine care. Physical functioning, social functioning, administration	Transitional care with 3 weekly telephone and 5 (minimum) home visits; patient education and counseling	Maternal: intervention group < antepartum rehospitalizations (p = 0.048) Infant: intervention group < birth weight babies (2 vs. 9, p = 0.56) and 378 g heavier

RCT = randomized controlled trial;

N = sample size;

CNS = clinical nurse specialist;

α = alpha coefficients;

IRR = interrater reliability.

Source: "Outcomes of Clinical Nurse Specialist Practice," by D. M. Doran, S. Sidani, & T. Di Pietro (in press), in J. Fulton (Ed.), *Essentials of Clinical Nurse Specialist Practice.* New York, NY: Lippincott Williams & Wilkins.

infection, drug overdose, fever (Forster et al., 2005; Gurka, 1991; Jacavone, Daniels, & Tyner, 1999; Wheeler, 2000), and endotracheal reintubation (Crimlisky et al., 1997). The majority of studies demonstrated a positive impact of CNS practice on early identification and prevention of complications, although it is important to note that many of these studies employed weaker study designs than an RCT. The one RCT study found no significant difference in hospital-acquired complications between general medical inpatients who received care from a CNS-supported multidisciplinary team and those who received care on general medical units (Forster et al., 2005). However, that RCT study had a relatively small sample size (175 patients in the intervention arm) and thus might have been too underpowered to detect significant differences.

Functional health outcomes encompass physical, psychological, and social functioning; self-management knowledge and skills; and modification of risky health behaviors. Under this category of outcome, we included studies that investigated the impact of CNS practice on functional health outcomes, quality of life, and self-management or adherence to treatment. Of the seven studies that investigated functional health outcomes, only two found a significant relationship between CNS practice and medical patients' self-reported functional health outcomes (Ryan et al., 2006; Tsay et al., 2005). This lack of evidence concerning the impact of CNS practice on functional health outcomes is somewhat puzzling; however, it could be a function of the way in which functional health was conceptualized and measured in those studies (Hurwitz et al., 2005; Naylor et al., 1999; Tijhuis et al., 2003; Vrijhoef et al., 2001; York et al., 1997). In our previous research, we observed that nurses have a significant influence on patients' functional health outcomes but for a specific sub-category only, namely, activities of daily living and instrumental activities of daily living (Doran, 2003). The studies investigating functional status outcomes of CNS practice have typically employed broad measures of patients' physical, social, and emotional role functioning, which might be less sensitive to CNS influence, especially within the context of a short hospital stay. Therefore, we suggest that further research is needed to investigate functional status as an outcome of CNS practice, with a particular focus on the conceptualization of appropriate indicators that will be amenable to change over relatively short periods of time. Functional health indicators that could be appropriately based on evidence from previous research include activities of daily living and instrumental activities of daily living.

Quality-of-life outcome is the most broadly conceptualized outcome under the functional health outcome category. Once again, the evidence in Table 4.4 indicates mixed findings, with one study reporting a significant relationship between CNS practice and quality-of-life outcome (Tijhuis et al., 2003) and one study reporting no significant relationship (Tranmer & Parry, 2004). Quality-of-life instruments typically combine into one measure the three dimensions of functioning: physical functioning, emotional functioning, and social functioning. That measure yields an assessment of general health status or health-related quality of life (McDowell & Newell, 1996). Such quality-of-life instruments have two characteristics that might make them insensitive to detecting the contribution of CNSs' practice to patient outcome. First, they often have a long-term time horizon, and thus, it is difficult to detect the influence of any particular direct-care activities from the influence of all the other events and circumstances that contribute to health and well-being. Second, because quality-of-life measures typically generate a global score, it is possible to miss the contribution of a clinician's practice if, for instance, the effect of that practice is only on a particular subdimension of the patients' quality of life. Based on these observations and the aforementioned evidence, we suggest that quality of life may be sensitive to CNS practice but that its relationship can be difficult to detect.

The third type of functional health outcomes identified in the empirical literature was *self-management* or *adherence to treatment*. Three studies were found that investigated self-management or compliance with treatment as an outcome of CNS practice (Capasso, 1998; De Jong & Veltman, 2004; Hall, Callow, Evans, & Johnston, 1994). In each of these studies, CNS practice was positively associated with patients' self-management and risk modification behavior.

Patient satisfaction with care is another category of outcome identified in Table 4.4. Four studies were identified that included patient satisfaction as an outcome of CNS practice (Charles, Le Vasseur, & Castle, 1999; Forster et al., 2005; Graveley & Littlefield, 1992; Naylor et al., 1999). Two of these found a significant relationship between the care provided by CNSs and patient satisfaction outcome (Charles et al., 1999; Forster et al., 2005). Charles et al. randomly assigned patients presenting to the ED who required suturing for minor lacerations to the services of a CNS or to a physician. Patients in the CNS arm reported higher satisfaction with their care than patients in the physician arm. In another RCT, Forster et al. reported higher satisfaction for patients admitted to the services of a CNS-supported medical team than for patients admitted to routine hospital services. In contrast, neither Naylor et al. nor Gravely and Littlefield found significantly higher satisfaction for obstetrical patients assigned to

CNS care than for patients assigned to routine care. Because these latter two studies involved women in an obstetrical setting, it is possible that the women were already predisposed to feel positive about their care, and that could have resulted in high satisfaction scores for women in both the intervention group and the control group. Previous research in the context of general nursing practice offers strong evidence of the sensitivity of patient satisfaction outcome to nursing care (Laschinger & Almost, 2003). It therefore seems reasonable to expect a similar sensitivity to CNS practice. However, it will be important to carefully assess the process mechanisms that explain how CNS practice affects patient satisfaction, something we say more about in the discussion that follows.

Organizational outcomes identified from the empirical literature investigating CNS practice were *unit length of stay, hospital length of stay*, and *total costs* for patient care. With only a couple of exceptions (Forster et al., 2005; Hurwitz et al., 2005), the research evidence suggests that CNS services can have a significant positive influence on cost outcomes (Ahrens, Yancey, & Kollef, 2003; Brooten et al., 2001; Graveley & Littlefield, 1992; Naylor et al., 1999; York et al., 1997). These findings were consistent across practice settings, including inpatient hospital settings (Ahrens et al., 2003; Naylor et al., 1999), ambulatory care (Graveley & Littlefield, 1992), and home care (Brooten et al., 2001; York et al., 1997). The CNS role activities in these studies included comprehensive discharge planning, case management, and home follow-up. These role activities had a significant impact on health care utilization and overall health care costs, demonstrating the CNSs' achievement of quality, cost-effective, patient-focused outcomes.

In summary, the following patient and organizational outcomes were found to be sensitive to CNS practice and are recommended as appropriate indicators for assessing the impact of CNSs within the health care system:

1. Patient Focused
   a. Disease/condition-specific outcomes
   b. Physical and psychosocial symptom outcomes
   c. Early identification and prevention of complications
   d. Self-management and adherence to treatment
   e. Patient satisfaction
2. Organization Focused
   a. Unit/hospital length of stay
   b. Total health care charges

In addition, functional status was identified as potentially sensitive to CNS practice; however, further research is needed to determine the most appropriate indicators for its measurement. These will likely be indicators that are amenable to change over a relatively short period of time, such as activities of daily living and instrumental activities of daily living.

DISCUSSION OF THE EVIDENCE

A systematic review of the theoretical and empirical literature was undertaken in order to describe the scope of CNS practice and to identify its impact on patient and organizational outcomes. The systematic review of the literature showed that the contribution of the CNS role to patient outcomes is variable and of a rather small magnitude. Most of the studies were not explicitly guided by a framework that clearly delineated the nature of the relationships between the CNS role functions or components and anticipated outcomes. The conceptualization of CNS practice, based on the NACNS (2004) statement and described earlier in this chapter, offers a potentially useful explanation of the observed variable and small effects of the CNS role on patient outcomes. As articulated in that statement, the CNS's contribution to patient outcomes encompasses both direct and indirect effects. While the direct effect may be small, the indirect effect, mediated by enhancements in the nurse and nursing care sphere of practice, may be more substantial. Such conceptualization could provide a comprehensive framework to guide future investigation and a more accurate understanding of the mechanisms underlying the impact of the CNS role.

The results of the review have implications for practice, quality monitoring, quality improvement, and future research. Each of these is discussed in turn.

With regard to practice, examples were found in the literature of CNSs engaged in the full range of practice roles described in the NACNS (2004) statement. The examples included directcare activities, such as advanced nursing assessment, intervention, and follow-up care. They also involved several examples of CNSs engaged in collaborative practice with the multidisciplinary team and in case management for patients in hospital and community settings. It was also noted that CNSs practice in a wide range of settings, including hospital-based, ambulatory care, and community-based settings. Such diversity of practice and demonstrated scope of practice provides strong evidence of the depth and breadth of the CNS role in our health care system today.

Roberts-Davis and Read (2001) conducted a Delphi study to establish similarities and differences between NPs and CNSs and found that the skills required for both roles are primarily nursing skills.

Their research demonstrated differences between NPs and CNSs in the area of systematic physical examination, systematic patient history taking, making diagnostic decisions, and prescribing treatment. However, Roberts-Davis and Read (2001) also concluded that both roles may evolve within the changing care context and may become more alike in some contexts. We found examples of this in the literature, such as CNSs assuming primary care management for patients admitted to the ED for suturing of minor lacerations (Charles et al., 1999) and of ambulatory care for patients with rheumatoid arthritis (Ryan et al., 2006).

The findings from our review have implications for selecting indicators for quality monitoring and quality improvement. Patient outcomes for quality monitoring and quality improvement are essentially the same types of outcomes that one would select for assessing the impact of any nursing role within our health care system. They are the types of outcomes that were identified in the American Academy of Nursing Expert Panel on Quality Health Care (Mitchell et al., 1989) and in the Nursing Role Effectiveness Model (Irvine et al., 1998). They include nurses' contribution to achievement of appropriate self-care, demonstration of health-promoting behaviors, functional status, perception of being well cared for, and symptom management to criterion (Irvine et al., 1998; Mitchell et al., 1989). In addition, CNSs contribute to quality outcomes at the organizational level, as articulated in the NACNS (2004) framework. This contribution is demonstrated in reduced health care costs, reduced rehospitalizations, and reduced length of hospital stay.

Future research is needed both to confirm some of the outcome indicators for which there is mixed evidence of sensitivity to CNS practice and to establish appropriate indicators for assessing the impact of CNS practice on patients' functional health outcomes. Furthermore, future studies should utilize research designs that both enable determination of causal inference and clarify the mechanisms by which CNS practice impacts patient and system outcomes. In doing so, we recommend a theory-driven approach to evaluating the quality of CNS practice (Sidani et al., 2004).

The world of practice is a complex system of multiple factors, multiple effects, and mutual causation (Hegyvary, 1993). Factors related to patients receiving care, to nurses providing care, to the setting or context in which care is provided, and to the nature of care provided interact and affect the outcomes expected as a result of care (Sidani & Braden, 1998). As a result, Sidani and colleagues (2004) recommended a theory-driven approach to evaluating the impact of nursing care by theorizing about the relationships among all the factors that affect outcomes. In adopting this approach to theorize about the contribution of CNSs to outcomes, it is important to identify the expected outcomes of CNS practice, to explain the processes responsible for producing the expected patient and organizational outcomes, and to identify the factors that influence the occurrence of these processes and, subsequently, the effectiveness of nursing care in achieving the outcomes (Sidani et al., 2004). In an evaluation study, the researcher will need to carefully identify and define the factors that influence the processes and outcomes. Sidani and Braden (1998) suggest there are five categories of factors. The first includes the personal, sociocultural, and health-related characteristics of the patients seeking and receiving care. The second category is the personal and professional characteristics of the nurse giving care. The third consists of the physical and social features of the setting in which care is delivered. The fourth is the type and dose of the interventions received by patients. The last category is related to the nature and timing of occurrence of outcomes expected as a result of the care provided. These five categories provide a comprehensive way of evaluating the impact of CNS practice within the health care system. We suggest that only through such careful theorizing will it be possible to effectively demonstrate the impact of CNSs on patient and organizational outcomes.

■ DISCUSSION QUESTIONS

- Consider your own practice as a CNS and identify which nurse-sensitive outcomes are appropriate for assessing the impact of your role in health care.
- Why do we often observe only small effects of the CNS practice on patient outcomes?
- Describe the different role mechanisms by which CNSs influence patient and organizational outcomes.
- Identify four key strategies for planning an evaluation of the CNS role in health care delivery.

REFERENCES

Ahrens, T., Yancey, V., & Kollef, M. (2003). Improving family communications at the end of life: Implications for length of stay in the intensive care unit and resource use. *American Journal of Critical Care, 12*(4), 317–330.

Arbour, R. (2003). A continuous quality improvement approach to improving clinical practice in the areas of sedation, analgesia and neuromuscular blockade.

Journal of Continuing Education in Nursing, 34(2), 64–71.

Barnason, S., Merboth, M., Pozehl, B., & Tietjen, M. J. (1998). Utilizing an outcomes approach to improve pain management by nurses: A pilot study. *Clinical Nurse Specialist, 12*(1), 28–36.

Bousfield, C. (1997). A phenomenological investigation into the role of the clinical nurse specialist. *Journal of Advanced Nursing, 25*, 245–256.

Brooten, D., Youngblut, J. A. M., Brown, L., Finkler, S. A., Neff, D. F., & Madigan, E. (2001). A randomized trial of nurse specialist home care for women with high-risk pregnancies: Outcomes and costs. *American Journal of Managed Care, 7*, 793–803.

Brooten, D., Youngblut, J. M., Deatrick, J., Naylor, M. D., & York, R. (2003). Patient problems, advanced practice nurse (APN) interventions, time and contacts among five patient groups. *Journal of Nursing Scholarship, 35*(1), 73–79.

Capasso, V. (1998). The theory is the practice: An exemplar. *Clinical Nurse Specialist, 12*(6), 226–229.

Carroll, D., Robinson, E., Buselli, E., Berry, D., & Rankin, S. H. (2001). Activities of the APN to enhance unpartnered elders for self efficacy after myocardial infarction. *Clinical Nurse Specialist, 15*(2), 60–66.

Charles, A., Le Vasseur, S. A., & Castle, C. (1999). Suturing of minor lacerations by clinical nurse specialists in the emergency department. *Accident & Emergency Nursing, 7*, 34–38.

Conger, M., & Craig, C. (1998). Advanced nurse practice: A model of collaboration. *Nursing Case Management, 3*(3), 120–127.

Crimlisky, J., Bernardo, J., Blansfield, J., Loughlin, M., McGonagle, E., McEachern, G.,…Farber, H. W. (1997). Endotracheal reintubation: A closer look at a preventable condition. *Clinical Nurse Specialist, 11*(4), 145–150.

Darmody, J. (2005). Observing the work of the clinical nurse specialist: A pilot study. *Clinical Nurse Specialist, 19*(5), 260–268.

De Jong, S., & Veltman, R. (2004). Effectiveness of a CNS led community based COPD screening and intervention program. *Clinical Nurse Specialist, 18*(2), 72–79.

Dickerson, S. S., Wu, Y. W. W., & Kennedy, M. C. (2006). A CNS facilitated ICD support group. *Clinical Nurse Specialist, 20*(3), 146–153.

Doran, D. M. (2003). Functional status. In D. M. Doran (Ed.), *Nursing-sensitive outcomes: State of the science* (pp. 27–64). Sudbury, MA: Jones & Bartlett.

Doran, D. M., O'Brien-Pallas, L., Sidani, S., McGillis Hall, L., Petryshen, P.,…Thompson, D. et al. (2003). An evaluation of nursing sensitive outcomes for quality care. *Journal International Nursing Perspectives, 3*(3), 109–125.

Forster, A. J., Clark, H. D., Menard, A., Dupuis, N., Chernish, R., Chandok, N.,…van Walraven, C. (2005). Effect of a nurse team coordinator on outcomes for hospitalized medicine patients. *The American Journal of Medicine, 118*, 1148–1153.

Fowler Byers, J., & Brunnell, M. L. (1998). Demonstrating the value of the advanced practice nurse: An evaluation model. *AACN Critical Issues, 9*(2), 296–305.

Froggatt, K., & Hoult, L. (2002). Developing palliative care practice in nursing and residential care homes: The role of the clinical nurse specialist. *Journal of Clinical Nursing, 11*(6), 802–808.

Gaston-Johansson, F., Fall-Dickson, J., Nanda, J., Ohly, K. V., Stillman, S., Krumm, S., & Kennedy, M. J. (2000). The effectiveness of the comprehensive coping strategy program on clinical outcomes in breast cancer autologous bone marrow transplantation. *Cancer Nursing, 23*(4), 277–285.

Graveley, E. A., & Littlefield, J. H. (1992). A cost-effectiveness analysis of three staffing models for the delivery of low-risk prenatal care. *American Journal of Public Health, 82*(2), 180–184.

Gurka, A. M. (1991). Process and outcome components of clinical nurse specialist consultation. *Dimensions of Critical Care Nursing, 10*(3), 169–175.

Hall, I. P., Callow, I. M., Evans, S. A., & Johnston, I. D. A. (1994). Audit of a complete home nebulizer service provided by a respiratory nurse specialist. *Respiratory Medicine, 88*, 429–433.

Harrington, L., & Smith, J. P. (2005). Program development: Role of the clinical nurse specialist in implementing a fast-track postanaesthesia care unit. *AACN Clinical Issues, 16*(1), 78–88.

Hays, R. D., Sherbourne, C. D., & Mazel, R. M. (1993). The RAND 36-item health survey 1.0. *Health Economics, 2*(3), 217–227.

Hegyvary, S. T. (1991). Issues in outcomes research. *Journal of Nursing Quality Assurance, 5*(2), 1–6.

Hegyvary, S. (1993). Patient care outcomes related to management of symptoms. *Annual Review of Nursing Research, 11*, 145–168.

Hurwitz, B., Jarman, B., Cook, A., & Bajekal, M. (2005). Scientific evaluation of community-based Parkinson's disease nurse specialists on patient outcomes and health care costs. *Journal of Evaluation in Clinical Practice, 11*(2), 97–110.

Irvine, D., Sidani, S., & McGillis Hall, L. (1998). Linking outcomes to nurses' roles in health care. *Nursing Economic$, 16*(2), 58–64, 87.

Jacavone, J. B., Daniels, R. D., & Tyner, I. (1999). CNS facilitation of a cardiac surgery clinical pathway program. *Clinical Nurse Specialist, 13*(3), 126–132.

Jenkinson, C., Peto, V., Fitzpatrick, R., Greenhall, R., & Hyman, N. (1995). Self-reported functioning and well-being in patients with Parkinson's disease: A comparison of the short-form health (SF-36) and the Parkinson's disease questionnaire (PDQ-39). *Age and Ageing, 24*, 505–509.

Jennings, B. M., Staggers, N., & Brosch, L. R. (1999). A classification scheme for outcome indicators. *Image: Journal of Nursing Scholarship, 31*, 381–388.

Lacko, L. A., Dellasega, C., Salernon, F., Singer, H., Delucca, J., & Rothenberger, C. (2001). The role of the advanced practice nurse in facilitating a clinical research study: Screening for delirium. *Clinical Nurse Specialist, 14*(3), 110–115.

Laschinger, H. K., & Almost, J. (2003). Patient satisfaction as a nurse-sensitive outcome. In D. M. Doran (Ed.), *Nursing-sensitive outcomes: State of the science* (pp. 243–281). Sudbury, MA: Jones & Bartlett.

Linck, C., & Phillips, S. (2005). Fight or flight? Disruptive behavior in medical/surgical services. *Nursing Management, 36*(5), 47–51.

Lohr, K. N. (1985). *Impact of Medicare prospective payment on the quality of medical care: A research agenda.* Santa Monica, CA: The Rand Corporation.

Martin, P. J. (1999). An exploration of the services provided by the clinical nurse specialist within one NHS trust. *Journal of Nursing Management, 7*, 149–156.

McAlpine, L. (1997). Process and outcome measures for the multidisciplinary collaborative projects of a critical care CNS. *Clinical Nurse Specialist, 11*(3), 134–138.

McCorckle, R., Benoliel, J. Q., Donaldson, G., Georgiadou, F., Moinpour, C., & Goodell, B. (1989). A randomized clinical trial of a home nursing care for lung cancer patients. *Cancer, 64*, 1375–1382.

McCreaddie, M. (2001). The role of the clinical nurse specialist. *Nursing Standard, 16*(10), 33–38.

McDowell, I., & Newell, C. (1996). *Measuring health: A guide to rating scales and questionnaires* (2nd ed.). New York, NY: Oxford University Press.

Mick, D., & Ackerman, M. (2000). Advanced practice nursing role delineation in acute and critical care: Application of the Strong Model of Advanced Practice. *Heart & Lung, 29*(3), 210–221.

Mitchell, P. H., Armstrong, S., Simpson, T. F., & Lentz, M. (1989). American Association of Critical-Care Nurses demonstration project: Profile of excellence in critical care nursing. *Heart & Lung, 18*, 219–237.

Mitchell, P. H., & Lang, N. M. (2004). Framing the problem of measuring and improving healthcare quality. Has the Quality Outcomes Model been useful? *Medical Care, 42*(Suppl. 2), II-4–II-11.

National Association of Clinical Nurse Specialists (NACNS). (2004). *Statement on clinical nurse specialist practice and education* (2nd ed.). Harrisburg, PA: Author.

Naylor, M. D., Bowles, K. H., & Brooten, D. (2000). Patient problems and advanced practice nurse interventions during transitional care. *Public Health Nursing, 17*(2), 94–102.

Naylor, M. D., Brooten, D., Campbell, R., Jacobsen, B. S., Mezey, M. D., Pauly, M. V., & Schwartz, J. S. (1999). Comprehensive discharge planning and home follow-up of hospitalized elders: A randomized clinical trial. *Journal of the American Medical Association, 281*(7), 613–620.

Phillips, J. (2005). Neuroscience critical care. The role of the advanced practice nurse in patient safety. *AACN Clinical Issues, 16*(4), 581–592.

Prevoo, M. I. L., van't Hof, M. A., Kuper, H. H., van Leeuwen, M. A., van de Putte, L. B. A., & van Riel, P. L. C. M. (1995). Modified disease activity scores that include 28 joint counts. Development and validity. *Arthritis Rheumatology, 38*, 44–48.

Raja-Jones, H. (2002). Role boundaries—research nurse or clinical nurse specialist? A literature review. *Journal of Clinical Nursing, 11*(4), 415–420.

Rankin, S. H., & Butzlaff, A. (2005). FAMISHED for support for recovering elders after cardiac events. *Clinical Nurse Specialist, 19*(3), 142–149.

Roberts-Davis, M., & Read, S. (2001). Clinical role clarification: Using the Delphi method to establish similarities and differences between nurse practitioners and clinical nurse specialists. *Journal of Clinical Nursing, 10*(1), 33–43.

Ryan, S., Hassell, A. B., Lewis, M., & Farrell, A. (2006). Impact of a rheumatology expert nurse on the well-being of patients attending a drug monitoring clinic. *Journal of Advanced Nursing, 53*(3), 277–286.

Savage, L. S., & Grap, M. J. (1999). Telephone monitoring after early discharge for cardiac surgery patients. *American Journal of Critical Care, 8*(3), 154–159.

Scott, R. (1999). A description of the roles, activities, and skills of clinical nurse specialists in the United States. *Clinical Nurse Specialist, 13*(4), 183–190.

Sidani, S., & Braden, C. J. (1998). *Evaluating nursing interventions: A theory-driven approach*. Thousand Oaks, CA: Sage.

Sidani, S., Doran, D. M., & Mitchell, P. (2004). A theory-driven approach to evaluating quality of nursing care. *Image: Journal of Nursing Scholarship, 36*, 60–65.

Siegert, C. D., Vleming, L. T., Vandenbroucke, J. P., & Cats, A. (1984). Measurement of disability in Dutch rheumatoid arthritis patients. *Clinical Rheumatology, 3*, 305–309.

Spielberger, C. G., Gorsuch, F., & Luchene, R. (1971). *STAI manual for the state trait anxiety inventory*. Palo Alto, CA: Consulting in Psychiatry Press.

Tijhuis, G. J., Zwinderman, A. H., Hazes, J., Breedveld, F., & Vliet, V. P. M. (2003). Two-year follow-up of a randomized controlled trial of a clinical nurse specialist intervention, inpatient, and day patient team care in rheumatoid arthritis. *Journal of Advanced Nursing, 41*(1), 34–43.

Tranmer, J. E., & Parry, M. J. E. (2004). Enhancing postoperative recovery of cardiac surgery patients: A randomized clinical trial of an advanced practice nursing intervention. *Western Journal of Nursing Research, 26*(5), 515–532.

Tsay, S. L., Lee, Y. C., & Lee, Y. C. (2005). Effects of an adaptation training programme for patients with end-stage renal disease. *Journal of Advanced Nursing, 50*(1), 39–46.

Tugwell, P., Bombardier, C., & Buchanan, W. W. (1987). Rehabilitation in people with rheumatoid arthritis. *Best Practices and Research Clinical Rheumatology, 17*(5), 847–861.

Vrijhoef, H. J. M., Diederiks, J. P. M., Spreeuwenberg, C., & Wolffenbuttel, B. H. R. (2001). Substitution model with central role for nurse specialist is justified in the care for stable type 2 outpatients. *Journal of Advanced Nursing, 36*(4), S46–S55.

Weisman, A. D., & Worden, J. W. (1976). The existential plight in cancer significance of the first 100 days. *International Journal of Psychiatry in Medicine, 7*(1), 1–15.

Wheeler, E. C. (2000). The CNS's impact on process and outcome of patients with total knee replacement. *Clinical Nurse Specialist, 14*(4), 159–172.

White, C. (1999). Changing pain management practice and impacting on patient outcomes. *Clinical Nurse Specialist, 13*(4), 166–172.

Willoughby, D., & Burrows, D. (2001). A CNS managed diabetes foot care clinic: A descriptive survey of characteristics and foot care behaviours of the patient population. *Clinical Nurse Specialist, 15*(2), 52–57.

Wojner, A. W., & Kite-Powell, D. (1997). Outcomes manager: A role for the advanced practice nurse. *Critical Care Nursing Quarterly, 19*(4), 16–24.

York, R., Brown, L., Samuels, P., Finkler, S. A., Jacobsen, B., Persely, C. A.,…Robbins, D. (1997). A randomized trial of early discharge and nurse specialist transitional follow-up care of high-risk childbearing women. *Nursing Research, 46*(5), 254–261.

5

Clinical Reasoning Model: A Clinical Inquiry Guide for Solving Problems in the Nursing Domain

Brenda L. Lyon

In watching disease, both in private houses and in public hospitals, the thing which strikes the experienced observer most forcibly is this, that the symptoms or the sufferings generally considered to be inevitable and incident to the disease are very often not symptoms of the disease at all, but of something quite different—of the want of fresh air, or of light, or of warmth, or of quiet, or of cleanliness, or of punctuality and care in the administration of diet, of each and all of these...If a patient is feverish, if a patient is faint, if he is sick after taking food, if he has a bed-sore, it is generally the fault not of the disease, but of the nursing. (Nightingale, 1860/1969, p. 8)

The ability to engage in rational and deliberate reasoning or clinical inquiry to effectively solve clinical problems in the *nursing* domain is one of the cornerstones of clinical nurse specialist (CNS) practice. Clinical reasoning is often thought to be synonymous with diagnostic reasoning; however, clinical reasoning, as used in this chapter, is more inclusive and

encompasses (a) the differential diagnostic process to identify etiologies requiring nursing intervention, also known as diagnostic reasoning; (b) therapeutic/interventional reasoning to select predictably effective interventions to alter the target etiology(ies); and (c) evaluation of outcomes. Although focused on the patient sphere of influence in this chapter, the clinical reasoning model (CRM) also has heuristic problem-solving value in both the nursing and system CNS spheres of influence because it is anchored in the identification of etiologies of problems.

CNS practice is focused on nursing's unique contributions to patient care while integrating, as appropriate, the care of other health care disciplines such as medicine. CNSs must be able to assess patient problems from a holistic *nursing perspective* to enable the accurate identification of problems that have etiologies requiring nursing interventions/therapeutics to achieve desired outcomes (National Association of Clinical Nurse Specialists [NACNS], 2004).

Knowledge informs perspective, that is, the perceptual lens through which clinicians assess, diagnose, and treat. Students often come to graduate programs preparing CNSs with a knowledge base grounded in and developed from educational as well as work/practical experiences that are predominantly disease focused. Knowledge and practical expertise regarding disease and the safe and therapeutic implementation

*Dr. Lyon gratefully acknowledges the permission from Wendy Unger, MSN, to use one of her CRM exemplars to demonstrate application of the CRM.

of medical therapeutics is critically important to caring for patients who have a condition requiring medical care. However, when knowledge of patient problems is principally embedded in knowledge about disease and disease-focused care, the result is that the "medical" perspective becomes the foreground of the nurse's perceptual lens. Consequently, nursing care needs can go unnoticed or thought to be less important. Additionally, without adequate knowledge of patient problems that require nursing interventions/ therapeutics, it is not possible to accurately rule in/ out etiologies that require nursing interventions/ therapeutics.

Effective CNS practice requires a highly developed perspective or perceptual lens that puts the nursing care needs of patients, when present, in the foreground of clinical reasoning, with medical problems and disease-focused care as critical background context. Central to the nursing perspective is the understanding that disease and illness are distinctly different phenomena and, furthermore, that the prevention and alleviation of illness experiences while promoting the experience of wellness is the essence of nursing.

The purpose of this chapter is to present the CRM developed for the pedagogical purpose of enhancing CNS students' clinical reasoning ability in identifying etiologies to solve clinical problems in the nursing domain. Prior to presenting the CRM, background information is presented, including brief discussions about clinical reasoning from a nursing perspective, phenomena of concern to nursing, nursing required etiologies (NREs), wellness as the target outcome of nursing care, and disease and illness as distinctly different phenomena. Then, the CRM is presented with an explanation of each of its components. The chapter concludes with a summary and implications for CNS education.

Although there are other CRMs, such as the Outcome-Present, State Test (OPT) Model of Clinical Reasoning developed by Pesut and Herman (1999), it is not the purpose of this chapter to present an overview of those models. Models such as the OPT rely heavily on the North American Nursing Diagnosis Association (NANDA), Nursing Intervention Classification (NIC), and Nursing Outcome Classification (NOC) language. Although identifying and using nursing language is important to make the work of the discipline visible, to date, the explicit link between problems, corresponding etiologies, and how etiologies determine what interventions are required is neglected. It is the insufficient attention to the criticality of identifying etiologies that require nursing interventions to effectively treat illness experiences and to promote wellness that compelled the development of the CRM.

CLINICAL REASONING FROM A NURSING PERSPECTIVE

What distinguishes clinical reasoning in nursing and CNS practice, in particular, from other disciplines such as medicine is not the reasoning process per se but the grounding in nursing's ontological and epistemological perspective with its focus on *phenomena of concern to nursing within a holistic contextual lens* (see Chapter 3). Additionally, what distinguishes clinical reasoning for CNSs from that of clinically skilled nurses prepared at the basic level is the expanded theoretical and research-based knowledge that informs practice. In addition to nursing research–generated knowledge, the expanded knowledge base encompasses knowledge generated by basic science disciplines pertinent to the phenomena of concern and to the intended effect of nursing interventions. An example would be knowledge generated from basic science research regarding the physiology of pain, inflammatory processes, nociceptive sensitization, and nociceptor recruitment that informs the identification of etiologies and nursing-generated knowledge of nonpharmacological therapeutics targeting the etiologies of pain to achieve relief.

Knowledge about phenomena of concern to nursing, along with the clinical expertise of the CNS in terms of patient population clinical experiences and outcomes, and skill in evaluating evidence and applicability to a patient population in terms of how evidence should be integrated into clinical decisions, informs CNS practice (Higgs & Jones, 2000; Victor-Chmil, 2013). The personal experience and clinical expertise of the CNS substantially contributes to the professional judgment required in the appropriate use of evidence in sound clinical reasoning.

Clinical reasoning from a nursing perspective has two focal points: (a) the types of problems that are of concern and (b) the types of etiologies of those problems. In the nursing perspective, the problems are expanded beyond disease, medical therapeutics, and/or side effects of medical therapeutics and are unique foci when compared with the perspectives of other health care providers such as physicians, physical therapists, psychologists, pharmacists, and nutritionists.

Diagnosing is discipline specific. [Emphasis added] Its focus derives from the categories of the phenomena central to that discipline. Thus, diagnoses are not medical because they are made by a physician but because they deal with phenomena in the medical domain. Similarly, nursing diagnoses are those which deal with phenomena central to the nursing domain. (Carnevali, 1987, p. 9)

Likewise, the etiologies of phenomena or problems central to nursing are expanded beyond disease and iatrogenic effects of treatments for disease to include other physical, psychosocial, and/or environmental etiologies that require nursing therapeutics/interventions to be altered. For the sake of conciseness, these etiologies for which nursing interventions are required are referred to as NREs versus non-disease-based etiologies.

Phenomena of Concern to Nursing

Nursing has struggled for years to clearly articulate its unique perspective and contribution to society—its phenomena of concern. As the pioneer of nursing, Nightingale (1860/1969) defined nursing as "[putting] the patient in the best condition for nature to act upon him" (p. 33). She was clear that different knowledge bases informed nursing practice and medical practice. Since Nightingale, multiple conceptual frameworks have been developed to capture nursing's discipline-specific perspective and phenomena of concern (Henderson, 1966; Johnson, 1980; King, 1989; Leininger, 1988; Neuman, 1989; Newman, 1986; Orem, 1985; Parse, 1989; Peplau, 1988; Rogers, 1970; Roy, 1984). Each framework reflects the respective author's conceptualization of phenomena that are of unique concern to nursing as well as implications for nursing actions in the context of the phenomena. Although every framework presents a somewhat different view, common threads consistent with Nightingale and the themes identified in Chapter 3 are (a) viewing the patient from a holistic perspective rather than a disease-focused perspective; (b) caring; (c) connecting, at some level, with the subjective or lived experience of the patient; and (d) meeting patients' needs for assistance in achieving wellness or well-being.

Phenomena of concern to nursing are articulated in the American Nurses Association's (ANA) *Nursing's Social Policy Statement* (ANA, 2010). The 2010 edition encompasses all previous editions of the social policy statement. Not surprisingly, examples of phenomena of concern are consistent with those identified in Nightingale's *Notes on Nursing* (1860/1969). Examples include, but are not limited to, self-care limitations; impaired functioning in the areas of rest, sleep, and breathing (e.g., shortness of breath); circulation problems; activity/inactivity problems (muscle weakness, balance problems, risk for falling, activity intolerance); nutritional problems, including dehydration; elimination (urinary incontinence, constipation, diarrhea); skin breakdown; sexuality problems; discomfort (pain); emotional problems such as anxiety, loss, loneliness, and grief; deficiencies in decision making; self-image changes; dysfunctional perceptual orientations to health; strains related to life processes such as birth, development, and death; and problematic affiliative relationships.

NREs

Importantly, phenomena central to the nursing domain are not grounded in disease or pathology but rather in the symptoms or sufferings and functional problems caused by or contributed to by factors other than disease-based etiologies, including physical, psychosocial, and environmental factors that require and are amenable to nursing interventions. NREs necessitate nursing interventions or therapeutics to be altered (lessened or alleviated). To be clear, disease and/or injury can cause symptoms or functional problems; however, on many occasions, even when caused by disease or injury, symptoms or functional problems are often intensified by NREs, thus requiring nursing interventions. Such is the case when awkward positioning strains an incision site or when extended dependent positioning of an extremity increases edema in a patient with congestive heart failure. Categories of NREs are outlined in Table 5.1.

In addition to intensifying symptoms or functional problems triggered by disease or injury,

TABLE 5.1

EXAMPLE CATEGORIES OF NURSING REQUIRED ETIOLOGIES (NRE)	
Person-Related NRE Categories	**Environmental-Related NRE Categories**
• Immobility	• Inadequate resources
• Improper positioning	• Noise
• Lack of knowledge	• Air pollution
• Inadequate nutrition	• Extreme temperatures
• Inadequate hydration	• Allergens
• Inappropriate body mechanics	• Social isolation
• Poor self-care	• Sources of friction
• Learned ineffective breathing pattern	• Dampness
• Stress	• Absence of self-care assistive devices
• Negative emotions	• Barriers, hazards
• Ineffective coping	

These lists are not all inclusive.

NREs are often the trigger for symptoms or functional problems in the absence of disease or injury. Some common examples of such experiences are (a) back pain caused by muscle strain resulting from lifting a heavy object using improper body mechanics, (b) back pain resulting from being in a supine position that strains back muscles, (c) headache caused from tensing neck and shoulder muscles while doing computer work, and (d) falling as a result of deconditioning while in the hospital. It has been estimated that 60% of all physician office visits are for illness experiences not caused by a disease, even in instances where there are multiple comorbidities (Fries, Koop, & Beadle, 1993; Hughner & Kleine, 2004; Sobel, 1995). There are also abundant examples in the literature of NREs that cause disease, complications, repeated hospital admissions, repeated visits to emergency rooms, and even death (e.g., lack of cleanliness, improper positioning, inadequate nutrition, over- or underhydration, immobility; Mokdad, Marks, Stroup, & Gerberding, 2004). Accurate identification of NREs plays a critical role in achieving positive results for nursing-sensitive outcomes and predictably will gain more attention nationally with the increased focus on value-based purchasing (see Chapter 24).

Nursing is concerned with preventing or alleviating NREs of symptoms and functional problems so as to promote the experience of wellness or well-being in the presence or absence of disease/pathology. Specifically, nursing's unique domain and, therefore, *nursing's unique contribution* to patient care is the focus on diagnosing and treating phenomena (problems/conditions) caused or contributed to by NREs.

Wellness/Well-Being

> Nursing is concerned with the human processes of well-being that are inherent among all human systems, whether individual, family or community. (Arslanian-Engorin, Hicks, Whall, & Algase, 2005, p. 318)

What is well-being, wellness, or the subjective experience of health? The terms *wellness* and *health* are often used interchangeably. An integrative review of the literature from 1983 to 2003 on lay views of health found that two critically important themes in describing the experience of health were the absence of symptoms and being able to function at an expected level (Hughner & Kleine, 2004). Unlike the medical perspective on health and wellness as objective phenomena, the subjective experience of health, or feeling "healthy," is proposed here to be synonymous with the subjective experience of wellness. *Wellness* is defined as the subjective experience of somatic comfort (physical and psychological) consistent with the person's normalized/expected comfort level *and* functional ability at or near perceived capability or expected level (Lyon, 1990). The physical dimension of wellness encompasses physical/somatic sensations, including the absence of any unexpected or normed discomforts, and the psychological dimension that encompasses emotional and spiritual aspects of self. The functional dimension encompasses all aspects of being able to "do" or behave consistent with the normalized or self-expected levels of functioning, including intellectual ability, self-care, daily activities, sleep/rest, and in all social/occupational roles.

Importantly, the experience of wellness is dynamic and can occur in the presence or absence of disease (Barsky, 1981, 1988; McMahon & Fleury, 2012). It is common for persons with chronic debilitating diseases such as rheumatoid arthritis to adapt to lower levels of function and comfort where the new levels become the expected normal. This is why it is also common to find that persons with long-standing chronic diseases will often describe themselves as very healthy or well (Faull et al., 2004; McKague & Verhoef, 2003). Wellness is the target goal of nursing care in the presence or absence of disease (Beech, Arber, & Faithful, 2011; Dunlop, 2010; Lyon, 1990, 2005; Mackey, 2009).

When wellness or health are defined as the absence of disease, disability, or symptoms, as it was by nurse researchers from 1977 to 1987 (Hwu, Coates, & Boore, 2001), then the logical extension is that persons with chronic diseases cannot experience wellness or health. Needless to say, this creates a practical problem for nurses because "health" is one of the major components of nursing's metaparadigm—and what to do if persons with a chronic disease cannot have it? Such usage also, in a practical sense, means the person with a chronic disease cannot experience wellness. Fortunately, nurse researchers from 1988 to 1998 increasingly recognized the subjective nature of health and, therefore, the experiences of both illness and wellness as well as the nonmedical causes of illness (Hwu et al., 2001). An understanding that disease, illness, and wellness are distinctly different phenomena is fundamentally important to nursing's unique perspective, unique contribution to patient care, and the CRM.

Disease and Illness as Distinctly Different Phenomena

In common lay and professional vernacular, the terms *disease* and *illness* are often used interchangeably.

When nurses view disease and illness as synonymous, the practical result is a limited search for potential etiological factors contributing to or causing symptoms and functional problems from any other model except the traditional medical model.

Disease

Disease is an abnormal condition including pathology of organ function or structure and abnormal behavior. *Disease* is defined in *Dorland's Medical Dictionary* as "a definite pathological process having a characteristic set of signs and symptoms. It may affect the whole body or any of its parts and its etiology, pathology, and prognosis may be known or unknown" (*Dorland's Medical Dictionary*, 2007, p. 469). Disease is an objective phenomenon with an identifiable group of signs and symptoms: It is observable and can be objectively measured. Therefore, the characteristics of a disease are the same across persons who have the disease; in other words, *diseases are normative phenomena*. Although there are a few exceptions, such as the attempt to label all obesity as a disease, for the most part the defining characteristic of disease is pathology (McConnell, 2007). As each disease has a normative set or template of signs and symptoms, the differential diagnosis of disease is principally accomplished through data collection (history, physical, lab tests), to identify patterns of signs and symptoms or "illness-scripts," and then "pattern-matching" of the revealed signs and symptoms to a prespecified template for a disease (Bowen, 2006; Norman, 2006; Schmidt, Norman, & Boshuizen, 1990). Thus, the differential diagnosis process in medicine is focused on identifying the pathology or disease that is causing symptoms and/or functional problems.

Medicine's social mandate and service to society is focused on the diagnosis and treatment of disease and the generation of knowledge regarding disease and its treatment. The physician's perspective, therefore, is necessarily focused on disease. That is, disease as the etiology or causal explanation of signs and symptoms is necessarily in the foreground of the physician's perceptual lens when working with patients.

Nursing's responsibility in the medical domain is to make judgments about the medical condition of the patient and to implement the delegated (authorized via physician orders, approved protocols, or guidelines) medical therapeutics safely and therapeutically (see Chapter 5). Similar to physicians, research has demonstrated that expert critical care nurses make rapid judgments about the need for intervention on physiological status problems (actual or potential) by quickly processing and grouping patient data/cues and then "pattern matching" with learned cues/indicators of physiological status (Baumann & Deber, 1987).

Illness

Illness is a distinctly different phenomenon than disease (Boorse, 1975; Eisenberg, 1976, 1980; Jensen & Allen, 1994; Long & Weinert, 1992; Loomis & Conco, 1991; Wikman, Marklund, & Alexanderson, 2005) and can have both disease-based and NRE causes (Figure 5.1). Importantly then, illness can be experienced in the presence or absence of disease. Illness, like wellness, is a subjective experience. Specifically, it is the experience of discomfort (physical and/or emotional) greater than the person's normalized or expected level and a functional ability (e.g., activities of daily living [ADLs], social role functioning, memory, decision making) below perceived capability or expected level (Lyon, 1990).

Even for patients who are unconscious, nurses are concerned with the subjective experience of symptoms and functional problems. As a subjective experience, illness is not normative like disease but instead is dynamic and often varies uniquely from person to person. Therefore, the differential identification of NREs that may be triggering or intensifying symptoms and functional problems is particularly challenging. Unlike medicine, where the differential diagnosis focus is on identifying the disease that is causing symptoms and/or functional problems, the differential diagnosis focus in nursing is on the identification of NREs causing symptoms and functional problems, often without preestablished templates. Thus, the CNS's advanced knowledge about phenomena of concern to nursing and possible etiologies, along with the ability to effectively search pertinent science-based literature to assist in identifying possible etiologies, is critical to reasoned speculation about possible NREs. The evidence-based differential diagnosis and treatment of illness caused by etiologies other than disease in the presence or absence of disease is identified as one of the hallmarks of CNS practice (Dayhoff & Lyon, 2009; NACNS, 2004).

EXPLANATION OF THE CRM AND ITS ELEMENTS

The CRM is used by the faculty in the Adult Health Nursing Department at Indiana University School of Nursing to facilitate CNS students' learning of the process of clinical inquiry while helping them shift

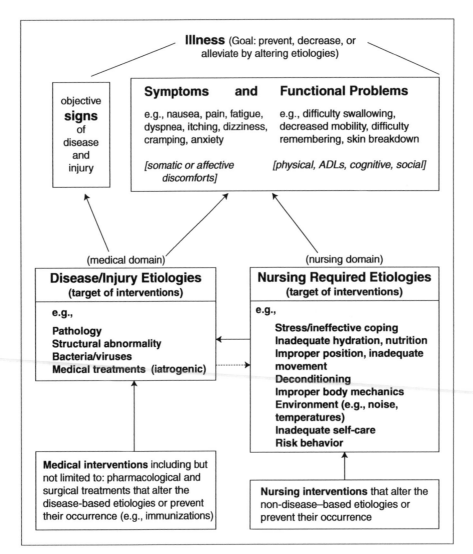

FIGURE 5.1 Etiologies of illness linked to treatment categories. The context in which a person is experiencing illness includes factors such as age, gender, development, and culture that may moderate or exacerbate etiologies or the illness experience.

Source: Used with permission from Brenda L. Lyon, Copyright© 1998.

their diagnostic perspective from a medically focused to a nursing-focused perspective. As an analytical heuristic model, the CRM is multidimensional. That is, it facilitates CNS students in

1. Differentiating diagnostic and interventional reasoning primarily informed by a medical perspective versus a holistic or context-rich nursing perspective that integrates disease and medical therapeutics as appropriate;
2. Appreciating that a clinician's knowledge of phenomena delimits the range of potentially relevant etiologies that can be hypothesized by the clinician to be ruled in or out;
3. Expanding their view of patient symptoms and functional problems by searching for possible NREs;
4. Valuing the critical role of target NREs in determining the intervention required to alter or change

the NRE and therefore effectively treat the problem or prevent a potential problem;
5. Evaluating evidence and developing a theory/ research-based rationale for selection and implementation of interventions;
6. Validating that the intervention acted as intended (manipulation check); and
7. Evaluating the efficacy of the intervention in achieving desired outcome(s).

Clinical problems in the patient sphere that need to be solved through nursing interventions typically focus on actual or potential symptoms, functional problems (including problems with skin integrity), and/or risk behaviors. The following examples represent common clinical problems: (a) how to decrease pain intensity that is not sufficiently relieved by analgesics in the context of disease or pathology, such as tissue/organ swelling or surgical incisions; (b) how to decrease the experience of dyspnea for a person with congestive heart failure or when weaning patients from ventilators; (c) how to prevent falls in persons who are at risk for falling; (d) how to reduce nausea in postoperative patients; and (e) how to prevent skin breakdown in persons who are at risk or how to treat early skin breakdown (Gordon, 1987; Lyon, 1990, 1996).

The CRM guides the reasoning process in a stepwise fashion, facilitating the identification of NREs in the context of disease and medical therapeutics when present, the rational selection of interventions to alter or resolve the etiologies, and the evaluation of intervention efficacy. The reasoning steps involved in diagnostic, therapeutic/interventional, and evaluation decisions contained in the CRM require the use of knowledge (theory/research/practical) about phenomena of concern to nursing. It is not possible for anyone to diagnose or recognize something that he or she does not understand (Carnevali, Mitchell, Woods, & Tanner, 1984). For example, if a registered nurse does not possess theoretical and evidence-based knowledge of symptoms and functional phenomena of concern to nursing and the corresponding NREs, his or her perceptual lens will be limited to misidentifying disease or iatrogenic affects of medical therapeutic as etiologies of patient problems.

It is imperative that the CNS be skilled in evaluating evidence. The challenge in applying evidence, particularly research evidence, into practice is that the scientific method focuses on a very limited number of variables at specified periods of time across many homogeneous subjects for the purpose of identifying generalizable findings. Clinical practice, in contrast, deals with a multitude of variables at a time within one patient in order to optimize a mix of outcomes intended to satisfy the particular patient's current needs and desires. It is, therefore, imperative that the CNS's professional judgments about the appropriate application of evidence be informed by the CNS's clinical expertise.

A pictorial representation of the CRM with exemplar content is presented in Figure 5.2. To promote understanding of the CRM, it is discussed here as a linear model. It is important to recognize that multiple problems often coexist and clinical situations are typically complex, so clinical reasoning must be appreciated as a complex iterative process. The components of the CRM are defined and discussed along with examples used in teaching the model, including content from an exemplar developed by Wendy Unger, MSN, when she was a student enrolled in the first Adult Health CNS course where pain was the symptom focus. Pain is used as the exemplar phenomenon because it is commonly experienced across populations of patients and is considered a nurse-sensitive

outcome (Doran, 2003; see Chapter 4). Additionally, focusing on one common phenomenon as an exemplar gives students the opportunity to appreciate that a thorough understanding of what is known about a symptom or functional problem is essential to identifying the full range of potentially relevant etiologies, thus guiding assessment in a meaningful manner.

Pertinent pain-related altered physiology, pharmacology, and assessment are integrated throughout the course. Each student selects a pain phenomenon that is common for his or her specialty area, for example, incisional pain, pain with endotracheal tube, pain from chest tubes on deep breathing, skin itching in dialysis patients, mobility-related pain, pain with turning, or pain in an extremity from dependent positioning.

Students learn, in depth, the physiology of pain and identify the pain pathway(s) for the particular type and context of pain experienced by patients in the specialty population. The learning experiences of students regarding the altered physiology of pain is enriched by the sharing of the commonalities of pain physiology across populations; they also gain knowledge from pain experiences unique to specialty populations (e.g., pain of mucositis in patients receiving chemotherapy, incisional pain in patients who have undergone a liver transplant, positional pain in a person undergoing a cardiac catheterization, back pain after lumbar surgery, pain experienced while deep breathing with chest tubes in place, phantom pain postamputation, incisional pain postsurgery, back pain during heart catheterization, pain on turning after hip replacement). Additionally, the students acquire an advanced understanding of the pathophysiology of any disease process or injury (e.g., incision) the patient may have along with the pharmacodynamics of pharmacological agents. For example, a student focused on mucositis in patients receiving chemotherapy must understand the nature of each patient's cancer and related pathophysiology along with the action, timing, and perfusion dynamics of the chemotherapeutic agent(s) so that appropriate interventions (e.g., use of popsicles, ice chips, or saline mouth washes) can be selected and appropriately implemented (timing, dose, duration). Knowledge of the pharmacodynamics of analgesics plays an important role in evaluating the separate effects of nursing interventions on pain relief, as patients more often than not are appropriately receiving analgesics for pain.

As students acquire additional knowledge of the phenomenon of pain, they begin hypothesizing about possible NREs that could be triggering or intensifying pain in the context of all that is relevant to patients experiencing the selected type of pain. The example shared in Figure 5.2 and developed by Wendy Unger, MSN, was focused on the common experience of

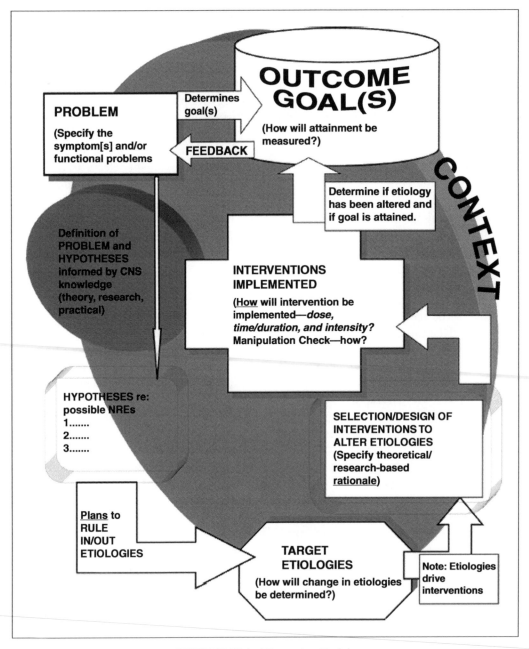

FIGURE 5.2 Clinical Reasoning Model.

post-open-heart surgery patients of "intensified pain at the triple lumen insertion (TLC) site during activity."

Context

The "context" is comprised of background information/data that, in addition to nursing domain knowledge, inform CNS clinical reasoning, while also assuring patient-centered care that encompasses all aspects of the person (Institute for Healthcare Improvement [IHI], 2011). The context contains nonvarying or slowly changing historical or current characteristics of the person and situation (Gordon, 1982). Dimensions of the context include, but are not limited to, age, gender, ethnicity, culture, education, patient and/or family preferences, personality/values, disease, medical therapeutics, and the situation (e.g., patient in critical care, outpatient, loss of loved one, loss of job).

The contextual background information provides the foundation for each of the remaining components of the model. Contextual variables for a patient often delimit the range of problems from a universe of possibilities. For example, some problems experienced by adults are not experienced by children; and some problems experienced by women are not experienced by men. Older adults may be more prone to certain types of problems than young adults. Likewise, persons who have diabetes are more prone to certain types of clinical problems than persons with arthritis. Context also influences the selection and implementation of a particular nursing intervention in terms of patient/family preferences, appropriateness, timing, dose, and frequency. The situational context for the exemplar presented here is adult patients in critical care after open-heart surgery.

Problem

The clinical problem—that is, the actual or potential symptom, functional problem, or risk behavior—is identified in the initial assessment. Clinical problems for patients who are unable to communicate are identified based on knowledge of the common types of uncomfortable sensations/symptoms or functional problems experienced by patients in a certain context. The clinical problem focused on in the CRM is caused by or contributed to by one or more NREs. That is, it is something that requires nursing interventions to alleviate or lessen and for which nursing is autonomously responsible and accountable (Gordon, 1987; see Chapter 7).

It is important that the clinical problem be precisely stated. For example, pain, postsurgery, needs to be clearly specified as incisional pain, or positional back pain at Level 8, or mouth pain in the context of receiving chemotherapy stated as mucositis pain at Level 6. A clearly stated clinical problem informs the identification of goals. The clinical problem focused on here is the common experience of post-open-heart surgery patients of "intensified pain above Level 3 at the TLC site during activity."

Goals (Desired Outcomes)

Goals are the predicted and desired outcomes (including indicators) of an intervention, which, if accomplished, represent a beneficial change in the problem. For example, incisional pain is alleviated or reduced to a two-pain level or mucositis pain is reduced to a two-pain level. It is also helpful to specify a time frame for when it is expected that the goal will be accomplished. For interventions that will not have an immediate effect, the time frame is critical because this affects the timing for evaluation. The goal in the exemplar was to *alleviate pain at the TLC site during activity during movement.*

Hypotheses Regarding NREs (Differential or Diagnostic Reasoning About Etiologies)

Hypotheses are reasoned speculations about possible etiologies that could be contributing to the problem. The speculations are tentative until validated (Carnevali, 1987). Unlike medical diagnoses that are normative and, therefore, only need to specify the disease, clinically relevant nursing diagnoses must identify the etiology(ies) causing or contributing to clinical problems, so that interventions can be effectively targeted to individual patients. The CNS's search for etiologies in a holistic assessment is expanded to include all relevant factors within the patient's context.

The essential question that is asked repeatedly during the speculation process about NREs is "What could be causing or contributing to this patient's symptom or functional problem other than disease or the iatrogenic effects of medical therapeutics?" For example, for a patient who is 24 hours postoperative from open-heart surgery who experiences breakthrough pain at the insertion site of chest tubes when using the incentive spirometer, what could be contributing to the pain over and above medical intervention–related causes? Identifying etiologies contributing to this pain is clinically important because the discomfort can preclude being able to deep breathe and could thus result in complications. Is it possible that the pain is being substantially contributed to by the patient not knowing how to do diaphragmatic deep breathing and, as a result, is moving the chest wall more than necessary?

Once the etiologies are hypothesized, the CNS moves to systematically collect data to rule in and rule out the probable etiologies. During the differential or diagnostic reasoning process, disease-based etiologies, including the iatrogenic effects of medical therapeutics (e.g., pharmacological agents), must be attended to because if the cause of the problem *is* limited to the pathology of the disease or injury (e.g., incision), or iatrogenic effects of medical therapeutics, then interventions must be surgical, complex mechanical, or pharmacological in nature. The CNS's ability to effectively identify probable etiologies and to conduct targeted assessment to rule in or out an etiology is delimited by the CNS's knowledge or evidence-based understanding of the phenomenon that is the problem. The accurate identification of etiologies is critical because there must be a good fit between the etiologies causing the problem and the interventions implemented, or the etiologies will not be altered or eliminated by the interventions. Implementing interventions to solve clinical problems without specifically identifying the etiologies to be targeted is like throwing darts at a dart board blindfolded.

A practical analogy is that upon trying to start your car to go home from work you discover that your car will not start. Your knowledge of the phenomenon "upon turning the key the car will not start" delimits the range of etiologies or causes that you can identify and rule in or out. If your knowledge is limited to two etiologies, such as "dead battery" and "out of gas," then those are the only two etiologies that you are capable of reasoning about. To rule out/in dead battery, if you understand that etiology, you might try to turn on the radio or notice if lights come on. If neither happens, then you "rule in" dead battery and get a jump start. Furthermore, in problem solving about the dead battery, you would most likely ask yourself, "Why did the battery die?" Upon reflection, you may also remember that you did not fully close the back door because you were in a hurry to grab your lunch bag—therefore, it's likely that the light was on during your entire 12-hour shift. Knowing that, a jump start would likely be sufficient, and you probably don't need a new battery. During the diagnostic reasoning process, if you discover that the radio plays and lights come on, then you might turn to the "out of gas" etiology and pay attention to the gas gauge—something that could be done simultaneously with the possibility of "dead battery." Remembering that you were running on fumes when you pulled into the parking lot at work, you think you will have to call to get someone to bring you some gas. If your gas tank is full and it is not a dead battery, your limited knowledge about the phenomenon does not permit you to diagnostically reason about a "bad starter" or "water in the carburetor," and therefore, you cannot identify the needed intervention and must refer the problem to someone else who has more knowledge.

There are times when the causal relationship between the etiology and the problem is clear. As in the previous simplistic example, when a car is out of gas there is a clear causal chain focused on one proximal cause. However, many times symptoms and functional problems are part of a complex set of etiologies, some of which are based in disease/pathology. For example, when there is a surgical incision, there is an obvious pathology in terms of tissue damage that is stimulating nerve endings and triggering the experience of "incisional pain," which requires pharmacological intervention. However, it is not uncommon for there to be breakthrough pain caused by other factors, such as improper positioning or mobilization that puts a strain on the incisional site and causes "intensified incisional pain."

Target Etiologies

Target etiologies are the validated, "ruled-in," likely causes or contributors to the problem and are amenable to nursing interventions. The ruling in or out of observable etiologies involves data collection and analysis and should be done prior to implementation of an intervention. Plans to rule in or out hypothesized etiologies are specified.

Clearly identifying the etiology (causative mechanism) is a requisite to guiding the clinician in choosing or designing an intervention that will most likely remedy the problem (Adelman, 1986; Eisenhauer, 1994). However, for an etiology that is not observable or cannot be validated a priori, the causative or contributing factors can only be confirmed with the implementation of an intervention intended to alter the etiologies and then evaluating the effectiveness of the intervention. When the deliberative intervention is effective in remedying the problem, the "action" of the intervention indirectly validates the presence of the hypothesized etiology. An example of hypothesized etiologies that cannot be validated prior to implementing an intervention would be a less than 30° head of bed elevation and inadequate mouth care as etiologies for ventilator-acquired pneumonia (VAP). These etiologies can only be confirmed when it is demonstrated that correcting them consistently eliminates the incidence of VAP.

Wendy's knowledge-based assessment searching for etiologies causing pain at the TLC site revealed that the catheter and sutures moved in the insertion site during activity and were likely causing mechanical tension/irritation at the TLC insertion site. It was hypothesized that the movement of the catheter and sutures was caused by *lack of securement of the TLC and increased weight of unused claves and stopcocks.* The presence of these etiologies was ruled in as the cause of the pain by applying a securement device and removing the unused claves and stopcocks and confirming the absence of discomfort with movement.

The physiological explanation for intensified pain from the tissue irritation caused by movement of catheter and increased weight of claves and stopcocks as a whole is that initial tissue injury occurs with the insertion of the TLC during surgery, causing initial nociceptor firing and sensitization. The catheter is left in place during and after surgery. Its presence leads to the inflammatory process and additional chemical release, nociceptive sensitization, and nociceptor recruitment. At the 48-hour postoperative mark, patients become more active, moving from bed to chair, and from chair to walking. When patients move, the lumens of the catheter fall, creating tension at the site, causing the sensitized nociceptors to fire, release more chemicals, and become further sensitized and further irritation and inflammation occurs. Resulting pain impulses travel along A-delta fibers to the dorsal horn of the spinal cord and, through tracts, to the thalamus and cortex where a sharp pain sensation is experienced. After the stimulus (tension) has been discontinued, the C fibers are involved in transmitting the burning, inflammatory pain that outlasts the stimulus (Phase 2 pain). Each tension episode leads to further chemical release, sensitization, and inflammation, putting the patient at risk for windup, hyperalgesia, and allodynia.

The diagnostic statement includes the validated problem and corresponding etiologies. For Wendy's exemplar, the diagnostic statement was *Pain at TLC site due to lack of securement of TLC and increased weight of unused claves and stopcocks*. Data regarding the effectiveness of using the securement device and removing unused claves and stopcocks in reducing or eliminating discomfort at the TLC site could contribute to the development of a "best practice" protocol for care of TLC sites.

Selection/Design of Interventions to Alter Etiologies

Sidani and Braden (1998) focus on a theory-driven approach to evaluating nursing interventions when doing interventional research. Although their work is focused on research, it offers an excellent overview of important factors to consider when selecting and/ or designing nursing interventions. *Interventions* are planned actions (treatments, therapies, procedures) into the life or environment of an individual, which are intended to bring about beneficial changes for the individual with minimal risk of adverse outcomes (McCloskey & Bulechek, 2004; Synder, Eagan, & Najima, 1996; Thomas, 1984). Assessment or monitoring activities are not interventions. The purpose of an intervention is aimed at altering the etiologies contributing to or causing a problem or preventing etiologies to prevent a potential problem. A few examples of nursing interventions are turning, repositioning, use of cold/warm, preoperative teaching, range of motion exercises, breathing exercises, counseling, and dietary management.

The selection or design of interventions is driven by the target etiology(ies) of the problem *and* the theoretical/research rationale, indicating that the planned action should alter the etiology. Comfort measures of choice, such as a wet wash-cloth to the forehead for nausea or pain, are often selected by registered nurses based on tradition and used on a trial-and-error basis without an understanding of the scientific rationale for why the intervention should work—that is, what is it that the intervention is altering? (Conn, Rantz, Wipke-Tevis, & Mass, 2001).

The interventions should fit the etiologies. For example, if the etiology of your "car won't start" is that it is out of gas, then the intervention is to put gas in the car. If the target etiology of intensified incisional pain is straining the abdominal area and incision cite because of turning technique, the intervention is to teach the patient a different technique for turning to avoid straining muscles in the incisional area. If a patient is unable to turn self, the nurse turns the patient using a known technique to avoid straining involved muscles.

Therapeutic/interventional reasoning encompasses appropriate matching of the intervention(s) with the validated target etiology(ies), selection of contextually appropriate implementation of the intervention, and evaluation of the intervention with respect to efficacy in achieving the desired outcome (Gordon, 1982, 1987). In addition to the target etiology, the selection of the intervention is grounded in a theoretical/research/practical or evidence-based rationale for being able to predict that the action will alter or remove the etiology, thereby linking the causal chain. The rationale is the logical basis for selection of the intervention; it makes use of the intervention legitimate, while avoiding anything that would be a contraindication for use of the intervention (Sidani & Braden, 1998).

In addition to matching the intervention to the etiology, it is imperative that consideration also be given to the potential for the intervention to create complications or unintended consequences. It is important to assure that use of the intervention will not counteract the intended effect of another intervention. An example would be not using cold on the skin or mucosal surface if a chemotherapeutic agent is intended to perfuse through dermal tissue.

Intervention Implementation

The implementation specifications include the "how" of delivery, including strength or dosage, when, and where. The specifications of a selected intervention are informed by theory/research (when available) or other evidence in addition to contextual factors (Sidani & Braden, 1998). Specifically, specifications identify the explicit activities of the intervention; detail the procedures, including timing, frequency, and duration; and identify patient preferences as well as the resources that would be needed to carry out the intervention.

The concept of *strength* of an intervention corresponds to the concept of *dose* of a medication. An example of strength of dosage is how cold a washcloth must be to effectively interrupt a pain pathway. *Timing* refers to when a treatment is done. An example would be waiting until the peak action of a pain medication to occur prior to implementing a mobility intervention. *Frequency* refers to how often an intervention needs to be done to either effectively treat the problem and/or maintain the desired effect. The duration of an intervention is the length of time the intervention takes or is applied (e.g., 15 seconds, 1 minute, 30 minutes, over a week). Many times the specifications for intervention implementation are informed through theory and empirical evidence; however, consistent with levels of evidence in evidence-based practice, expert opinion can guide the CNS.

After implementation of the intervention, or during if the duration is long, it is important to validate that the intervention was implemented as intended. If it is not possible to implement the intervention with an adequate dose or frequency, then it is quite probable that the intended effect will not occur.

Nursing interventions used by Wendy in her exemplar with patients were directed at preventing or reducing mechanical tissue tension at the TLC insertion site (aligning intervention with hypothesized etiology). The first intervention was use of a securement device. A Stat-Lock brand TLC securement device was applied per the manufacturer's instructions to achieve securement of the TLC and its lumens. Manufacturer's instructions indicate to place the device, which is a piece of adhesive foam with four small plastic prongs on top of it, to achieve securement, which may vary given differing patient anatomy (usually 2.5 to 3 inches from insertion site). Securement is indicated when patient can turn head left to right without causing tension and when all lumens are in place and immobile between prongs on the device. Dose: NA; Amount: 1 device; Frequency: Once and as needed if device soiled; Duration: As long as TLC in place. The second intervention was removal of superfluous claves and stopcocks from TLC lumens. All claves and stopcocks were removed until only one clave per lumen existed. Dose/Amount: Removal of all claves and stopcocks until only one clave per lumen exists; Frequency: Once; Duration: As long as TLC in place. The interventions were implemented at the peak action time of any pain medication that had been administered.

Manipulation Check

A manipulation check is done to determine if the intervention acted as intended. That is, "Was the washcloth really cool, did the music really distract the patient, or did the wedge under the knees when the patient was lying flat really tilt the pelvis up to a 30° angle?" It cannot be assumed that an intervention created the effect for which it was intended. If patient-selected music was used for the intended effect of distracting the patient because the etiology of his intensified pain is that he is focused on the pain, then it cannot be assumed that the patient experienced the music as a distraction. To be able to draw a valid conclusion about whether or not the intervention worked to alleviate or lessen the target etiology, the effective action of the intervention must be validated because there might be myriad reasons why the music did not work as a distraction. The patient must be asked if the music helped him take his mind off the pain to validate that the music acted as intended.

Wendy's manipulation check for securement involved examining all devices after application and during activity to determine if they did indeed *secure* the TLC and its lumens. For removal of superfluous claves and stopcocks, it *was* ascertained that extra claves and stopcocks are indeed removed.

Evaluation of Outcomes

Absence of a problem (actual or potential) is the generic goal or desired outcome of nursing interventions. Outcomes of nursing interventions are referred to as nurse-sensitive outcomes. Outcomes can be objective or subjective in nature (see Chapters 4 and 10).

To effectively evaluate the impact of nursing interventions on outcomes, the evaluation plan (data collection plan) should be set prior to implementation of the intervention and should include the what (desired outcome), when it is measured, where it is measured, and how it is measured. Some outcomes are immediately evident, while others take time to evolve. The specifications of the intervention and the theoretical/research-based causal chain of how the intervention should work will inform the timing of the evaluation. Consideration needs to be given to ensure as much as possible that the data (e.g., measurement tool) has construct validity and will be reliable and sensitive enough to pick up the desired change, for example, assessing physical functioning outcomes resulting from a cardiac exercise program (Sidani & Braden, 1998).

For Wendy's patients, the outcome goal was elimination of intensified pain at TLC insertion site during activity in the population. Achievement of the outcome was measured by comparing the preintervention pain intensity rating on a valid pain scale ranging from 0 to 10 with the postintervention pain intensity rating on the same scale before and during activity.

Additional considerations in the evaluation of interventions are particularly important when considering patient population needs and developing best-practice guidelines for populations to prevent or alleviate NREs. These considerations include objective capability, adequacy of the intervention procedure, unintended consequences, and ethical suitability. Objective capability encompasses considerations in terms of the objective nursing work requirements (time and effort) and cost considerations in terms of material resources and nursing time. Adequacy of the intervention procedure, in addition to answering the question of whether or not the intervention is effective, includes considerations discussed earlier, such as strength/dose and frequency, that would be applicable across patients. It is important to anticipate and prevent unintended consequences of interventions such as possible interference with a medical therapy or creation of unrealistic patient expectations for adherence. Ethical suitability entails ensuring that patients are fully informed about the intervention and that they participate, when able and as appropriate, in decisions pertinent to the intervention.

> Wendy informed patients regarding the application of the securement device and the removal of unnecessary claves and stopcocks; there were no risks involved in implementing the interventions. The interventions were easy to administer and would not burden the nursing staff. The securement device was readily available and the cost was minimal, and the interventions are applicable across patient populations with a TLC.

Additionally, it is imperative to inform patients of any risk or possible negative consequence of the intervention and to seek verbal consent (Thomas, 1984). As always, adherence to the American Nurses Association Code of Ethics is of paramount importance (ANA, 2001).

SUMMARY

Graduate programs preparing CNSs have a societal obligation to prepare graduates in the *advanced practice of nursing*. The focus of this chapter has been on the use of a CRM as a guide for solving clinical problems in the nursing domain. The CRM is anchored in the differential diagnosis of etiologies (NREs) for clinical problems that require nursing interventions.

Critical to the advanced practice of nursing by CNSs in the nursing domain is the understanding that disease and illness are different phenomena and that illness can be caused or contributed to by etiologies other than disease or the iatrogenic effects of medical therapeutics. Use of the CRM facilitates learning the process of clinical inquiry in the patient sphere focused on nursing's unique contribution to patient care. Furthermore, experience with using the CRM helps students to shift their perceptual lens so that disease and medical therapeutics are viewed as critical parts of the "context" or background of the patient's experience and NREs are moved to the foreground in differential diagnosis. The importance of disease and its treatment are not minimized, just placed in the background and incorporated as appropriate in the differential determination of etiologies. Students often describe the experience of conducting a clinical inquiry using the model as transformational.

For patients to benefit from multidisciplinary practice, members of each discipline, while open to the perspective of other disciplines, must bring to the clinical situation a discipline-related bias in clinical reasoning—thereby collectively expanding the range of etiologies addressed. The emphasis by some organizations on, and their requirement that curriculums include for all APNs, including CNSs, the generic and primary care focused three "Ps" (physical assessment, pathophysiology, and pharmacology), without mention of other content areas critical to informing CNS practice focused on phenomena of concern to nursing, limits the acquisition of essential knowledge for CNS practice. "For too long, CNS education has included courses on physical assessment, physiology, pathophysiology, and pharmacology inconsistent with CNS practice—focusing not on illness and risk behaviors but on primary care diagnosis and management of disease" (Fulton, 2006, p. 114). Although many physical symptoms have corresponding altered physiology, the pathology of disease does not help us understand what is happening with phenomena of concern to nursing. The CNS's knowledge of phenomena of concern to nursing enables the types of clinical inquiries that will result in the identification of best-practice guidelines that will promote the experience of wellness.

How to use language when communicating the results of clinical reasoning in terms of diagnostic statements and inclusion of target etiologies that guide interventions is particularly challenging. Although there are substantial benefits to the use of standardized nursing language, including ease of documentation in computerized records, communication of nursing care nationally and internationally, and reimbursement of nursing care services (Rutherford, 2008), the profession has not yet identified how to identify target etiologies within standardized diagnoses or interventions. There is still considerable work to be done.

▓ DISCUSSION QUESTIONS

- Identify common symptoms and functional problems within your specialty populations that might be caused or contributed to by NREs, and discuss with your peers.
- Select one symptom or functional problem that is experienced across different patient populations and identify contextual factors that would influence both NREs and what type of nursing interventions might be effective. Identify theory and research-based sources that would need to be retrieved and evaluated to explain how the NRE may be causing or contributing to the problem and that would contribute to the rationale for the type of intervention needed.

▓ ANALYSIS AND SYNTHESIS EXERCISE

- Conduct your own clinical inquiry using the CRM as a guide to resolve a clinical problem frequently experienced by patients in your specialty population.

REFERENCES

Adelman, H. S. (1986). Intervention theory and evaluating efficacy. *Evaluation Review, 10*(1), 65–83.

American Nurses Association (ANA). (2001). *Code of ethics for nursing with interpretive statements.* Washington, DC: Author. Retrieved January 21, 2009, from http://nursingworld.org/books/anps earchdetail.cfm?PubNum=9781558101760&thedesc=Code%20of%20ethics%20for%20n&DisNum=10&StartRow=1

American Nurses Association (ANA). (2010). *Nursing's social policy statement: The essence of the profession* (3rd ed.). Silver Spring, MD: Author.

Arslanian-Engorin, C., Hicks, F. D., Whall, A. L., & Algase, D. L. (2005). An ontological view of advanced practice nursing. *Research and Theory for Nursing Practice: An International Journal, 19*(4), 315–322.

Barsky, A. J. (1981). Hidden reasons some patients visit doctors. *Annals of Internal Medicine, 94*(Pt. 1), 492–498.

Barsky, A. J. (1988). *Worried sick: Our troubled quest for wellness.* Boston, MA: Little, Brown.

Baumann, A., & Deber, R. (1987). Decision making in critical care: Implications for future development. In K. J. Hannah, M. Reimer, W. C. Mills, & S. Letourneau (Eds.), *Clinical judgement and decision making: The future with nursing diagnosis* (pp. 371–375). New York, NY: Wiley.

Beech, N., Arber, A., & Faithful, S. (2011). Restoring a sense of wellness following colorectal cancer: A grounded theory. *Journal of Advanced Nursing, 68*(5), 1134–1144.

Boorse, C. (1975). On the distinction between disease and illness. *Philosophy and Public Affairs, 5,* 49–68.

Bowen, J. L. (2006). Educational strategies to promote clinical diagnostic reasoning. *New England Journal of Medicine, 355*(21), 2217–2225.

Carnevali, D. L. (1987). Diagnostic reasoning: Nursing and medicine compared. In K. J. Hannah, M. Reimer, W. C. Mills, & S. Letourneau (Eds.), *Clinical judgement and decision making: The future with nursing diagnosis* (pp. 29–32). New York, NY: Wiley.

Carnevali, D. L., Mitchell, P. H., Woods, N. F., & Tanner, C. A. (1984). *Diagnostic reasoning in nursing.* New York, NY: J. B. Lippincott.

Conn, V. S., Rantz, M. J., Wipke-Tevis, D. D., & Mass, J. L. (2001). Designing effective nursing interventions. *Research in Nursing & Health, 24*(5), 433–442.

Dayhoff, N., & Lyon, B. L. (2009). Assessing outcomes in clinical nurse specialist practice. In R. M. Kleinpell (Ed.), *Outcome assessment in advanced nursing practice* (2nd ed., pp. 191–218). New York, NY: Springer.

Doran, D. M. (2003). *Nursing-sensitive outcomes: The state of the science.* Sudbury, MA: Jones & Bartlett.

Dorland's Medical Dictionary Disease. (2007). St. Louis, MO: Elsevier.

Dunlop. S., R. (2010). Towards an antological theory of wellness: A discussion of conceptual foundations and implications for nursing. *Nursing Philosophy, 11*(3), 223.

Eisenberg, L. (1976). Disease and illness distinctions between professional and popular ideas of sickness. *Culture, Medicine and Psychiatry, 1*(1), 9–23.

Eisenberg, L. (1980). What makes persons "patients" and patients "well." *The American Journal of Medicine, 69,* 277–286.

Eisenhauer, L. A. (1994). A typology of nursing therapeutics. *Image: Journal of Nursing Scholarship, 26*(4), 261–264.

Faull, K., Hills, M. D., Cochrane, G., Gray, J., Hunt, M., McKenzie, C., & Winter, L. (2004). Investigation of health perspectives of those with physical disabilities: The role of spirituality as a determinant of health. *Disability and Rehabilitation, 26*(3), 129–144.

Fries, J. F., Koop, C. E., & Beadle, C. E. (1993). Reducing health care costs by reducing the need and demand for medical services. *New England Journal of Medicine, 329,* 321–325.

Fulton, J. S. (2006). In search of advanced clinical nurse specialist education. *Clinical Nurse Specialist, 20*(3), 114–115.

Gordon, M. (1982). *Nursing diagnosis, process and application.* New York, NY: McGraw-Hill.

Gordon, M. (1987). The nurse as a thinking practitioner. In K. J. Hannah, M. Reimer, W. C. Mills, & S. Letourneau (Eds.), *Clinical judgement and decision making: The future with nursing diagnosis* (pp. 8–17). New York, NY: Wiley.

Henderson, V. (1966). *The nature of nursing.* New York, NY: Macmillan.

Higgs, J., & Jones, M. (2000). Clinical reasoning in the health professions. In J. Higgs & M. Jones (Eds.), *Clinical reasoning in the health professions* (2nd ed., pp. 3–14). Oxford, UK: Butterworth Heinemann.

Hughner, R. S., & Kleine, S. S. (2004). Views of health in the lay sector: A compilation and review of how individuals think about health. *Health: An*

Interdisciplinary Journal for the Social Study of Health, Illness and Medicine, 8(4), 395–422.

Hwu, Y. J., Coates, V. E., & Boore, J. R. P. (2001). The evolving concept of health in nursing research: 1988–1998. *Patient Education and Counseling, 42*(2), 105–114.

Institute for Healthcare Improvement (IHI). (2011). *Across the chasm aim #3: Health care must be patient centered.* Retrieved April 4, 2013, from http://www.ihi.org/IHI/Topics/PatientCenteredCare

Jensen, L. A., & Allen, M. N. (1994). A synthesis of qualitative research on wellness-illness. *Qualitative Health Research, 4*(4), 349–369.

Johnson, D. E. (1980). The behavioral system model for nursing. In J. P. Riehl & C. Roy (Eds.), *Conceptual models for nursing practice* (2nd ed., pp. 207–216). Norwalk, CT: Appleton-Century-Crofts.

King, I. M. (1989). King's general systems framework and theory. In J. Riehl-Sisca (Ed.), *Conceptual models for nursing practice* (3rd ed., pp. 149–158). Norwalk, CT: Appleton & Lange.

Leininger, M. M. (1988). Leininger's theory of nursing: Cultural care diversity and universality. *Nursing Science Quarterly, 1*(4), 152–160.

Long, K. A., & Weinert, C. (1992). Descriptions and perceptions of health among rural and urban adults with multiple sclerosis. *Research on Nursing and Health, 15,* 335–342.

Loomis, M., & Conco, D. (1991). Patients' perceptions of health, chronic illness, and nursing diagnoses. *Nursing Diagnosis, 2*(4), 162–170.

Lyon, B. L. (1990). Getting back on track: Nursing's autonomous scope of practice. In N. Chaska (Ed.), *The nursing profession: Turning points* (pp. 267–274). St. Louis, MO: CV Mosby.

Lyon, B. L. (1996), Meeting societal needs for CNS competencies, . *Online Journal of Nursing Issues, 1*(1).

Lyon, B. L. (2005). Reflecting on "Getting back on track": Nursing's autonomous scope of practice. *Clinical Nurse Specialist, 19*(1), 25.

Mackey, S. (2009). Towards an ontological theory of wellness: A discussion of conceptual foundations and implications for nursing. *Nursing Philosophy, 10,* 103–112.

McCloskey, J. C., & Bulechek, G. M. (2004). *Nursing Intervention Classification (NIC)* (4th ed.). St. Louis, MO: CV Mosby.

McConnell, T. (2007). *The nature of disease: Pathology for the health professions.* Baltimore, MD: Lippincott, Williams & Wilkins.

McKague, M., & Verhoef, M. (2003). Understandings of health and its determinants among clients and providers at an urban community healthy center. *Qualitative Health Research, 13*(5), 703–717.

McMahon, S., & Fleury, J. (2012). Wellness in older adults: A concept analysis. *Nursing Forum, 47*(1), 39–51.

Mokdad, A. H., Marks, J. S., Stroup, D. F., & Gerberding, M. D. (2004). Actual causes of death in the United States, 2000. *Journal of the American Medical Association, 291*(10), 1238–1245.

National Association of Clinical Nurse Specialists (NACNS). (2004). *Statement on clinical nurse specialist practice and education* (2nd ed.). Harrisburg, PA: Author.

Neuman, B. (1989). *The Neuman systems model* (2nd ed.). Norwalk, CT: Appleton & Lange.

Newman, M. A. (1986). *Health as expanding consciousness.* St. Louis, MO: Mosby-Year Book.

Nightingale, F. (1860/1969). *Notes on nursing.* New York, NY: Dover.

Norman, G. (2006). Building on experience—The development of clinical reasoning. *New England Journal of Medicine, 355*(21), 2251–2252.

Orem, D. E. (1985). *Nursing: Concepts of practice* (3rd ed.). New York, NY: McGraw-Hill.

Parse, R. R. (1989). Man-living health: A theory of nursing. In J. Riehl-Sisca (Ed.), *Conceptual models for nursing practice* (3rd ed., pp. 253–257). Norwalk, CT: Appleton & Lange.

Peplau, H. E. (1988). The art and science of nursing: Similarities, differences and relations. *Nursing Science Quarterly, 1,* 8–15.

Pesut, D. J., & Herman, J. (1999). *Clinical reasoning: The art and science of critical and creative thinking.* Boston, MA: Delmar.

Rogers, M. E. (1970). *An introduction to the theoretical basis of nursing.* Philadelphia, PA: F. A. Davis.

Roy, C. (1984). *Introduction to nursing: An adaptation model* (2nd ed.). Englewood Cliffs, NJ: Prentice Hall.

Rutherford, M. A. (2008). Standardized nursing language: What does it mean for nursing practice? *The Online Journal of Nursing Issues, 13*(1). Retrieved January 19, 2009, from http://www.nursingworld.org/MainMenuCategories/ANAMarketplace/ANAPeriodicals/OJIN/TableofContents/vol132008/No1Jan08/ArticlePreviousTopic/StandardizedNursingLanguage.aspx

Schmidt, H. G., Norman, G. R., & Boshuizen, H. P. S. (1990). A cognitive perspective on medical expertise: Theory and implications. *Academic Medicine, 65*(10), 611–621.

Sidani, S., & Braden, C. J. (1998). *Evaluating nursing interventions: A theory-driven approach.* Thousand Oaks, CA: Sage.

Sobel, D. S. (1995). Rethinking medicine: Improving health outcomes with cost-effective psychosocial interventions. *Psychosomatic Medicine, 57,* 234–244.

Synder, M., Egan, E. C., & Najima, Y. (1996). Defining nursing interventions. *Image: Journal of Nursing Scholarship, 28*(2), 137–142.

Thomas, E. J. (1984). *Designing interventions for the helping professions.* Thousand Oaks, CA: Sage.

Victor-Chmil, J. (2013). Critical thinking versus clinical reasoning versus clinical judgement: Differential diagnosis. *Nurse Educator, 38*(1), 34–36.

Wikman, A., Marklund, S., & Alexanderson, K. (2005). Illness, disease, and sickness absence: An empirical test of differences between concepts of ill health. *Journal of Epidemiology and Community Health, 59,* 450–454.

Managing the Change/ Innovation Process

Jeannette Richardson

The clinical nurse specialist (CNS), regardless of practice setting, must always be alert to the need for maintaining or improving the quality of care for his or her defined population, whether it be individual patients, families, groups, or communities (National Association of Clinical Nurse Specialists [NACNS], 2004). Continual surveillance activities and focused assessments can help identify the need for practice changes. Once a need is identified, a detailed and methodical approach is utilized to establish the current evidence base, set a goal for future practice, and create a plan for how to achieve this change.

A critical component of any planned change project is the choice of optimal intervention strategies. An inappropriate intervention could result in failure to effect the practice change and, ultimately, suboptimal patient care. The CNS, as project leader, is responsible for the outcome of the project and any resulting impact on patient care. Consequently, he or she must be knowledgeable about which interventions apply best to different practice situations.

An intervention may follow a tried-and-true methodology familiar to those in the targeted practice setting, or it might be based on an innovative idea specifically created to address the project goal, personnel, and/or setting. The Agency for Healthcare Research and Quality (AHRQ, 2013) defines *health care innovation* as "the implementation of new or altered products, services, processes, systems, policies, organizational structures, or business models that aim to improve one of more domains of health care quality or reduce health care disparities." An

innovative intervention, therefore, would be an application of a new strategy or a new twist on an old intervention for the purpose of achieving desired outcomes. It presents an intriguing combination—to take a standardized base of clinical knowledge and apply it to a specific practice setting in a way that has been tailored to work best in that practice arena. Use of highly innovative interventions may help to improve the chance for success and endurance of a practice change in our current complex health care environment (Strom, 2001).

Given the leadership responsibility, how does the CNS best guide the project team in choosing implementation strategies for their project? Which methods would be most effective and enduring? And what does it mean to be innovative in choosing interventions? This chapter explores how the CNS plays a key role in planning, developing, and encouraging innovative interventions for better patient care outcomes.

BACKGROUND/LITERATURE REVIEW

The health care system in the United States encourages a culture of evidence-based practice (EBP) in all aspects of patient care. Nursing, medicine, pharmacy, and other disciplines are using similar methodologies to examine traditional and intuition-driven practice and move toward a culture based on research-gleaned evidence. Numerous guidelines and practice statements have been established based on meta-analyses of clinical research studies, and the strength of a recommendation is related to the strength of the research.

As the diligent CNS strives to examine practice in his or her area of expertise, he or she will note that many validated, published guidelines exist that articulate exactly what is needed for optimal patient care in specific clinical scenarios. However, in many cases, health care team members have not successfully achieved either compliance with the recommended process, or desired patient outcomes. Translating research into practice is a complex science and should be based upon scientific evidence.

Moving from the current state of health care to a desired state requires a change in practice; multiple factors related to clients, the health care team, and the setting must be considered. Many different change interventions may be available to the CNS, but it is most efficient and reasonable to choose strategies that have been formally researched and shown to have positive outcomes. This philosophy of investigating and choosing specific interventional strategies on the basis of research-related evidence and for the purpose of promoting the translation of research findings into practice is relatively new. This field is referred to as Implementation Science and can be defined as "the study of methods to promote the integration of research findings and evidence into health care policy and practice" (Fogarty International Center, n.d.). The current body of knowledge is limited but, over time, more rigorous research studies will generate further information. In the meantime, the CNS can use the evidence that is available, in addition to some recognized generalities, to provide guidance when choosing optimal interventions for a given project.

Current Knowledge Related to Interventional Strategies

Alexander and Hearld (2011) proposed that implementation of most new, innovative practices requires sustained leadership, extensive training and support, robust measurement and data systems, realigned incentives and human resource practices, and cultural receptivity to change. Within the profession of nursing, Sandström, Borglin, Nilsson, and Willman (2011) completed a literature review on the implementation of nursing-related EBP. They describe characteristics mostly strongly associated with successful implementation, including:

- Characteristics of the leader—Role modeling and support
- Characteristics of the organization—Policy revisions, resource allocation, education, human, and material support
- Characteristics of the culture—Valuing research, incorporating research utilization in performance appraisals

Several researchers have found that the strength of evidence based on published guidelines and clinical trials alone cannot be expected to change behavior—in fact, disagreement with the interpretation of reported trials is a key barrier to implementation (Rello et al., 2002). Likewise, a passive approach, such as targeted mailing of guidelines, is not likely to result in a behavior change. Didactic lectures are also generally ineffective (Grimshaw et al., 2001; Grol & Grimshaw, 1999).

One critical strategy for success lies in assembling a valuable team of key individuals who are dedicated to the project and considered thought leaders among their peers. Creating a workgroup of these exceptional people increases the probability of the social acceptance of change (Thompson, Estabrooks, Scott-Findlay, Moore, & Wallin, 2007).

Educational outreach sessions have also proved successful and involve having a trained topic expert with setting-specific information meet with health care team members within their practice arena. Providing clinicians with face-to-face conversation, the ability to ask and answer questions, and real-time problem solving improves the likelihood of project acceptance. Additionally, the use of multiple, varied, and targeted strategies to enhance compliance and avoid specific potential barriers was generally effective (Grimshaw et al., 2001).

Some health care team members are motivated to change practice through the use of a rewards system. These incentives may be either financial or of a nonfinancial nature such as paid time off or professional recognition (Joshi & Bernard, 1999). The CNS who wishes to provide rewards may need to negotiate with administrative personnel regarding budgetary or union concerns, staffing levels, and so forth. To be accepted, a change strategy must deliver some type of perceived benefit—enough benefits to make change worthwhile. It may be that the benefit is altruistic in nature and reflected in improved patient care outcomes. It is the responsibility of the CNS to guide the health care team members to recognize and value the benefit of the specific project implementation.

Electronic medical records systems and informatics-based approaches to improving patient care can assist in working with both individual patients and large patient populations. Innovative strategies have included the use of population registries, decision support at the time of a patient visit, and web-based communication between patients and providers. Some research has shown that identification of patients at risk, coupled with a web-based alerting system for physicians, has not impacted patient outcomes

(Grant & Meigs, 2006). Alternatively, other trials have indicated that intensive, protocol-driven, nurse practitioner–run clinics have resulted in significant improvement in risk factor modification for hyperglycemia, hypertension, or hyperlipidemia (New et al., 2003). Suggestions for future trials recommend consideration for the use of clinical support staff (such as nurses), administrative staff (such as secretaries), or even direct patient-centered outreach to maximize interventional impact (Grant & Meigs, 2006).

Providing for clinical decision support in real time at the point of care through an electronic or even a paper mechanism can provide support for change with immediate and round-the-clock access to necessary information in multiple formats (protocols, published guidelines, pocket cards, intranet information, telephone hotlines, etc.; Joshi & Bernard, 1999). Other potential interventional strategies could include the use of the following (White, 2004):

1. Clinical reminders and prompts
2. Feedback on performance
3. Interactive computer-based learning
4. A continuous quality improvement (CQI) process

CQI is a formal and structured process involving the use of data analysis tools and change strategies to bring about ongoing, positive outcomes. Many facilities utilize specific CQI processes (e.g., Six Sigma and Lean methodologies) for ensuring the quality of care for their patient populations; to enhance multidisciplinary and multidepartment communication, the CNS should be aware of and utilize those strategies sanctioned by his or her employer. CQI principles provide a powerful framework for project planning and have been used in health care over the last several decades to provide a systematic approach to health care reform.

Although the use of multiple, targeted interventions simultaneously can improve the chance for success, this process should be used cautiously and accompanied by sound rationale. It has been noted by several investigators that implementing *all* interventions at the same time is neither desirable nor practical. Furthermore, the evaluation of the interventions will be challenging due to the inability to determine which strategy caused the practice change. Making several small changes in a care process can be more easily effected and more effective than one larger action (Strom, 2001). Additionally, the innovation strategy should be accessible, useful, and dependable. Cost must be considered—if the intervention does not yield the desired results, then the strategy has been both costly and useless (Crow, 2006).

Examples of innovative thinking and strategies exist throughout health care and in other industries.

The Institute for Healthcare Improvement (IHI) is credited with the conception and initial implementation of improving clinical outcomes through the use of care bundles. A *bundle* is a collection of interventions related to a specific disease process that are implemented together to significantly improve patient care outcomes. Each bundle is generally made up of three to five specific interventions. Each intervention must be supported by irrefutable scientific evidence, and all elements of the bundle have to be executed in the same space and time to ensure that clinical improvement occurs (The Joint Commission on the Accreditation of Healthcare Organizations [JCAHO], 2006). This concept of achieving quality by reducing variation has been widely established in industry (Strom, 2001). Since its creation, the bundle concept has helped to implement critical care EBP in facilities throughout the United States, and it is spreading to multiple other patient care projects in other settings.

In multiple industries, innovative thinking in resource management has led to the advent of *crowdsourcing*—a method of web-based advertising to locate talent outside immediate company walls and capitalize on the limitless talent provided by the Internet. Challenges in software programming, business, chemistry, engineering, life sciences, math, and physical sciences are posted, and Internet users of all backgrounds, talents, and specialties are encouraged to submit innovative solutions to the prescribed problems. Various levels of financial compensation are rewarded to the consultants who compete with and expand upon each others' work. Examples of crowdsourcing in health care include sites that monitor and manage infectious disease outbreaks, problem-solve difficult patient diagnoses, or offer diagnostic opinions to patients for a fee (Strohmeyer, 2013). This strategy may one day prove to be a highly successful means for promoting quality and cost-effectiveness of health care in our country.

Cullen and Adams (2012) acknowledge that implementation can be the most difficult step in the implementation of EBP. They have published a comprehensive guide to implementation strategies for EBP to help practitioners and clinical teams move recommendations into practice (Exhibit 6.1). They break out the different implementation strategies into four phases; Create Awareness and Interest, Build Knowledge and Commitment, Promote Action and Adoption, and Pursue Integration and Sustained Use. This tool provides a valuable resource for the CNS to use in considering different options for implementation strategies.

In addition to considering those items that promote innovation, it is equally important to examine those characteristics that limit innovation. Once identified, effort can be channeled toward reversing

EXHIBIT 6.1

Implementation Strategies for Evidence-Based Practice

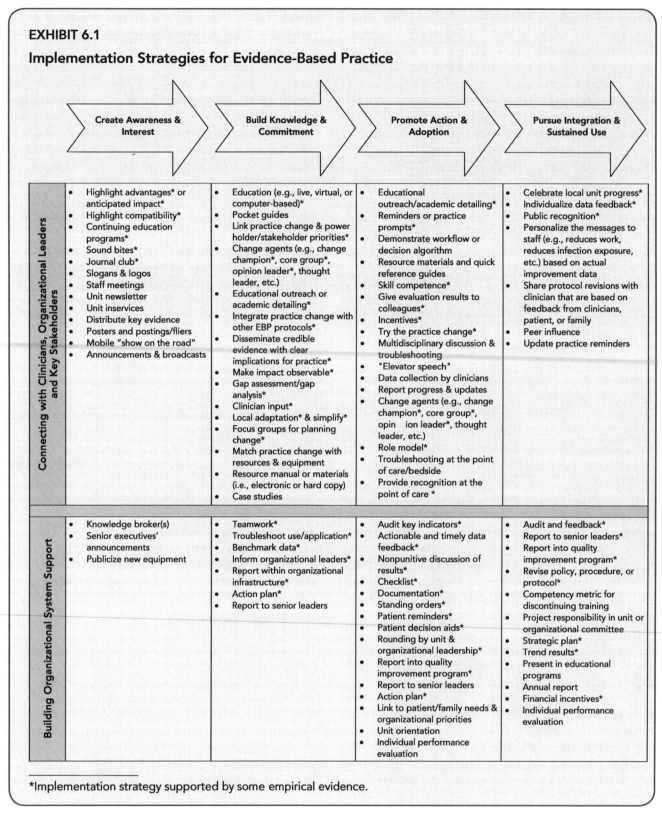

	Create Awareness & Interest	Build Knowledge & Commitment	Promote Action & Adoption	Pursue Integration & Sustained Use
Connecting with Clinicians, Organizational Leaders and Key Stakeholders	• Highlight advantages* or anticipated impact* • Highlight compatibility* • Continuing education programs* • Sound bites* • Journal club* • Slogans & logos • Staff meetings • Unit newsletter • Unit inservices • Distribute key evidence • Posters and postings/fliers • Mobile "show on the road" • Announcements & broadcasts	• Education (e.g., live, virtual, or computer-based)* • Pocket guides • Link practice change & power holder/stakeholder priorities* • Change agents (e.g., change champion*, core group*, opinion leader*, thought leader, etc.) • Educational outreach or academic detailing* • Integrate practice change with other EBP protocols* • Disseminate credible evidence with clear implications for practice* • Make impact observable* • Gap assessment/gap analysis* • Clinician input* • Local adaptation* & simplify* • Focus groups for planning change* • Match practice change with resources & equipment • Resource manual or materials (i.e., electronic or hard copy) • Case studies	• Educational outreach/academic detailing* • Reminders or practice prompts* • Demonstrate workflow or decision algorithm • Resource materials and quick reference guides • Skill competence* • Give evaluation results to colleagues* • Incentives* • Try the practice change* • Multidisciplinary discussion & troubleshooting • "Elevator speech" • Data collection by clinicians • Report progress & updates • Change agents (e.g., change champion*, core group*, opin ion leader*, thought leader, etc.) • Role model* • Troubleshooting at the point of care/bedside • Provide recognition at the point of care *	• Celebrate local unit progress* • Individualize data feedback* • Public recognition* • Personalize the messages to staff (e.g., reduces work, reduces infection exposure, etc.) based on actual improvement data • Share protocol revisions with clinician that are based on feedback from clinicians, patient, or family • Peer influence • Update practice reminders
Building Organizational System Support	• Knowledge broker(s) • Senior executives' announcements • Publicize new equipment	• Teamwork* • Troubleshoot use/application* • Benchmark data* • Inform organizational leaders* • Report within organizational infrastructure* • Action plan* • Report to senior leaders	• Audit key indicators* • Actionable and timely data feedback* • Nonpunitive discussion of results* • Checklist* • Documentation* • Standing orders* • Patient reminders* • Patient decision aids* • Rounding by unit & organizational leadership* • Report into quality improvement program* • Report to senior leaders • Action plan* • Link to patient/family needs & organizational priorities • Unit orientation • Individual performance evaluation	• Audit and feedback* • Report to senior leaders* • Report into quality improvement program* • Revise policy, procedure, or protocol* • Competency metric for discontinuing training • Project responsibility in unit or organizational committee • Strategic plan* • Trend results* • Present in educational programs • Annual report • Financial incentives* • Individual performance evaluation

*Implementation strategy supported by some empirical evidence.

or eliminating these obstacles. Potential barriers to innovation include (Idea Champions, n.d.)

1. Lack of a shared vision
2. Lack of commitment/ownership by leaders
3. Constantly shifting priorities
4. Short-term thinking
5. Focus on intervention rather than customer
6. Focus on past successes
7. Unwilling to change without significant benefit
8. Political barriers protecting entrenched interests
9. Reactive rather than proactive philosophy

Barriers to EBP implementation in nursing also include lack of access to relevant research evidence, inadequate database searching skills, difficulty understanding research articles, time and resource constraints, lack of mentoring and organizational support, and lack of authority to change practice (Oman, Duran, & Fink, 2008). By recognizing and working with or around potential barriers, the CNS can improve his or her potential for a positive and enduring change.

CONCEPTUAL FRAMEWORK

A Model for Practice, Planned Change, and Innovative Interventions

Change theory concepts encourage use of a step-by-step methodology to plan for, implement, and maintain an intervention in order to achieve specific goals. Use of a detailed plan can help break down a complex and overwhelming project into bite-sized manageable pieces. Additionally, it can help to set a realistic timeline, which is helpful not only for the workgroup team but also for administrators who might be anxious to see the project reach fruition.

There is no single best way to understand change management because each individual brings his or her own experiences and worldviews to each unique project. But many change agents find that the use of a model can assist in planning and following through with the various aspects of a change project (Shanley, 2007). The Johns Hopkins Nursing Evidence-Based Practice Model (JHNEBP) was developed specifically for nurses and reflects the three essential cornerstones that are the foundation for professional nursing: practice, education, and research (Exhibit 6.2). Use of this model can support end-user adoption of evidence and assist in embedding EBP into the organizational culture (Dearholt & Dang, 2012).

The JHNEBP model acknowledges that nursing practice is the basic component of all nursing activity. Nurses need to question the basis of their practice and use an evidence-based approach to validate or change current practice. Education reflects the acquisition of nursing knowledge and skills; EBP is now a core competency for all health care professionals (IOM, 2003). Nursing research uses qualitative and quantitative systematic methods directed toward the study and improvement of patient care, care systems, and therapeutic outcomes (Dearholt & Dang, 2012).

The core of the JHNEBP model contains the evidence itself. Research produces the strongest type of evidence but is not always available or applicable to

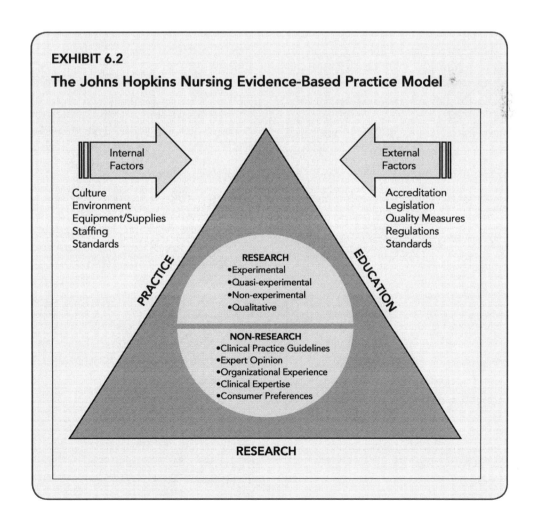

EXHIBIT 6.2

The Johns Hopkins Nursing Evidence-Based Practice Model

all clinical practice settings. Consequently, nurses also need to consider nonresearch sources of evidence when examining a particular practice. Guidelines, expert opinion, and clinical judgment are sources of nonresearch evidence and need to be examined and evaluated. Patient values, beliefs, and preferences regarding health care treatments may be one of the most influential factors in the determination and implementation of new practices.

Finally, the JHNEBP model represents an open system model that is influenced by both external and internal factors. External factors can include regulatory organizations, such as The Joint Commission or the Office of Inspector General, whose standards of practice and quality greatly impact nursing practices. The availability of resources and the process for disbursement within the organization is an internal factor that can modify plans for the implementation of an EBP intervention (Dearholt & Dang, 2012).

Taking the practice model a step further, the JHNEBP process encourages scientific inquiry and investigation by providing a systematic procedure for the examination of current practice and the implementation of EBP. This schema occurs in the three phases of Practice Question, Evidence, and Translation (see Exhibit 6.3). These phases are further broken down into 18 detailed steps and assembled in a management guide to assist the user through the process (Exhibit 6.4; Dearholt & Dang, 2012).

The CNS as team leader or change agent for the project is critical to guiding the choice of EBP innovational strategies and interventions for change. A review and plan for project progression through the 3 phases and 18 steps of this model includes intervention-related components at numerous times throughout project planning, implementation, and evaluation.

Practice Question

As noted earlier, scientific inquiry and questioning of practice are to be encouraged to promote an EBP culture. In response to a clinical question, Steps 1 to 5 of the JHNEBP Project Management Guide prescribe the recruitment of an interprofessional team and the development of a succinct and answerable question. Based upon the scope of the question, the CNS can facilitate formation of a team that should include clinical staff from all professions who may be most impacted by a change in practice. Other stakeholders to be included are personnel from departments controlling resources and managers with the authority to impact decision making at higher administrative levels; group members may need dedicated time and resources to participate in the required work sessions, and this will require administrative sanctioning. Evidence indicates that successful organizational change requires senior leadership support (Gustafson et al., 2003). In some teams, it is appropriate to include a patient representative.

Responsibilities of the team are to determine project leadership and set ground rules for the scheduling and format of team meetings. Based upon educational competencies, the CNS is an ideal project manager and can lead the team through project completion. During group meetings, the CNS should utilize group process techniques such as brainstorming, flowcharts, and multivoting techniques to promote group ownership and buy-in.

Formalizing the clinical question may be one of the most difficult aspects of a project. However, developing and refining a specific question at the outset is critical to all subsequent phases of the project. Determination of an appropriate precise question can optimize the review of evidence and guide the team in the choice of interventions and outcome measures. The JHNEBP Question Development Guide was developed to assist the team in constructing a good clinical question using the PICO format (Exhibit 6.5; Sackett, Straus, Richardson, Rosenberg, & Haynes, 2000).

Evidence

The second phase of the PET process (Steps 6 to 10) deals with the search for, appraisal of, and synthesis of the best available evidence (Dearholt & Dang, 2012). During this stage, the CNS needs to guide the team in collecting current information available on the practice in question. There should be a thorough review of the literature relating to the identified problem. The CNS has experience in the use of systematic literature reviews, through the course of academic study and in the work setting. He or she can draw

---

EXHIBIT 6.3

The JHNEBP Practice Question, Evidence, and Translation (PET) Process

JHNEBP, Johns Hopkins Nursing Evidence-Based Practice Model.

EXHIBIT 6.4

The JHNEBP Project Management Guide

Initial EBP Question:
EBP Team Leader(s):
EBP Team Members:

Activities	Start Date	Days Required	End Date	Person Assigned	Milestone	Comment / Resources Required
PRACTICE QUESTION :						
Step 1: Recruit interprofessional team						
Step 2: Develop and refine the EBP question						
Step 3: Define the scope of the EBP question and identify stakeholders						
Step 4: Determine responsibility for project leadership						
Step 5: Schedule team meetings						
EVIDENCE:						
Step 6: Conduct internal and external search for evidence						
Step 7: Appraise the level and quality of each piece of evidence						
Step 8: Summarize the individual evidence						
Step 9: Synthesize overall strength and quality of evidence						
Step 10: Develop recommendations for change based on evidence synthesis ☐ Strong, compelling evidence, consistent results ☐ Good evidence, consistent results ☐ Good evidence, conflicting results ☐ Insufficient or absent evidence						
TRANSLATION:						
Step 11: Determine fit, feasibility, and appropriateness of recommendation(s) for translation path						
Step 12: Create action plan						
Step 13: Secure support and resources to implement action plan						
Step 14: Implement action plan						
Step 15: Evaluate outcomes						
Step 16: Report outcomes to stakeholders						
Step 17: Identify next steps						
Step 18: Disseminate findings						

JHNEBP, Johns Hopkins Nursing Evidence-Based Practice Model.

EXHIBIT 6.5

The JHNEBP Question Development Tool

1. What is the problem and why is it important?

2. What is the current practice?

3. What is the focus of the problem?

☐ Clinical   ☐ Educational   ☐ Administrative

4. How was the problem identified?   (Check all that apply)

☐ Safety/risk management concerns
☐ Quality concerns (efficiency, effectiveness, timeliness, equity, patient-centeredness)
☐ Unsatisfactory patient, staff, or organizational outcomes
☐ Variations in practice within the setting

☐ Variations in practice compared with external organizations
☐ Evidence validation for current practice
☐ Financial concerns

5. What is the scope of the problem?

☐ Individual   ☐ Population   ☐ Institution/system

6. What are the PICO components?

P – (Patient, population, problem):

I – (Intervention):

C – (Comparison with other interventions, if applicable):

O – (Outcomes that include metrics for evaluating results):

7. Initial EBP question:

8. List possible search terms, databases to search, and search strategies:

9. What evidence must be gathered?   (Check all that apply)

☐ Literature search
☐ Standards (regulatory, professional, community)
☐ Guidelines
☐ Expert opinion

☐ Patient/family preferences
☐ Clinical expertise
☐ Organizational data

JHNEBP, Johns Hopkins Nursing Evidence-Based Practice Model.

upon this expertise to help guide team members to the appropriate databases and/or guideline clearinghouses. The medical librarian in many larger health care organizations is an invaluable ally and should be consulted for assistance if available.

Patient preferences and dissatisfaction, quality improvement (QI) metrics, clinical practitioner expertise, and clinical patient outcome data all need to be considered as well. Data on current internal practices should be collected and compared to external sources to benchmark any differences noted from community or more global standards (Pipe, 2007).

Once evidence on the identified problem is collected, it must be evaluated for its usefulness. An inexperienced team can benefit greatly from the use of a structured worksheet for literature review. This worksheet should include criteria for reference inclusion and strengths and weaknesses of the publications. Many examples of worksheets for review of the evidence are available in the literature.

Analysis of the literature review is completed by synthesizing the best evidence and combining that information with contextual data and the potential for project viability in the current practice setting. All possible benefits, risks, and costs should be considered. Finally, the group must make a recommendation on whether or not sufficient evidence exists to support the practice change in the proposed setting.

Translation

The final phase of project management completes the determination of whether the practice change is feasible and a good fit for clinical practice area. If the team decides to proceed with the practice change, an action plan is developed. Implementation and evaluation of the practice change and the results are communicated both internally and externally (Dang & Dearholt, 2012).

At this point, the CNS and his or her workgroup should consider and clarify potential interventions and activities while identifying the impact of barriers and potential obstacles. If it has not already been done, there should be a thorough review of the literature now relating to the potential intervention(s), and the outcome indicators.

The group should be encouraged to "think outside the box" and to be creative in their approach to various options. Examples of innovations may be provided by the CNS to help jump-start idea formation, which will be based primarily on clinical judgment, systems priorities, and resources.

Innovative thinking itself can be fostered by the CNS through a model based on encouraging childlike creativity of expression. The KIDS approach to innovative thinking gives the CNS general principles as guidance to foster creative thinking among staff (Shirey, 2007):

Kindle a culture of innovative thinking and doing
Inspire others to discover and utilize the available tools of innovation
Disseminate innovation by using tested frameworks
Sustain the momentum for innovation—for innovation to be sustainable, it requires attention, focus, and the allocation of resources

The workgroup also has the responsibility to select potential outcome indicators at this time. The CNS can help the team decide what the project goals might be in terms of specific practice changes and patient outcome measurements. When facilitating group discussion and decisions regarding planned outcome measurements, the CNS should encourage the use of standardized classification systems and language whenever possible. By adhering to customary patient identifiers/descriptors, such as diagnosis-related groups (DRGs), or nursing classifications systems, such as nursing interventions classifications (NICs), for instance, the ability for different individuals to communicate on the same terms is greatly enhanced. In addition, the ability to compare like data with outside facilities will be improved.

Once the decision has been made to proceed with a practice change, clear articulation of that change is needed. All stakeholders should be involved in the description of all the detailed steps of how that change will influence practice for the specified population. This process improves the likelihood that all the necessary steps and personnel who may be affected by the change have been included. It also keeps the team members engaged and focused on the specific practice change. The step-by-step process that has been clarified is often written in the format of a protocol, procedure, or standard and can be presented visually as a flowchart or algorithm. All components of the document must be supported by the evidence base.

Any resources that may be needed, either in the implementation process or for the practice change itself, should be identified. Costs of any type—personnel, equipment, and/or capital expenditure—must be presented to administrators for clarification and support.

At this point, the CNS can lead the team in planning for implementation of the practice change. If the proposed change is large, a pilot study can help with adaptation to practice settings and enhance ownership by team members for a smoother transition. The team will need to define both desired and undesired outcomes and any specific goals for a pilot study. Creation of an evaluation form to be used along with or after implementation can help clarify process and outcome criteria and increase interrater reliability through the use of objective performance measures.

Approvals from institutional review boards, QI forums, research oversight committees, and other regulatory bodies may be necessary and need to be pursued prior to implementation. Waivers and expedited reviews can often be utilized in CQI-style projects to decrease workload.

Finally, it is time for implementation of the planned intervention. If a pilot study is to be used, that will be the initial step. The CNS must closely monitor the progress of the pilot and must be available to answer questions for successful implementation. Evaluation of the implementation process and the specified outcomes should occur at the desired stages of project implementation. Occasionally, patient and staff opinion surveys and CQI methods can be used to collect evaluation data. After the evaluation data is collected, the CNS should coordinate data analysis. Computer graphics such as charts and bar graphs can be used to visually present the results back to the workgroup.

Based on results of the pilot project, the team now needs to decide to adapt, adopt, or reject the practice change for the entire practice area. The following questions should be considered: Did the intervention result in the desired practice change as expected? What were the patient outcomes? What were the costs and feasibility data? What was the feedback from the stakeholders?

Maintaining the Change. Once the recommended practice change is accepted as appropriate, it needs to be communicated to all stakeholders. The CNS should consider which methods for communication are appropriate to each practice setting. He or she should consider the culture of the practice setting and the optimal strategy for enacting a change; some organizations function through top-down enforcement of change, others value multilevel collaboration. Shared governance organizations will most likely require formal committee approval of the change. The CNS must consider which mechanisms exist in the setting to permanently integrate the new practice. Formal policies, procedures, and standards of care can help to maintain the change.

The CNS can enhance ownership and encourage professional development by enlisting the help of the workgroup to present staff in-service education on the practice change. This also helps to reinforce the value of a health care culture based on EBP. Incorporating the practice into orientation manuals and processes for new staff helps to establish ongoing education of the practice.

Depending upon the practice change, ongoing monitoring of process and outcome criteria may be warranted. Intermittent or continuous CQI data collection can be used to evaluate continued compliance or the need for reinforcement strategies. Either upon the completion of project implementation or while maintaining the change, the CNS can consider incentives or rewards for performance.

Despite the fact that it can be both effective and efficient to view a plan for change in a rational and linear fashion, the successful CNS must appreciate the complex nature of change. He or she should be aware that the aforementioned processes are not truly linear; there is much overlap and backtracking and certain items might be omitted, while other unexpected aspects are included (Shanley, 2007).

Conceptual Approaches to Interventions. When considering innovative interventions as part of a specific practice change, the CNS should consider the complex individual and group professional behaviors in his or her practice setting in addition to the project plan. Different theoretical approaches can help elucidate rationales for behavior change and can assist the CNS in choosing appropriate interventions. Categorizing an intervention as related to a specific approach while planning for a varied group of approaches may provide a strategy that would appeal to multiple people on different levels. Some of these approaches overlap, but each has a slightly different emphasis (Grol & Grimshaw, 1999).

1. Educational Approach—Includes learning in small interactive groups and problem-based strategies. This strategy appeals to individuals who are internally motivated to strive for professional excellence and achievement. It enhances the feeling of "ownership" of the process. By choosing a project team as a resource workgroup, the CNS can maximize the empowerment aspect as well as outreach potential of an educational strategy.
2. Epidemiologic Approach—Includes the development and dissemination of evidence-based guidelines or decision-making tools. This "common sense" approach assumes that humans will make rational decisions when given information on costs, benefits, harms, and preferences.
3. Marketing Approach—Focuses on the development and marketing of an attractive product or message that is tailored to the targeted group. Innovative approaches that address various needs should be spread through multiple channels (use of key opinion leaders, mass media, etc.).
4. Behaviorist Theory Approach—Based on behavior modification through conditioning, which emphasizes that most people seek reinforcement and rewards. Review of performance, provision of feedback, and various other incentives or sanctions act as positive reinforcement.
5. Social Influence Approach—Learning and changing are often achieved through interactions within social networks. The CNS who follows the tenets of this approach will use respected peers, opinion leaders, and role models to promote use of the innovation.
6. Organizational Approach—Based upon the belief that the system guides the practices within it. Systemwide CQI strategies, including assessment of organizational barriers, are used to promote change.
7. Coercive Approach—Change occurs through regulatory pressure and control. Contracts, licensure, and standards provide authoritative power and may provide the impetus to change in a setting of organizational inertia.

Conceptualizing that a change in professional behavior can be linked to a theoretical approach can assist the CNS in guiding the choice of a related innovative interventional strategy. In addition, the project team may better understand the rationale for a particular intervention when framed by one or more of these approaches.

APPLICATION TO CNS PRACTICE

The CNS is uniquely poised to effect change throughout and across the health care continuum. Within a health care organization, he or she is often charged with directly or indirectly monitoring the quality of patient care and acting on discrepancies. CNS educational curricula provide coursework on change theory and program development (NACNS, 2004). The CNS can integrate advanced knowledge on change theory, adult learning principles, organizational psychology, expertise in clinical specialty area, managing electronic information systems, patient safety organizations, EBP, regulatory bodies, and stress/coping theories to plan for change.

Historically, CNS practice was broken down into the subroles of expert practitioner, educator, researcher, change agent, administrator, and consultant (Hamric, 1989). These subroles are now conceptually integrated throughout the three spheres of CNS practice: (a) direct client care, (b) nurses and nursing practice, and (c) organizations and systems (NACNS, 2004). The change agent role remains an important part of CNS practice, and awareness of the characteristics of successful change agents can assist the CNS in achieving successful project implementation (Sullivan & Decker, 2001; White, 2004; Exhibit 6.6).

The CNS as change agent must consider the impact on all three spheres of influence. This conceptual model not only describes the focus of CNS practice as centering on clients, nurses, and systems, but it also elucidates the challenges in fulfilling this role (NACNS, 2004). When planning for a complex multidisciplinary QI project or simply a reinforcement of current practice regimens, it is not unusual to strategize interventions that have to address direct client care, nurses and nursing practice, and organizations and systems sequentially or simultaneously.

Much of this chapter has described working with clients and their primary caregivers. However, the CNS–nurse interface is not only critical to patient care but also a major source of personal and professional satisfaction for the CNS. In addition to being one of the spheres of influence, nurses are often the largest group of employees in many different types of health care settings. They represent a population that has a key role in steering the health care industry on many fronts, including the use of health information technology (Geibert, 2006). The relationship between the CNS and the staff nurse is based upon common interests and practice and can be a strong influence for change (Rogers, 2003).

When considering the systems perspective, the CNS must be aware that certain organizational factors can be major determinants of project success. Multiple different qualities of the practice setting must be considered. In today's health care environment, a flexible and participative climate is most likely to yield the desired results. Other organizational characteristics that are associated with positive change include (Crow, 2006):

1. Openness to change
2. Level of staff support for the change
3. Ease of past change implementation
4. Flexibility and adaptability
5. Optimism
6. The organization's capacity to cope over time

The CNS is often charged with ensuring the quality of patient care and the use of EBP in many different practice settings, and so he or she frequently functions as a combination of team leader, change agent, and project manager. Treating all members as valuable contributors and collaboratively troubleshooting helps in team building. The CNS is responsible for keeping the project on schedule while still allowing for flexibility to adjust plans as needed and to stimulate creative thinking. It behooves the CNS to encourage an environment of intellectual curiosity. Working within a team that questions traditional methods of care and the rationale that "we have always done it that way" creates a mindset for positive and innovative change.

Encouraging innovation might seem to be at odds with the detailed work of project management, but it is possible for the CNS to fulfill both criteria. Innovation in diagnosis and treatment to improve practice is considered to be a hallmark of CNS practice (NACNS, 2004). Individuals who utilize innovative strategies

---

EXHIBIT 6.6

Characteristics of Successful Change Agents

1. Ability to combine unrelated ideas
2. Ability to energize others
3. Skill in human relations
4. Integrative thinking; big-picture focus, and detail-oriented
5. Flexibility to modify ideas
6. Persistence to resist nonproductive tampering
7. Confidence; not easily discouraged
8. Realistic thinking regarding timelines
9. Trustworthiness; history of previous successes
10. Ability to articulate a vision
11. Ability to handle resistance

share certain qualities. The CNS who wishes to cultivate an innovative style can consider the following attributes (Ditkoff, 2004). The successful CNS incorporates gained experiential knowledge, literature, outcomes, and benchmarking data to promote teamwork and creative thinking for innovative change techniques (Kaplow, 2007). He or she is aware that monumental organizational changes are often interprofessional and team-oriented in nature and that such changes may arise from people straying outside the normal bounds of their specialties (Exhibit 6.7).

Following a well-designed and comprehensive template for change (as described in the conceptual framework), the CNS helps the team to set reasonable timelines and to visualize their progress (Strom, 2001). Structured agendas should be created and followed for each meeting, and minutes should be distributed afterward to reinforce any work assignments. Meeting times should be established early on, and each session should be used efficiently (Strom, 2001). Supervising for follow-up and holding people accountable for their individual responsibilities helps keep the team positive-minded and moving forward. Finishing the feedback loop with administrative recognition for individual accomplishments and pride in performance can serve to keep staff interested in progressive improvements in their work arena.

The CNS who takes on this challenging role as change agent, team leader, and project manager often serves as the cornerstone of effective and lasting change within dynamic systems and multidisciplinary groups. Although the project workload can feel Herculean at times, expertise and skills earned by experience and developed over time can serve to flatten subsequent learning curves and decrease project anxiety. Professional, interpersonal, and economic rewards reinforce job satisfaction and prepare the CNS for the next project at hand.

> Genius is one percent inspiration and ninety-nine percent perspiration. Accordingly, a "genius" is often merely a talented person who has done all of his or her homework. Opportunity is missed by most people because it is dressed in overalls and looks like work. (Thomas Edison)

EVALUATION

Leading change efforts can be a frustrating challenge that might sometimes feel as if you will never be finished. After considerable experience with project leadership and change management, the CNS can still be surprised by the fact that even when an innovation appears to have obvious advantages, it can still prove difficult for the strategy to be adopted. Change takes time—innovations may take many years from the time they become available until they are widely adopted (Rogers, 2003).

Different rates of adoption may be due to any or all of five characteristics of innovations (Rogers, 2003):

1. *Relative advantage*: The "perceived" value of an innovation has more to do with its adoption than the "objective" value. Each individual asks, "What is in it for me?"
2. *Compatibility*: Adoption of an innovation is related to the degree that individuals perceive the idea to be consistent with their values, past experiences, and needs.
3. *Complexity*: Innovations perceived to be more complex or that require the development of new skills will be adopted more slowly.
4. *Trialability*: Implementing an innovation in a phased approach may allow for enhanced value and decreased complexity of the strategy.
5. *Observability*: When individuals can easily see the results of an innovation, it is more likely to be adopted.

Evaluation of a project is necessarily done upon project completion. If very complex, use a pilot study first—evaluate—then move to the next phase.

As noted in Rosswurm and Larrabee's (1999) model for change toward EBP, evaluation of an innovative intervention begins with the initial planning for

---

EXHIBIT 6.7

Qualities of a Successful Innovator

Flexible/adaptive	Takes risks
Curious	Self-motivated
Visionary	Situationally collaborative
Persevering	Resilient
Playful and humorous	Self-accepting
Makes new connections	Reflective
Recognizes patterns	Committed to learning
Balances intuition and analysis	Formally articulate
Challenges status quo	Entertains the fantastic
Peripatetic	Tolerates ambiguity

the change itself. Data should be collected on both the process used for implementation and the outcome of the intervention. As noted earlier, building in a method for objective evaluation of both process and outcome can aid in data analysis by increasing interrater reliability. Additionally, the use of standardized nomenclature improves the ability to compare data between practice areas and even different facilities.

According to Gawlinski (2007), evaluation criteria of both process and outcome should include:

1. The outcomes that are expected to change after implementation of the innovation or practice change,
2. The outcomes or dependent variables evaluated in prior research on the issue, and
3. The outcome data already available in the institution (accessible without expending more time, energy, and money).

As alluded to earlier, multifaceted interventions are often more successful than one individual strategy. Unfortunately, it is difficult to separate the outcomes related to any specific intervention when multiple processes are applied simultaneously, so the group needs to be evaluated as a grouped intervention. One difficulty associated with implementing multiple interventions within the CQI approach is identifying which intervention had the greatest impact on improving outcomes (Strom, 2001).

In addition to using evaluation data to make determinations on the current project, the CNS will be able to use every interventional experience when planning for future changes. Publishing both process and outcomes from planned interventions for EBP can add to the body of knowledge regarding process and program effectiveness.

ADVANCED PRACTICE NURSING

In a role delineation study (Kenward, 2007), CNS respondents rated the following as those professional activities that they practiced most often:

1. Demonstrate critical thinking and diagnostic reasoning skills in clinical decision making.
2. Assess, plan, implement, and evaluate health care with other health care professionals/primary care providers to meet the comprehensive needs of patients.
3. Identify and analyze factors that enhance or hinder the achievement of desired outcomes for patients and family members.

The CNS carries out these activities within the context of ensuring the quality of care for his or her targeted patient or population. Critical thinking, individualizing a plan for care, and analysis of factors influencing outcomes all could contain QI initiatives.

The ability of CNSs to act as leaders is also influential in determining their ability both to facilitate change and to encourage others to regard best-practice statements as a priority for implementation. Nurses who were most effective in promoting local implementation of best-practice statements adopted facilitator and leadership roles within their organizations. It would appear that nurses who act as local facilitators and leaders are most effective in promoting EBP (Ring, Malcolm, Coull, Murphy-Black, & Watterson, 2005).

CNSs do not typically have supervisory responsibility for employees and so may not be able to mandate changes. But consistently partnering with the nurse manager can greatly enhance the potential for success in any project. In addition, the CNS can capitalize on this nonauthoritative relationship to coach staff nurses in activities that improve patient care. Coaching, which provides a focus on improving skills rather than providing education, can be a very rewarding and productive role for the CNS. Clinical coaching has been proposed as a comprehensive approach to achieve and maintain a culture of EBP (Ervin, 2005). The literature offers some additional guidance on specific actions to consider when creating an EBP culture (Crow, 2006; Exhibit 6.8).

EXHIBIT 6.8

Specific Actions to Consider When Creating an Evidence-Based Practice Culture

Build an intricate understanding of the business side of health care and nursing

Manage and lead from the future

Create relentless discomfort for the status quo in administrative and clinical practice

Rearrange the power and authority structure using Velcro hooks (easily rearranged again as required)

Frame all activities before taking action

Manage the emotions of change

Ensure that commitment for the change is abundant in both administration and staff

Keep the changes simple and concrete

Source: From Crow (2006).

The CNS should also consider the emotional impact of a practice change on the staff. The potential for sustained change depends on the clinician's responses to project efforts. The change itself is not usually the problem; it is the reaction to the change. Organizations are emotional environments. Research suggests that individuals make choices based on estimates of what they expect to experience with any given change. Anxiety and fear can lead to inertia and distrust of leaders and change agents. Emotions can often be interpreted as resistance and lead to further breakdown of trust (Crow, 2006).

Eight lessons learned regarding overcoming resistance to change and on strategies and practices to facilitate improvement include the following (Joshi & Bernard, 1999):

1. *Don't reinvent the wheel.* Clinical guidelines and best-practice techniques are widely published, so don't waste time in program development.
2. *Start with the usual suspects.* Look for areas that are ripe for improvement and where it will be easy to demonstrate substantial impact on patient outcomes.
3. *Pilot programs should be just that, pilots.* The focus of a pilot should be on content and process, not outcomes. Programs should be piloted for 3 months or less.
4. *Research data can sometimes be a barrier, not an enabler.* Do not wait for results from studies to implement a current best approach to care; expert opinion is an acceptable way to establish practice until research data is available.
5. *Guidelines by themselves have little impact in changing behavior.* Intensive effort and energy must be placed on effective strategies.
6. *One-on-one academic detailing is very effective, but resource intensive.* This may be used sparingly in appropriate situations.
7. *Clinical champions are instrumental in leading change.* Key thought leaders play a critical role in influencing colleagues.
8. *Change is constant!*

ETHICAL CONSIDERATIONS

The CNS who leads initiatives that improve the quality of patient care must always have an eye toward patient protection and privacy. Diligent appraisal of planned changes for the appropriate evidence-base and application site are required to ensure that translation is put into the correct practice setting. If project outcomes are not met or are suboptimal, an immediate change in care processes may be necessary for safe patient care.

Although projects for improvement should be scrutinized for any ethical dilemmas, in many cases it is not acceptable for those improvements *not* to happen. In fact, members of the health care team are ethically responsible to participate in CQI initiatives for their patient population in order to improve care. Consider known effective interventions that can save lives, prevent disabilities, and improve quality of life. It would not be appropriate for a patient care area to withhold clinical practices supported by an evidence base.

In the course of project implementation and evaluation, structured collection and analysis of individual patient data elements are often required. Additionally, some information on clinicians may also be needed to fully evaluate a process. All this data must be treated in a highly confidential manner. The data must be completely deidentified prior to any discussions and presentations of project information. All individuals involved in the collection and analysis of the data most likely need facility-specified education on patient privacy and human subject research. In addition, confidential data must be stored in a locked location and destroyed after a designated use date.

It is not always clear which activities are classified as QI and which are considered human subjects research. Most QI activities are not human subjects research and do not require review by an institutional review board. However, because such activities may still put patients at risk, some other review may be necessary.

Specialists in the conduct of human subjects research believe that it involves the "intent" of the project. The general belief is that QI projects are created to bring about immediate improvements in health care activity and, as such, are an intrinsic normal part of health care operation. Usually, the knowledge resulting from QI activities is most applicable to the local practice arena as an effort to improve care in that particular setting.

Studies classified as research are designed to develop or contribute to generalizable knowledge and applicable to other people or situations (Lynn et al., 2007). It may require the institutional review board (IRB) within a facility to determine whether or not a project qualifies as QI or research. Some facilities have created worksheets to help project leaders determine whether or not a project should be submitted to the IRB.

■ DISCUSSION QUESTIONS

- Consider a practice change that has occurred recently in your work environment. Who were the leaders of the change? Which interventions did they use? Were the interventions novel and innovative, or did the team choose tried-and-true strategies? Do you think that the change will still be in effect a year from now? Why or why not?
- You may have heard the expression "If we continue to do what we've always done, we will get the results we have always gotten." Can you think of a situation in health care in which a practice change was desired but just never happened? Were interventions attempted but ultimately proved unsuccessful? What were the barriers in that situation? Do you think that another intervention might have been more successful?
- By its very nature, innovation can be inefficient. During economic downturns, health care systems often downsize by laying off those personnel who are not considered necessary for direct patient care. This might include the CNS and other leaders who are experienced change agents. Do you think that this is a fiscally responsible strategy? If you were the CNS, how might you justify the retention of your position?

■ ANALYSIS AND SYNTHESIS EXERCISES

- Think about a clinical question in your field of expertise. Perform a literature search to determine the level of evidence and any patient care recommendations that exist. Is the care in your health care system consistent with the recommendations? Design a plan to make any necessary changes and choose interventions based on the characteristics of your practice arena.
- The Institute of Medicine (IOM) estimates that the time that it takes to integrate research findings into routine practice can be as long as 17 years (IOM, 2001). Although this may be hard to believe, the change agents within many facilities can understand why this is true. Engage a CNS in a discussion on this topic to brainstorm strategies to increase the rate of research translation into practice.
- Various health care disciplines have turned to industry and engineering/informatics as sources of important and emerging innovations. Search the Internet for examples of industrial research that has now been applied to nursing and/or medicine. (Hint: the airline industry has heavily influenced our current practices for avoiding errors to enhance patient safety.)

REFERENCES

Agency for Healthcare Research and Quality (AHRQ). (2013, March 6). *Innovations exchange*. Retrieved from http://www.innovations.ahrq.gov/faq.aspx

Alexander, J. A., & Hearld, L. R. (2011). The science of quality improvement implementation. *Medical Care*, 49, S6–S20.

Crow, G. (2006). Diffusion of innovation: The leaders' role in creating the organizational context for evidence-based practice. *Nursing Administration Quarterly*, 30(3), 236–242.

Cullen, L., & Adams, S. L. (2012). Planning for implementation of evidence-based practice. *Journal of Nursing Administration*, 42, 222–230.

Dearholt, S. L., & Dang, D. (Eds.). (2012). *Johns Hopkins nursing evidence-based practice: Model and guidelines* (2nd ed.). Indianapolis, IN: Sigma Theta Tau International.

Ditkoff, M. (2004). *Qualities of an innovator*. Retrieved August 25, 2013, from http://ideachampions.com/downloads/qualities_of_an_innovator.pdf

Ervin, N. E. (2005). Clinical coaching: A strategy for enhancing evidence-based nursing practice. *Clinical Nurse Specialist*, 19(6), 296–301.

Fogarty International Center. (n.d.). *Implementation science information and resources*. Retrieved August 24, 2013, from http://www.fic.nih.gov/researchtopics/pages/implementationscience.aspx

Gawlinski, A. (2007). Evidence-based practice changes: Measuring the outcome. *AACN Advanced Critical Care*, 18(3), 320–322.

Geibert, R. C. (2006). Using diffusion of innovation concepts to enhance implementation of an electronic health record to support evidence-based practice. *Nursing Administration Quarterly*, 30(3), 203–210.

Grant, R. W., & Meigs, J. B. (2006). Overcoming barriers to evidence-based diabetes care. *Current Diabetes Reviews*, 2, 261–269.

Grimshaw, J. M., Shirran, L., Thomas, R., Mowatt, G., Fraser, C., Bero, L.,...O'Brien, M. A. (2001). Changing provider behavior: An overview of systematic reviews of interventions. *Medical Care*, 39(8 Suppl. 2), II2–II45.

Grol, R., & Grimshaw, J. (1999). Evidence-based implementation of evidence-based medicine. *Joint Commission Journal on Quality Improvement*, 25(10), 503–513.

Gustafson, D. H., Sainfort, F., Eichler, M., Adams, L., Bisognano, M., & Steudel, H. (2003). Developing and testing a model to predict outcomes of organizational change. *Health Services Research*, 38, 751–776.

Hamric, A. B. (1989). History and overview of the CNS role. In A. B. Hamric & J. A. Spross (Eds.), *The clinical nurse specialist in theory and practice* (pp. 3–18). Philadelphia, PA: W. B. Saunders.

Idea Champions. (n.d.). *Culture of innovation*. Retrieved August 25, 2013, from http://www.ideachampions.com/creating_coi.shtml

Institute of Medicine (IOM). (2003). *Health professions education: A bridge to quality*. Washington, DC: National Academies Press.

The Joint Commission on the Accreditation of Healthcare Organizations (JCAHO). (2006). Raising the bar with bundles. *Joint Commission Perspectives on Patient Safety*, 6(4).

Joshi, M. S., & Bernard, D. B. (1999). Classic CQI integrated with comprehensive disease management as a model for performance improvement. *Joint Commission Journal on Quality Improvement, 25*(8), 383–395.

Kaplow, R. (2007). Synergy model: Guiding the practice of the CNS in acute and critical care. In M. G. McKinley (Ed.), *Acute and critical care clinical nurse specialists: Synergy for best practices* (pp. 29–47). St. Louis, MO: Saunders Elsevier.

Kenward, K. (2007). *Report of findings from the role delineation study of nurse practitioners and clinical nurse specialists* (Research Brief Vol. 30). Chicago, IL: National Council of State Boards of Nursing, Inc.

Lynn, J., Baily, M. A., Bottrell, M., Jennings, B., Levine, R. J., Davidoff, F.,…James, B. (2007). The ethics of using quality improvement methods in health care. *Annals of Internal Medicine, 146*(9), 666–673.

National Association of Clinical Nurse Specialists (NACNS). (2004). *Statement on clinical nurse specialist practice and education* (2nd ed.). Harrisburg, PA: Author.

New, J. P., Mason, J. M., Freemantle, N., Teasdale, S., Wong, L. M., Bruce, N. J.,…Gibson, J. M. (2003). Specialist nurse-led intervention to treat and control hypertension and hyperlipidemia in diabetes (SPLINT): A randomized controlled trial. *Diabetes Care, 26*(8), 2250–2255.

Oman, K., Duran, C., & Fink, R. (2008). Evidence-based policy and procedures. *The Journal of Nursing Administration, 38*(1), 47–51.

Pipe, T. B. (2007). Optimizing nursing care by integrating theory-driven evidence-based practice. *Journal of Nursing Care Quality, 22*(3), 234–238.

Rello, J., Lorente, C., Bodi, M., Diaz, E., Ricart, M., & Kollef, M. H. (2002). Why do physicians not follow evidence-based guidelines for preventing ventilator-associated pneumonia? *Chest, 122*(2), 656–661.

Ring, N., Malcolm, C., Coull, A., Murphy-Black, T., & Watterson, A. (2005). Nursing best practice statements: An exploration of their implementation in clinical practice. *Journal of Clinical Nursing, 14*, 1048–1058.

Rogers, E. M. (2003). *Diffusion of innovations*. New York, NY: Free Press.

Rosswurm, M. A. & Larrabee, J. H. (1999). A model for change to evidence-based practice. *Image: Journal of Nursing Scholarship, 31*, 317–322.

Sackett, D. L., Straus, S. E., Richardson, W. S., Rosenberg, W., & Haynes, R. B. (2000). *Evidence-based medicine: How to practice and teach EBM*. Edinburgh, UK: Churchill.

Sandström, B., Borglin, G., Nilsson, R., & Willman, A. (2011). Promoting the implementation of evidence-based practice: A literature review focusing on the role of nursing leadership. *Worldviews on Evidence-Based Nursing, 4*, 212–223.

Shanley, C. (2007). Management of change for nurses: Lessons from the discipline of organizational studies. *Journal of Nursing Management, 15*, 538–546.

Shirey, M. R. (2007). Leadership and organizational strategies to increase innovative thinking. *Clinical Nurse Specialist, 21*(4), 191–194.

Stanley, D. (2006). Role conflict: Leaders and managers. *Nursing Management, 13*(5), 31–37.

Strohmeyer, K. (2013, July 9). Not alone in a crowd: Crowdsourcing for healthcare. *Healthcare IT News*. Retrieved from http://www.healthcareitnews.com/blog/not-alone-crowd-crowdsourcing-healthcare

Strom, K. (2001). Quality improvement interventions: What works? *Journal for Healthcare Quality, 23*(5), 4–14.

Sullivan, E., & Decker, P. (2001). *Effective leadership and management in nursing*. Upper Saddle River, NJ: Prentice Hall.

Thompson, D. S., Estabrooks, C. A., Scott-Findlay, S., Moore, K., & Wallin, L. (2007). Interventions aimed at increasing research use in nursing: A systematic review. *Implementation Science, 2*, 15–31.

White, A. (2004). Change strategies make for smooth transitions. *Nursing Management, 35*(2), 49–52.

Evaluating Interventions

Kelly A. Goudreau

The process of disciplined evaluation permeates all areas of thought and practice.... It is found in scholarly book reviews, in engineering's quality control procedures, in the Socratic dialogues, in serious social and moral criticism, in mathematics, and in the opinions handed down by appellate courts.... [I]t is the process whose duty is the systematic and objective determination of merit, worth or value. Without such a process, there is no way to distinguish the worthwhile from the worthless. (*Scriven, 1991, p. 4*)

*E*valuation of nursing interventions is a key component of what nursing does in each and every practice, process, or procedure—yet in many instances it is left to interpretation rather than definitive discussion. Typically in practice, nursing interventions are poorly documented and are not described in measurable terms, making it almost impossible to evaluate them effectively. Additionally, the process of evaluation is haphazard and poorly documented at best, or nonexistent at worst. As an action-oriented discipline, we often move very quickly to identify an intervention from our repertoire, implement it, and then change the plan of care and subsequent interventions due to a perception that the intervention was not working as intended. But have we determined exactly what the etiology of the problem was in the first place? Do we know for certain that the intervention was not effective, or was it just that the cause of the problem was different than we initially thought, making the intervention inert? Action without thought or thorough

evaluation is the plague of our profession. Evaluation is given short shrift in spite of the increasing focus on evidence-based practice. How is it that we can implement an intervention without truly taking the time to think about, reflect on, and evaluate its effectiveness?

The documentation to affirmatively support what we are doing is also often lacking. The rigor, reliability, and validity of what we are doing is not measurable because we have not documented what we were doing in a sufficient manner and, therefore, cannot link the causal chain and *prove* that the intervention was either working or not working or that the changes we made had some impact of a measurable nature. We simply move to act and change the intervention even before we have thoroughly considered the etiology of the need that requires intervention, the effect of the intervention, and its outcome. It is time to change that perspective and bring to bear the tools that have been created over the past few years in support of the work of nurses and nursing. Tools added to that list include such things as research, evidence-based practice, and the science of evaluation. It is time to be proactive rather than reactive, and it is the role of the clinical nurse specialist (CNS) to do this.

The nursing process has been in place for as long as many can remember (Orlando, 1961). It is an integral component of the manner in which nurses function and understand one another as they communicate regarding patient care initiatives and programs. Unfortunately, evaluation is also the least documented, effectively utilized, and understood component of the nursing process. According to the Centers for Disease Control and Prevention (2012), evaluation is "[t]he systematic collection of information about the activities, characteristics, and outcomes of programs (which may include interventions, policies, and specific projects) to make judgments about that program, improve program effectiveness, and/or inform decisions about future program development" (see the appendix to this chapter).

Many times, the focus of the nursing and health care professional staff and the CNS is the assessment of the needs of the patient, his or her family or support system, and the health care environment in which the care is being provided. In the flurry of activity surrounding establishment of a new care plan that is assumed will meet identified needs, or ensuring that the assessment is thorough and evidence based, evaluation of a measurable intervention is not well established. As a result, from the outset, evaluation of the interventions is often not well documented either. Although evaluation may be done informally or is evidenced indirectly through actions taken to modify the plan of care when interventions do not demonstrate the desired outcomes, it is not clearly documented and thoroughly examined. As nurses and CNSs, we do, of course, evaluate the care given and modify the care given in order to increase the likelihood that the patient will achieve the intended outcomes. What we frequently do not do is fully document what the intervention consisted of and the outcomes and reasons for changes in the plan of care.

Although the direct patient interaction is the foundation of evaluation for both nursing and CNS practices, the CNS is expected to take evaluation to an advanced level as he or she interacts with all three spheres of influence: the patient, the nursing and health care professional staff, and the system (National Association of Clinical Nurse Specialists [NACNS], 2004, 2010). It is in the interaction with all three spheres that the CNS enacts the advanced nature of his or her role. It is up to the CNS to bring the thought process back into the selection or creation of an intervention, documentation of the intervention in measurable steps, and evaluation of the outcomes of that intervention. The CNS is the bridge between research, evaluation, and application to practice in every environment he or she touches.

Interventions performed by CNSs must include all three spheres of influence (NACNS, 2004, 2010) and are, therefore, broader than just direct application to patients. The work that is done with the nursing and allied health personnel and the system interventions is equally important. It is the synergy created by the interaction of all three spheres that creates the greatest impact to the patient and the outcomes of care that meet his or her needs. Evaluation of the outcomes of care is essential in today's health care environment, as is the evaluation of the effectiveness of interventions conducted within the nursing/health care personnel sphere of influence (educational programs and product evaluation) and systems sphere interventions (projects and quality improvement) that are implemented in an effort to increase patient safety.

This chapter provides a brief overview of nursing interventions and how an intervention should be designed to facilitate effective evaluation. It also discusses the background and history of evaluation processes, including the theoretical foundation both within and external to nursing and the application of evaluation to interventions within the patient sphere of CNS practice. Interventions in the nursing/health care workers sphere have been discussed to some extent in the chapter by Doran, Sidani, and DiPietro (Chapter 4) and Pacini (Chapter 9). Doran et al. also discuss evaluation of systems level/systems sphere interventions, as does O'Malley in her discussion of product evaluation (Chapter 25) and Benton in her discussion of quality improvement (Chapter 12). Although Lyon touches on the evaluation of interventions, in her chapter on the clinical reasoning model (Chapter 5), what has not been thoroughly discussed is the work of the CNS in evaluation itself. The CNS plays a specific role in working directly with the patient/client and his or her family, the nursing and health care worker, and the system, as interventions are thoroughly evaluated. This chapter provides background to all three spheres (the patient, the nursing and health care professional staff, and the system) but focuses on the patient/client and the interventions nurses and CNSs develop and ultimately should evaluate.

BRIEF HISTORICAL BACKGROUND

To truly provide a frame of reference for evaluation of interventions, it is important to first give voice to the intervention itself. In Chapter 6, Richardson outlines the means by which the CNS develops innovation, change, and interventions in a very practical sense through the collaborative efforts of the change process. By taking interventions of the past and using change theory to create innovation, she describes an "on the ground" approach to how the CNS can innovate and generate changes in the clinical environment through application of evidence-based practice and changes in interventions over time. How does one develop an intervention in the first place, however, and then subsequently bring to bear the evaluative measures needed to determine its effectiveness?

According to Conn (2007), interventions must be clearly defined in measurable terms for two reasons: (1) so that they may be used in a replicable way and effectively in practice, and, more importantly, (2) so they can be studied for their effectiveness. The World Health Organization (2012) also identified that

> no matter how small your project you need to develop evaluation measures in order to learn. In an evaluation, you gather the monitoring information you have collected based on your indicators.... You can use the clues the indicator data provide to make an assessment of how successful you were in carrying out your activities and meeting your objectives. (p. 32)

The measurability of the intervention is often lost on the day-to-day practitioner and is a concept that we struggle with on a constant basis. How can we slow down enough to truly incorporate the concepts of research and evaluation into the day-to-day practice when patients are so much more complex, with comorbidities and care issues that previously would have placed them in an intensive care environment but now are in the home or nursing skilled care units? This increased complexity creates an aura of urgency in provision of care and, therefore, it could be argued, does not allow as much time for consideration and reflective thought as interventions are developed and implemented (Resnick et al., 2005).

The theory of the nursing process was first articulated by Orlando in the 1950s (Faust, 2002), with first discussion of the theory in the literature in 1961 (Orlando, 1961). In the nursing process theory, Orlando does not clearly delineate the use of the five-step process of assessment, diagnosis, planning, implementation, and evaluation, which we know today as the nursing process. Instead, she described her observations of the manner in which nurses interacted with their patients. Orlando (1961) discussed three elements in every nursing encounter: the behavior of the patient, the reaction of the nurse, and the nursing action undertaken to benefit the patient. It is an iterative process whereby the nurse clearly modifies his or her behavior based on the behavior of the patient. Orlando's theory is seen as a middle-range theory by some (Fawcett, 1995) because it does not clearly define the four elements of the metaparadigm of nursing: person, environment, nursing, and health. What it does, however, is set the tone and expectation that the scientific process will be used in the day-to-day operations of nursing, and it is considered a seminal work in the foundations of nursing practice. It is a concept that is unfortunately lost in today's hustle and bustle of daily care. It ought to see a resurgence, however, as nurses and patients now are going to be far more collaborative in the new era of "patient-centered care" and all that it entails (Agency for Healthcare Research and Quality [AHRQ], 2013).

Years later, these foundational concepts were taken by other nursing theorists, such as Abdellah, Henderson, and Orem, and developed over time as an adaptation of the scientific process for experimentation (Meleis, 1991). The theory was immediately seen as a way to frame the manner in which nurses thought about the care they provided to patients in all settings. The universality of the nursing process as an explanation for the way in which nurses thought and then interacted with their patients provided a scientific basis for their day-to-day activities. When the American Nurses Association (ANA) adopted the model and integrated it into all documents that defined the professional role of nursing, it became a fundamental way in which to describe what nurses do. Now, the implementation of evidence-based practice emphasizes even further the need to thoroughly evaluate the interventions that are being used with various patient populations and to question why a method has been used, whether or not it should continue to be used, and what evidence supports its continued use. This daily application of the scientific method brings to light the increasing need for nursing and all health care staff to understand how to thoroughly evaluate the care they are providing.

The purpose of evaluation is, of course, broader than just nursing and the nursing process. Stufflebeam and Shinkfield (2007) describe evaluation as a distinct profession with specific models and theories that guide and support the appropriate implementation of the specific discipline. Ultimately, evaluation should determine whether or not an intervention (individual, group, or regional/national) has achieved the desired outcome.

Within nursing, *evaluation* has been defined as the final step in an iterative process where an assessment of needs was conducted, a diagnosis and a plan were formulated and implemented, and then an assessment was conducted to determine the effectiveness of the intervention. Any intervention at any level should to be evaluated. This general description can apply equally to any of the three spheres of CNS influence: the nursing and health care staff, the system, or the patient.

Nursing/Health Care Staff

There are key areas that the CNS evaluates when working with the nursing and health care staff. These areas include product evaluation, cost-to-benefit ratio savings measures across interventions conducted by the staff, evaluation of aggregate clinical care outcomes, and direct educational interventions.

Product evaluation is the consideration of various types of products that the staff will be using in day-to-day operations and interactions with patients. The

CNS performs the function of seeking stakeholder input, feedback, and buy-in for any new products that will be used in the clinical environment (Goudreau, 2010; U.S. Food and Drug Administration [USFDA], 2013). Will this particular product provide the safest, most efficient, and cost-effective method of care for the patients in the context in which it is intended to be used? Product evaluation must take into consideration many factors, including the ergonomics of the environment; the demographics of the staff in terms of educational preparation, age, gender; and demographics of the patient population to be served. The CNS often uses his or her knowledge of evaluation processes to create a tool that outlines the criteria to be evaluated and then provides the summation of the outcomes for those who will make the final decisions.

This assessment of stakeholder feedback on the proposed product and buy-in to its use in the clinical environment must also include the cost/benefit ratio and analysis of both the objective and subjective data relative to a product and how the staff interacts with the product. If a product is cost-effective and efficient but is not used by the staff, it can be as costly as, or more costly than, a product that is a little more expensive but is used effectively by the staff. Safety considerations and the costs associated with injury management must also be factored into the cost/benefit ratio if the data are to present a full and comprehensive picture of the overall effectiveness and efficiency of a particular product.

The evaluation of interventions by the health care staff in aggregate form for overall assessment of attainment of desired outcomes for patients is a data analysis component of the CNSs interaction with the health care staff. The CNS must identify overall patterns and trends in care outcomes so that the staff can take further action or be lauded for the efforts made to improve care (Dickerson, Wu, & Kennedy, 2006). Examples of this are explicitly detailed in the Institute for Healthcare Improvement (IHI) "bundles" and measures of clinical outcomes (Resar, Griffin, Haraden, & Nolan, 2012). Issues such as ventilator-associated pneumonia (VAP) are known to be impacted and prevented as a result of the very specific nursing interventions of mouth care and positioning. The CNS can increase nurses' awareness related to these relatively simple nursing interventions and their overall impact on patient care outcomes.

From these aggregate analyses of outcomes come the focused educational interventions that are developed, implemented, and evaluated by the CNS. These educational interventions with the nursing staff can range from new procedures to information about illness states that are new to the staff in the patient population they care for or existing knowledge that should be reinforced. The evaluation of an educational intervention must take into consideration the adult learning principles and learner preferences in the clinical and educational environments or the context of care for these populations; it typically includes measurements of the learning achieved through pre- and posttesting of knowledge, as well as value judgments and informal observation of behavior in the posteducational intervention period by the CNS, the learner's self-reflection on his or her learning, and peer review of changes in activities and behaviors (Miller, Linn, & Gronlund, 2008). The role of the CNS is to collect these data and analyze the outcomes of the educational intervention so that it can continue to be reinforced or so that it can be modified to attain the desired results.

The System

Within the system sphere of influence, CNSs can have broad-reaching effects and should, therefore, have strong evaluative effects. Evaluation of programs at a unit, facility, regional, or national level is in many instances the driving factor behind CNS practice. The assessment of specific needs on a unit can often be identified and acknowledged as essential across an entire facility. The CNS uses his or her skills to address the needs of the staff and patients from a broad perspective, which can frequently extend across multiple care units and environments. The current acknowledged fractioning of the health care system is increasing the demand for use of systems-level skill sets that are inherent in CNS practice (Institute of Medicine [IOM], 2001). As a result, CNSs are in greater demand than ever before. These skills are even more important as individuals look to redesign systems and increase patient safety in all aspects of care. CNSs have a clear role in guiding, leading, and facilitating the change efforts that must take place in today's health care system in order to increase patient safety and the quality of nursing care. Systems- or programmatic-level evaluation has been discussed in the literature for many years (Casper, Kenron, & McDaniel, 2005; Daponte, 2008; Rossi & Freeman, 1993; Wood, 1998). Unfortunately, however, although systems-level interventions are key to the CNS role and evaluation is a key component of CNS practice, evaluation of systems-level interventions has had little attention in the nursing or CNS literature (Goudreau, 2010).

The W. K. Kellogg Foundation (1998, 2008) describes a process whereby project-level evaluation takes into consideration the context of the project or program, evaluation of the implementation of the program or project in its various stages of implementation, and the final outcomes assessment whereby the intended outcomes are compared to the actual outcomes. This logical flow model can best be described in a pictorial manner and allows for action-oriented changes to the plan as the intervention unfolds and both intended and unintended outcomes are realized. Kellogg (2008) identified that "a logic model presents program information and progress toward goals in ways that inform, advocate for a particular program approach, and teach program stakeholders" (p. 5). Perhaps this tool can and should be added to the CNS toolkit when looking at the development, implementation, and subsequent evaluation of programs- and system-level interventions. Through the description of factors (resources or barriers to implementation of a program), activities (including products, services, and infrastructure needed to implement the program), outputs (direct results of the program), outcomes (changes in behaviors as a result of the program), and finally impacts (the ripple effect in the targeted community as a result of the program), the logic model provides both a framework for the establishment of a program or project as well as the evaluative model. By specifically describing the outputs, outcomes, and intended impacts at the beginning of a project or program, the CNS can clearly identify the evaluative measures that will be used as the program unfolds and is completed. The framework also provides the logical model for reporting the results of the program to stakeholders, thereby reducing the potentially duplicative work involved in trying to reframe evaluation information for reporting purposes.

Stufflebeam and Shinkfield (2007) identify a number of theoretical foundations for evaluation that would most likely be considered midrange theories if they were within nursing. Stufflebeam's Context, Input, Process, and Product (CIPP) model of evaluation is described along with Stake's 1967 responsive/client-centered evaluation, Patton's utilization-focused evaluation, and Scriven's 1967 model of formative and summative evaluation processes (cited in Stufflebeam & Shinkfield, 2007). Each of the described models defines a specific process for evaluation that would inform the CNS of the outcomes of system-level programs or educational processes if used within the context of health care. Each has its strengths and weaknesses and so it is left to the CNS to explore the feasibility of use within his or her specific environment.

The Patient

The interaction of the patient and the nursing intervention is a key focus and essentially a primary raison d'être for the function and role of the CNS. The influence of the CNS in day-to-day practice and interventions with the patient and the staff who support the patient derives from the focus of CNS practice origination, "from nursing and for nursing."

Unfortunately, much like the nursing staff that the CNS works with, the documentation of the evaluative process is not always easily traced in the charting system or in documents that clearly articulate the outcomes of care from a nursing perspective. Typically, evaluation is not documented in a formal process but instead is reflected in the changes to the plan of care in an implicit versus explicit manner. When a notation is made to change the plan of care from one nursing intervention to another, it is assumed that the nurse evaluated the impact of the initial or previous intervention and determined that it was either ineffective or not working as well as intended and, therefore, had to be modified or removed in lieu of an alternative intervention that will subsequently be evaluated for its effectiveness.

Documenting the effectiveness of an intervention requires a thoughtful process of establishing the etiology of the issue or need that is the indication for an intervention, crafting an intervention that is measurable and will meet that issue or need, and then evaluating the effectiveness of that intervention in addressing the issue or need. It must be based on subjective evidence that is contained within the data collected. The evidence must be validated with the patient and added to objective evidence that is available both in the chart and through observation of the patient in the context of his or her care. Key to all of these elements is that the need or problem can be addressed through the application of a nursing intervention and not a medically delegated intervention. Many times, the nurse will look to the medical interventions that are easily pulled from a list of delegated tasks rather than look to the ways in which the nurse can use his or her skills to meet the patient's needs. For some reason, the nursing skill set and ability to intervene is downplayed or seen as less important than the delegated medical tasks that nurses carry out. It is not clear why that happens, and the issue has been a constant struggle for nurse educators for many years (Fulton, 2003).

The difficulties with the articulation of the nursing plan of care and subsequent concurrent updating and modification of the nursing interventions on the plan of care are well known throughout the history of nursing. The reality of nursing care on a day-to-day basis, mixed with the need to document that care in a manner that is unobtrusive to the care process itself, is nearly impossible to balance or integrate. Some consider the nursing care plan to be a purely academic exercise not based in reality. How, then, does nursing reconcile the need to document and provide evidence for the foundations of care and the actual provision of care in an extremely active environment while still staying true to the fact that our autonomous focus for nursing interventions should not be only the delegated medical tasks ordered by our physician peers?

CONCEPTUAL AND/OR THEORETICAL FRAMEWORKS FOR EVALUATION OF NURSING INTERVENTIONS

The foundation of evaluation of interventions is difficult to determine because evaluation has been a component of the research process for generations. Aside from the background within nursing (Meleis, 1991; Orlando, 1961) that defines evaluation from the perspective of nursing interventions and assessment of outcomes, there are many different disciplines that have clearly defined the process of evaluation (Fitzpatrick, Sanders, & Worthen, 2003; Goudreau, 2010; Rossi & Freeman, 1993; Stufflebeam & Shinkfield, 2007).

It is clear, however, that in order to get beyond the day-to-day volatility of the nurses' world, one needs to slow down and think about the process of intervention and subsequent evaluation. Truly, evaluation should be the foundation of clinical practice for all nurses, but it is especially important in the advanced practice role that the CNS carries. It tends to be lost, however, in the flurry of activity that is patient care, working with the nursing and allied health staff, and "fixing the system," which is the day-to-day reality of the CNS in clinical practice. Frankly, most CNSs would indicate that they do not have time to be thoughtful and methodical in the evaluation of interventions. However, it is through this thoughtful application of evaluation that mirrors the research process that we can attain the best understanding of the interventions we are carrying out.

CNSs and nurses must look at the interventions they are implementing and assess whether or not they are *nursing* interventions, whether or not they are measurable, and whether or not they can be reliably and accurately evaluated for their effectiveness. The intervention should be grounded in theory and should have a conceptual framework that supports the foundation of the intervention. Finally, in addition to the intervention having a conceptual framework, the evaluation itself must have a conceptual framework upon which it is based.

Conn, Rantz, Wipke-Tevis, and Maas (2001) describe the attributes to be considered when designing or selecting interventions, including "What is the conceptual basis of the intervention?" "Have previous descriptive studies been conducted on the intervention?" "What does the related intervention research show?" "Has the intervention been designed for a specific population?" "Is the specificity or generality of the intervention consistent with the conceptual framework?" "Are the interventions singled or bundled, and if either, is this consistent with the conceptual framework?" "What is the method of delivery of the intervention?" and finally, "What is the dose of the intervention, and is it also supported by the conceptual framework?" In each case, the intervention must be consistent with the literature and the conceptual framework that supports it. If these attributes are not in alignment with the framework, then it is extremely difficult to draw any conclusions in the evaluative stage as to effectiveness of the intervention (Sechrest, West, Phillips, Redner, & Yeaton, 1979). In this era of evidence-based practice, it is extraordinarily important to the CNS and the staff nurse alike that the selection or design of the intervention be grounded in a conceptual framework founded on subjective and objective data gained from research, as well as the patient/client and the particular context at the time that the intervention is needed. This foundation is essential if the nurse wants to be able to predict that the action will alter or remove the etiology, thereby linking the causal chain and upholding his or her hypothesis as to the etiology of the actual or perceived need.

Sidani and Braden (1998) also identified this point when they concluded that "knowledge of the critical inputs (component, mode of delivery, and dosage) and the chain of processes linking the intervention to outcomes are necessary for delineating the outcomes' pattern of change" (p. 141). Clearly, one cannot effectively evaluate an intervention without first designing the intervention to be measurable and linking those measures through a conceptual framework back to the interventions. In other words, in order to look at the conceptual framework for evaluation, it is also necessary to look at the intervention and the conceptual framework for the intervention (Conn et al., 2001). In many instances, the conceptual framework of the evaluation is a mismatch to the interventions and, therefore, it is not possible to measure effectively the outcomes attained. As an example, Lyon states in Chapter 5 that a nursing intervention is proposed only to alter the hypothesized etiologies contributing to or causing a problem. Alternatively, an intervention is intended to prevent etiologies and, therefore, prevent a potential problem from becoming an actual problem. It is up to the individual who is attempting to determine the most effective intervention and then measure the effectiveness of that intervention to ensure that it has been constructed in such a way as to be measurable in the evaluation phase. If it has not been constructed effectively, it will be difficult at best to determine whether or not it was the intervention that actually created the outcome that was noted and/or desired.

This thoughtful processing of interventions is often lacking in the day-to-day hustle and bustle of work on the unit, in the facility overall, and in general in the practice of the nursing and health care worker today. It is the role of the CNS to bring it back to the fore where it belongs.

APPLICATION TO CNS PRACTICE

With so many potential midrange theories on evaluation, where does a CNS begin to assist the patient and the staff who care for them to ensure that the intervention has been constructed in such a way as to facilitate the evaluative process? It is important to think about whether or not there is a conceptual framework for the care being provided when looking at and thinking about innovative ways to interact with patients/clients within the practice environment. If there is a framework that can be used in the care of a patient, then it is the role of the CNS to bring the theoretical perspective back to the day-to-day work of the nursing and health care staff. It is also the role of the CNS to increase the visibility of the evidence base in the care of patients and to bring his or her experience and expertise in the field to the care of each patient/client and population. A quick and easy way to address this is to look at what has already been done and to adapt the content of a project to the needs of the patient population or facility culture. A ready resource is available for all clinicians that describes a number of focused interventions that have been evaluated and rated by the IHI (2013).

A focus on the nursing aspects of care is an essential aspect of the overall management of the patient that is often lost in the daily activities of a busy unit. It is up to the CNS as the advanced practice nurse to bring the spotlight back onto the aspect of nursing care, which is essential to the improved outcomes that patients achieve while in the health care system.

According to Thomas (1984), "the fashioning of an intervention plan calls for consideration of suitable alternatives, given available methods, as well as new approaches that might be adopted to meet the problem in question" (p. 21). Daponte (2008) outlines a specific process that can be used fairly universally and incorporates many of the previously described evaluation theories (Stufflebeam & Shinkfield, 2007). Although not specifically designed for nursing care or CNS practice, Daponte describes an evaluation framework that can be modified to meet nursing needs as follows:

• Assess whether or not there is a conceptual framework that has either been explicitly or implicitly used to create the intervention. Make it explicit if it is not.

• Determine whether or not the intervention will likely impact the etiology of the problem that the patient is articulating or that the nurse has identified and validated with the patient.
• Identify whether any current evaluative activities are formative (focused on improvement of the intervention as it is being enacted) or summative (conclusions regarding the outcomes).
• Define all the possible questions that could be asked about this intervention and its effectiveness.
• Rigorously describe the intervention by developing the theory and using a logic model that is interactive and iterative.
• Revisit the evaluation questions that could be asked.
• Only after the previous steps have been completed, develop the evaluation plan.
• Collect the data, analyze it, and write the evaluative report.

This modification of the research process specific to evaluation of interventions can be implemented fairly quickly. With easier access to nursing databases and literature searches, the CNS can model these behaviors for the nurses and health care workers.

Key to evaluation of interventions is not only that the intervention has been clearly articulated and that the evaluation is outlined very specifically as it relates to the conceptual framework of the intervention, but also that the manner in which the data are collected is reliable (consistent and replicable) and valid (able to clearly address the original problem, show change that can be attributed to the intervention, and be validated by more than just one measure; C. Beausang, personal communication, February 12, 2009).

A final consideration for evaluation in action is the potential of the Hawthorne Effect. In any formal evaluation there will be an effect simply because you are formally evaluating the care being provided. The staff will become more acutely aware of the processes and, therefore, will improve their processes, whether that was the intent or not. A notable change will take time, but by incorporating the processes and procedures into daily activities within the unit or area, the overall outcomes of care will ultimately be impacted in a measurable, reliable, and valid manner.

It is possible to implement a formal evaluation process for the care provided on a unit or with a patient population as demonstrated by Allen, Bockenhauer, Egan, and Kinnaird (2006). These administrative nurses described a 10-year process whereby nursing practice was tied directly to patient outcomes. The result was increased satisfaction from the nursing staff, an increased awareness of how their practice impacts the patient care, an ability to critically analyze he data from patient care outcomes, and, most importantly, increased patient satisfaction with the care provided.

ETHICAL CONSIDERATIONS

Ethics have always been an important aspect of care for nurses and health care workers. Fortunately, in today's society, ethics are becoming an explicit component of care and are being discussed freely and openly in the context of care. Evaluation of interventions has a key ethical component and should be focused on the aspects of care that are intended to provide benefit to the patient/client. When any intervention is being developed, three key things should be considered: (1) the patient/client is fully informed of the implications of the intervention, both positive and negative, and gives consent to the treatment; (2) the benefits must be assumed to outweigh the risks associated with the intervention; and (3) the patient/client is assured of confidentiality in all aspects of the care (Thomas, 1984).

Further, nurses are bound by the ANA Code of Ethics as a statement of values for the profession. The ANA has clearly articulated key ethics statements in the care of patients/clients across the continuum of care provided by nurses in general, inclusive of CNS practice.

As the evaluative process mirrors the research process in many aspects, it is important to take into consideration the needs of the patient/client and the issue of whether or not there would be potential harm to the patient/client as a result of the intervention or the evaluation being proposed. It is important to consider all aspects of the treatment and care of patients/clients from the perspective of the protection of human subjects regardless of whether or not the treatment is part of a research protocol.

SUMMARY

Evaluation of nursing interventions is an area of nursing that has been considered for generations but poorly implemented within the day-to-day activities of the nursing and health care staff. The reality of the busy unit, or large number of patients/clients that the nurse or allied health worker must see on a daily basis, means that there is often a loss of the reflective thought process that should be elemental to the care provided.

It is the role of the CNS as the advanced practice nurse to model the behaviors that all nurses and health care workers should be exhibiting as we care for our patients/clients and populations. Key to this is

the establishment or clear articulation of the evidence base and conceptual framework supporting the interventions that are carried out and the evaluations that must be enacted. Only through clear statement of the intervention in measurable terms can we then in turn evaluate the care provided and determine whether or not the intervention carried out was in fact effective in ameliorating the problem articulated and validated by the patient/client and the data collected by the nurse.

Not only does the intervention have to be clearly articulated and measurable, but it also must be linked appropriately to the etiology of the problem that the patient/client is experiencing. Nursing too often falls into the perception that the best intervention is one that has been delegated by medicine to nursing. Delegated medical interventions, such as medications to manage pain, rather than nursing interventions of positioning, distraction, or touch and presence are often used and assumed to be within the realm of nursing as interventions. There is a need to reclarify the role of nursing and the autonomous domain of nursing interventions and their overall value and worth. There is a need to evaluate the care provided by nurses other than the delegated medical authority that seems to be forefront. CNSs have a primary role in assisting nursing and health care workers to shift their perspective and evaluate the care they are providing.

As a result of the loss of focus on nursing interventions, so too has the documentation of interventions and their evaluation suffered. Orlando (1961) first articulated the role of the nurse in providing that supportive and relationship-based interface between the health care system and the patient/client. We now have many more tools we can bring to bear on further describing that unique contribution of nursing to the health care system. Evidence-based practice, midrange theory, and a far better understanding of the research process and how it can be applied to daily activities of nursing are just a few examples of what we have today that our predecessors did not.

CNSs must lead the way for the nursing staff and, through doing so, can impact the overall satisfaction of the staff, the patients/clients, and the patient/client outcomes. Evaluation is key to attaining those outcomes.

■ DISCUSSION QUESTIONS

- Discuss the differences between nursing interventions and medically delegated interventions. Do you think there is greater value to one versus the other? How well do we document the medical interventions? The nursing interventions? Does nursing need to reevaluate nursing interventions as a process and outcome?

- The author has proposed that in order to have evidence of outcomes that are causal from the intervention to the evaluation, there should be concrete evidence that the intervention has created the outcome. Discuss how that does or does not apply to your current practice as a nurse or CNS.
- Discuss how you presently use evaluation in the three spheres of influence of CNS practice.

ANALYSIS AND SYNTHESIS EXERCISES

- A CNS working with a staff nurse has noted that the patient who has a chest tube is complaining of pain to the chest wall when breathing and states he cannot do the deep breathing and coughing exercises that are needed to maintain and expand his lung tissue. Describe the potential etiologies of the pain (include physiologic, psychologic, and medical reasons). Describe potential *nursing* interventions that are specific, measurable, and based on a conceptual framework. Define how you would evaluate these interventions.
- It was noted that staff were having difficulty with identifying cardinal signs of impending failure in patients on a cardiac unit. The CNS determined that there was need for a case-based high fidelity simulation (HFS) exercise to improve recognition of the cardinal signs and ultimately improve the staff response to those signs. Outline the conceptual framework you would use to ground this intervention. What would be some of the measurable interventions used in this case? What would be measurable outcomes that could be attributed to the HFS? What other issues/evaluative measures would you need to consider?

APPENDIX

Types of Evaluation

Grantees may conduct evaluations for a variety of reasons. Different types of evaluations can be used to answer different types of questions. The following descriptions provide an overview of four of the primary types of evaluations.

Process Evaluation. This form of evaluation assesses the extent to which a program is operating as it was intended. It typically assesses program activities' conformance to statutory and regulatory requirements, program design, and professional standards or customer expectations.

Short-Term	Mid-Term	Long-Term	Ultimate
Awareness and uptake of environmental health messages; Additional grant funding; More efficient and effective individuals and organizations; Stronger partnerships	Individual changes in behavior; Secondary transfer of messages; Increased capacity to leverage resources; Changes in environmental policies and regulation; Project reach extended; New projects developed	Social behavior change and informed decision making; Sustainability; Future research collaborations; Improved local environment; Reduced exposure to environmental hazards; Safer workplaces; Safer/healthier communities	Decrease in disease and other adverse health outcomes; Increased quality of life; Increased worker productivity; Healthier environment and ecosystem; Increase in gross national product

IMPACTS — 0 Grant Award, 2, 3, 4, 5, 6, 7 (Complete Project), 8, 9, 10, 20, 50 or More Years (Post-Project Period)

Source: U.S. Government Accountability Office (GAO) (2011).

Impact Evaluation. Impact evaluation is a form of outcome evaluation that assesses the net effect of a program by comparing program outcomes with an estimate of what would have happened in the absence of the program. This form of evaluation is employed to isolate the program's contribution to achievement of its objectives when external factors are known to influence the program outcomes.

Outcome Evaluation. This form of evaluation assesses the extent to which a program achieves its outcome-oriented objectives. It focuses on outputs and outcomes (including unintended effects) to judge program effectiveness but may also assess program process to understand how outcomes are produced.

Cost-Benefit and Cost-Effectiveness Analyses. These analyses compare a program's outputs or outcomes with the costs (resources expended) to produce them. When applied to existing programs, they are also considered a form of program valuation. Cost-effectiveness analysis assesses the cost of meeting a single goal or objective and can be used to identify the least costly alternative for meeting that goal. Cost-benefit analysis aims to identify all relevant costs and benefits, usually expressed in dollar terms.

REFERENCES

Agency for Healthcare Research and Quality (AHRQ). (2013). *Patient centered medical home.* Retrieved October 20, 2013, from http://www.pcmh.ahrq.gov/portal/server.pt/community/pcmh__home/1483/pcmh_defining_the_pcmh_v2

Allen, D. E., Bockenhauer, B., Egan, C., & Kinnaird, L. S. (2006). Relating outcomes to excellent nursing practice. *Journal of Nursing Administration, 36*(3), 140–147.

Casper, G. R., Kenron, D. A., & McDaniel, A. M. (2005). Information technology and the clinical nurse specialist: A framework for technology assessment. *Clinical Nurse Specialist: The Journal for Advanced Nursing Practice, 19*(4), 170–174.

Centers for Disease Control. (2012). *Improving the use of program evaluation for maximum health impact: Guidelines and recommendations.* Retrieved October 19, 2013, from http://www.cdc.gov/eval/materials/FinalCDCEvaluationRecommendations_Formatted_120412.pdf

Conn, V. S. (2007). Intervention? What intervention? *Western Journal of Nursing Research, 29*(5), 521–522.

Conn, V. S., Rantz, M. J., Wipke-Tevis, D. D., & Maas, M. L. (2001). Focus on research methods: Designing effective nursing interventions. *Research in Nursing and Health, 24*, 433–442.

Daponte, B. O. (2008). *Evaluation essentials: Methods for conducting sound research.* San Francisco, CA: Jossey-Bass.

Dickerson, S. S., Wu, Y. B., & Kennedy, M. C. (2006). A CNS-facilitated ICD support group. *Clinical Nurse Specialist: The Journal of Advanced Nursing Practice, 20*(3), 146–153.

Faust, C. (2002). Orlando's deliberative nursing process theory: A practice application in an extended care facility. *Journal of Gerontological Nursing, 28*(7), 14–18.

Fawcett, J. (1995). *Analysis and evaluation of conceptual models of nursing* (3rd ed.). Philadelphia, PA: F. A. Davis.

Fitzpatrick, J. L., Sanders, J. R., & Worthen, B. R. (2003). *Program evaluation: Alternative approaches and practical guidelines.* New York, NY: Addison Wesley Longman.

Fulton, J. S. (2003). Nursing interventions vs. interventions delivered by a nurse: Similar words, different meanings. *Clinical Nurse Specialist: The Journal of Advanced Nursing Practice, 17*(5), 227–228.

Goudreau, K. A. (2010). Evaluating interventions. In J. S. Fulton, B. L. Lyon, & K. A. Goudreau (Eds.), *Foundations of clinical nurse specialist practice* (pp. 87–98). New York, NY: Springer.

Institute for Healthcare Improvement (IHI). (2013). *Improvement map.* Retrieved October 30, 2013, from http://app.ihi.org/imap/tool/#Process=0ce038f1-fcde-4afc-8ffd-f0a83c7c9de7

Institute of Medicine (IOM). (2001). *Crossing the quality chasm: A new health system for the 21st century.* Washington, DC: Author.

Kellogg, W. K. (1998). *W. K. Kellogg Foundation evaluation handbook.* Battle Creek, MI: Author.

Kellogg, W. K. (2008). *W. K. Kellogg Foundation evaluation handbook & logic model development guide.* Battle Creek, MI: Author.

Meleis, A. I. (1991). *Theoretical nursing: Development and progress* (2nd ed.). New York, NY: J. B. Lippincott.

Miller, M. D., Linn, R. L., & Gronlund, N. E. (2008). *Measurement and assessment in teaching* (10th ed.). New York, NY: Macmillan.

National Association of Clinical Nurse Specialists (NACNS). (2004). *Statement on clinical nurse specialist practice and education* (2nd ed.). Harrisburg, PA: Author.

National Association of Clinical Nurse Specialists (NACNS). (2010). *CNS core competencies.* Retrieved October 19, 2013, from http://www.nacns.org/docs/CNSCoreCompetencies.pdf

Orlando, I. J. (1961). *The dynamic nursing-patient relationship: Function, process and principles of professional nursing practice.* New York, NY: G. P. Putnam's Sons.

Resar, R., Griffin, F. A., Haraden, C., & Nolan, T. W. (2012). *Using care bundles to improve health care quality.* IHI Innovation Series white paper. Cambridge, MA: Institute for Healthcare Improvement.

Resnick, B., Inguito, P., Orwig, D., Yahiro, J. Y., Hawkes, W., Werner, M., . . . Magaziner, J. (2005). Treatment fidelity in behavior change research: A case example. *Nursing Research, 54*(2), 139–143.

Rossi, P. H., & Freeman, H. E. (1993). *Evaluation: A systematic approach* (5th ed.). Newbury Park, CA: Sage.

Scriven, M. (1991). Beyond formative and summative evaluation. In M. W. McLaughlin & D. C. Phillips (Eds.), *Evaluation and education: At quarter century* (pp. 19–64). Chicago, IL: National Society for the Study of Education.

Sechrest, L., West, S., Phillips, M., Redner, R., & Yeaton, W. (1979). Some neglected problems in evaluation research: Strength and integrity of treatments. In L. Sechrest, S. West, M. Phillips, R. Redner, & W. Yeaton (Eds.), *Evaluation studies review annual* (vol. 4, pp. 15–35). Newbury Park, CA: Sage.

Sidani, S., & Braden, C. J. (1998). Outcomes related factors. In S. Sidani & C. J. Braden (Eds.), *Evaluating nursing interventions: A theory driven approach* (pp. 138–160). Thousand Oaks, CA: Sage.

Stufflebeam, D. I., & Shinkfield, A. J. (2007). *Evaluation theory, models and applications.* San Francisco, CA: Jossey Bass.

Thomas, E. J. (1984). *Interventions for the helping professions.* Beverly Hills, CA: Sage.

U.S, Food and Drug Administration (FDA). (2013). *Medical devices: Product evaluation.* Retrieved October 6, 2013, from http://www.fda.gov/MedicalDevices/DeviceRegulationandGuidance/PostmarketRequirements/QualitySystemsRegulations/MedicalDeviceQualitySystemsManual/ucm122653.htm

U.S. Government Accountability Office (GAO). (2011). *Performance measurement and evaluation.* GAO 11–646SP. Retrieved February 15, 2012, from http://www.gao.gov/new.items/d11646sp.pdf

Wood, M. J. (1998). Evaluative designs. In P. J. Brink & M. J. Wood (Eds.), *Advanced design in nursing research* (2nd ed., pp. 124–141). Thousand Oaks, CA: Sage.

World Health Organization. (2012). *Youth and road safety action kit.* Retrieved October 19, 2013, from http://www.youthforroadsafety.org/uploads/tekstblok_bijlagen/printable_yours_youth_and_road_safety_action_kit_1.pdf

Using Complex Adaptive Systems Theory to Guide Change

Kathleen Chapman

Clouds are not spheres, mountains are not cones, coastlines are not circles, and bark is not smooth, nor does lightning travel in a straight line. (*Benoit Mandelbrot, n.d.*)

This chapter focuses on the transformational leadership role of the clinical nurse specialist (CNS) at the systems and organizational level. Transforming practice requires adeptness in change management. The tools of change include the competencies of leadership, persuasion, influence, and negotiation. The focus of many articles and books about change is on the tools, rather than on the foundational step of thoroughly evaluating as many of the aspects of the involved system as possible. An appreciation of the myriad parts affected by the systems and their real or potential impact on the change is an essential first and ongoing step. This discernment will make the formulation of strategies that enhance the positives and mitigate the negatives possible so the desired change can be accomplished.

The goal of this chapter is to stimulate introspection and awareness of the questions that must be answered while the CNS engages in the various phases of change management. To apply the tools of change effectively, the dynamics of the system to which the tools are applied must be fully evaluated and well understood. Using complex adaptive theory as a framework for posing questions, the CNS will be positioned to groom the environment for successful and enduring change.

CHANGE AGENT

The advanced practitioner educates, challenges policy with new evidence, takes on clinical issues that are in search of a solution, and innovates—that is, effects change. There is no lack of opportunity for change at any level of the organization or across the continuum of care. Change might be reactionary, that is, a necessary response to maintain equilibrium when other things change (e.g., economic downturns and upturns, system mergers, war, evolving patient demographics, presence of new disease entities, and staff shortages), or it may be an intentional disruption of equilibrium so that continuous improvement can occur (e.g., new technology, emerging evidence, new health care roles, and new scopes of practice).

Change has been defined as the product of the interactions or interconnections between different systems or different people from which new behaviors emerge (Penprase & Norris, 2005). The definition is expressive of the daunting task involved in successfully managing the process of change. Interactions and interconnections imply many potential paths to simultaneously consider, control, empower, enhance, and mitigate.

CNSs achieve systemic change in many ways. They lead multidisciplinary teams through the selection and implementation of new technology; develop new approaches to the care of patient populations with new clinical guidelines and new staff roles; chair magnet steering committees; organize colleagues to form new professional organizations; change medical center policies, procedures, and by-laws; and form local and university partnerships with physicians and nurses to enhance the education of students and residents.

Practice is transformed through specialist involvement in the clinical, professional, political, and educational arenas. The human and health care systems the CNS interacts with are complex, the variables are many, and the subsequent potential outcomes are diverse. To be successful, many elements have to converge harmoniously so that change is adopted and sustained. Complex adaptive systems (CAS) theory provides a framework within which change can be anticipated, understood, embraced, and designed (Zimmerman, Lindberg, & Plsek, 2001).

COMPLEX ADAPTIVE SYSTEMS

Three principles central to CAS are *relationships, self-organization,* and *nonlinear predictability.* Several definitions of CAS appear in the literature. A definition provided by Plsek and Greenhalgh (2001) is that a CAS is a collection of individual agents "whose actions are interconnected" (*web of relationships*) "so that one agent's actions changes the context for other agents" (*self-organization*) "with freedom to act in ways that are not always totally predictable" (*nonlinear*).

Relationships

CAS theory emerged from the physical sciences of mathematics and physics in three phases. The first phase occurred in the early decades of the 20th century with the description of the principle of relationships. It is the concept that the whole is more than merely the sum of its parts. A CAS is made up of a web of relationships. Everything impacts everything else.

While exploring the subatomic world, physicists discovered that matter could not be adequately described just by naming its parts, that is, protons, neutrons, and electrons. They found that the same combination of subatomic particles did not guarantee the same physical outcome. Instead, identical ratios of the same protons, neutrons, and electrons existed in varying forms.

Capra (1982) observed that whether an electron was a wave or a particle depended on the electron's relationship with other subatomic particles. He said that as we penetrate into matter, nature does not show us any isolated basic building blocks, but rather appears as a complicated web of relations between the various parts of a unified whole.

Self-Organization (Emergence)

The second phase emerged from the science of thermodynamics. Scientists discovered that heating a thin layer of liquid resulted in the organization of new structures. They found that if enough energy flowed from the outside, a new pattern of complex structures spontaneously organized.

Experimentation demonstrated that as heat reached a certain critical value, convection replaced conduction and a pattern of hexagonal, honeycomb-shaped cells appeared. Heating the liquid moved it from equilibrium. There no longer was a uniform temperature throughout. The unstable form reorganized into an ordered hexagonal pattern. This principle was defined as self-organization (Capra, 1996). In more contemporary literature, the principle is also referred to as emergence (Penprase & Norris, 2005).

In self-organization, order is created without direction from the top; there is no focal point, no "centralized" clearinghouse for ideas. The ability of a system to self-organize is a function of the number of agents included within it and the intensity of its connections.

Nonlinear Predictability (Coevolution)

The third phase involved the concept of nonlinear relationships and actions, also referred to as chaos. CAS have multiple positive and negative feedback loops, the influence of external constraints, and exquisite sensitivity to initial conditions. Because of this nonlinearity and sensitivity to initial conditions, the details of the new behavior are inherently unpredictable (Penprase & Norris, 2005).

To illustrate, Holden (2005) describes meteorology experiments in which only a few decimals in a weather modeling computer program were changed. Even though the changes were minimal, the resulting weather prediction was very different. Small changes in the initial characteristics of an active system were found to dramatically affect the long-term behavior of that system.

CAS coevolve. Coevolution means that small changes can have a large impact. When one thing changes, it all changes. The system boundaries are open or fuzzy, not fixed. Depending on what the system is, they are open to the flow in or out of matter, energy, and information. Members in a system are not static. Each can be a member of different systems at the same time (Minas, 2005).

Living Systems Versus Machines

Prior to these scientific discoveries, the world was described in a mechanical, predictable, cause-and-effect manner. Machines move in a consistent way, are made up of consistent parts, and remain static in size and function. Living systems behave differently than machines. Living systems flow, move, adapt, become, burst, and morph. They are complex and adaptive.

There are many examples from nature, for example, flocking birds, ant colonies, and schools of fish. Cilliers (1998) described fish behavior to illustrate the concept of nonlinear relationships. He said that the condition of the fish being observed would depend on a large number of factors, including the availability of food, the temperature of the water, the amount of oxygen and light, the time of the year, and so forth. As these conditions varied, the size of the school of fish adjusted itself optimally to suit prevailing conditions, despite the fact that each individual fish could only look after its own interests. The system of the school of fish as a whole organized itself to ensure the best match between the system and the environment.

This organization of fish was also adaptive in the same sense that the school would be sensitive to changing conditions in the light of past experience. There was no agent that decided for the school what should happen, nor did each individual fish understand the complexity of the situation. The organization of the school emerged as a result of the interaction between the various constituents of the system and its environment.

Within a framework of CAS, health care organizations and systems of care are characterized as living entities. Health care systems are adaptive. Unlike mechanical systems, they are composed of individuals who have the capacity to learn and change as a result of experience. The components (individuals) react to internal and external stimuli, and adapt in response (Plsek, 2001; Rowe & Hogarth, 2005).

Health care systems, like all living systems, cannot be broken into simple parts. The complex cannot be made simple, cannot be understood in simple terms, and cannot be solved in simple ways (Lindstrom, 2003). Complex systems are nonlinear and not completely predictable. It is not known whether the complex system will unfold in a trajectory, a bifurcation, self-organize, emerge, or coevolve. The causal incident is a change in the value of one or more parameters. Even at the point of bifurcation, as an example, there is unpredictability as to which branch the system will follow.

Systems with even a minute amount of uncertainty in their current condition are likely to behave unpredictably in their next condition due to different reactions to negative and positive feedback. In addition, the behavior of a CAS is time dependent. The direction the system may take at any point is a function of how it behaved in the past, but it is not possible to predict the trajectory based on its past behavior alone. Rowe and Hogarth (2005) summarize key features of CAS in Exhibit 8.1.

USING CAS THEORY TO INFORM CNS PRACTICE IN MANAGING CHANGE

Observations from nature can be applied to human behavior and organizational systems. Advanced practice nurses learn to view the health care environment

---

EXHIBIT 8.1

Key Features of Complex Adaptive Systems

Complex adaptive systems will be self-organizing, and new elements will emerge at various points. These changes may be incremental or dramatic as they adapt to reactions between subsystems and with other systems.

Uncertainty is inevitable in an evolving system, rendering top-down control impossible. The views and experiences of those at a variety of points in an organization are necessary to gain an understanding of it.

Spontaneous change occurs more readily where there is a range of different behavior patterns (microdiversity).

Agents within an organization act according to their own internal rules or mental models. Attractor patterns within the system will "frame" and limit change.

Simple rules or guiding principles can lead to innovative emergent changes.

Change can be stimulated by the encouragement of new generative relationships. These can produce new insights and solutions into complex problems.

There will be simultaneous stability and instability at the edge of chaos, this being a requirement for the emergence of novelty.

Source: Adapted from Zimmerman et al., Olsen and Eoyang, and Stacey, as discussed and cited in Rowe and Hogarth (2005).

through a number of lenses, including the system and policy-setting level that drives the quality of patient care. To ensure success, the change agent must consciously step back and up, always viewing the issue from the balcony and through the added lens of complexity science.

Minimum Specifications (Self-Organization)

It may seem counterintuitive, but complexity science research demonstrates that relatively simple rules lead to complex, innovative system behavior. Plsek cites studies of the flocking of birds and the schooling of fish to avoid predators: "These studies and computer models have confirmed that a few simple rules can guide complex behavior toward a goal. Such systems move toward their goals by having (a) a common purpose (avoiding predators), (b) internal motivation (surviving another day), and (c) some simple rules that guide behavior (keeping up with the group, moving toward the center of mass of the group, and avoiding collisions)" (2001, p. 63).

The tendency is to do the opposite, that is, to specify in great detail what is to be done at all levels of the system so the desired goal (the change) is accomplished. This overspecification can result in inefficiency, that is, steps that are not necessary, unnecessary additional handoffs, lower quality, lower satisfaction, and higher costs.

Minimum specifications, on the other hand, leave room for self-organization and emergence, creativity, and innovation. Rather than lengthy, defined process and implementation steps, the system undergoing change is given a few simple and flexible rules and a statement of desired outcome.

Minimum specifications invite discussion about how the change is to be achieved and, in so doing, increase connectedness and a shared vision among the component parts. If minimum specifications focus on broad outcomes, they will encourage generative relationships and the emergence of solutions that are relevant to local conditions (Minas, 2005).

Attractors Versus Resistance

Resistance is often cited as the reason change comes slowly, or not at all. Minas (2005) asserts that if resistance is seen as the reason, then the concluded solution is to battle against, and to overcome, resistance wherever it is found. CAS theory, however, informs us that behavior follows the attractors in a system. Managing change within the context of CAS involves a paradigm shift. In CAS, change is viewed as a "drawing toward" rather than as a "pushing against."

To be successful, the CNS must understand how a change in system parameters can shift the system from one attractor pattern to another that is more desirable. In other words, what are the nonpunitive incentives for changing behavior? The change agent needs to deliberately set the stage by making compelling, evidence-based arguments for the desired outcome in a way that will be viewed as deserving of the time and effort of those impacted.

Considerations could include incentives that are patient-related, profession-related, process-related, or financial, as well as incentives that are individually based or team based. Something is an attractor if involved members of the change are able to meaningfully fill in the blank, "If A becomes B, the benefit will be _____."

Surprise!

The edge that lies between order and chaos is where creativity and flexibility thrive. At the edge of chaos,

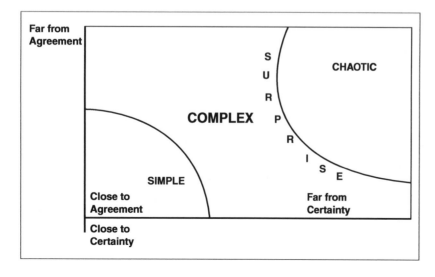

FIGURE 8.1 Complexity matrix.

Source: Modified from Stacey, Hassey, and Brown as cited in Brown (2006).

the environment is unpredictable, exciting, and bursting with new ideas and innovation (Penprase & Norris, 2005). It is at this edge of surprise where change occurs (Figure 8.1) (Brown, 2006).

In the daily work of health care, moments of surprise occur regularly. We are surprised by our patients, by our colleagues, by our systems, and by our own reactions. Attempts to eliminate surprise are futile. The complexity lens suggests that surprise is not necessarily the result of any one factor, but rather is the result of the fundamental nature of the system being observed (McDaniel, Jordan, & Fleeman, 2003). We are not machines that operate in linear and predictable ways.

We simply need to come to terms with the notion that uncertainty and unpredictability cannot be mapped out in advance. In human ecosystems, the only predictable element is lack of predictability. Therefore, surprise is inevitable because it is part of the natural order and cannot be avoided, eliminated, or controlled.

CAS allows us to capitalize on the surprises that confront our work lives using the strategies of creativity and learning. The change agent's role is to identify patterns and trends, assist staff to accept and adjust to changes, support coordination of the various elements of change, and help staff maintain focus and identity as they experience a turbulent health care environment (Begun & Kaissi, 2004). Change agents need to anticipate, develop a capacity for, and invite surprise on a daily basis. In the words of McDaniel, "It is not a question of, 'How can I keep this from happening,' but rather, 'How can I make creative use of what is happening?'" (McDaniel et al., 2003, p. 272). In fact, the system and its components should be moved regularly to the edge of chaos so that creativity and flexibility can thrive. At the edge of chaos, self-organization can only result from interactions between people. As a change agent, the CNS encourages new ideas and supports risk-taking by presenting evidence, challenging rituals, and asking questions. The CNS is instrumental in contributing to an environment in which relationships reflect trust, comfort, acceptance, inquiry, celebration, and flexibility.

Because the edge of chaos is unstable, the environment is ripe for an infinite number of new behaviors and new ideas to spontaneously emerge. The Institute of Medicine (IOM) report states, "In complex adaptive systems...the parts...have the freedom and ability to respond to stimuli in many different and fundamentally unpredictable ways.... Such behavior can be for better or for worse, that is, it can manifest itself as either innovation or error" (Plsek, 2001, p. 322). The challenge for the CNS, of course, is to intervene by leading innovation.

CAS THEORY AND COMPLEXITY LEADERSHIP

Leadership competency and execution of the leadership role is essential for leading innovation, developing new approaches to care, initiating new programs and services, and, in general, advancing health (IOM, 2010). Historical styles that reserve leadership roles for specific titles in a hierarchical structure assume a knowable and predictable world view with top-down power dynamics and centralized decision making (Uhl-Bien, Marion, & McKelvey, 2008). Traditional leadership assumes that workers are mechanistic and task-focused. This "traditional" leadership style is rigid and regimented, with tightly specified operating procedures (overspecification). There is little room for new ideas, new behaviors, risk-taking, or innovation. The style is not sufficient to meet the complex problems currently facing health care (Weberg, 2012).

Leading change requires a different approach. CAS theory informs us that living systems need the space to move, emerge, and adapt. Living systems are not predictable or constant. The complexity leader is successful when an environment of inclusion, acceptance, and openness is created. Complexity leaders invite input from team members using shared governance principles and interact with team members using interviews, conversation, and observation to gather information about issues, work streams, barriers, perceptions about the change needed and potential solutions. Complexity leadership is associated with the bottom-up emergent dynamics within organizations and is defined as a dynamic, interactive influence process among individuals and groups. The ultimate goal is that the members of the group will lead one another to adaptability, innovation, and learning (Exhibit 8.2) (Uhl-Bien et al., 2008; Weberg, 2012; and Center for the Study of Healthcare Management, n.d.).

THE VIEW FROM HERE: PREPARING FOR CHANGE

While embarking on a change process, the CNS needs to thoughtfully consider a series of questions so that the entire CAS is appreciated. The competencies defined in the *Statement on Clinical Nurse Specialist Practice and Education* (Exhibits 8.3–8.6 and 8.8) provide a conceptual framework for evaluating the complexity of the environment (National Association of Clinical Nurse Specialists [NACNS], 2004). Formulating answers to the questions suggested by the competencies can be used as a strategy to inform a template for action.

EXHIBIT 8.2

Comparison of Leadership Styles

Traditional Leaders	Complexity Leaders
Are controlling, mechanistic	Are open, responsive, catalytic
Repeat the past	Offer alternatives
Are in charge	Are collaborative
Are autonomous	Are connected
Are self-preserving	Are adaptable
Resist change, bury contradictions	Acknowledge paradoxes
Are disengaged; nothing ever changes	Are engaged; continuously emerging
Value position and structure	Value persons
Hold formal position	Are shifting as processes unfold
Set rules	Prune rules
Make decisions	Help others
Are knowers	Are listeners

Source: Adapted from Center for the Study of Healthcare Management (n .d.).

Assessment: Identifying and Defining Problems and Opportunities

Each and every step within the change process is equally important. The questions for assessment presented here are neither intended to be complete, nor used once. Instead, the questions should evolve and should be asked again and again as circumstances self-organize, new relationships emerge, or surprise is encountered. Each step in the CAS change process is not a one-time event.

What organizational structures and functions exert impact?

Are levels of approval required? Does the desired change impact other functions and organizational entities? What organizational data are accessible? What are the tools available to collect additional relevant organizational data?

What is the professional climate and the level of multidisciplinary collaboration?

Is the group of stakeholders a unified team? A high-level functioning group will facilitate the change process. Is the group dysfunctional? Lack of multidisciplinary functioning will require additional preparation of the environment involving attention to communication and team building.

What are the system-level variables?

What is the state of the organization's financial health? Does the desired change cost anything? What are the indirect costs? What is the opportunity cost? In what ways can the desired change be matched to the organization's strategic plan? What are the other things that the system is dealing with that will add energy or drain energy?

What are the relationships within and external to the organization/system that are facilitators or barriers?

What is the organization's past history relative to staff cooperation and follow-through? Who are the external stakeholders—external to the CNS group, external to nursing, external to the organization? Is each a facilitator or a barrier? In what way?

What are the effects of organizational culture on departments, teams, and groups?

Does the CNS have position power, expert power, or other informal power? Does the culture consist of traditional leaders who expect formal designation, or is the culture supportive of complexity leaders? Does the organization celebrate risk taking and change? Is the culture bureaucratic? Is there a charge letter for the initiative that is widely distributed?

What legislative and regulatory health policies provide impact?

EXHIBIT 8.3

CNS Competencies: Organization/System Sphere of Influence

Assessment: Identifying and Defining Problems and Opportunities

Uses/designs system-level assessment methods and instruments to identify organization structures and functions that impact nursing practice and nurse-sensitive patient care outcomes.

Assesses the professional climate and the multidisciplinary collaboration within and across units for their impact on nursing practice and outcomes.

Assesses targeted system-level variables, such as culture, finances, regulatory requirements, and external demands that influence nursing practice and outcomes.

Identifies relationships within and external to the organization/system that are facilitators or barriers to nursing practice and any proposed change.

Identifies effects of organizational culture on departments, teams, and/or groups within an organization.

Monitors legislative and regulatory health policy that may impact nursing practice and/or CNS practice for the specialty area/population.

Source: From National Association of Clinical Nurse Specialists (NACNS), 2004.

Are there scope of practice considerations, The Joint Commission (TJC) considerations, or payor considerations? What are the implications for existing medical center policies and procedures?

Diagnosis, Outcome Identification, and Planning

After each assessment, the CNS is ready to interpret findings and identify options. Priorities, feasibility, and minimum specifications are considered.

What are the facilitators and barriers?

Who are the supporters of the change and who are the process owners? Are they on board? Could the initiative be considered controversial, provocative, or otherwise anxiety producing? What are the nonhuman facilitators and barriers, (e.g., time, space, location)?

What are the variations in organizational culture that exert influence?

What are the values, attitudes, and beliefs of the affected group about the proposed initiative? What are the values, attitudes, and beliefs of the affected group about change, in general? Are the values, attitudes, and beliefs among the affected group of patients and/or staff homogeneous or heterogeneous? What is the impact of age and experience? What are the positive influences and the negative influences of each? How can the positives be enhanced and negatives minimized?

What variations across the organization exert influence?

What is the organizational structure? Is it centralized, decentralized, matrix, product line? Are staff empowered to participate? Is the manager hands-on or hands-off? What are the implications for communication, socialization, and permission? How does that vary for each of the potentially affected groups? Is the platform burning equally for each of the impacted groups—that is, does everyone believe change is needed? If not, what strategies can be used to turn up the heat?

What will achieve intended systemwide outcomes while avoiding or minimizing unintended consequences?

What groundwork is needed? Are the desired outcomes specifically defined and measurable? If the initiative fails, what is the worst-case scenario for patients, staff, and the organization? How does the initiative potentially impact the conditions of work? What are the obligations to the union and how will they be met?

What is the impact to legislative and regulatory policy?

Are legislative stakeholders involved? What are the funding implications? Are there any role boundary or scope of practice issues? Are there state certificate of need regulations that must be considered? Will the initiative impact the organization's scope or level of services? If so, what are the potential reporting obligations to external regulatory entities, and what new systems will have to be put in place to meet new regulations? Does this result in additional cost to the organization?

Intervention: Developing and Testing Solutions

An overarching consideration in this section is whether the testing of the potential solution will be a process improvement or research. Discussion of the differences is not within the scope of this chapter. Because the distinction can be gray, it is recommended that the local nursing research resource be consulted. Depending on the intervention method and how the outcomes are intended to be reported to the professional community, the initiative will require addressing the related ethical considerations and may require institutional review board approval.

What innovative solutions can be generalized across differing units, populations, or specialties?

Does the innovation have potential for application to other situations? Is the initiative under consideration generic enough to work across the continuum of care? What variations may be necessary? How can others from different units, populations, or specialties be invited to shape the intervention?

How will resulting innovations be deployed across the full continuum of care for different population groups and/or specialties?

Is it realistic for implementation in other areas? Will customization be needed? How will the innovation be communicated to other audiences? What are the deployment issues and options?

What are the implications for the development of multidisciplinary standards of practice and evidence-based guidelines for care, such as pathways, care maps, and benchmarks?

What additional development is needed? Should the innovation be tested with other patient or staff populations? What tools be developed to assure consistent implementation and permanence?

How can system-level barriers to change be targeted and reduced?

What are the identified barriers? What are the attractors? How can the attractors be enhanced and communicated? How can trust and openness be enhanced? How can necessary relationships be garnered? How can the environment be encouraged to ask questions and express concerns? What is the best way to communicate answers so everyone feels informed?

What are the paths for developing system-level policies that affect innovation and programs of care?

How should the required policies be developed, tested, and/or revised? Who should be involved? What does the evidence suggest? What amount of consensus is reasonable? Which are the minimum specifications?

How can the factors to effect program-level change be facilitated?

How will the system/organizational factors impact the change at the program level? What are the attractors at the program level? Are they consistent with the attractors at the organizational level?

What strategies are needed to sustain and spread change and innovation?

How can change be stabilized? What will move the edge from the upper right quadrant toward the lower left quadrant? What structures can be put in place to ensure continuing relationships, and how can the attractors be made more permanent?

What methods and processes will ensure that evidence-based changes will be sustained?

What are the success factors? What is the plan to update the evidence over time? How will

---

EXHIBIT 8.4

CNS Competencies: Organization/System Sphere of Influence

Diagnosis, Outcome Identification, and Planning

Diagnoses facilitators and barriers to achieving desired outcomes of integrated programs of care across the continuum and at points of service.

Diagnoses variations in organizational culture (i.e., values, beliefs, or attitudes) that can positively exert influence.

Draws conclusions about the effects of variance across the organization that influences outcomes of nursing practice.

Plans for achieving intended system-wide outcomes, while avoiding or minimizing unintended consequences.

Draws conclusions about the impact of legislative and regulatory policies as they apply to nursing practice and outcomes for specialty populations.

Source: From National Association of Clinical Nurse Specialists (NACNS), 2004.

EXHIBIT 8.5

CNS Competencies: Organization/System Sphere of Influence

Intervention: Developing and Testing Solutions

Develops innovative solutions that can be generalized across differing units, populations, or specialties.

Leads nursing and multidisciplinary groups in implementing innovative patient care programs that address issues across the full continuum of care for different population groups and/or specialties.

Contributes to the development of multidisciplinary standards of practice and evidence-based guidelines for care, such as pathways, care maps, benchmarks.

Solidifies relationships and multidisciplinary linkages that foster the adoption of innovations.

Develops or influences system-level policies that will affect innovation and programs of care.

Targets and reduces system-level barriers to proposed changes in nursing practices and programs of care.

Facilitates factors to effect program-level change.

Designs methods/strategies to sustain and spread change and innovation.

Implements methods and processes to sustain evidence-based changes in nursing practice, programs of care, and clinical innovation.

Provides leadership for legislative and regulatory initiatives to advance the health of the public with a focus on the specialty practice area/population.

Mobilizes professional and public resources to support legislative and regulatory issues that advance the health of the public.

Source: From National Association of Clinical Nurse Specialists (NACNS), 2004.

the policy issues? What are the current legislative opportunities? What is the relevant professional group that can be contacted with information about the innovation? Are professional committee membership opportunities available?

How can professional and public resources be mobilized to support legislative and regulatory issues that advance the health of the public?

What are the grants and other funding streams available to support initial, current, and developing innovation? How can colleagues be informed of relevant pending legislation and opportunities for educating policy makers? What volunteer opportunities are available to position the CNS for future influence?

Evaluation of the Effects

Evaluation tools and methods must be considered at the beginning of the change process, much like discharge planning must begin at patient admission.

What evaluation methods or instruments can be used to identify system-level outcomes of programs of care?

Will the evaluation be formal or informal? Are standardized tools available? Will permissions be required? Who will be responsible for the collection of data? How often? Where will the results be reported?

How will system-level clinical and fiscal outcomes of products, devices, and patient care processes using performance methods be evaluated?

Who will the audience be? How will effectiveness be defined? Is the definition the same for the patient, the nurse, the physician, the administrator, and the chief financial officer? How will modeling be used? How can a dashboard or balanced scorecard be developed to demonstrate effectiveness?

How can the organizational structure and existing organizational processes be used to provide feedback about the effectiveness of nursing practices and multidisciplinary relationships in meeting identified outcomes of programs of care?

What are the typical reporting formats and frequencies at the organization level? How can the innovation and its impact be made visible to the organization? Can updates be added to the agendas of key medical and administrative committees? How can opportunities be created to publicize the outcomes in internal and external medical center communication?

What organizational policies should be evaluated for their ability to support and sustain outcomes of programs of care?

Are there policies that are in conflict with the innovation? Does the new evidence provide a path for

incremental success be celebrated? What are the ongoing person, money, and space resource implications? How will access to needed resources be guaranteed?

How can the CNS provide leadership for legislative and regulatory initiatives to advance the health of the public with a focus on the specialty practice area/population?

How should the innovation inform legislation, regulations, or professional standards? What is the role of the change in ensuring public safety? What are

EXHIBIT 8.6

CNS Competencies: Organization/System Sphere of Influence

Evaluation of the Effects

Selects evaluation methods and instruments to identify system-level outcomes of programs of care.

Evaluates system-level clinical and fiscal outcomes of products, devices, and patient care processes using performance methods.

Uses organizational structure and processes to provide feedback about the effectiveness of nursing practices and multidisciplinary relationships in meeting identified outcomes of programs of care.

Evaluates organizational policies for their ability to support and sustain outcomes of programs of care.

Evaluates and documents the impact of CNS practice on the organization.

Documents all outcomes in a reportable manner.

Disseminates outcomes of system-wide changes, impact of nursing practices, and CNS work to stakeholders.

Source: From National Association of Clinical Nurse Specialists (NACNS), 2004.

revision? Who are the stakeholders of the existing policy? What additional policies are needed to provide the structure to support the desired outcome? Are there union bargaining obligations involved?

How will the impact of CNS practice on the organization be evaluated and documented?

What are the organization's stated and unstated expectations regarding the change? What are the ways the expectations can be shaped (for example, targets established, timeline identified, and work products defined)? Who will evaluate the change? What did the CNS personally bring to the value equation? Where will the CNS's leadership role in the change be acknowledged and documented?

How will outcomes be documented, ensuring a reportable format?

Some of the report customization issues for the various reports include who will read it; report details such as length, language, and technical level; and verbal or written format. Additional considerations include "what are the quantifiable and objective outcomes?" and "what additional calibration is needed to refine the measurement as the change process stabilizes?"

How will outcomes of systemwide changes, impact of nursing practices, and CNS work be disseminated to stakeholders?

Who are the various stakeholders? How do the attractors vary among stakeholders? What information is most compelling for each group? What were the nonlinear impacts? What was the value of the change on the system? What was the impact of the change on the nursing process?

THE BUSINESS CASE

The CNS may need the organizational hierarchy to formally embrace and endorse a change. Organizational-level initiatives that require resources in the six figures, or detailed computer programming, or the establishment of a new service or program, for example, will have to compete for limited institutional resources. To compete successfully, a written proposal that demonstrates a thorough analysis of the issue, thoughtful consideration of options, data-driven recommendations, and financial projections will be required.

Each organization will likely have its own customized template for presenting the business case. CAS theory provides a firm foundation for developing comprehensive and compelling arguments. A disciplined consideration of the questions suggested in the previous section will enable the CNS to convey a comprehensive and credible proposal. The questions asked can be customized to the scope and complexity of the desired change.

An example of a business template that lends itself well to incorporating the CAS perspective is displayed in Exhibit 8.7. The Executive Decision Memorandum is an example of a formal format that has been used by the Department of Veterans Affairs (n.d.; Exhibit 8.7) to describe recommended changes and request approval for implementation.

Each of the content areas is completed, considering impact of the change on a number of complex system elements: stakeholders, dissenting opinions, impact on existing programs and facilities, legal or legislative impact, budget or financial impact, public relations or media considerations, and congressional or public officers or public agency considerations. In the example, Option 1 is typically status quo. Pros and cons of each are outlined, and the recommended option is indicated.

EXHIBIT 8.7

Executive Decision Memorandum

I. Summary of facts/background

II. Synopsis of significance of related issues

III. Criteria for decision making

IV. Stakeholder involvement

V. Options and arguments

A. Option 1

1. Argument pro

2. Argument con

B. Option 2

1. Argument pro

2. Argument con

C. Option 3

1. Argument pro

2. Argument con

VI. Recommended option

VII. Dissenting opinions regarding recommended option

VIII. Effect of recommended option on existing programs and/or facilities

IX. Legal or legislative considerations of the recommended option

X. Budget or financial considerations of the recommended option

XI. Public relations or media considerations of the recommended option

XII. Congressional or other public official or agency consideration of the recommended option

XIII. Implementation considerations

Source: Department of Veterans Affairs (n.d.).

EXHIBIT 8.8

Organization/System Sphere of Influence

Outcomes of CNS Practice

Clinical problems are articulated within the context of the organization/system structure, mission, culture, policies, and resources.

Patient care processes reflect continuous improvements that benefit the system.

Change strategies are integrated throughout the system.

Policies enhance the practice of nurses individually as members of multidisciplinary teams.

Innovative models of practice are developed, piloted, evaluated, and incorporated across the continuum of care.

Evidence-based, best-practice models are developed and implemented.

Nursing care and outcomes are articulated at organizational/system decision-making levels.

Stakeholders (nurses, other health care professionals, and management) share a common vision of practice outcomes.

Decision makers within the institution are informed about practice problems, factors contributing to the problems, and the significance of those problems with respect to outcomes and costs.

Patient care initiatives reflect knowledge of cost management and revenue enhancement strategies.

Patient care programs are aligned with the organization's strategic imperatives, mission, vision, philosophy, and values.

Staff comply with regulatory requirements and standards.

Policy-making bodies are influenced to develop regulations/procedures to improve patient care and health services.

Source: From National Association of Clinical Nurse Specialists (NACNS), 2004.

ADVANCED NURSING PRACTICE

The advanced practice nurse is well positioned by education and by role to exert a positive influence on the organization and on the system. A complexity leadership style and utilization of CAS theory to create change moves the nurse beyond the realm of expert clinical practitioner to new arenas of major organizational impact. Specific outcomes of CNS practice at the organization and system level are displayed in Exhibit 8.8.

Complexity theory appears largely in the computer science, physics, biology, medicine, and management literature (Brown, 2006; Goldberger, 1996; Kernick, 2002). The lack of literature describing how CAS theory is manifest in the clinical nursing arena and

in CNS practice, however, provides an abundance of research opportunities. In addition to research, it is important that the CNS contribute to CAS literature by describing successes and failures. Often the most valuable insights are gained from what did not work well and from the lessons learned.

CAS theory informs the CNS that there is no formula guaranteeing successful change. Furthermore, the same combination of staff and/or resources that led to successful change in one setting does not guarantee the same results in another setting. In each case, the approach must be customized to account for all of the unique characteristics of the individuals, the situation, and the physical and emotional environment.

CAS theory challenges us to embrace uncertainty and to support self-organization. The goal is to create the environmental conditions within which an innovation can emerge, not to engineer the change. The CNS complexity leader creates the conditions in a number of ways, through reflection, debate, challenge, fostering development of multiple new relationships, education, and validating new skills.

CAS provides insight into how organizations are sustained, how they self-organize, and how outcomes emerge. CAS theory informs us that organizations learn, adapt, and change through behavioral processes. As an agent of change, the CNS understands and unravels relationships, fosters new interconnections, and facilitates new solutions—all at the edge of chaos.

■ DISCUSSION QUESTIONS

- The following two quotes were retrieved from a complexity website (Plexus Institute, 2013): "Life will never surrender its secrets to a yardstick," attributed to Dee Hock, and "As humans we are complex and chaotic when healthy and rigidly orderly when ill," attributed to Stuart Davidson. What does each statement tell you about CAS theory and/or change? How do the statements relate to CNS practice?

- Research has demonstrated that 75% of all change initiatives fail (Bunker & Wakefield, 2005). Does this figure surprise you? Why do you think this might be the case? In your opinion, what are the most difficult aspects of leading change?

- Think of an example of a well-known change that has been sustained over time and another of a well-known change that has not lasted. From a CAS perspective, what could the different outcomes be attributed to? What are the hallmarks of enduring change?

- Data are an essential component of demonstrating value. What are examples of the types of data that could be used to measure the impact of change? How would you collect or retrieve that data? What resources do you have in your organization to develop your skills in accessing, analyzing, and displaying data for your various audiences?

■ ANALYSIS AND SYNTHESIS EXERCISES

- Using an example from your personal experience, analyze a change in terms of self-organization, emergence, and coevolution. What was the change? What was your role in the change? How did self-organization, emergence, and coevolution each present? Was the change successful? Why or why not?

- Analyze a failed change that you experienced from the CAS principle of "web of relationships." What are the different types of relationships that you can identify in your example? How did each contribute to the change? What relationships were ignored but should have been addressed? What could you have anticipated that would have made a difference in the outcome? What relationships should have been created?

- Visit a complexity, change, or innovation website. What elements of surprise did you discover there? How do the concepts relate to CNS practice at the organization level?

- Interview a CNS about a successful change led at the organization level. Use a subset of questions suggested by CNS system/organization-level competencies to form the interview tool. How did each step develop? What insights did the CNS gain? What were the lessons learned? What other questions did you formulate from a CAS and change perspective under the categories of assessment, diagnosis, intervention, and evaluation? What were the attractors? What does the CNS cite as the key success factor? How did the CNS celebrate the success?

REFERENCES

Begun, J., & Kaissi, A. (2004). Uncertainty in health care environments: Myth or reality? *Health Care Management Review*, 29(1), 31–39.

Brown, C. (2006). The application of complex adaptive systems theory to clinical practice in rehabilitation. *Disability and Rehabilitation*, 28(9), 587–593.

Bunker, K., & Wakefield, M. (2005). *Leading with authenticity in times of transition*. Greensboro, NC: CCL Press.

Capra, F. (1982). *The turning point*. Toronto, Ontario, Canada: Bantam Books.

Capra, F. (1996). *The web of life*. New York, NY: Anchor Books.

Center for the Study of Healthcare Management. (n.d.). *Applying complexity science to health and healthcare*. University of Minnesota: Author. Retrieved October 16, 2013, from http://c.ymcdn.com/sites/www.plexusinstitute.org/resource/collection/6528ED29–9907-4BC7–8D00–8DC907679FED/11261_Plexus_Summit_report_Health_Healthcare.pdf

Cilliers, P. (1998). *Complexity and postmodernism: Understanding complex systems*. London, UK: Routledge.

Department of Veterans Affairs. (n.d.). *Attachment J. EDM format*. Retrieved October 31, 2013, from http://www.va.gov/VHAPUBLICATIONS/ViewPublication.asp?pub_ID=1725

Goldberger, A. (1996). Non-linear dynamics for clinicians: Chaos theory, fractals, and complexity at the bedside. *The Lancet, 347*(9011), 1312–1314.

Holden, L. (2005). Complex adaptive systems concept analysis. *Journal of Advanced Nursing, 52*(6), 651–657.

Institute for Healthcare Improvement (IHI). (n.d.). *Transforming care at the bedside*. Retrieved October 29, 2013, from http://www.ihi.org/IHI/Programs/StrategicInitiatives/TransformingCareAtTheBedside.htm

Institute of Medicine (IOM). (2010). *The future of nursing: Leading change, advancing health*. Washington, DC: Author.

Kernick, D. (2002). Complexity and healthcare organizations. In K. Sweeney & F. Griffiths (Eds.), *Complexity and healthcare, an introduction* (pp. 93–121). Abingdon, UK: Radcliffe Medical Press.

Lindstrom, R. (2003). Evidence-based decision-making in healthcare: Exploring the issues through the lens of complex adaptive systems theory. *Healthcare Papers, 3*(3), 29–35.

Mandelbrot, B. (2010). In J. Challoner. *How Mandelbrot's fractals changed the world*. BBC News, October 18. Retrieved October 15, 2013, from http://www.bbc.co.uk/news/magazine-11564766

McDaniel, R., Jordan, M., & Fleeman, B. (2003). Surprise, surprise, surprise! A complexity science view of the unexpected. *Healthcare Management Review, 28*(3), 266–278.

Minas, H. (2005). Leadership for change in complex systems. *Australasian Psychiatry, 13*(1), 33–39.

National Association of Clinical Nurse Specialists (NACNS). (2004). *Statement on clinical nurse specialist practice and education* (2nd ed.). Harrisburg, PA: Author.

Penprase, B., & Norris, D. (2005). What nurse leaders should know about complex adaptive systems theory. *Nursing Leadership Forum, 9*(3), 127–132.

Plexus Institute. (2013). Retrieved October 15, 2013, from http://www.plexusinstitute.org/page/edgeware/?

Plsek, P. (2001). Redesigning health care with insights from the science of complex adaptive systems. In Committee on Quality of Health Care in America & Institute of Medicine (Eds.), *Crossing the quality chasm: A new health system for the 21st century* (pp. 61–88). Washington, DC: National Academies Press.

Plsek, P., & Greenhalgh, T. (2001). The challenge of complexity in health care. *British Medical Journal, 323*, 625–628.

Rowe, A., & Hogarth, A. (2005). Use of complex adaptive systems metaphor to achieve professional and organizational change. *Journal of Advanced Nursing, 51*(4), 396–405.

Uhl-Bien, M., Marion, R., & McKelvey, B. (2008). Complexity leadership theory: Shifting leadership from the industrial age to the knowledge era. In M. Uhl-Bien & R. Marion (Eds.), *Complexity leadership part 1: Conceptual foundations* (pp. 185–224). Charlotte, NC: Information Age Publishing.

Weberg, D. (2012). Complexity leadership: A healthcare imperative. *Nursing Forum, 7*(4), 268–275.

Zimmerman, B., Lindberg, C., & Plsek, P. (2001). *Edgeware: Insights from complexity science for health care leaders* (2nd ed.). Irving, TX: VHA, Inc.

Engaging Staff in Learning

Christine M. Pacini

Change in health care as a microcosm of the broader world experience is occurring at a rate that makes it almost impossible to keep up. Mechanisms for delivering service, generating relevant products and processes, and reconfiguring systems are becoming increasingly complex. Some of the most formidable characteristics of these systems are that they are inherently uncontrollable and unpredictable, thereby requiring new models and approaches for responsive intervention. For example, concepts such as shared leadership, healing sanctuaries, servant leadership, communities of caring, collaborative innovation, and self-managed work teams are evolving in support of values related to patient–family centrality, accountable care, customer-focused behavior, process improvement, safety, and high-quality clinical and behavioral outcomes.

The publication of the Institute of Medicine (IOM) Report in 2011 related to the future of nursing documents several key requirements that frame the transformation of nursing development, education, and practice (IOM, 2011). A panel of 18 key leaders who value and advocate for the contributions of nursing to the well-being of citizens in the United States crafted eight recommendations and four key messages to address possible solutions for the multitude of complex health concerns that face the United States and the world. To this end, the report articulates that developmental/educational work in nursing needs to incorporate collaboration, residency programs, ongoing academic preparation (doctor of nursing practice [DNP], master of science in nursing [MSN], doctoral studies), lifelong learning, and leadership with respect to change.

In light of the IOM report (IOM, 2011) and in concert with the spheres and competencies that characterize clinical nurse specialist (CNS) practice (National Association of Clinical Nurse Specialists [NACNS], 2004), it is evident that CNSs have a key role in leading and realizing the charges articulated in the IOM Report. The work of providing patient-centered care, collaborating within interprofessional teams, utilizing evidence-based practice (EBP) principles, applying QI frameworks, and utilizing informatics are essential to framing the practice of a CNS and enhance favorable clinical outcomes. The CNS has the obligation to step up and take the stance of authority for leading transformation in practice. Excellence in health care requires someone with clinical expertise (i.e., the CNS) to work with a variety of providers and shape the direction for clinical nursing excellence in any given delivery scenario.

One of the key problems is that past approaches to leading, managing, and learning are far less relevant in environments characterized by values associated with newer knowledge about how change occurs and how individuals think and behave (Ancona & Bresman, 2007; Goleman, 1995, 1998; Greenleaf, 1996; McCrimmon, 2010; Parris & Peachey, 2013; Porter-O'Grady & Malloch, 2003, 2010). In particular, traditional approaches to teaching and learning with regard to aims, content, and methods may now serve as impediments to organizational growth and understanding models of transformation. The work of transformation requires a movement away from outdated, linear, industrial and/or hierarchical thinking toward a focus on integration, outcome, flexibility, responsiveness, holism, contingency thinking, and anticipatory openness to possibility.

As has been the case for several decades, CNSs engage and function within this dynamic context providing "expertness representing advanced or newly developed practices [in nursing]" (Peplau, 1965/2003). The *Statement on Clinical Nurse Specialist Practice and Education* (NACNS, 2004) clearly articulates a practice paradigm whereby the application of clinical expertise may occur either directly or by influencing nurses and nursing personnel through evidence-based standards and programs of care. As such, CNSs, in addition to their foundational obligation to provide expert nursing practice in the patient/client sphere, further advance nursing practice and improve patient outcomes through role modeling, consultation, education, and advocacy as they engage in work with other nurses (nursing and nursing practice sphere) and the broader organization or system.

As is evident in the description of CNS outcomes and competencies (NACNS, 2004), the work of translating clinical expertise may take many forms in the daily life of a CNS. However, the obligation to consistently and creatively transmit knowledge and skill development is most clearly apparent in the sphere of influence dedicated to nurses and nursing practice. Therein, key outcomes represent the dimension of CNS performance necessarily dedicated to the functions of instruction and facilitation of learning:

- Knowledge and skill development needs of nurses are delineated
- Nurses engage in learning experiences to advance or maintain competence
- Career enhancement programs are ongoing, accessible, innovative, and effective
- Educational programs that advance the practice of nursing are developed, implemented, evaluated, and linked to EBP and effects on clinical and fiscal outcomes

Furthermore, specific competencies demonstrate expectations that the CNS

- Utilizes and designs appropriate methods and tools to assess knowledge, skills, and practice competencies of nurses and nursing personnel to advance the practice of nursing;
- Identifies desired outcomes of continuing or changing nursing practices;
- Mentors nurses to critique and apply research evidence to nursing practices;
- Develops and implements educational programs that target the needs of staff to improve nursing practice and patient outcomes; and
- Evaluates the ability of nurses and nursing personnel to implement changes in nursing practice.

CONCEPTUAL/THEORETICAL SUPPORT

The Context of Change

Several organizing frameworks serve to enhance an understanding of the trajectory for facilitating learning in the service of nurses and nursing practice. Foundational to all tenets of instruction and education is the incorporation of a meaningful context about change. In the 21st century, the work of teaching and learning in our health care settings consistently occurs within environments characterized by complexity, variety, activity, variability, patterned chaos, and ever-present change. As soon as one has the time to consider the nuances and details of the most recent changes, new changes transpire. Porter-O'Grady and Malloch (2003, 2010) vividly depict the context wherein health care and clinical practice occur. They describe a "new vessel" where leaders, clinicians, educators, and others must exercise their intellect and demonstrate productivity in entirely new ways. Using quantum theory as the basis for their analysis, they further explicate that change is not a thing or an event, but rather a "dynamic that is constitutive of the universe" (2003, p. 6). As such, it is entirely impossible to avoid change because it is everywhere. Instead, the appropriate work or response is to influence the circumstances and consequences of change. Providing direction is the work of leading change. As Steven Hawking has stated, "Change is." Chaos, complexity, and change are not things but forms of dynamic activity, and they are the only constants in the universe. This represents a substantive paradigm shift from previous change models that prescribed a movement to and away from "freezing" (Lewin, 1951; Millay, 1995; Reinhard, 1988).

Incorporation of this current perspective regarding change should transform and revolutionize processes that de facto impede or delay innovation. It is imperative that creativity, applied knowledge, responsiveness, and openness be expected and prevail as normative behavior. It is a fundamental requisite of life to be able to adapt to ever-changing conditions. Science and technology are altering every aspect of our lives. The challenge is to embrace the new circumstances and then sort out their implications and applications as we go.

Principles of Teaching and Learning: Focus on Adults

As change represents a major contextual entity for the function of education, several principles of teaching and learning serve to frame the actual work of engaging with others to accomplish knowledge transfer and skill development. The literature is replete with a variety of philosophical perspectives and theories related to learning (Bandura, 1977; Clark, 1993; Cross, 1981; Dewey, 1938; Galbraith, 1990; Knowles, 1980; Maslow, 1987; Merriam & Brockett, 1997; Rogers, 1994; Skinner, 1974; Thorndike, Bregman, Tilton, & Woodyard, 1928). Rather than providing summative descriptions of the various theories, several principles are delineated that have been derived from an analysis of several key references (Abruzzese, 1996; Alspach, 1995; Avillion, 2008; Bastable, 2014; Bastable, Gramet, Jacobs, & Sopczyk, 2011; Billings & Halstead, 2012; Bruce, 2009; Spath, 2002) and highlight principles that address the requirements of adult learners.

Adults Need a Reason for Learning and Are Problem-Centered Learners.

Adult learners want to know why it is important for them to participate in an educational activity. They more readily engage in work-related learning activities to solve anticipated or actual problems. Their interests tend to focus on immediate application of that which has been learned in order to more effectively fulfill required role expectations or responsibilities. Motivation and readiness are enhanced to the degree that adult learners perceive that the instruction is relevant to their work. Furthermore, adults more readily place a high value on their time, given their many personal and professional obligations.

Most Adults Are Self-Directed in Their Pursuit of Learning.

It is commonly documented that adults demonstrate a preference to exercise some degree of control over what they learn and how they learn it. In addition, they typically exhibit both the need and desire to participate in determining when and where they will engage in learning activities and what kinds of activities those will be.

Adults Bring a Variety of Life and Work Experiences to Any Learning Situation.

One's personal and professional experiences enhance any learning situation and, even if not directly relevant, may serve to complement the learning process. Adults place value on their own experiences as well as those of others. Furthermore, adults expect that others, most notably the individual(s) engaged in the work of teaching/instruction, will recognize and value those past and current experiences.

An Adult Is Not an Adult Is Not an Adult.

Adults are heterogeneous as learners and deserve respect as mature individuals. Unlike school-age children who experience a strong pressure to conform, adults more commonly value their independence in thought and behavior. In addition, adult learners have considerably more diverse backgrounds and, as such, may require varying degrees of support in learning. Developmental stages vary across the trajectory of the adult life span and flexibility may fluctuate concomitantly. For example, habits, attitudes, values, and behaviors evolve over many years of life experience and may be more deeply embedded in the older adult learner than in those who are younger.

Adults Are Voluntary Learners.

The option of seeking employment and subsequently engaging in required learning activities may occur for any number of reasons. Some individuals will present with altruistic motivation and high levels of professional commitment. Others may primarily be interested in securing a paycheck, obtaining improved benefits, or changing to a new employer after having been downsized from a more prestigious position. The possibilities and motivations are almost limitless. Nonetheless, the essential understanding is that learner engagement is likely affected by the situation that precipitates voluntary entry into the learning process.

Principles Related to Learning

Having given consideration to the reality that adults are the key recipients of learning interventions in the sphere of influence related to nurses and nursing practice, it is also necessary to delineate other evidence-based learning principles that should be incorporated as CNSs exercise their leadership in the development of others. These fundamental precepts represent a synthesis of theoretical and empirical literature that presently guides best practice in the realm of instruction and facilitation of learning (Abruzzese, 1996; Alspach, 1995; Avillion, 2008; Barkley, 2010; Bastable, 2014; Bastable et al., 2011; Billings & Halstead, 2012; Bruce, 2009; Cannon & Boswell, 2012).

Learning Occurs as a Consequence of Self-Activity.

Learners will learn more, retain more, and achieve more effectively when they are actively involved in the learning experience. Thus, learning requires active participation by the learner. Dewey's (1916) axiom that "we learn by doing" is as true today as it was when first documented in the early 20th century. Learning is a dynamic process that requires active participation in order to more readily accomplish educational aims.

Learning Is Influenced by the Environment Within Which It Occurs.

Both physical surroundings and psychological climate impact instruction and learning. Understandably, the process may be further influenced by virtue of the nature of clinical environments wherein CNSs and their clinical colleagues practice. Pace, volume, and acuity provide the context for new learning and application of principles in real time.

Complexity and variability in processes, environment, and personnel further complicate one's trajectory for learning, whether new to the profession, new to the organization, or new to the focus for requisite instruction.

Empirical evidence demonstrates that physical environment can facilitate learning when it includes adequate lighting, temperature control, and acoustics; when media can be readily seen and heard; and when learners are comfortable in their seating and workspace (Bastable, 2014; Galbraith, 1990). The dilemma of crafting this type of ideal environment in the midst of a clinical reality characterized by "just-in-time" learning needs, complexity, and extraordinary demands to preserve patient safety and sustain high-quality outcomes becomes readily evident.

Learning Is Social and Interactive. Similar to the perspective that links learning outcomes with environmental appropriateness, it is also essential to understand that the psychological environment impacts learning as well. Learning is substantively enhanced in an environment characterized by consistent and supportive interpersonal interactions, engaged responsiveness, acknowledgment of existing knowledge and competence, and a spirit of inquiry, fairness, and openness. Learning is a responsibility shared between teachers and learners. Thus, CNSs can facilitate learning by way of their social interactions with staff by relating to them as trustworthy colleagues who deserve recognition and by welcoming them to the process of growth and enhanced understanding. Interpersonal skill and application of emotional intelligence on the part of the CNS are critical to the process of engaged, interactive learning. The degree to which one postures in a hierarchical way gravely diminishes any potential for free expression of learning needs or any openness to the wisdom of the CNS. Learners will actively avoid individuals who project an "aura" of hierarchy, thus defeating any opportunity for CNS influence in the early development of excellence in practice.

Learning Is Intentional and Is Influenced by the Motivation and Readiness of the Learner. In concert with the understanding that adults are most commonly self-directed in their pursuit of learning, it stands to reason that learning is most effective when it is directed at objectives or aims that the learner interprets as being meaningful and useful. Motivation is enhanced when learners can participate in identifying their needs and in the planning activities that would meet those needs. It is important to note that motivation to learn waxes and wanes in response to stress, fatigue, demands, hassle factors, and/or perception about the relevance (or lack thereof) of learning activities. Evidence further suggests that positive intrinsic

motivators (e.g., a personal sense of accomplishment, self-satisfaction, feelings of competence, and subsequent role security) enhance the process of learning more than negative extrinsic motivators (e.g., threats, criticism, punishment for "noncompliance"). As the old adage suggests, "Success breeds success." Thus, one of the strongest motivators for continued interest and engagement in learning is the experience of success. Similarly, readiness to learn is shaped by an individual's personal state of physical, psychological, social, and intellectual preparedness for learning and is an intrinsic characteristic that influences learning outcomes.

Learning Is Facilitated by Positive and Immediate Feedback. As noted previously, successful performance of a newly learned or improved skill provides a strong motivating stimulus for continued learning. Thus, timely recognition of successful achievement of a learning outcome is critical to sustain the momentum for ongoing growth and development. The impact of positive feedback is well described as a critical element that enforces optimal performance (Alspach, 1995; Fitzgerald & Keyes, 2014; Wlodkowski, 1990). It may take many forms, including verbal recognition, encouragement, or written comments. As such, CNSs can be very influential in terms of noticing and intentionally/publically acknowledging positive outcomes and/or success of individuals, teams, units, or organizations.

Learning Is Retainable and Can Be Transferred to New Situations. Despite the pressure exacted by many learners requiring new information or knowledge, retention and transference of learning are best accomplished by preliminarily introducing general principles (e.g., standards, guidelines, concepts, norms) before exceptions to general principles are introduced. The habit of eagerly introducing a new learner to all the "shortcuts" or exceptions that one has acquired over years of previous experience adds no value whatsoever to the attainment of an appropriate understanding of the phenomenon of interest. The ability to tolerate ambiguity or variance requires a higher level of cognitive interpretation and evolves as one acquires more *experiential* knowledge accumulated over time. Thus, it is reasonable to expect that as one is learning a new process, it is easier to learn the *usual* process before attempting to learn how the process may differ for emergent situations, atypical patients, or some other type of variable. Premature instruction related to exceptions or variation tends to provoke a sense of personal distress about limited capacity or evoke a crisis of trust about others and their level of understanding or support. At the very least, precipitous attention to variation and exceptions tends to confuse learners who may experience a sense of being overwhelmed by unnecessary details provided too soon.

Learning Is Inferred Rather Than Observed. The fundamental manifestation that learning has occurred is the subsequent observation that behavior has changed. These changes may be demonstrated in actual work performance (which is ideal and preferred), in a simulated experience, in documentation, or by way of verbal or written evidence. Embedded in this premise is the understanding that there are three essential domains of learning: cognitive, affective, and psychomotor. As such, observations of behavioral change as a consequence of learning are correlated with these domains. That is, psychomotor performance related to fine motor, manual, or gross motor skills is best assessed in a situation that requires demonstration of the ability to manipulate equipment, coordinate physical movements around a task, or exercise gross body movement to accomplish a requirement. Evidence that affective learning has occurred is revealed when learners manifest attitudes, beliefs, and values that are compatible with the aims of the learning experience or, more broadly, with the philosophy of the sponsoring organization. Thus, observation of individual performance *in context* is more likely to provide verification of affective learning, though that is not the only method to confirm that values or beliefs have been changed as a consequence of an instructional intervention. Behavioral changes in the cognitive domain are manifested in a variety of ways. Often written tests are used to determine if learners possess adequate knowledge requisite for their position. It is important to note, however, that distinction among levels of cognitive performance (e.g., knowledge, comprehension, application, analysis, synthesis, and evaluation) may mandate different approaches to verify integrated/internalized behavioral manifestation of learning.

Learning Is Influenced by the Nature of the Learning Experience. Given that learning is a continual and dynamic process of integrating new information or skills with existing knowledge or competence, learners are continually adding, subtracting, modifying, or changing what they previously held to be true. As such, it is critical that instructional interventions be suitable for the content and skills that are to be learned and vary in response to learners' progress and development. The burden of success rests with the instructor's sensibility about the relevance and utility of the learning experience and his or her correlated response to modify learning experiences in order to sustain the momentum of discovery and accomplishment. There is nothing less helpful than iterating and reiterating the same message or technique in light of evidence suggesting that the experience is not moving learners to change anything. The fun part of the work of instruction and learning is engaging in the interactive and dynamic exchange with learners and implementing creative instructional solutions to accomplish learning outcomes. It is also important to note that the business of *unlearning* also is relevant to this analysis. That is, as organizational change precipitates new performance requirements or new technology or any other phenomenon that generates a necessity for new learning, it may also render obsolete previous customary procedures or standards of care. Thus, experienced learners may have considerable amounts of knowledge to unlearn if new procedures, products, or processes differ considerably from what they have been accustomed to. This reality may also provoke a stance of resistance when new learning expectations conflict with prior experience or understanding. Correspondingly, less experienced staff have less of a need to unlearn because their experience is limited.

Finally, it is evident that learning proceeds best when it is organized and clearly communicated (Alspach, 1995). Instructional organization of principles to be delivered facilitates the transfer, acquisition, and integration of knowledge to new situations. Furthermore, clear communication of the purpose, aims, objectives, and outcomes of the learning experience establish the context and expectations for behavioral change, performance, and normative standards. It is also important to note that every learning experience should be targeted and focused toward accomplishing a delineated set of outcomes. Often there is a tendency to be sure that every possible nuance of a learning topic is "excavated" and addressed. Retention and mastery of content is enhanced when clear delineation of realistic expectations are articulated and instructional interventions correlate with a sensible scope of expectation.

Novice to Expert

An extraordinarily useful developmental framework of how individuals come to know and engage in clinical practice has been developed and empirically validated by Patricia Benner (1984) and colleagues (Benner, Tanner, & Chesla, 1996, 2009). This paradigm has substantive implications for reforming instructional interventions in the clinical world. A fundamental construct is that practice without theory cannot alone produce fully skilled behavior in the complex working situations experienced by nurses. This is a common professional belief that is well understood and valued in nursing. The critical consideration articulated by Benner et al. (1996, 2009) that leads to a more accurate understanding of the nature of progression in practice is that theory without practice experience has even a lesser chance of producing fully realized success in the field. Thus, it is critical to understand that theory and experience intertwine in a mutually supportive process as nurses continually develop their skills. Only when both dimensions are cultivated and valued can full expertise be realized.

Five stages of development have been described: novice, advanced beginner, competent, proficient, and expert (Benner, 1984; Benner et al., 1996, 2009). Each stage is characterized by manifestations that should direct those charged with instruction and development to respond and design appropriate interventions that make sense and have logical congruity with the prevailing behaviors and learning needs exhibited at that stage. For example, the term *novice* is typically and mistakenly used to describe anyone who is new to a situation. More accurately, the term refers to individuals who have virtually no background, understanding, or *experience* of a given clinical situation. Thus, the term more appropriately describes the stage of practice manifested by nursing students who have no previous experiential or practical knowledge upon which to base their judgments or interventions. Thus, through instruction, the novice requires and acquires *rules* for drawing conclusions or determining actions based upon facts of the situation that are recognizable without experience in the skill domain that is being learned. For example, if one is learning to drive a car and has never done so before, the novice driver is given a rule or formula for the safe distance at which to follow another car at a given speed. From an experiential perspective, instructional time is not spent describing what a car looks like because this knowledge is assumed to have been already acquired. Rather, the emphasis is placed on the targeted rule that will frame safe performance. It is important to note that nuances related to safe distance and safe speed as they are applied in varying environmental conditions (e.g., snow, sleet, rain) cannot be fully understood or learned until there is a concomitant experiential learning event where the three interactive variables occur simultaneously.

In contrast to the context-free *rules* that are taught to novices, advanced beginners require extensive, guided experiences with patients so that they can readily identify components of recurring patient situations. Advanced beginners in nursing typically include new graduates or experienced nurses who have transferred to a setting where they have no previous *experiential knowledge* (e.g., staff nurse from an inpatient general practice unit transferring to the OR to work as a circulating nurse). Clinical situations present to advanced beginners as a set of *tasks* that must be accomplished. The task requirements

are central at this stage, and all other aspects of the clinical situation, such as the patient's changing condition or the family's concerns or distress, do not form the background for their focus. It is critical to understand that this is not a flaw in the individual. This is a normal developmental stage in the journey to acquiring expertise across a broad range of aspects of practice. It is suggested that everyone who engages in staff development of any kind reflect back on his or her early practice and recall how personal success was perceived and measured. Recall the thrill and relief associated with getting through a shift, completing every task that needed to be done, starting an IV, finishing report on time, and managing to avoid incurring the wrath of a more seasoned colleague. This represents an appropriate trajectory and focus for individuals early in their career. Personal distress is rampant during this stage and is only exacerbated by arrogant and insensitive posturing by more experienced individuals who express concerns about progression and expectations that are unrealistic and unfair.

Competence in practice is typically demonstrated by nurses who have been in the same or similar clinical practice for 18 months or more. Nurses practicing at this level differ from advanced beginners in their improved organizational ability and technical skills. This increase in skill opens up possibilities for noticing and developing new clinical knowledge so that in *familiar situations* they have an increased ability to anticipate a likely course of events and respond appropriately. The work of the nurse at this stage is typically organized around the work of planning for and anticipating likely events in the given course of a patient situation. The language of the nurse is more process focused, and one detects a commitment to setting and accomplishing goals. It is at this stage that one also begins to see the manifestation of disillusionment because the nurse is more able to detect the fallibility of other providers and recognize gaps in scientific knowledge. This can provoke a sense of crisis as the realization grows that not everyone is as competent or supportive as was previously thought. Furthermore, at this stage, nurses realize that they are responsible not only for task accomplishment but also for subsequent outcomes. This growing awareness that one has actual authority for a defined scope of practice and is accountable for patient outcomes can provoke a sense of personal distress about limited capacity. Constructive, supportive, and caring developmental support by the CNS at this stage is critically important and can influence a trajectory of ongoing success and progression of the nurse. If the CNS, manager, or other more experienced nurses on the unit are unable to discern the nature of "tension" within the intellect of a competent nurse at this stage and take up a judgmental or punitive stance, they likely will delay or interfere with the nurse's progression to proficiency and expertise. In the worst case scenario, inappropriate interpretation of competency in practice and negative judgment/criticism thereof can contribute to the evolution and development of disengagement in the developing competent nurse.

Proficiency is a stage of transition between competency and expertise. Benner and her colleagues (1996, 2009) describe that practice is transformed in five major ways:

1. Development of engaged reasoning in transitions;
2. Emotional attunement to a situation—doing what needs to be done;
3. Ability to recognize changing relevance of aspects in the clinical situation;
4. Socially skilled sense of agency; and
5. Improved and more differentiated skills of involvement with patients and families.

Increased perceptual acuity and responsiveness to a *particular* situation are hallmarks of this stage. Performance at this level requires an experiential base with a *particular* patient population because the skills noted previously depend on having a perceptual grasp of qualitative distinctions, which can only be acquired by seeing and contrasting patterns of clinical manifestations in a variety of situations as they evolve over time.

Expert nurses have extensive experience and possess an intuitive grasp of clinical situations. They identify critical problem areas without having to review multiple alternatives. They are smooth and fluid in the initiation of appropriate interventions. Expert nurses detect subtle changes, and their performance is characterized by a fusion of thought and action. They are able to see the big picture and accurately derive salient features from the clinical situation, and they demonstrate embodied "know-how." The practice of expert nurses is further characterized by strong moral agency and an overt commitment to the preservation of personhood, patient attunement, and respect for the dignity and integrity of patients and families.

Given that most organizations invest the vast majority of their nursing developmental dollars in the work of onboarding, early orientation, residency programs, and/or annual competency validation, it becomes essential for CNSs to take up the work of higher level development of nurses progressing from competency to proficiency or proficiency to expertise. In these instances and in accordance with the documented outcomes of CNS practice within the sphere of nurses and nursing practice (NACNS, 2004), the experienced CNS who demonstrates clinical mastery with respect to a particular patient population or domain of practice

has the obligation to delineate the "knowledge and skill development needs of nurses" and engage nurses in "learning experiences to advance or maintain competence" (pp. 31–32). Understanding the context and language of Benner and her colleagues (1996, 2009; Benner, Hooper-Kyriakidis, & Stannard, 2011), the CNS needs to be instrumental in facilitating the development of nurses beyond competency. Experiential knowing and development in the clinical world is best guided by those who have accomplished proficiency, expertise, or mastery in the care of patients/families/ groups and who are able to see, discern, and manage the unique phenomena (particulars) that present in varying clinical situations.

Leadership Principles

The NACNS *Statement on Clinical Nurse Specialist Practice and Education* (2004) clearly identifies that leadership is an essential CNS characteristic required for effective practice in all spheres of influence. In order to accomplish an educational agenda and facilitate learning outcomes, the NACNS statement articulates a set of leadership skills that are critical for delineating and analyzing a problem, formulating a strategic vision and plan, deriving creative solutions and possibility for change, and inspiring others to action. These include

- Interpersonal skills of listening, validating, reflecting, providing constructive feedback, and conveying a caring attitude;
- An ability to formulate and logically convey ideas while being sensitive to the needs and feelings of others;
- Utilization of nursing science and knowledge generated by related disciplines;
- Creation of innovations in patient care;
- An ability to think critically, make decisions, and synthesize scientific knowledge for application to practice;
- Participation in research, clinical inquiry projects, and research utilization including cost analysis;
- Creation and implementation of evidence-based change to improve safety, quality, and cost-effectiveness;
- Collaborative systems thinking that detects that which is working well, that which requires revision, and that which will best predict the successful accomplishment of high-quality and cost-effective outcomes;
- A shared decision-making philosophy that encourages strong working relationships among nurses and other multidisciplinary health care providers.

As a corollary to these identified skills, it is also important to recall the perspective advanced by

Porter-O'Grady and Malloch (2003, 2010). It is their thesis that leadership is fundamentally concerned with adaptation to change. Given the assumptions and realities exhibited in the present-day health care arena, leaders need to be fluid and adaptable because their role changes in concert with the ever-changing conditions.

> Leaders are aware that it is in the pursuit of meaning that the direction of change can best be discerned. They continually look past the real and the present toward the unformed and potential to better evaluate the present and the direction of transformation. The subtle themes and ebbs and flows that lie just beneath the surface of events and experiences have more to say to leaders than the events themselves. (2003, p. 36)

This represents a vastly different paradigm than that espoused less than one generation ago when leadership meant being a good manager, guiding one's peers and subordinates like a good parent, and directing their activities in the interest of the organization. The critical skills were those required for planning, organizing, directing, and controlling (Marriner, 1980). In the current context of complexity and change, *authentic* leaders are motivated by the connections that give meaning and value to the current reality. For example, motivated leaders focus on potential, share the work, understand that new kinds of work are evolving and requisite, and do different work differently. Unmotivated leaders focus on the present, wallow in the negative, project that things consistently are getting worse, and manifest a disengaged stance.

Leadership skills are learned, and their mastery does not require extraordinary intellectual capability. As is evident from even a basic/fundamental review of world history, leaders emerge in a wide variety of circumstances and manifest an extensive range of talents and personalities. There is no one "correct" pattern of behavior or personality type that is most suitable for the leadership role. What leaders have in common, however, is the ability to understand the complexities and nuances of human interactions and relationships. They appreciate patterns revealed in a chaotic and ever-changing world and are able to "straddle" that which is current and that which is evolving. Furthermore, they are optimistic, energetic, and able to engage others in the journey of progress toward a visionary and preferred future. Even though one may hear in practice that some characterize competencies related to emotional intelligence, shared leadership, interpersonal skills, and relationship-based practice as "soft skills," there is substantive evidence (Cadmus, 2013; Lyon, 2010; Porter-O'Grady & Malloch, 2003, 2010; Zuzelo, 2010) demonstrating

that these types of abilities related to preserving personhood and engaging in humane practices are central and essential to crafting a role of influence and leadership as a CNS. Relationships and relationship building are central to the construct of "influence" that characterizes the work of CNS practice.

STRATEGIES FOR ENGAGING STAFF IN LEARNING: APPLICATIONS TO CNS PRACTICE

It is essential to preface the subsequent discussion with the fundamental disclaimer that educational intervention is absolutely *not* the universal solution to every problem or practice gap that may be detected in a clinical setting. Far too often, the standard response to any demonstrated need, less than desirable clinical outcome, or performance gap is to first and foremost set out on a quest to "educate them." Perhaps even more distressing is the notion that gathering nurses together in some kind of a collective herd for a staff development program is necessarily the preferred method for imparting wisdom and leading the masses to the "promised land." Wright (2004) reports that only 10% to 15% of all problematic issues in nursing practice are due to knowledge or skill deficits. She identifies that several other factors may better serve to explain undesirable variance in outcomes such as system problems, communication barriers, attitudinal issues, individual performance patterns, unavailability of necessary tools or equipment, or departmental barriers. Indeed, there is a vast body of literature demonstrating that breakdown or errors in practice are frequently associated with phenomena that have nothing to do with the intellect, knowledge, or cognitive grasp of the nurse engaged in the situation (Ebright, 2010; Ebright, Patterson, & Render, 2002; Ebright, Patterson, Chalko, & Render, 2003; Zuzelo, 2010). Yet, the solutions that are frequently articulated in formal root cause analyses routinely prescribe educational (telling/teaching) interventions despite documented evidence therein that nurses knew/understood what they should have done. It is critical that CNSs discern the fine distinctions among well-reasoned advocacy, system barriers, and knowledge deficit when they work to develop nurse colleagues as a dimension of their role. It is critical that CNSs exercise appropriate leadership within the organizational/system sphere to assure that practices "in the larger system facilitate nursing practice for improvement of quality cost-effective outcomes" (NACNS, 2004, p. 20).

In any case, it is clearly the obligation of those exercising clinical leadership to participate in the careful analysis of these problems and to accurately assess why they occurred. An educational intervention should be designed and implemented only when there is clear evidence that a lack of knowledge or skill was the underlying reason for the problem.

Facilitating Learning by Creating Opportunity

In light of the conceptual and theoretical support presented thus far, the development of strategies to engage staff in learning must necessarily be framed within a context of creativity and encouragement. As a clinical leader and expert, the CNS's role is to create opportunity that encourages employees' personal and professional growth. The American Nurses Association (ANA, 2010) has outlined the scope and standards of practice for nursing professional development. Several philosophical statements direct one to interpret that the creative work of professional development requires a substantive commitment far beyond obligations associated with meeting regulatory or task-focused requirements. The work of facilitating the development of fully engaged nursing professionals transcends a notion of something "nice to do" to something essential and necessary to do. Again, there exists an abundance of literature that recommends and describes a wide range of strategies to accomplish staff learning outcomes (Abruzzese, 1996; Alspach, 1995; Avillion, 2008; Bastable, 2014; Bastable, Gramet, Jacobs, & Sopczyk, 2011; Billings & Halstead, 2012; Bruce, 2009; Spath, 2002). The subsequent focus is targeted to address those strategies that are most consistent with a realistic picture of current practice environments where one is essentially "building the bridge as one walks on it" (Quinn, 2004).

Mentoring and Coaching

There is substantial evidence that supports and prescribes mentorship and coaching as strategies that facilitate the development and transformation of nurses in practice (Benner et al., 1996, 2009, 2011; Cadmus, 2013; Cunningham & McNally, 2003; Dracup & Bryan-Brown, 2004; Ervin, 2005; Goudreau, 2010; Grossman, 2012; Penn, 2008; Robinson-Walker, 2004; Waddell & Dunn, 2005; Wilson & Porter-O'Grady, 1999). The NACNS (2004) standards specifically identify mentoring as a necessary competency in the sphere of influence related to nurses and nursing practice.

Merriam-Webster's Online Dictionary (2013) defines *mentor* as a "trusted counselor or guide" (2013b), *preceptor* as a "teacher, tutor" (2013c) and *coach* as "one who instructs or trains a performer, or team of performers" (2013a). The role of *preceptor* is usually limited in time, to orientation or validation of competency for a specific required skill (Penn, 2008). In contrast, a *mentor's* role is ongoing and requires a higher level of knowledge and expertise because a mentor not only serves as a role model and resource but also assists an individual in acquiring new knowledge and skills. The role is formalized when the mentor also creates a formal educational plan with an individual to assist him or her in developing his or her practice, including a range of competencies or aspects of practice. The mentor and protégé meet regularly to discuss progress toward identified goals and any new needs that have arisen (Cadmus, 2013; Cannon & Boswell, 2012).

Coaching can be either formal or informal. It is characterized as a process in which the *learner* sets the agenda, identifies the challenges or needs that are present, and postulates strategies and pathways that will facilitate growth and accomplishment. At its root, coaching is about change. The coach is a partner who can enhance the learner's understanding of his or her present reality. The coach is a "guide on the side" or a "guide from behind" who is skilled in the process of sorting out what is working well, letting go of what is no longer serving well, and assisting in the development of new skills and practices that are required for future success.

Coaching provides "just-in-time" learning. It is listening and focused facilitation that is 100% dedicated to the agenda of the staff member in transition. In the healthiest of situations, the coach is somewhat like a friend in that he or she is dedicated to the learner's needs and is genuine in his or her interest and care. The coach is unlike a friend in that he or she is guided by objectivity, is external to or "outside" of the personal experience, and has a primary stake in the outcome of the relationship such that the learner demonstrates forward progress and expresses satisfaction thereof (Cannon & Boswell, 2012; Klein, 2007; Penn, 2008). Given the span of responsibility that is embedded in the definition of the CNS role (NACNS, 2004), it is apparent that coaching as a behavior is requisite and foundational to interactions and relationships with nursing staff. The actions and intent associated with coaching and mentoring should be obvious and prevalent in the day-to-day practice of any CNS.

Facilitating Development Around Stages of Practice

Advanced Beginners. In most instances, the work of developing the practice of advanced beginners is assigned to preceptors. However, there are common misconceptions about how best to frame the learning experience of our newest colleagues in practice.

The strategies described may be directly applied by CNSs as they make rounds and encounter orientees in practice. Another possibility is that the strategies could be reinforced among preceptors who most likely assume the bulk of responsibility for local orientation. In either instance, the principles are critical for ensuring an appropriate learning intervention that facilitates the transition toward competence (Benner et al., 1996, 2009).

Benner and her colleagues (1996, 2009) articulate that beginners require a historical context and some kind of dialogue about the possible future course of any given patient situation. They simply have not had adequate experience to see a given population of patients with varied disease processes through complete illness trajectories. Thus, it is useful to provide a *context* for presenting symptoms as they arise and to let the learner know what is and is not to be expected with particular categories of patients or illnesses. Dialogue about typical expectations in the course of a normal experience is helpful. The advanced beginner can then begin to "see" or detect routine presentations and achieve some level of security about his or her observations. Without context or a grasp of normal clinical expectations, how would anyone with limited experiential knowledge about patterns be able to discern a variation from normal in context?

Because the clinical world of the advanced beginner revolves around tasks and procedures and the patient situation more frequently shows up as background, it is helpful then to assist the learner by linking together the sometimes disjointed components of report, the chart, and clinical presentation of the patient into a meaningful whole. This will facilitate the learner's ability to detect some kind of order in the immense and sometimes conflicting information that exists for each patient and fluctuates from moment to moment.

Providing care in other ways than "by the book" requires practical reasoning gained by experience over time. Thus, it is *not* helpful to divert beginners from the rules or standards by which they were taught. Instead, it is more affirming and encouraging to recognize that the learner is replicating the standard process and to acknowledge his or her accomplishment when he or she has completed it.

Advanced beginners live in a world of insecurity and concern about the adequacy of their performance overall. They can be assisted by offering opportunities to review and contemplate situations that did not go particularly well. Questions about why a particular patient died or why certain actions were or were not taken frequently go unanswered. It is useful to review complex or interesting cases by specifically examining the decisions and actions that were documented in a patient chart. This approach distances the learner from some of the emotion faced in the situation and provides an opportunity to learn from experience that is grounded in a specific case.

It is critical to assist the advanced beginner in knowing how to safely "delegate up." Sadly, not everyone in a clinical setting is motivated to be supportive and helpful to new employees or learners. Similarly, not all experienced individuals demonstrate sufficient competency with all of the skills and knowledge required for clinical practice. Thus, a key strategy early in the trajectory of development for the beginner is to identify safe, knowledgeable, and willing persons who will assist him or her through any dilemmas he or she may encounter. In this capacity, it is the obligation of every CNS to assume a stance of availability and openness that welcomes the questions and accepts the vulnerability of someone new to a setting.

There is a substantial teaching role in helping advanced beginners manage aspects of nursing that occur away from direct patient care. Included in this are issues such as obtaining appropriate physician response and managing interactions with other services such as laboratories, dietary, and pharmacy. Because the advanced beginner is characteristically so focused on patient care (e.g., getting through the shift, task completion), the smooth acquisition of skill related to problem resolution with the larger system should not be the focus of instruction at this phase. Rather, interventions should be targeted toward assisting this learner with requisite skills associated with working with physicians. Learners benefit from information about fundamental situations that require questioning. It is helpful to reinforce beginners' correct judgments about situations when they are in conflict with physicians' assessments or plans. Most importantly, it is essential to coach the learner in formulating a "script" for proposing something that will more likely evoke a responsive action. For example, the utilization of the situation–background–assessment–recommendation (SBAR) communication approach provides a useful framework for organizing one's thoughts during a situational briefing (Institute for Healthcare Improvement [IHI], 2006).

It is imperative that advanced beginners work in environments where they feel secure asking questions. In order to maintain a safe clinical experience for patients, it is essential that beginners' inexperience not be judged as personal inadequacy but recognized as an expected phase in the development of clinical judgment. Most hazardous to patients are environments that are interpersonally threatening, that punish early mistakes, or that set up barriers to the free exchange of questions from advanced beginners. Despite the reality that "official" orientation may conclude after 6, 8, 10, or 12 weeks, it is crucial to sustain some type of mentoring or coaching relationship for at least 6 months. Giles and Moran (1989) discovered that the option of maintaining a recognized relationship between each advanced beginner and one experienced nurse for the full duration was most efficacious. In reality, the need for support and continuing orientation does not automatically end on the day that someone is counted in staffing.

Becoming Competent

Benner and colleagues (1996, 2009) note that nurses practicing at the competent stage differ primarily from advanced beginners by their increased clinical understanding, technical skill, organizational ability, and the ability to anticipate the likely course of events. This stage is further characterized by a degree of disillusionment because nurses begin to detect fallibility in the system, gaps in scientific knowledge, and the existence of nonaltruistic motivation in others. Unfortunately, it is common to observe that responses to nurses at this stage may be dismissive in nature and suggestive that their concerns are a symptom of adjustment problems rather than legitimate observations of systems issues that require intervention and resolution. One of the most supportive strategies at this stage is to truly listen to their struggles rather than insisting that they cope or get along. This can be a mechanism for creating institutional renewal that can break the cycle of disillusionment and departure or disengagement from the profession. It is personally very compelling to recall the extreme pain and disillusionment expressed by a competent nurse about 2 years into her practice in a large perioperative service where she routinely observed and experienced verbal abuse secondary to an excessive system of authority gradient. More tragic was the complacency of others and their inability to take action to bring a halt to this long-standing pattern of violence. Needless to say, this nurse with exceptional intellect and potential left the setting and struggled with her career decision thereafter. Fortunately, a CNS and clinical educator on her new unit collaborated to debrief and design an intervention that combined instructional requirements with consistent interpersonal support that facilitated her transition to proficient practice after another period of 18 months.

Because competent nurses rely heavily on goal setting and planning, they can further benefit from ongoing practice in problem identification. Exercises in determining which of many competing problems is the most salient can increase their capability with respect to discernment. Similarly, practice in seeing the "big picture," through detailed case analysis or following patterns of patient responses as depicted in the electronic record or flow sheet, can enhance

understanding of the relationship between patient response and related therapy. It is also useful at this stage to share personal narratives, stories, or exemplars that reveal mistakes or things that went wrong. Often dramatic and emotional, yet very memorable, these types of shared experiences can be more effective in modifying behavior than procedural accounts of standard practice or that which *should* be done.

As one reflects on typical instructional patterns in clinical settings, it is common to observe a monumental investment in orientation and staff development during the early phase of employment or internal transfer. Additional instructional investment is routinely provided in order to accomplish mandatory competency requirements on an annual basis. Despite evidence that suggests that the stage of competency represents a highly vulnerable period in the transition to proficiency and expertise (Benner et al., 1996, 2009), one rarely hears of interventions designed to manage this developmental stage of skill acquisition in terms of debriefing disillusionment, clarifying manifestations of hyperresponsibility, or learning about skill of involvement with patients and families. CNSs are uniquely prepared to facilitate this type of intervention, given their expert grasp of clinical phenomena, ability to see the larger picture, and aptitude for providing nurses with a venue for articulating their concerns. More importantly, because the CNS is engaged in the organization and system sphere, he or she can advocate for appropriate reform and resolution of issues at a higher level. The degree to which the CNS seriously takes up the phenomena of concern experienced by advanced beginners and competent nurses in any organization is correlated with the reality that patients in that setting will experience care delivery that is congruent with documented best practices. CNSs are in a unique position to organize, analyze, and integrate grounded data and institutional data related to negative outcomes in the system. As such, they have a moral and ethical obligation to advocate for substantive changes that improve/enhance the experience of both patients and providers. Avoidance and/or a stance that dismisses legitimate issues as "the way it is around here," are not congruent with the principles of CNS practice (NACNS, 2004).

Proficiency: A Transition to Expertise

Benner et al. (1996, 2009) suggest that new kinds of staff development be implemented for nurses who are becoming proficient. Narratives of learning told in small groups that focus on changing one's perspectives and expectations in a clinical situation can be very instructive and support the advancement of skill development in problem identification and responsiveness to salient patient manifestations. It is important for the individual who is leading this exercise to publicly recognize the learner's detection of changing clinical relevance and acknowledge the thinking as being legitimate and astute. This is a very different instructional stance than being critical that the individual had the incorrect perception or plan from the outset. Instead, the developmental and instructional work is to flesh out the thinking and judgment exhibited by the nurse that changes with evolving clinical data.

At this stage of practice, it is critical that nurses become more skilled at negotiating with physicians (Benner, 1996, 2009). As they become more adept at detecting changing relevance in the patient's circumstances, the capacity to adequately communicate that to those who are often functioning away from the actual situation becomes ever more essential. Negotiating clinical knowledge requires interpersonal skill, trust in one's own grasp, and a capacity to see the situation from a different vantage point. That being the case, instructional strategies that simulate responses characterized by skepticism, intellectual challenge, acceptance, or complacency can assist the learner in targeting his or her communication so that the risk to patients is minimized.

Saliency is a key phenomenon of interest in communication. Nurses growing into proficiency require validation from clinical experts and masters that their "hypothesis" or interpretation of that which is most prominent or "conspicuous" is accurate. CNS engagement and dialogue regarding these higher levels of thinking are critical to facilitating the development of proficiency and expertise.

Perhaps the most important consideration in facilitating learning with proficient nurses or those transitioning to that level of practice is the reality that one's *authentic* engagement, support, acceptance, and receptivity can actually contribute to the individual's formation around moral agency. This is a very powerful obligation, and the work of assisting nurses to know what things can and cannot wait has substantive implications for the well-being of patients and families. The courage associated with exercising appropriate judgment and intellect for the benefit of others, and sometimes with some degree of real risk, can only be achieved when supported by those who are similarly committed to role modeling their own response-based practice in concrete situations. That is, the CNS must "walk the talk." If the developing nurse observes that the CNS "tells" one story about what is best practice and "acts" very differently, all credibility is lost. The work of development with more proficient/expert clinicians demands authenticity and integrity.

Expertise in Practice

Perhaps the most important intervention related to working with nurses at the expert stage is to study and learn from their practice. Indeed, their frame of reference is extraordinarily valuable, as they are able to provide experiential evidence and observations that inform a grounded perspective in terms of patient/family trajectory and clinical manifestations. Implications from this type of analysis should arm the CNS with information to bring forward in larger organizational venues. Narrative evidence suggests that all too often expert nurses must engage in Herculean efforts to overcome organizational impediments to their practice (Benner et al., 1996, 2009, 2011). Typically, structures and processes are geared toward minimal expectations, "pushing excellence to the unacknowledged and unaccommodated margins" (1996, p. 169). Leveling organizational structures and policies to the *minimal* standards of performance only serves to mask the very examples of excellence that should be highlighted and perpetuated in practice. Consequently, this handicaps leaders in the organization by forcing an emphasis on fixing deficits rather than designing for excellence. Simple compliance is not the answer for movement toward fully engaged and empowered practice. It is essential, then, to study the patterns of expert nursing practice demonstrated in our organizations/systems and to redesign structures and processes that remove barriers and facilitate a reality whereby these nurses are able to exercise the full complement of their skills and knowledge.

Instructional Strategies

Role Modeling. It is suggested (Alspach, 1995; Fitzgerald & Keyes, 2014) that CNSs are ideally suited for effectively demonstrating their expertise by role modeling key behaviors, especially in complex patient/family situations. They are able to exemplify through behavior and observable action how a particular role is assumed. Other nurses can enhance their clinical competence by observing and emulating the practice that was observed. For example, complex communication with several players exhibiting a range of intellect and emotion is a common reality in practice. Think of insecure, frightened, and frustrated families who have difficulty navigating the environment and the phenomena impacting their loved one. Add to the mix a group of service line physicians who may have a different agenda or demands and may be perceived to be in a hurry or not adequately attentive. This has the potential for evoking strong responses and interactions that only further compromise the well-being of the family. In these types of situations, it is common to call upon a CNS to facilitate the management of this type of encounter. However, the key *developmental* intervention is to purposely bring a staff nurse to the encounter and subsequently engage in a moment or two of debriefing about the key communication principles that were operationalized in the situation. This facilitates an ability to link principles with action, behavior, and outcome.

Rounds. There are many conceivable purposes for engaging in clinical rounds. Often CNSs function as partners in multidisciplinary rounds where case presentations occur and plans are crafted for transitioning patients/families toward desirable outcomes. In these instances, it goes without saying that the CNS should include the staff nurse in the process and engage him or her in participation while preserving his or her integrity and safety if the individual is at a stage where he or she is just beginning to demonstrate agency in the context of multidisciplinary communication.

More importantly, however, it is recommended that CNSs, in the course of their routine individual rounds and interactions with patients, staff, and families, use this opportunity as a vehicle for detecting exceptional practice and acknowledging progress thereof. These circumstances provide wonderful options for extending growing practice to the next stage of development. Positive feedback and reinforcement are strong motivators for continued personal investment in ongoing practice improvement. The credibility of one's expertise in the field is enhanced by relating and applying knowledge in concrete and visible ways. Concomitantly, as one engages in what may be considered to be an "environmental scan," trends, themes, and patterns of less than desirable practice may be detected as well. It is critical to confront the practice, relate the observed variance to the applicable standard/principle, provide instruction regarding the appropriate alternative, and offer concrete rationale.

Mini In-Service. In the current world of clinical practice characterized by high acuity, staffing demands, and fast pace, it is almost impossible to implement planned instructional in-services where nurses leave their environment and engage in a more formal learning encounter. However, almost every day a challenging patient/family situation will reveal itself as an opportunity for development. Because one may be required to implement a complex intervention, it would be useful to use this as a just-in-time occasion to bring a few staff together for a few minutes to demonstrate a particular skill or engage in a creative solution. Subsequently, patients will benefit from

staff learning and learners benefit because they can see the immediate application of theory to practice. Needless to say, patients and families must agree to participate in this exercise.

Family as "Faculty." The mini in-service mechanism can also set the stage for engaging patients or family as "faculty." Many patients present with long-term chronic conditions where they have achieved mastery around their ability to manage devices, navigate the health system, and vividly depict the experience of being a recipient of health care and nursing services, some that is good and some that is problematic. The personal account of a patient or family member as an instructional intervention can be extraordinarily powerful and profound. Furthermore, their acquired psychomotor skills in light of their own unique characteristics can provide nurses with enhanced understanding about modifying interventions.

Critical Incident. Davis (1995) and Abruzzese (1996) describe the critical incident teaching/learning strategy as being useful for the purpose of exploring events in the learner's own life that have relevance to a particular clinical situation. Commonly, learners initiate this type of opportunity when they reveal a personal experience that provokes a response, emotion, or crisis. In this instance, it is essential to assess the degree to which this revelation and response may impact patient care. More often, this situation affords an opportunity for learners to share clinical information and apply previously learned knowledge to the current situation. The CNS can take advantage of this by framing differences and similarities or deriving principles that are transferable to the current patient situation.

In light of the big-picture thinking that characterizes CNS practice, it is more reasonable to expect that the clinical leader will *initiate* a critical incident intervention in the face of tragic outcomes. For example, the sudden and unanticipated loss of a hospitalized child can provoke much personalization and emotion. Many nurses in the setting may be parents, and their attunement to the pain and suffering experienced by another parent will enhance their ability to connect and engage in extraordinary ways. Others at earlier developmental stages of practice may not yet have the capacity to respond in such a sensitive and involved manner. In those instances, the CNS must extend outward to include individuals in dialogue about the trajectory of engaging with patients and families in crisis. Timely, responsive, flexible, and sensitive coaching around critical incidents can foster an engaged stance required for humane and personalized care.

Strategies and Activities Linked to Principles of Adult Learning

Previously, several general learning principles and others more specific to adult learning were delineated as a theoretical/conceptual frame of reference for implementing the instructional or developmental role in CNS practice. Table 9.1 correlates these principles with relevant learning strategies and activities that could be applied in practice.

EVALUATION

There is an abundance of literature regarding the importance of evaluating learning outcomes in practice (Abruzzese, 1996; Alspach, 1995; Avillion, 2008; Bastable, 2014; Bastable et al., 2011; Billings & Halstead, 2012; Bradshaw & Lowenstein, 2011; Cannon & Boswell, 2012; JCAHO, 2008; Kirkpatrick, 1999; Oermann & Gaberson, 2009;

TABLE 9.1

TEACHING/LEARNING STRATEGIES AND ACTIVITIES CORRELATED WITH PRINCIPLES OF ADULT LEARNING	
Principle	**Strategies and Activities**
Adults need a reason for learning and are problem-centered learners	• Ask adult learners to identify problems that they perceive as most important and immediate in their work
	• Focus instruction on that which is essential for successful job performance
	• Initially, attend to learning needs and issues that are likely to be experienced on a daily basis; limit content to those areas with immediate applicability
	• Use realistic case studies and actual work scenarios
	• Provide meaningful rationale that supports the purpose for acquiring any given skill or knowledge
Most adults are self-directed in their pursuit of learning	• Provide resources and learning aids that are readily available and support the learner's quest for "just-in-time" information
	• Use a contract or timetable that articulates clear learning outcomes, yet allows the learner flexibility and options for accomplishing those aims
Adults bring a variety of life and work experiences to any learning situation	• Use critical incident methodology to link personal experience with actual learning foci. Seek out and assess the background of learners to create meaningful teaching/learning interventions
	• Design methods using small group discussion, rounds, case studies, or simulated role play to enable learners to link their past experience with current learning and facilitate transfer of understanding
Adults are heterogeneous as learners and deserve respect as mature individuals	• Expect differences in opinions, interpretations, values, and viewpoints. Use this rich diversity of thinking to progress innovative learning options
	• Avoid taking a dogmatic stance
	• Relate to learners as adults and avoid hierarchical positioning as teacher over students. Take the stance of being the "guide at the side"
	• Limit the use of arbitrary or unnecessary rules and policies in teaching/learning situations
Adults are voluntary learners	• Engage in conversation about what an individual aspires to accomplish by working in a given setting or organization
	• Detect behavioral cues (e.g., apathy, failure to complete required assignments, etc.) suggesting that the learner's needs may not be adequately addressed. The default interpretation is that there is something wrong with the learner. Instead, probe to detect the utility of the instructional intervention
	• Collaborate with the learner to brainstorm other options to accomplish the learning outcome

(continued)

TABLE 9.1

TEACHING/LEARNING STRATEGIES AND ACTIVITIES CORRELATED WITH PRINCIPLES OF ADULT LEARNING (CONTINUED)	
Principle	**Strategies and Activities**
Learning occurs as a consequence of self-activity	• Whenever possible, be sure to use active learning methods
	• Avoid overutilization of passive observational learning experiences
	• Facilitate action, thinking, reflecting, doing, practicing, talking, utilizing repetitive opportunities for psychomotor skill acquisition, and so forth
Learning is influenced by the environment within which it occurs	• Encourage staff to ask questions and challenge current practice
	• Avoid the "blunting" phenomenon by suppressing enthusiasm that comes with accomplishment. It is not helpful to suggest that a newly acquired task or skill is really "no big deal" or to suggest that "after 100 times," one will get disenchanted or jaded
	• Portray an impression of openness, acceptance, sensitivity, and care
	• Adopt a nonjudgmental stance in working with learners. Avoid threatening language
	• When engaged in an instructional activity, minimize distractions and fully attend to the learner
Learning is social and interactive	• Use realistic case studies that require learners to think, apply principles, detect subtle changes, problem-solve, and so forth
	• Bring together a small group of staff at differing stages of practice to interact around an interesting or challenging patient
	• Exercise patience
	• Be constructive when delivering a critique
	• Use humor, have fun!
Learning is intentional and is influenced by the motivation and readiness of the learner	• Suggest that learners keep a "tic" card in their pocket to jot down any intriguing findings for future instructional follow-up or dialogue
	• When rounding, ask about employee-learning goals as well as their patient care goals. Correlate any potential learning opportunities with their assignment
	• Influence assignment making that fosters intrinsic motivation by assuring that learners achieve some consistent degrees of success
	• Counsel learners to keep performance expectations realistic. The work of the advanced beginner is a normal developmental trajectory and one should not ever be made to feel badly about his or her practice
Learning is facilitated by positive and immediate feedback	• Be generous in offering support, approval, and praise
	• Provide criticism by first noting that which was done accurately/properly and then clarifying how to improve other aspects of performance
	• Plan or interject opportunities for learners to experience as much success as possible. This requires an ability to detect learner strengths and manipulate within the clinical environment to provide unique and interesting options
	• Remember that development does not end when individuals complete orientation. It is affirming to detect progress and accomplishment among *all* levels of staff

(continued)

TABLE 9.1

TEACHING/LEARNING STRATEGIES AND ACTIVITIES CORRELATED WITH PRINCIPLES OF ADULT LEARNING (CONTINUED)	
Principle	**Strategies and Activities**
Learning is retainable and can be transferred to new situations	• Review new concepts shortly after introduction
	• Summarize key instructional messages frequently and before proceeding to a new concept
	• Limit content to that which is necessary in a given situation. Do not overwhelm learners with unnecessary detail
	• Provide for adequate practice
	• Build learning activities on previous experiences
	• Progress from simple to complex; or from concrete to abstract
Learning is influenced by the nature of the learning experience	• Avoid reliance on any one instructional method, especially passive activities
	• Include learners' suggestions and preferences regarding learning activities and options
	• Inquire about discrepancies that may exist between old and new practices. Provide rationale for local differences. Avoid adopting a defensive posture
Learning proceeds best when it is organized and clearly communicated	• Use appropriate sequencing principles: easy to hard, simple to complex, concrete to abstract, first to last step
	• Use retrievable learning aids to supplement content
	• Develop small units of instruction that are organized around one major principle or construct

Penn, 2008; Spath, 2002). The critical element about evaluation in practice is an ability to detect in real terms and in real time the learners' capacity to apply principles in practice. Recall that learning is evidenced only when one observes a change in behavior. Alspach (1995) describes four steps in an evaluation process that confirm that the learner is able to translate principles into action: (a) measurement, (b), comparison, (c), appraisal, and (d) decision.

For example, at the first level, one could evaluate performance by detecting a learner's ability to simply measure. Using body weight as an example, it is easy to think about ways that one could evaluate a learner's ability to accomplish that skill. The second step of the process then suggests that the learner would be able to compare a measured outcome against an established standard for weight that is expressed in pounds or kilograms for different heights and ages. Next in the process, one would evaluate to determine if the learner can appraise the outcome. For example, he or she would interpret that the measured weight reveals that a patient is overweight, underweight, or within normal range for his or her height and age. At the final stage of the process, the learner would be able to utilize the information acquired through the first three steps to make a decision or take some

action about the finding. For example, he or she would be able to decide that someone needed to gain weight and subsequently take action to establish a nutritional consult or engage in patient teaching.

Kirkpatrick (1999) provides another framework for guiding evaluation. This model is useful in that it directs the evaluator to get to a level of validating behavioral change and impact on outcomes. Kirkpatrick describes four levels of evaluation reaction, learning, behavior, and results. Table 9.2 summarizes the key elements and characteristics of each level.

LEADING TO OUTCOME: THE UNIQUE MANIFESTATIONS OF CNS LEADERSHIP IN THE DEVELOPMENT OF OTHERS

One of the most unique features of the CNS role is the prevailing requirement and expectation that all action leads to outcome. Every assessment, plan, intervention, and consultation is directed toward enhancing quality, patient safety, and EBP. Thus, the work of engaging staff in learning is necessarily driven by these obligations and responsibilities.

TABLE 9.2

A SUMMARY OF LEVELED EVALUATION APPROACHES	
Level of Evaluation	**Characteristics of Evaluation Approach**
Reaction	• Reaction data are a measure of customer satisfaction
	• Data have applicability for improving instructional methods and program revision
	• End-of-program evaluation instruments are frequently used to assess what is commonly referred to as the "happiness factor"
	• Evaluation questions address presenter requirements (i.e., style, use of instructional aids, class timeliness, etc.)
	• Data are often gathered to assess the degree to which the instructor met the learning objectives
	• Open-ended questions are included to solicit additional comments and suggestions
	• Posttraining measurement may also be designed to occur several weeks after training has been conducted. This allows the learner to evaluate the instruction using his or her subsequent experience in practice as a context for satisfaction
Learning	• Serves to detect if the learner has actually learned anything as a consequence of the instructional activity
	• Common methods include paper-and-pencil tests to validate cognitive knowledge, skill performance validation to assess psychomotor competency, or field observation to discern application of values or organizational beliefs/standards
	• Best practice requires that there be a pre- and posttest, ideally validated with a control group
Behavior	• Determines whether learned knowledge and skill are actually applied in the workplace; also known as knowledge transfer
	• Chart reviews and audits serve to verify if learned behaviors actually occur and are documented
	• Other resources for data regarding behavior include measurement of employee performance during drills and simulations; performance measured by 360° surveys; performance reported on annual evaluation instruments; or review of other records such as code cart checklists, quality control logs, and so forth
	• Best practice requires that baseline data be collected and compared with measures subsequent to instruction
	• Unscheduled observations provide a more realistic evaluation of internalized behavior
Results	• Common indicators include time savings, better quantity, improved quality, or personnel data (e.g., fewer injuries, less absenteeism, etc.)
	• Results evaluation can only be linked to instructional intervention when an appropriate and relevant terminal program objective is imbedded in the program
	• Best practice requires that baseline data be collected and compared with measures subsequent to intervention

Quality

The identification of nursing-sensitive and multidisciplinary quality indicators has reframed the context of practice over the past few decades. Initially, the emphasis was placed on the study of processes and improvement thereof. Presently, the concern of providers, health care organizations, insurers, payers, recipients of health care, and others is focused on outcomes. This reality manifests its impact every day and in every setting where nursing and health care are delivered. Significant debate persists concerning the appropriate identification and measurement of quality indicators. The numerous ways of considering indicators can lead to confusion and frustration with quality-improvement (QI) activities, especially as it relates to measurement and resource utilization. Yet, the prevailing interest among all involved parties is that the quest for quality is essential. It is further understood that nursing makes a profound contribution to the well-being of patients and families.

How, then, does the CNS transcend the chasm between true interest and motivation toward improvement and the often prevailing sense of threat or frustration associated with measurement, tracking, and auditing? The dissonance represented by this question provides a focus for developmental intervention on the part of the CNS. The literature is replete with evidence that the CNS has a major role with respect to influencing quality processes and outcomes in practice (Benton, 2010; Duffy, 2002; Finkelman, 2013; Girouard, 2013; Saks, 1998; Zuzelo, 2010). In this capacity and with the requisite skill set and preparation, the CNS is viewed as a credible practitioner who can favorably influence clinical outcomes. From this power base, team members will be more apt to follow recommendations and suggestions. CNSs can set the tone for expected behaviors of team members in terms of open-mindedness and professionalism by way of their own demeanor. It is suggested that through mentoring, the CNS can help staff nurses develop the skills to take on additional responsibilities in the continued identification of quality indicators.

Evidence-Based Practice

Nothing appears more essential to the CNS competencies than exhibiting a fully realized commitment to the utilization of evidence in practice. Repeatedly, the NACNS (2004) statement articulates the obligation to translate clinical expertise into nursing care provided either directly or via influence of nurses and nursing personnel through evidence-based nursing. This emphasis is a key feature that distinguishes the practice of CNSs from other clinical experts and is well documented and described in the literature (Campbell & Profetto-McGrath, 2013; Ervin, 2005; Ferguson & Day, 2004; Heitkemper & Bond, 2004; Hopp, 2010; Messecar & Tanner, 2013; Newhouse, Dearholt, Poe, Pugh, & White, 2005; Stevens, 2005). Inherent in the literature are suggestions and direction with respect to the corollary developmental requirements that accompany the implementation of EBP strategies. Ervin (2005) identifies that CNSs typically have staff positions in which they interact with nurses in everyday practice. Because they usually do not have supervisory responsibilities for employees, this organizational relationship may be capitalized on to assist individual nurses to improve their skills through the mechanism of coaching and for the purpose of enhancing the use of empirical rationale for practice. Ervin suggests that a CNS can assist individuals or groups of nurses to establish plans for review of current literature. Another approach is for the CNS

to organize a group of nurses to read a specific article or journal each month and prepare a written summary for the entire staff. It is also the role of the CNS to assist staff nurses in discriminating between evidence that has been accumulated using sound methods and analysis from that which is not as robust. In this capacity, the CNS may ask targeted questions that guide thinking about the implications of information for practice within the context of patients in the particular setting. CNSs serve as role models and motivators for others to become interested in seeking answers to complex problems. Analyzing and synthesizing literature are approaches to address these problems and enhance critical thinking and judgment. Any exercise that fosters healthy discourse and debate around evidence and best practice serves to enhance the intellect of those caring for patients. Embedding a stronger sensibility around asking better questions rather than sustaining an ideology of "dogma worship" will go far to facilitate the development of an informed workforce motivated by consistent attention to inquiry. Wisdom and improved intellectual capacity are not outcomes associated with being right at all times. Instead, wisdom is fostered by open dialogue and intellectual exchange of thoughts, ideas, and informed propositions.

Safety

One of the most compelling and current requirements in clinical settings across the country is the necessary attention and effort required to ensure that patients are safe while they are recipients of nursing and health care. Ebright and colleagues (2002, 2003, 2010) have provided convincing evidence to suggest that a major developmental domain for CNS leadership is essential in four key areas: changing to a nonpunitive culture, learning about system complexity, learning about health care worker resiliency, and introducing change. They suggest that the CNS is in an excellent position to change the traditional culture of blame that typically surrounds error. An essential behavior in CNS practice is building and maintaining trust through relationships on a daily basis with patients, staff, and leadership. These relationships can serve to increase understanding from near-miss or adverse events. The key objective is to learn from these events and work collaboratively to eliminate those systems issues that precipitate the probability for error.

It is readily apparent that there exist gaps and disconnections that contribute to a practice environment characterized by complexity, hazards, and workarounds. Identification of these gaps at the point of care is essential for improving safety. To accomplish this, the CNS can contribute by leading near-miss and adverse-event investigations. In this capacity, the CNS can influence others to view these processes as opportunities for learning rather than assigning blame. He or she can role model for all health care staff *the acknowledgment and then* the setting aside of hindsight and bias. Multidisciplinary collaboration should incorporate human factors science and the New Look Model (Ebright et al., 2002), which provide an easy-to-use framework for educating others about concepts related to complex system failure as well as new approaches to safety.

CNSs are well positioned in organizations to study and detect how staff manage to navigate the complexity of the actual work environment. In the course of leading near-miss or adverse-event investigations, data can be derived that explain how staff react effectively and successfully to prevent an adverse event or minimize negative outcomes. These data can be used to design educational interventions or forums that highlight practitioner thinking, recognition, and actions. The utilization of storytelling, especially as the stories relate to successful "rescues," provides a powerful basis for studying the interface of systems processes.

Finally, it is suggested that CNSs are in a key position not only to respond to data and events. but also to anticipate and articulate the potential contribution of planned organizational changes that carry some degree of risk for creating new system gaps or latent failures (Ebright et al., 2002). Anticipating and preparing for how change might introduce new forms of complexity or latent failures is also needed to maintain safe environments.

SUMMARY

Given the current demands of the health care environment, CNSs are optimally positioned to apply their leadership, collaboration, and consultative competencies to the work of staff development. This work is consistent with standards set forth by the NACNS. The obligation to consistently and creatively transmit knowledge and skill development is most clearly apparent in the sphere of influence dedicated to nurses and nursing practice.

Theoretical and conceptual models related to the context of change, principles of teaching and learning, and leadership serve to frame strategies for engaging staff in learning as it relates to unique dimensions of CNS practice. Key interventions related to creating opportunities, coaching, mentoring, facilitating development around stages of practice, and utilizing specific strategies derived from fundamental adult learning principles are introduced to provide options for targeted learning needs. Two frameworks for evaluation are provided that validate learning outcomes

and applicability in practice. Finally, the essential work of "leading to outcome" is described as a phenomenon that distinguishes CNS practice in health care settings.

■ DISCUSSION QUESTIONS

- How does transformation differ from or relate to change?
- Chaos theory and complexity science require leaders to alter their understanding of how change works. In this context, how does the CNS operationalize his or her role in relationship to change, the larger system, the staff, and the challenges that lie ahead? Frame the discussion in light of engaging staff in learning.
- Identify at least three current educational practices or common instructional interventions that are counterproductive to facilitating learning among advanced beginners.
- How can the CNS collaborate with education specialists, clinical educators, and expert nurses to accomplish learning outcomes?
- What factors commonly contribute to an outcome where education is used inappropriately to resolve a problem, issue, need, or gap?
- What three evaluation strategies are least likely to be utilized in practice? How can the CNS go about implementing those strategies more effectively?

■ ANALYSIS AND SYNTHESIS EXERCISES

- Relate CNS competencies as described in the NACNS (2004) statement to the work of facilitating learning among clinical staff. What are the priorities in this domain of practice?
- Analyze how the recommendations documented in the IOM report on the "Future of Nursing" impact the role of the CNS in day-to-day practice.
- Relate the IOM "Future of Nursing" recommendation No. 7 (Prepare and enable nurses to lead change to advance health) to the NACNS Core competencies and outcomes (NACNS, 2004).
- Reflect on the current environment where you work. Analyze the physical surroundings and psychosocial climate in terms of facilitating a successful learning encounter. Identify modifications or adjustments that are requisite for accomplishing meaningful learning outcomes.
- Identify two different circumstances where you would engage in the work of mentoring or coaching. Analyze how the relationships would differ in each circumstance.

▓ CLINICAL APPLICATION

- Using the principles of teaching and learning, develop a learning intervention to resolve observed variability in the nursing care of a circumscribed population of patients. Assume that there exists a knowledge or skill deficit. *For example*, design a just-in-time learning intervention that reduces variability in the management of pain.
- Reflect on the talents and competencies of the nursing staff where you currently practice, and apply novice-to-expert theory to managing observed disillusionment among competent nurses.
- Apply relevant learning principles that would enhance the development of a proficient nurse in terms of improving communication with physicians.
- Construct a collaborative rounding model, including a CNS and a nursing administrator, that would facilitate learning outcomes for new graduates.

REFERENCES

Abruzzese, R. S. (1996). *Nursing staff development: Strategies for success* (2nd ed.). St. Louis, MO: Mosby.

Alspach, J. G. (1995). *The educational process in nursing staff development.* St. Louis, MO: Mosby.

American Nurses Association (ANA). (2010). *Scope and standards of practice for nursing professional development.* Washington, DC: Author.

Ancona, D. G., & Bresman, H. (2007). *X-teams: How to build teams that lead, innovate and succeed.* Cambridge, MA: Harvard Business School.

Avillion, A. E. (2008). *A practical guide to staff development: Evidence-based tools and techniques for effective education* (2nd ed.). Marblehead, MA: HCPro.

Bandura, A. (1977). *Social learning theory.* Englewood Cliffs, NJ: Prentice Hall.

Barkley, E. F. (2010). *Student engagement techniques: A handbook for college faculty.* San Francisco, CA: Wiley.

Bastable, S. B. (2014). *Nurse as educator: Principles of teaching and learning for nursing practice* (4th ed.). Boston, MA: Jones & Bartlett.

Bastable, S. B., Gramet, P., Jacobs, K., & Sopczyk, D. L. (2011). *Health professional as educator: Principles of teaching and learning.* Sudbury, MA: Jones & Bartlett.

Benner, P. (1984). *From novice to expert: Excellence and power in clinical nursing practice.* Menlo Park, CA: Addison-Wesley.

Benner, P., Hooper-Kyriakidis, P., & Stannard, D. (2011). *Clinical wisdom and interventions in acute and critical care: A thinking-in-action approach* (2nd ed.). New York, NY: Springer.

Benner, P., Tanner, C. A., & Chesla, C. A. (1996). *Expertise in nursing practice: Caring, clinical judgment, and ethics.* New York, NY: Springer.

Benner, P., Tanner, C. A., & Chesla, C. A. (2009). *Expertise in nursing practice: Caring, clinical judgment, and ethics* (2nd ed.). New York, NY: Springer.

Benton, N. (2010). Creating a culture of quality. In J. S. Fulton, B. L. Lyon, & K. A. Goudreau (Eds.), *Clinical nurse specialist practice* (pp. 159–168). New York, NY: Springer.

Billings, D. M., & Halstead, J. A. (2012). *Teaching in nursing: A guide for faculty* (4th ed.). St. Louis, MO: Elsevier/Saunders.

Bradshaw, M. J., & Lowenstein, A. J. (2011). *Innovative teaching strategies in nursing and related health professions* (5th ed.). Sudbury, MA: Jones & Bartlett.

Bruce, S. L. (2009). *Core curriculum for staff development* (3rd ed.). Pensacola, FL: National Staff Development Organization.

Cadmus, E. (2013). Leadership for APNs: If not now, when? In L. A. Joel (Ed.), *Advanced practice nursing: Essentials for role development* (3rd ed., pp. 387–401). Philadelphia, PA: Davis.

Campbell, T. D., & Profetto-McGrath, J. (2013). Skills and attributes required by clinical nurse specialists to promote evidence-based practice. *Clinical Nurse Specialist, 27*(5), 245–254.

Cannon, S., & Boswell, C. (2012). *Evidence-based teaching in nursing: A foundation for educators.* Sudbury, MA: Jones & Bartlett.

Clark, M. C. (1993). Transformational learning. In S. Merriam (Ed.), *An update on adult learning theory* (pp. 47–56). San Francisco, CA: Jossey-Bass.

Cross, K. P. (1981). *Adults as learners: Increasing participation and facilitating learning.* San Francisco, CA: Jossey-Bass.

Cunningham, L., & McNally, K. (2003). Improving organizational and individual performance through coaching. *Nurse Leader, 1*(6), 46–49.

Davis, B. G. (1995). *Tools for teaching.* San Francisco, CA: Jossey-Bass.

Dewey, J. (1916). *Democracy and education.* New York, NY: Macmillan.

Dewey, J. (1938). *Education and experience.* New York, NY: Collier.

Dracup, K., & Bryan-Brown, C. W. (2004). From novice to expert to mentor: Shaping the future. *American Journal of Critical Care, 13*(6), 448–450.

Duffy, J. R. (2002). The clinical leadership role of the CNS in the identification of nursing-sensitive and multidisciplinary quality indicator sets. *Clinical Nurse Specialist, 16*(2), 70–76.

Ebright, P. R. (2010). Newer thinking about patient safety. In J. S. Fulton, B. L. Lyon, & K. A. Goudreau (Eds.), *Clinical nurse specialist practice* (pp. 169–182). New York, NY: Springer.

Ebright, P. R., Patterson, E. S., Chalko, B. A., & Render, M. L. (2003). Understanding the complexity of registered nurse work in acute care settings. *The Journal of Nursing Administration, 33*(12), 630–638.

Ebright, P. R., Patterson, E. S., & Render, M. L. (2002). The "new look" approach to patient safety: A guide for clinical nurse specialist leadership. *Clinical Nurse Specialist, 16*(5), 247–253.

Ervin, N. E. (2005). Clinical coaching: A strategy for enhancing evidence-based nursing practice. *Clinical Nurse Specialist, 19*(6), 296–301.

Ferguson, L. M., & Day, R. A. (2004). Supporting new nurses in evidence-based practice. *Journal of Nursing Administration, 34*(11), 490–492.

Finkelman, A. (2013). The clinical nurse specialist: Leadership in quality improvement. *Clinical Nurse Specialist, 27*(1), 31–35.

Fitzgerald, K., & Keyes, K. (2014). Instructional methods and settings. In S. B. Bastable (Ed.), *Nurse as educator: Principles of teaching and learning for nursing practice* (4th ed., pp. 469–515). Burlington, MA: Jones & Bartlett.

Galbraith, M. W. (1990). *Adult learning methods.* Malabar, FL: Kreiger Publishing.

Giles, P. F., & Moran, V. (1989). Preceptor program evaluation demonstrates improved orientation. *Journal for Nurses in Staff Development, 5*(1), 17–24.

Girouard, S. (2013). Measuring advanced practice nurse performance: Outcomes indicators, models of evaluation, and the issue of value. In L. A. Joel (Ed.), *Advanced practice nursing: Essentials for role development* (3rd ed., pp. 404–428). Philadelphia, PA: Davis.

Goleman, D. (1995). *Emotional intelligence.* New York, NY: New York Times.

Goleman, D. (1998). *Working with emotional intelligence.* New York, NY: Bantam.

Goudreau, K. A. (2010). Mentoring. In J. S. Fulton, B. L. Lyon, & K. A. Goudreau (Eds.), *Clinical nurse specialist practice* (pp. 259–266). New York, NY: Springer.

Greenleaf, R. K. (1996). *On becoming a servant leader.* San Francisco, CA: Jossey-Bass.

Grossman, S. C. (2012). *Mentoring in nursing: A dynamic and collaborative process* (2nd ed.). New York, NY: Springer.

Heitkemper, M. M., & Bond, E. F. (2004). Clinical nurse specialists: State of the profession and challenges ahead. *Clinical Nurse Specialist, 19*(3), 135–140.

Hopp, L. (2010). Shaping practice: Evidence-based practice models. In J. S. Fulton, B. L. Lyon, & K. A. Goudreau (Eds.), *Clinical nurse specialist practice* (pp. 131–147). New York, NY: Springer.

Institute for Healthcare Improvement (IHI). (2006). *SBAR.* Retrieved January 12, 2009, from http://www.ihi.org/ihi.

Institute of Medicine (IOM). (2011). *The future of nursing: Leading change, advancing health.* Washington, DC: National Academies Press.

JCAHO. (2008). *The Joint Commission guide to staff education.* Oakbrook Terrace, IL: Author.

Kirkpatrick, D. L. (1999). *Evaluating training programs: The four levels.* San Francisco, CA: Berrett-Koehler.

Klein, D. G. (2007). From novice to expert: CNS competencies. In M. G. McKinley (Ed.), *Acute and critical care clinical nurse specialists: Synergy for best practices* (pp. 11–28). St. Louis, MO: Saunders/Elsevier.

Knowles, M. S. (1980). *The modern practice of adult education: From pedagogy to andragogy* (Rev. ed.). New York, NY: Associated Press.

Lewin, K. (1951). *Field theory in social science.* New York, NY: Harper & Row.

Lyon, B. L. (2010). Transformational leadership as the clinical nurse specialist's capacity to influence. In J. S. Fulton, B. L. Lyon, & K. A. Goudreau (Eds.), *Clinical nurse specialist practice* (pp. 149–157). New York, NY: Springer.

Marriner, A. (1980). *Guide to nursing management.* St. Louis, MO: Mosby.

Maslow, A. H. (1987). *Motivation and personality* (3rd ed.). New York, NY: Harper & Row.

McCrimmon, M. (2010, July/August). A new role for management in today's post-industrial organizations. *Ivey Business Journal Online. Retrieved from iveybusinessjournal.com/ibj_issue/july-august-2010*

Merriam, S. B., & Brockett, R. G. (1997). *The profession and practice of adult education: An introduction.* San Francisco, CA: Jossey-Bass.

Merriam-Webster's online dictionary. (2013a). Springfield, MA: Merriam-Webster. Retrieved August 1, 2013, from http://www.merriam-webster.com/dictionary/coach

Merriam-Webster's online dictionary. (2013b). Springfield, MA: Merriam-Webster. Retrieved August 1, 2013, from http://www.merriam-webster.com/dictionary/mentor

Merriam-Webster's online dictionary. (2013c). Springfield, MA: Merriam-Webster. Retrieved August 1, 2013, from http://www.merriam-webster.com/dictionary/preceptor

Messecar, D.C., & Tanner, C.A. (2013). Evidence-based practice. In L. A. Joel (Ed.), *Advanced practice nursing: Essentials for role development* (3rd ed., pp. 242–259). Philadelphia, PA: Davis.

Millay, C. S. (1995). Planned change. In A. Marriner-Tomey (Ed.), *Case studies in nursing management: Practice, theory and research* (2nd ed., pp. 93–116). St. Louis, MO: Mosby.

National Association of Clinical Nurse Specialists (NACNS). (2004). *Statement on clinical nurse specialist practice and education* (2nd ed.). Harrisburg, PA: Author.

Newhouse, R., Dearholt, S., Poe, S., Pugh, L. C., & White, K. M. (2005). Evidence-based practice. *Journal of Nursing Administration, 35*(1), 35–40.

Oermann, M. H., & Gaberson, K. B. (2009). *Evaluation and testing in nursing education* (3rd ed.). New York, NY: Springer.

Parris, D. L., & Peachey, J. W. (2013). A systematic literature review of servant leadership theory in organizational contexts. *Journal of Business Ethics, 113*(3), 377–393.

Penn, B. K. (2008). *Mastering the teaching role: A guide for nurse educators*. Philadelphia, PA: Davis.

Peplau, H. (1965/2003). Specialization in professional nursing. *Clinical Nurse Specialist, 17*(1), 3–9.

Porter-O'Grady, T., & Malloch, K. (2003). *Quantum leadership: A textbook of new leadership*. Sudbury, MA: Jones & Bartlett.

Porter-O'Grady, T., & Malloch, K. (2010). *Quantum leadership: Advancing information, transforming health care* (3rd ed.). Sudbury, MA: Jones & Bartlett.

Quinn, R. E. (2004). *Building the bridge as you walk on it: A guide for leading change*. San Francisco, CA: Jossey-Bass.

Reinhard, S. C. (1988). Managing and initiating change. In E. J. Sullivan & P. J. Decker (Eds.), *Effective management in nursing* (2nd ed., pp. 93–119). Menlo Park, CA: Addison-Wesley.

Robinson-Walker, C. (2004). Coaching: A tool for excellence in nursing leadership. *Voice of Nursing Leadership, 2*(11), 8–9.

Rogers, C. (1994). *Freedom to learn* (3rd ed.). New York, NY: Merrill.

Saks, N. (1998). Developing an integrated model for outcomes management. *Advanced Practice Nursing Quarterly, 4*(1), 27–32.

Skinner, B. F. (1974). *About behaviorism*. New York, NY: Knopf.

Spath, P. L. (2002). *Guide to effective staff development in health care organizations*. San Francisco, CA: Jossey-Bass.

Stevens, R. R. (2005). *Essential competencies for evidence-based practice in nursing*. San Antonio, TX: Academic Center for Evidence-Based Practice.

Thorndike, E. L., Bregman, E. D., Tilton, J. W., & Woodyard, E. (1928). *Adult learning*. New York, NY: Macmillan.

Waddell, D. L., & Dunn, N. (2005). Peer coaching: The next step in staff development. *Journal of Continuing Education in Nursing, 36*(2), 84–89.

Wilson, C. K., & Porter-O'Grady, T. (1999). *Leading the revolution in healthcare: Advancing systems, igniting performance* (2nd ed.). Gaithersburg, MD: Aspen.

Wlodkowski, R. J. (1990). Strategies to enhance adult motivation to learn. In M. W. Galbraith (Ed.), *Adult learning methods: A guide for effective instruction* (pp. 97–117). Malabar, FL: Krieger Publishing.

Wright, D. (2004). Is education the answer? *Trend Lines, 15*(1), 1, 8.

Zuzelo, P. R. (2010). *The clinical nurse specialist handbook* (2nd ed.). Sudbury, MA: Jones & Bartlett.

Shaping Practice: Evidence-Based Practice Models

Lisa Hopp

Evidence-based practice (EBP) became the mantra of health care in the first decade of the 21st century. In fact, some authors have declared that EBP is one of the most significant themes ever to develop in global health care (Rycroft-Malone, Bucknall, & Melynk, 2004). The forces driving the world's preoccupation with EBP include recognition that large margins of people do not receive recommended care and that more than a decade can pass before new discoveries become routine practice, as well as a number of sociopolitical factors. These include the following:

- Governments need to contain escalating health care costs
- Recognition that reform must occur to change care processes and human resource management
- Systems must change to enable the way clinical knowledge is produced, critiqued, implemented, and evaluated in practice
- Health care systems must refocus on patient safety and patient-centeredness

Like many movements, there are true, pseudo, and false claims of health care providers "doing EBP." Because of their skills and competencies in the patient, nurses/nursing practice, and organization/system spheres of influence, clinical nurse specialists (CNSs) are particularly well suited to authentically implement evidence in their own and others' practice.

Many authors and disciplines have defined EBP, but most definitions include three elements that inform and contribute to making decisions in clinical practice. That is, EBP occurs when clinicians make decisions using the best available evidence, their clinical expertise, and patient preferences. Sackett, Rosenberg, Gray, Haynes, and Richardson (1996) wrote that evidence-based medicine is

the conscientious, explicit, and judicious use of current best evidence in making decisions about the care of individual patients. The practice of evidence-based medicine means integrating individual clinical expertise with the best available external clinical evidence from systematic research. (p. 71)

DiCenso, Cullum, and Ciliska (1998) expanded upon this definition to include four elements that should inform clinical decision making in nursing practice: best available evidence from research, patient preferences, clinical expertise, and available resources. Each element of this definition provides opportunities for CNSs to influence the health outcomes of patients. They need to develop competencies in the systematic search, retrieval, appraisal, synthesis, transfer, implementation, and evaluation of the best available evidence while integrating their tacit clinical knowledge and the preferences of the patient.

HISTORICAL BACKGROUND

EBP has both a long and short history, beginning with Florence Nightingale but taking on "movement" status in the mid-1990s. For nursing, its origins can be attributed in part to Nightingale's work in the years after the Crimean war. She advocated for the proper generation, interpretation, and implementation of findings from research. Her knowledge of the scientific method and statistical procedures informed her efforts to influence how policy makers could use epidemiologic data to make decisions. She complained that the governmental ministers' lack of proper understanding of the data they collected contributed to their failure to use the results to make decisions (McDonald, 2001).

The next significant activity occurred in the late 1970s and 1980s when nursing leaders focused on models of research utilization. The CURN and WICHE projects were large-scale efforts aimed at increasing nurses' use of research, but they did not emphasize exhaustive search and synthesis of the best available evidence, nor did they stress the integration of patient preferences and clinical expertise in the equation.

Nightingale's frustration with decision makers' neglect of the evidence was echoed some 80 years later when Archie Cochrane, a British epidemiologist and physician, criticized the medical community for its failure to use rigorous systematic reviews of available evidence to inform the decisions (Cochrane Collaboration, n.d.). Like Nightingale, he recognized that preventable infant deaths could be improved on a large scale if physicians based their decisions on the unused, but consistent, findings from several randomized controlled trials. Indeed, the subsequent efforts of the collaboration named after Cochrane were first aimed at assembling a registry of trials involving perinatal health. Cochrane emphasized the supremacy of the randomized controlled trial for determining the effect of treatments, publishing two hard criticisms of medicine in 1972 and 1979. He campaigned for the wide availability of systematic reviews and meta-analyses of multiple randomized controlled trials to inform treatment decisions (Cochrane Collaboration, n.d.). Although he died in 1988 before his ideas became reality, the Cochrane Center, later renamed as the Cochrane Collaboration, launched in 1992. It has rapidly grown to be a multinational collaboration that includes the largest library of systematic reviews of effect, a database of controlled trials, and a variety of entities working to support EBP. During the same time period, York University established the Center for Research Dissemination [CRD] with a similar purpose of developing systematic reviews of evidence of treatment effectiveness. The CRD has continued to grow and has close links with the Cochrane and Campbell Collaborations, the latter being a collaboration aimed at evidence synthesis relevant to the social sciences.

Although the Cochrane library contains some evidence that is directly related to the effects of nursing interventions, another organization evolved to more directly address problems relevant to nursing and nurse midwifery. In 1996, Alan Pearson and colleagues founded the Joanna Briggs Institute (JBI) in Adelaide, South Australia. JBI is the research and development arm of the School of Translational Sciences at the University of Adelaide. Prior to becoming part of the University, it was affiliated with the tertiary care medical center, the Royal Adelaide Hospital, on the same campus. The institute was so named to pay homage to the first matron of nursing at the Royal Adelaide Hospital that provided the institute's initial funding and continued support (JBI, 2013). Like the Cochrane Collaboration, JBI's purpose was to develop a worldwide collaboration to address global health priorities through synthesis and dissemination of systematic reviews of evidence. But the founders took a broader view of what constitutes legitimate evidence, to include findings from rigorous quantitative and qualitative research as well as from experience and expertise. They advocated that health care and nursing practice would benefit from syntheses of studies of feasibility, appropriateness, and meaningfulness as well as effectiveness. The collaboration now includes 70 centers and thousands of members distributed throughout six continents of the world in both developed and developing nations. The work of the Institute and collaborating centers continues its strong focus on nursing and nurse midwifery but embraces multiple health care disciplines. All of the JBI centers are developed on a framework of academic–clinical partnerships within their regional jurisdictions as well as research and development linkages among the international collaboration (JBI, 2013). CNSs can consult the JBI web pages to find a center near their area; at the time of this publication, seven centers exist in North America.

In 1997, the Agency for Healthcare Research and Quality (AHRQ) began its initiative to support EBP in the United States. While the mission of AHRQ is broad and includes all aspects of supporting health care quality and safety, it began awarding 5-year contracts to EBP centers in the United States and Canada to produce technology assessment, health reports, and systematic reviews that have particular clinical, social, or economic importance (AHRQ, n.d.). The completed electronic reports are freely available on the AHRQ website (http://www.ahrq.gov/research/findings/evidence-based-reports/index.html).

The Institute of Medicine (IOM) series of reports about the safety of patients in the hospital had profound impact on accelerating interest in EBP in the United States. The authors estimated that on the whole, only about 55% of Americans received recommended care, that inadequate care resulted in 18,000 unnecessary deaths annually from myocardial infarction, and that on average, it takes 17 years before a new discovery becomes routine practice (IOM, 2003). Subsequent to these reports, the IOM and other organizations have called for significant changes to accelerate the integration of evidence into practice.

CNSs are poised to play a significant role in the next chapter of EBP in North America and other countries where this model of advance practice exists. Many health care agencies continue to struggle with the transfer of evidence from its generation and synthesis to the everyday practice of clinicians. CNSs practice nursing at the intersections of disciplines, of science, clinical expertise, patients, and other nursing professionals; thus, they are the ideal candidates to accelerate the complex and messy process of evidence implementation and utilization.

CONCEPTUAL/THEORETICAL SUPPORT FOR EBP AND CNS PRACTICE

Many models have emerged to guide EBP. Most of them reflect five basic steps—posing a question, searching for evidence, critically appraising the evidence, implementing the recommendations of the evidence, and evaluating the outcomes. These steps are parallel to the nursing process (Table 10.1). The models can be differentiated based on their focus

and scope, their degree of conceptual and empirical support, and how they can be operationalized (Table 10.2).

Two of these models, Promoting Action on Research Implementation in Health Services (PARIHS) and JBI, are particularly fitting for CNS practice and are discussed in more depth here. To learn more about other models, readers can refer to the original publications or descriptions in texts focused specifically on EBP and their models (e.g., Rycroft-Malone & Bucknall, 2010).

PARIHS Model

Kitson, Harvey, and McCormack (1998) introduced the PARIHS model in an effort to describe the complexities of implementing evidence into practice while offering a practical framework for evidence implementation. They argued that superficial, linear models were inadequate to help clinicians successfully drive the change process. The model emerged from their work with clinicians as they tried to improve their nursing practice through guideline implementation. The research and development team at the Royal College of Nursing Institute in London have continued to refine the model based on a series of concept analyses addressing each of the elements of the model, retrospective data analysis, and a descriptive study to evaluate its content validity (Rycroft-Malone, 2004). In addition, a number of investigators, including Health Services Research and Development Services project teams within the U.S. Department of Veterans Affairs, have used the model to frame evidence implementation studies (Quality Enhancement Research Initiative [QUERI] project; Brown & McCormack, 2005; Doran & Sidani, 2007; U.S. Department of Veterans Affairs, 2006). Subsequently, Kitson et al. (2008) conducted

TABLE 10.1

COMPARISON OF THE NURSING AND EBP PROCESS	
Nursing Process	**EBP Process**
Assess	Gather data to identify the magnitude and nature of the problem
Diagnose	Formulate question based on baseline data/situation analysis
Plan	Transfer evidence by designing interventions and systems based on best available evidence, patient preference, and clinical expertise
Implement	Implement these interventions using evidence-based strategies
Evaluation	Measure outcomes

TABLE 10.2

COMPARISON OF SELECT EBP MODELS DEVELOPED OR REVISED SINCE 1990				
Model	**Focus/Scope**	**Empirical/Theoretical Support**	**Operational Tools**	**Comments**
ACE Star		Used to guide clinical implementation projects but limited published empirical or theoretical support	EBP competency statements derived from iterative consensus process of invited U.S. clinical and academic experts in progress. Testing of an inventory of EBP readiness in progress	A practical model that describes the steps commonly associated with the evidence-based process. Competency statement and inventory may be helpful in guiding CNSs in their own and others' development. Model would be stronger with greater empirical and theoretical support
Iowa	• A schematic algorithm that begins with problem or knowledge-focused triggers and decision algorithm leading to development and implementation of guidelines • Aimed at facilitating decisions of teams	Developed based on experiences; pragmatic approach that has been used extensively to run unit-based projects and to guide development activities	Toolkit available for purchase	A practical model that helps structure the decisions relevant to evidence implementation; represents process in a highly linear manner. Model is very popular for its ease of practical application; would be stronger with greater empirical and theoretical support
Stetler (2001)	• Refinement of research utilization model to include individual and groups as well as organizational use of evidence • Phased approach with focus on critical thinking throughout the process and a greater emphasis on synthesis	Pragmatic model that integrated a variety of theoretical underpinnings; refined in collaboration with CNSs and reflects the shift from research utilization (RU) to EBP; broad application to all forms of practice	Detailed explanation and tips for each phase included in publication	Assumptions well-explicated; revised model reflects evolution of thinking about RU; bears the wisdom of experiences long involved in bridging research–practice gap
Rosswurm & Larrabee (1999)	• Blends steps of EBP process and Rogers's diffusion of innovation theory • Aimed at organizational diffusion of change	Theoretical support based on Rogers's diffusion theory; used to guide implementation projects	Critical Appraisal work sheet cited provided in original article	This model appeals to many who understand Rogers's Diffusion of Innovations model; has been used in evaluation work

(continued)

TABLE 10.2

COMPARISON OF SELECT EBP MODELS DEVELOPED OR REVISED SINCE 1990 (CONTINUED)				
Model	**Focus/Scope**	**Empirical/Theoretical Support**	**Operational Tools**	**Comments**
Dobbins, Ciliska, Cockerill, Barnsley, & DiCenso (2002)	• Aimed at dissemination and utilization of research findings in clinical decision making and health policy • Built on Rogers's five-stage Diffusion of Innovations model	Incorporates Rogers's theoretical work with evidence from systematic reviews of research implementation	Lists of strategies based on systematic reviews	Model appealing for changing health policy; strength is in the incorporation of synthesized evidence from implementation research
PARIHS	• Comprehensive organizational model aimed at describing interactions and complexities of changing practice and moving evidence into practice • Weighs factors that contribute to the relative strength and relationships among evidence, context, and facilitation	Extensive concept analyses for the three major elements of the model; validation study; used to guide a variety of implementation studies and practice development	Context Assessment Tool available to assess qualities of the environment that aid or inhibit implementation	This model has particular appeal for CNS practice and warrants consideration. CNSs are prepared to move organizations toward the high end of evidence, context, and facilitation; model fits how CNSs advance nursing practice via the three spheres of influence
JBI	• Comprehensive, cyclical model that reflects the iterative nature of EBP. Incorporates diverse types of evidence to answer many types of clinical questions • Aim is to improve global health through tools available to aid EBP implementation at multiple levels from individuals to countries	Based on examination of literature and broad experience in leading global efforts in the research and development of EBP; research in progress to evaluate the effectiveness of tools	Robust, comprehensive toolset for each stage of the EBP process, including software for systematic reviews, critical appraisal, preappraised sources of evidence, systematic reviews, best-practice sheets, implementation and evaluation tools, and searching and providing evidence sources to evaluation of evidence utilization	

Sources: ACE, Academic Center for Evidence-Based Practice website (www.acestar.uthscsa.edu/); Iowa; Iowa, from Titler et al. (1994); Stetler, from Stetler (2001). Rosswurm & Larrabee, from Rosswurm & Larrabee (1999). Dobbins et al., from "Dobbins et al. (2002); PARIHS, Promoting Action on Research Implementation in Health Services, from Rycroft-Malone (2004); JBI, Joanna Briggs Institute, from Pearson et al. (2005).

an evaluation of how the model has shaped implementation with recommendations for the next phase of development. Finally, Stetler, Damschroder, Helfrich, and Hagedorn (2011) proposed a revision of the framework based on a critical synthesis of the literature and their experiences with the QUERI project. They proposed to modify subelements, integrated Rogers's characteristics of innovation into the assessment of the evidence to highlight its practical attributes (e.g., relative advantage, observability, compatibility, complexity, trialability), and offered a guide and tools for using the framework to structure and guide implementation efforts.

The original model predicts that successful implementation of research is a function of a dynamic relationship of three elements: evidence, context, and facilitation. These elements exist on a low to high continuum within a health system; success is more likely when all three elements are strong. CNSs can impact all three elements and their subelements if they employ competencies to shift or maintain evidence, context, and facilitation toward the high end of the continuum.

Rycroft-Malone, Seers, et al. (2004) conducted a concept analysis of evidence and presented a convincing argument that legitimate evidence includes not only the findings from research but also local data, professional knowledge and clinical experience, and patient experience and preference. The interaction among these forms of evidence is complex and untidy. Rycroft et al. stressed that nurses must assess the value and weight of each information source according to criteria before entering these into the decision-making process, in order to legitimize each source. In addition, health care providers must strive to use the most robust evidence to inform practice.

Research is generally regarded as the most important source of information for EBP. Indeed, some equate EBP with research-based practice and regard the randomized controlled trial as the only believable source of evidence. Rycroft-Malone, Seers, et al. (2004) and many others have argued for a far more pluralistic view that endorses many other forms of research evidence. Nonetheless, health care providers must critically appraise and weigh the quality and strength of the research and its applicability. Examples of criteria embedded in the PARIHS model characteristic of low-level research-based evidence criteria include poorly conceived, designed, or executed research or when research is seen as certain or unequivocal proof. On the other hand, examples of high-level research-based evidence criteria include studies that are well-conceived, designed, and executed and studies in which research evidence is seen as one part of a decision, when it is judged as relevant, and when

investigators acknowledge the lack of certainty inherent in research (Rycroft-Malone, 2004).

Less consensus exists related to the role and strength of clinical expertise. Rycroft-Malone (2004) acknowledged that the discipline is in the early stages of explicating and testing the meaning of clinical expertise. For individual expertise to be considered credible, this knowledge must be consciously explicated, analyzed, exposed to external sources of critique, and affirmed by consensus.

Like clinical expertise, the discipline does not yet fully understand the role of patient/client preferences as a source of evidence or its influence in evidence-based decision making. Nurses and CNSs have the moral and ethical obligation to meld the patient/client's interest into the design of any assessment, intervention, or evaluation process, but the mechanisms to do this are more reliant on the expertise of the caregiver than hard and fast rules. In addition, CNSs can use syntheses of qualitative studies of patient experiences to inform their understanding of patient preferences. In some countries, mechanisms exist to engage consumers in the development of clinical practice guidelines (CPGs) and systematic reviews. As CNSs analyze and appraise CPGs, they should judge the degree to which developers involved patients as stakeholders in the construction of the guideline (Brouwers et al., 2010). According to the PARIHS model, criteria indicating a low level on the patient preference continuum include patient preferences not valued as evidence or seen as the only type of evidence; those indicating a high level include multiple biographies used, partnerships with health care professionals in place, and patient preferences judged as relevant and importance weighted.

The second major theme of the PARIHS model is context, which is defined as the setting where people receive their health care services or where individuals and teams implement the EBP change. In their concept analysis, McCormack et al. (2002) contended that when organizations are strong in culture, leadership, and evaluation they more likely support getting evidence into practice. For example, cultures will be more successful if they promote learning; can self-define prevailing beliefs and values; allocate human, financial, and equipment resources; and align initiatives with strategic goals. Leadership rated on the high end of the continuum would be characterized by transformational styles; role clarity; effective teamwork; effective organizational structures; democratic decision making; and enabling and empowering in the teaching, learning, and managing processes. Similarly, leaders who are autocratic, unclear about roles, lack team-building skills, and are didactic in their teaching, learning, and management skills will be less successful in evidence implementation. The third component of context is evaluation. Organizations that use multiple sources and methods (clinical, performance, economic, experience evaluations) to give feedback to individuals, teams, and systems will be more successful than those that use narrow, single-method approaches or none at all (Rycroft-Malone, 2004). The model suggests that CNSs who lead and support other leaders to move toward the high end of the leadership continuum will promote a culture conducive to getting evidence into practice.

The third theme of the PARIHS model is facilitation, defined as enabling others or making easier the process of implementing evidence (Harvey et al., 2002). CNSs can directly act as facilitators to implement evidence into practice. The model predicts that they will be most successful when they act more holistically (as opposed to focused on a specific task) to enable others through sustained partnerships and use adult learning approaches to teaching and a wide range of skills to support and enable others. Skilled facilitators adjust their role based on the needs of the learners and the phase of the project (Rycroft-Malone, 2004). In the PARIHS group's latest work, they recommend that when users apply their model, they use it in two phases (Kitson et al., 2008). That is, CNSs might first assess the qualities of the evidence and context and then plan a tailor-made and effective approach to facilitation. Critical appraisal tools allow appraisal of the evidence. McCormack, McCarthy, Wright, Slater, and Coffery (2009) have completed preliminary psychometric analysis of the Context Assessment Index that CNSs could use to engage staff and other stakeholders in the assessment of context.

In summary, the PARIHS model suggests that CNSs will be more successful when they select the most robust evidence to inform practice; support a learning culture that is characterized by strong, transformational leadership with a capacity to appropriately evaluate outcomes of change and implementation; and act to facilitate implementation of evidence in a skillful, fluid, and holistic manner (see Table 10.3; Rycroft-Malone, 2004).

JBI Model

The second model that merits further discussion is the JBI model. This model is quite different from the PARIHS framework because it aims to improve global health rather than implement evidence in a local situation and has multiple tools to make the model operational. Its developers define EBP in a manner consistent with previously stated definitions. That is, EBP is clinical decision making that incorporates the best available evidence, the context of care, client preference, and professional judgment (Pearson, Wiechula, Court, & Lockwood, 2005). The model represents EBP as a four-component process of evidence generation, synthesis, transfer, and utilization to achieve global health. Clinicians and/or consumers identify questions, concerns, or interests relevant to health care, and evidence and knowledge are generated to effectively meet these needs in feasible and meaningful ways. The evidence is then synthesized and transferred to health care providers who use and evaluate the impact on health outcomes. CNSs can play a role in each phase of the cycle, from generating knowledge through research; synthesizing research through systematic reviews; transferring knowledge through education; advocating for and planning information systems; and facilitating evidence utilization through practice change, evaluation of process, systems, and outcomes, and embedding changes within the system. The model is based on the premise that consumers and health care providers are interested in questions that relate to the feasibility, appropriateness, meaningfulness, and effectiveness of interventions (Pearson et al., 2005).

APPLICATION TO CNS PRACTICE

According to all conceptual models, the EBP process begins when health care providers question the usual and standard approaches to practice. Regardless of the sphere of influence or stage in the nursing process, CNSs continuously reflect upon their practice and look for opportunities for improvement. One can argue that nearly every stage of the nursing process and most of CNS competencies can be related to EBP. For example, when conducting assessments of the patient, nursing personnel, or organizational problems, CNSs use tools and methods based on the best available evidence of sensitivity, specificity, positive and negative predictive value, and reliability. Their choices are also affected by the feasibility and understanding of the resources and context. The interventions that they choose are based on the best available evidence from research, their clinical expertise, and the patient or client preferences. In the nursing personnel and organizational spheres of influence, the meaning of client preferences includes the preferences and needs of nurses and the system. When they implement the evidence-based interventions directly or indirectly, they consider the evidence that supports particular strategies to facilitate change, the context that influences the probability of success, and the tools and skills to facilitate changing practice. Finally, they use valid and reliable measurements of outcomes

TABLE 10.3

STRATEGIES FOR CNS IMPLEMENTATION OF EVIDENCE—APPLICATION OF PARIHS MODEL
Evidence
• Select questions that are highly relevant to the population and/or care unit
• Seek highest quality synthesized evidence sources when available
• Consider all legitimate sources of evidence (feasibility, applicability, meaningfulness, and effectiveness), matching type of evidence and clinical question
• Use standardized tools to appraise all sources
• Provide preappraised sources to frontline staff
• Consider the magnitude of the evidence
• Develop mechanisms to incorporate patient preference into decision making, including evidence from systematic reviews of meaningfulness
• Maintain openness to discussing tacit clinical knowledge; seek critique from and consensus with others
Context
• Participate and advocate for transformational leadership models
• Advocate for adequate staff access to computers and the Internet
• Build relationships with nurse researchers to facilitate a climate of investigation
• Develop programs that are keenly relevant to staff to ignite their interest in EBP
• Use audit and feedback to build a culture of evidence and evaluation
• Advocate for and request information system support to enable data mining prospectively and retrospectively
• Develop EBP skills of key leaders
• Collaborate with administrators to develop appropriate skill mixes to support EBP
• Provide outcome feedback to nursing leaders to demonstrate capacity and outcomes of EBP
• Advocate for information systems that have the capacity to bring evidence summaries to the point of care as well as cues and prompts within electronic plans of care
Facilitation
• Use multiple strategies to build staff skills that are highly interactive; avoid passive didactic strategies
• Assess and enhance search skills of databases that are appropriate for the point of care
• Build mechanisms to enhance access to librarian resources and professional services of library scientists
• Develop peer experts who are recognized for their EBP skills
• Provide concise preappraised summaries of evidence on the burning topics, making the evidence quality and source explicit
• Incorporate cues and prompts to remind providers of key interventions
• Build policies that incorporate the best available evidence; make the evidence source and quality explicit

and generate local data to feedback into the EBP cycle (see Table 10.4).

Both the PARIHS and JBI models provide a framework and tools that are compatible and useful to this cycle of evidence-based improvement and innovation.

An Attitude of Inquiry and Asking Questions

This attitude of clinical curiosity and skepticism is critical to advanced nursing practice. Examples of CNS patient/client sphere competencies that relate to

TABLE 10.4

SELECT CNS OUTCOMES AND COMPETENCIES RELATED TO EBP		
CNS Outcomes	**CNS Competencies**	**EBP Application/Examples**
Patient/Client Sphere		
1. Diagnoses are accurately aligned with assessment data and etiologies	Conducts comprehensive, holistic wellness and illness assessments using known or innovative evidence-based techniques, tools, and methods	Selects and uses (e.g., fall, pressure ulcer, venothrombosis) risk assessment tools based on critical appraisal of measurement qualities (sensitivity, specificity, positive and negative predictive ability)
2. Nursing interventions target specified etiologies	Selects evidence-based interventions that target etiologies of illness or risk behaviors	Identifies specific modifiable risk factors (e.g., balance, gait, immobility) based on application of risk assessment tool
3. Prevention, alleviation, and/ or reduction of symptoms, functional problems, or risk behaviors are achieved	Incorporates evidence-based nursing interventions within a specialty population	Selects interventions (e.g., medication modification, bed surface, mobility program) to modify specific risk based on a critical appraisal of sources, transparency in methods, and fit with patient preferences
4. Unintended consequences and errors are prevented	Develops interventions that enhance the attainment of predicted outcomes while minimizing unintended consequences	Uses internal and external data (e.g., documentation of risk modification or observational data) to identify common rates and sources of errors or complications to develop preventative approaches
5. Predicted and measurable nurse-sensitive patient outcomes are attained through evidence-based practice	Before designing new programs, identifies, collects, and analyzes appropriate data on the target population that serve as the basis for demonstrating CNS impact on program outcomes	Identifies a need for change and establishes a baseline by conducting a baseline audit of process and outcome or analyzing available baseline data (e.g., used JBI's PACES and POOL audit/feedback tool to identify nursing process and patient outcomes related to falls, pressure ulcer, catheter-related infections). Compares institutional data with available external data or benchmarks (e.g., compares fall, pressure ulcer and catheter infection rates with national and international benchmarks)
	Selects, develops and/or applies appropriate methods to evaluate outcomes of nursing interventions	Uses valid, reliable, specific, and sensitive measures of outcomes (e.g., CDC criteria for hospital-acquired infections, National Pressure Ulcer Prevention Advisory Panel staging criteria)
	Documents and disseminates the results of innovative care	Presents poster/paper in collaboration with staff at local, regional, national, or international event to share findings. Writes publication based on project
Nurses/Nursing Practice Sphere		
1. Evidence-based practices are used by nurses	Uses/designs methods and instruments to assess patterns of outcomes related to nursing practice within and across units of care	Gathers process and outcome data using valid and reliable tools; develops charts and data displays to determine patterns (e.g., develops run-charts to relate process and outcome trends related to venothrombosis, pressure ulcers, etc.)

(continued)

TABLE 10.4

SELECT CNS OUTCOMES AND COMPETENCIES RELATED TO EBP (CONTINUED)		
CNS Outcomes	**CNS Competencies**	**EBP Application/Examples**
2. The research and scientific base for innovations is articulated, understandable, and accessible	Mentors nurses to critique and apply research evidence to nursing practice	Conducts EBP rounds with small groups of nurses to specify PICO questions; uses rapid appraisal checklists to appraise synthesized sources of evidence or individual reports of research when synthesized sources are unavailable; advocates for Internet access and/or creates space on intranet for staff access to preappraised sources such as JBI's Best Practice Sheets
	Anchors nursing practice to evidence-based information to achieve nurse-sensitive outcomes	Attends systematic review training and conducts a systematic review related to a relevant problem; collaborates with others to design policies based on synthesized evidence; imbeds sources and levels of evidence with policy recommendations; conducts audit and feedback cycles to determine care unit's effectiveness
3. Educational programs that advance the practice of nursing are developed, implemented, evaluated, and linked to evidence-based practice and effects on clinical and fiscal outcomes	Develops and implements educational programs that target the needs of staff to improve nursing practice and patient outcomes. Assists staff in the development of innovative, cost-effective patient/ client programs of care. Creates an environment that stimulates self-learning and reflective practice. Mentors nurses to acquire new skills and develop their careers. Disseminates results to stakeholders	Uses an "academic detailing" approach to engage staff in learning evidence-based practice innovations (e.g., offering one-on-one and small group sessions based on unit of care needs, providing short summaries of evidence and tips for implementation via a monthly EBP newsletter). Provides consultation on costs/benefits of changing a nursing practice based on a comprehensive systematic review that includes an economic evaluation. Designs a merit-based system of reward that includes recognition of staff's participation in self-learning activities (e.g., criteria include participation in PICO and EBP rounds, rapid appraisals of evidence sources, evidence-based policy development, etc.); designs or makes accessible distance learning self-learning modules about EBP (e.g., collaborates with librarian to create an online module about searching for evidence). Mentors small groups of nurses of varying expertise to develop EBP skills; leads team to develop, implement, and evaluate an EBP quality improvement practice change and helps publish and present the findings
Organization/System Sphere		
1. Patient care processes reflect continuous improvements that benefit the system	Contributes to the development of multidisciplinary standards of practice and evidence-based guidelines for care, such as pathways, care maps, and benchmarks	Evaluates multidisciplinary EBP resources; collaborates to develop a proposal to integrate information systems to enhance access to EBP resources at the point of care; implements plan to integrate these EBP systems into daily decision-making processes (e.g., considers systems such as JBI Connect™, InfoPOEMS™, and Pepid™)
2. Evidence-based, best practice models are developed and implemented	Develops or influences system-level policies that will affect innovation and programs of care	Develops systemwide guideline for policy development that requires transparency in methods and information sources; advocates that developers of major practice changes study the impact of the change on nursing work flow and patterns before sustaining the change (e.g.., pilot test and evaluate impact of evidence-based handoff process change before implementing it systemwide)
3. Change strategies are integrated throughout the system	Implements methods and processes to sustain evidence-based changes to nursing practice, programs of care, and clinical innovation	Develop a proposal for a EBP practice council within a shared governance model to influence implementation of EBP within a system; frame implementation of the EBP practice council with a model such as PARIHS and/or JBI

Source: Outcomes and competency statements are verbatim from the *NACNS Statement on Clinical Nurse Specialist Practice and Education* (2004); statements and examples are selected as illustrations and are not meant to be a comprehensive list.

clinical inquiry include identifying the need for new assessments, selecting evidence-based nursing interventions that target etiologies, and choosing appropriate methods to evaluate outcomes. Similarly, the nurse and organizational spheres of influence require CNSs to question standard and usual practice. Examples of nurses and nursing practice–related competencies include using/designing methods and instruments to assess outcomes related to nursing practice within and across units of care; using/designing appropriate methods and instruments to assess knowledge, skills, and practice competencies of nurses; and identifying needed changes in equipment or other products based on evidence, clinical outcomes, and cost-effectiveness. Examples of organization and system sphere of influence competencies include using and designing system-level assessment methods and instruments to identify organization structures and functions that impact nursing practice and nurse-sensitive outcomes, diagnosing variations in organizational culture that positively or negatively affect outcomes, and developing or influencing system-level policies that affect innovation and programs of care. These competencies require that CNSs first pose questions that lead to the search, selection, and application of evidence in order to use the best assessment tools to assess, intervene, and evaluate outcomes.

CNSs employ an attitude of clinical inquiry to formulate a specific question that will drive the rest of the EBP process. These so-called foreground questions are those that are searchable and lead to particular types of evidence sources. Foreground questions address issues related to diagnosis, prognosis, harm, effects of interventions, and economic impact. Background questions are those that are broader, more descriptive in nature, and more likely addressed by information found in textbooks or similar resources. For example, a background question related to the patient sphere of influence might be, "How does smoking lead to chronic bronchitis and emphysema?" and a foreground question might be, "What is the effect of inspiratory muscle training versus general exercise on inspiratory muscle strength and endurance in patients with chronic bronchitis and emphysema?" The CNS would most likely answer the background question with a summary of the basic science and theory about how smoking leads to destruction of lung parenchyma and the subsequent mechanical impact of thoracic hyperinflation. However, the foreground question about effectiveness of treatments is best answered by a systematic review with meta-analysis of randomized controlled trials. Questions related to the effect of interventions can be specified using a PICO format, where P corresponds to the population of interest, I represents the intervention or exposure in question, C is the comparison intervention or control, and O is outcome.

Other foreground questions relate to the meaning of health and illness as experienced by patients. These questions are best answered with metasyntheses of qualitative studies or within a comprehensive systematic review. An example of a meaningfulness question might be, "What is the meaning of breathlessness in patients with chronic obstructive pulmonary disease who experience an exacerbation?" These questions are best formed using a PIC format, where P represents participants, I corresponds to the phenomena of interest, and C represents context or, alternatively, a two-part approach framed by situation and population (Dicenso, Guyatt, & Ciliska, 2005). Readers can consult many excellent textbooks and other references for templates to help formulate searchable questions.

Searching and Appraising the Evidence

The next phase of the EBP process is to search and critically appraise the evidence. The PARIHS model predicts that when the evidence from research is strong, evidence is more likely to become part of practice. Therefore, CNSs need to know what types of evidence will answer their questions, where and how to search for the evidence, and how to critically appraise the evidence to inform their selection. The search strategy is structured by keywords and synonyms derived from the PICO question and conducted in a stepwise manner that will most likely lead to the highest level of evidence. That is, they would first search for a high-quality CPG based on meta-analyses or systematic reviews. If no high-quality guideline exists, they would search for a systematic review. If no synthesized sources exist, they would seek individual reports of research.

Unfortunately, no single search strategy or database exists to find the best available evidence. Rather, CNSs need to know where to look and how to search. CPGs are inventoried at the Agency for Healthcare Quality's website (www.guidelines.gov). Because these guidelines vary in quality, users must take care to critically evaluate them by first screening the many guidelines that may exist for a particular condition or problem, using the "compare" tool to screen, and then closely appraising those they select from the first-pass screening. The Registered Nurses Association of Ontario (RNAO) has published many high-quality CPGs relevant to both general and specialized nursing practice, and electronic versions are freely available to the public at www.rnao.org under its best-practice guideline pages. Other global organizations produce quality CPGs, such as the National Institute for Clinical Excellence in the United Kingdom (www.nice.org.uk) and the New Zealand Guidelines Group (www.nzgg.

org.nz/index.cfm). In the United States, many professional societies create guidelines that can be found online. However, because these organizations have no standard criteria or approach, readers must critically appraise the rigor of these CPGs. Links to many organizations that produce guidelines throughout the world can be found on the links page of the JBI website (http://www.joannabriggs.org/). CNSs can look for systematic reviews using bibliographic databases or at sites that publish systematic reviews, such as the Cochrane, JBI, and AHRQ websites.

Both the PARIHS and JBI models of EBP stress a pluralistic view of what constitutes legitimate evidence. However, both models address the dual need to be comprehensive in the search and to judge the strength of the evidence in order to determine the *best available* evidence. These models both underline the importance of selecting and blending the types of evidence that will appropriately answer a particular question. For example, questions related to effectiveness of an intervention will best be answered by a systematic review of randomized controlled trials (usually ranked at the top of any evidence hierarchy), but questions related to the appropriateness of an intervention may be better answered with local data in conjunction with the consensus of local experts. Regardless of the type of best available evidence, it is imperative that the methods, source, quality, and strength of the evidence be transparent to the users.

Because evidence sources vary widely in quality, CNSs need to use standardized approaches to critically appraise the evidence they find. Clinical practice guidelines can be evaluated using the Appraisal of Guidelines Research and Evaluation (AGREE) instrument developed by an international collaboration of researchers and policy makers (Brouwers et al., 2010). Systematic reviews and individual reports of research can be appraised with tools developed by the JBI Rapid Appraisal Program (RAPid; www.joannabriggs.edu.au/services/rapid.php) or the Critical Appraisal Skills Programme (CASP) tools developed by the Public Health Research Unit of the United Kingdom National Health Service (www.phru.nhs.uk/Pages/PHD/resources.htm). Essential criteria for any synthesized source are that the methods are transparent and there is proof of the evidence. For example, if an organization or author makes a claim of "best practice" or that they have published a guideline but do not include a discussion of the protocol for the search or mention criteria for including and excluding evidence, the source cannot be judged for how it could be considered "best available." Similarly, if a guideline does not identify the level of the evidence using a ranking system, one cannot judge the quality of information supporting the guideline.

Evidence Synthesis and Transfer

If the search and appraisal process has produced an excellent CPG or systematic review, the next step is to transfer the evidence to practice. If the search does not net a synthesized source, CNSs may rely upon the next best available source or plan to conduct a systematic review. In order to conduct systematic reviews, CNSs and other investigators should seek appropriate training and will likely need software to aid the process. The JBI and its collaborating centers offer periodic systematic review training. In addition, JBI has published a suite called the System for the Unified Management of the Review and Assessment of Information (SUMARI), which allows users to develop a protocol; manage bibliographic references; and analyze quantitative, qualitative, and economic evidence, and text and opinion through its four analytical applications. If users wish to submit protocols for peer review and publish systematic reviews through JBI, they must first be certified by successfully attending a training workshop. The Cochrane Collaboration also has freeware available to conduct meta-analyses of randomized controlled trials with an accompanying user's manual and resources. Visitors can find links to a variety of workshops and resources on the Cochrane website. Alternatively, JBI includes use of the Cochrane freeware, Review Manager (RevMan), in its training. In order to conduct a Cochrane review, authors must submit protocols and reports for peer review to a specific Cochrane Review Group. Other entities produce and publish high-quality systematic reviews using other methods and tools.

The transfer of evidence into practice is one of the more challenging aspects of EBP. Tools for transfer include CPGs or other condensed information sources such as the Oncology Nursing Society's Putting Evidence into Practice (PEP) series, JBI's Best Practice Information Sheets, the American Association of Critical Care Nurse's Practice Alerts, or other commercially available products such as POEM™—Patient-Oriented Evidence that Matters. These transfer tools must meet quality criteria, including transparency in methods and evidence quality ratings, but they help solve the issue of putting the evidence in the hands of clinicians at or near the point of care—a key issue in moving EBP forward. CNSs may find that having CPGs available via a handheld device is helpful to inform their practice. This has yet to become a broadly used technology by frontline nurses.

CNSs play a key role in the transfer of evidence. They fit the role of "knowledge broker" through multiple competencies. A CNS incorporates evidence into nursing interventions within specialty populations (patient sphere); draws conclusions about the evidence base and outcomes of nursing practice that require change, enhancement, or maintenance (nurses and nursing practice sphere); and contributes to the development of multidisciplinary standards of practice and evidence-based guidelines of care (organization/system sphere; National Association of Clinical Nurse Specialists [NACNS], 2004). CNSs can advocate for technological solutions to help transfer evidence to the point of care. For example, they can advocate for Internet access for frontline nurses; participate in planning information systems that support easy access to condensed, preappraised evidence; evaluate quality of information sources; work in transdisciplinary teams to examine the impact of information systems on workflow, and so forth.

Implementation/Utilization

Implementation of evidence makes or breaks the EBP process. This step may be most dependent upon CNS facilitation skills and is likely highly dependent upon context. However, the empirical evidence to support what nursing organizational infrastructure best supports implementation of evidence is underdeveloped. Foxcroft and Cole (2006) conducted a systematic review of randomized controlled trials, controlled clinical, and interrupted time series (updated to include literature through 2002) aimed at determining the effectiveness of nursing organizational infrastructures on promoting EBP. They defined nursing infrastructure as the "underlying foundation or basic framework through which clinical care is delivered and supported" (p. 3). They classified elements in a taxonomy that included management framework, work patterns, skill mix, information strategies, nurse development structures, research infrastructure, clinical supervision programs, quality monitoring systems, and "other." They were unable to make any recommendations because of the poor quality of the research that they found. That is, none of the studies met the rigor of their original criteria. They relaxed selection criteria to include any study that included an evaluation of infrastructure on outcomes in order to describe the baseline science. They found that authors tended to make claims of success without providing adequate evidence to support their conclusions. They made no recommendations for practice but concluded that investigators need to conduct more research using high-quality interrupted and complex interrupted time series designs.

Meijers et al. (2006) conducted a systematic review aimed at assessing the relationships between contextual factors and research utilization in nursing, using the PARIHS model to frame the review. They used less conservative criteria in order to capture existing research, albeit lacking sufficient controls to make cause–effect claims. They excluded studies of poor methodological quality using a standardized set of appraisal criteria and found 10 papers that met their inclusion criteria. They found statistically significant relationships between research utilization and multiple modes of research education and training; access to library resources, CNSs, or nurse researchers; extent of research-related role responsibility and sustained involvement in change teams; the degree of research climate; perceived support of colleagues, physicians, and key administrators; time spent studying while on and off duty; support for involvement in research and data collection; and material support.

Other systematic reviews of CPG implementation studies have examined interventions aimed at increasing physician use of guidelines. The interventions that showed the more consistent improvements in provider compliance with guidelines included reminders (median improvement of 14.1% improvement in 14 randomized cluster comparisons), dissemination of educational materials (8.1% improvements in four randomized cluster comparisons), audit and feedback (7.0% improvements in four randomized cluster comparisons), and multifaceted interventions involving educational outreach (6.0% improvements in 13 randomized cluster comparisons) with no relationship between the number of components and the effects of multifaceted interventions (Grimshaw et al., 2006).

While there may be no evidence from experimental designs, descriptive data exist that point to barriers to implementing evidence in nursing practice. CNSs can address these barriers within a conceptual framework such as PARIHS or JBI to facilitate and strengthen the context for EBP. Pravikoff, Tanner, and Pierce (2005) surveyed 3,000 American nurses using a stratified random sample with a net response rate of 37%. There were 760 clinical nurse respondents, with 39% holding baccalaureate degrees, 51% holding diplomas or associate's degrees, and only 9% with master's degrees. They found that the most common method of seeking information was from a colleague, and respondents seldom sought journal articles, research reports, or hospital libraries to answer their questions. Only 46% were familiar with the term *EBP*. Among the top 10 individual barriers (other than time) were lack of value for research in practice, lack of understanding of the structure of electronic databases, difficulty accessing research materials, lack of computer skills, difficulty understanding research articles, lack of access to a computer, lack of library access, and lack of search skills. The top institutional barriers included other goals taking higher priority, difficulty recruiting and retaining staff, organizational budget for acquisition and training in information resource use, organizational perception that nursing staff are not eager to incorporate or pursue EBP, and a persistent perception that EBP is not achievable in the real world.

These findings and the theoretical frameworks suggest a number of implications for CNS practice (see Table 10.3). When designing interventions within the patient sphere of influence, CNSs implement the recommendations from the best available evidence from research but negotiate these interventions in collaboration with the patient/client and other providers, while blending their clinical expertise with the decision.

When influencing nursing practice and personnel, CNSs use facilitation skills to break barriers. When educating nurses, they need to conduct interactive sessions rather than passive, didactic sessions and use an "academic detailing" approach where they engage in development through EBP rounds and one-on-one sessions in the midst of care delivery as the context allows. They should preassess the staff's information management skills and build them where necessary and provide them with concise, straightforward summaries of the best available, preferably synthesized, evidence sources. They can increase access to evidence by providing it at the point of care and helping nurses interpret the findings so they may be empowered to negotiate with patients and other disciplines.

CNSs influence context via the system/organizational sphere. These interventions are complex and require collaboration with others. CNSs can provide transformational leadership through direct and indirect strategies. Though the evidence is evolving, the theoretical framework suggests that when CNSs occupy line administrative roles they can have profound impact by building the skill mixes that support EBP, building relationships with nurse researchers in academic settings if none exist in their own settings, and promoting a culture of evidence. CNSs in traditional roles contribute to context by building teams to address EBP in their settings. These teams need to include key stakeholders such as the frontline staff. CNSs can advocate for staff to have time on the job to participate in evidence-based initiatives by exploring innovative strategies to cover staffing needs for patient care while releasing staff to engage in evidence-based initiatives. CNSs can work with information system workers to develop data-mining systems to gather both prospective and retrospective data to enable diagnosis of problems and their etiologies as well as outcome measurements.

EVALUATION AND OUTCOME MANAGEMENT

Evaluation is the final step of both the nursing and EBP process. Most of the CNS outcomes listed in the NACNS Statement relate to the impact of EBP. But those that explicitly address EBP are as follows:

- Predicted and measurable nurse-sensitive patient outcomes are attained through EBP (patient sphere)
- EBPs are used by nurses
- Evidence-based, best practice models are developed and implemented (NACNS, 2004).

In order for evaluation of outcomes to be meaningful, CNSs need to select measurement tools that are valid and reliable and fit the question at hand. Both process and outcome measurements are necessary to enable analysis of the effects of evidence-based initiatives. The reality of the clinical setting can pose barriers to obtaining these data. For example, electronic documentation methods may not provide adequate data to monitor critical aspects of a care process or even to capture the outcome precisely. Though proxy measures may be the more feasible, they usually come at some cost to measurement quality.

CNSs should strive to capture data in a way that is simple to understand but revealing. A complete discussion of how best to represent data is outside the scope of this chapter. However, the metric must allow for adequate precision to detect differences. For example, infrequent events may be better tracked by measuring days between occurrences rather than rates. When tracking rates, the denominator must provide a meaningful metric. For example, when measuring catheter-related infections, it is more meaningful to index incidence with those at risk, that is, those with catheters inserted, than all patients regardless of exposure.

Finally, like any quality management process, outcomes have to be fed back into the cycle of improvement. In addition, key stakeholders must be informed of performance and engaged in the continuous cycle of improvement. Particularly successful and unsuccessful approaches to implementation merit dissemination via journals, agency events, and national and international meetings.

ADVANCED NURSING PRACTICE

CNSs often address practice issues that are quite fundamental to nursing practice, but the methods of advancing the practice of nursing and using evidence to support these fundamental practices are complex. Pravikoff et al. (2005) concluded that nurses in the United States are not ready for EBP. Very few respondents in Pravikoff's sample were master's-prepared nurses, so it is unlikely that this conclusion can be extended to CNSs. Certainly, nursing educators need to prepare their graduates at all levels of practice to move from a tradition-based discipline toward an evidence-based discipline. The data underline a great need for frontline nursing staff development, and CNSs are already positioned to move this agenda forward through facilitation and context building. This will happen best in the midst of practice where CNSs work with their sleeves rolled up, side-by-side with the bedside nurse.

Not all nurses are or will be prepared for every step of the EBP. Nurses prepared at the technical level can collaborate with professional and advanced practice nurses to identify clinical issues and assist with the practical aspects of evidence implementation. Professional nurses prepared at the baccalaureate level have the skill to search literature and do rapid appraisals of research and CPGs, recommend practical solutions for implementation, and participate in evaluation audits. CNSs participate and lead all aspects of EBP, including conducting systematic reviews. Their critical appraisal skills are more sophisticated, and they understand the complexities of the implementation process. They use data to diagnose and specify etiologies of problems within all three spheres and manage all aspects of using evidence to solve these problems. These competencies set them apart from nurses prepared at the undergraduate levels.

ETHICAL CONSIDERATIONS

EBP is aimed at "doing the right thing." That is, it is about acting with beneficence to achieve the best possible patient outcomes. The ethical principles of beneficence, justice, and respect all play a role in evidence-based decision making (Ledbetter, 2000).

In some cases, data exist to quantify the benefit of treatment to help inform decisions related to beneficence and harm. In fact, the probability of benefit and harm can be estimated by calculating the numbers needed to treat (NNT) from frequency data and the potential harm of a treatment using numbers needed to harm (NNH); (DiCenso et al., 2005). For example, if an intervention has a NNT of five (95% confidence interval [CI], [3, 7]), then five people would need to receive the intervention to benefit one person, with the true value falling between three and seven (DiCenso et al., 2005). Similarly, a NNH of 100 (95% CI [90, 120]) means that 100 people would need to receive a treatment before 1 more person would be harmed by the adverse effects of a treatment, with the true number falling between 90 and 120. When these data exist, they may help systems and individuals weigh the benefits and harm of interventions and their adverse effects. The magnitude of the treatment effect, the type and probability of adverse effect, and the nature of the decision itself will contribute to how CNSs engage patients' autonomous preferences. CNSs can learn more about using patient decision aids to help staff use these aids (DiCenso et al., 2005).

The principles of justice, beneficence, and respect must be upheld when CNSs make decisions about what type of EBP efforts require human subject committee oversight. CNSs should seek institutional review board (IRB) approval for projects when they plan to collect data and disseminate the findings of the project. If they are involved in quality improvement cycles where all data are deidentified, the project may not require IRB approval, but they should discuss the project with the chair of the human subjects committee before launching any EBP project.

Ethical issues are likely to dominate discussions related to evidence-based health policy and new health care resource allocation schemes. CNSs need to remain actively engaged in these deliberations, advocating for the responsible use of health care dollars as well as for patient interests.

SUMMARY

EBP is the burning issue of the decade. Since the advent of advanced nursing practice, CNS practice and education have focused on using theory and research to advance the practice of nursing. CNSs use evidence in their individual clinical decisions in the patient sphere of influence and facilitate and lead other nurses, and organizations to use evidence to achieve the best outcomes. They are uniquely positioned to ask the questions, find and appraise the evidence, and design, implement, and evaluate innovations. In short, they are and will be the catalyst for evidence-based nursing practice.

■ DISCUSSION QUESTIONS

- What are the key elements of the definition of evidence-based nursing practice? What are the implications of these elements for CNS practice?
- How has the EBP movement developed throughout the world? How have sociopolitical factors influenced EBP among nations that have largely private-pay health care systems and those that are largely nationalized?
- What are some examples of false, pseudo, and authentic claims of EBP that you have seen in your practice or education? What factors differentiate these claims?

- How do the nursing process and EBP process compare?
- What requirements are necessary for a model to help CNSs implement EBP in all spheres of influence? How do the various EBP models compare in their support of CNS implementation of evidence?
- What CNS competencies and outcomes as described in *NACNS's Statement on Practice and Education* speak directly to promoting EBP among the three spheres of influence? Which address EBP indirectly?
- How and why do the following sources of evidence compare in terms of their breadth, strength of control of bias, and role in EBP: systematic reviews of RCTs, systematic reviews of non-RCTs, CPGs, single RCTs, cohort studies, before and after single group studies, consensus statements by a specialty organization, and metasynthesis of qualitative studies. In what circumstances might these be the "best available evidence"?
- According to Rycroft-Malone, Seers, et al. (2004), clinical expertise must be consciously explicated, analyzed, exposed to external sources of critique, and affirmed by consensus. How might CNSs affirm their clinical expertise to meet these criteria?
- According to the PARIHS model, what conditions should the CNS promote to increase the probability of successfully implementing an evidence-based innovation?
- Based on the findings of Pravikoff et al. (2005) and evidence from systematic reviews of implementation strategies, how can CNSs influence nursing personnel to further EBP in the United States?
- What tools will facilitate getting evidence into practice, and where might they be found? What type of approaches to implementation are ineffective? How can CNSs promote technical solutions to break down barriers to evidence implementation?

■ ANALYSIS AND SYNTHESIS EXERCISES

- Search for a systematic review on a particular topic of interest to your specialty practice. Find a single research study about the same issue. Compare the findings from the systematic review and the individual study. Are the conclusions similar or different? How does your confidence in the bottom-line recommendation compare?
- Select a clinical topic of interest to your specialty practice. Go to www.guidelines.gov/ to search for CPGs. Use the "compare" tool to compare three of them at a time. How do the guidelines compare in terms of the rigor of their development, the transparency in methods, and supporting evidence?

Select one and apply the AGREEII instrument to complete the critical appraisal. Would you consider facilitating its implementation? Why or why not?
- Select a model to consider in depth. How does the model fit the complexity of EBP? How does it help direct CNS practice in the three spheres of influence?
- Find five different systems for ranking levels of evidence (e.g., Centers for Disease Control, U.S. Preventive Services Task Force, etc.). Create a comparison chart and summarize the similarities and differences. What are the implications of the lack of a standard leveling system for CNS practice?
- Search and analyze systematic reviews related to implementation of guidelines or other sources of evidence (begin by searching the Effective Practice and Organization of Care [EPOC] database of systematic reviews at www.cochrane.org). Create three lists: strategies that consistently work, strategies that may work, and strategies that consistently do not work. How might you use this list to design implementation interventions?

■ CLINICAL APPLICATIONS

- Develop a clinical implementation project in collaboration with a clinical team; use a conceptual model to frame the process to include the following:
  a. Identify a potential problem.
  b. Brainstorm potential etiologies, and gather assessment data to support or refute the diagnosis.
  c. Generate a PICO question related to the effectiveness of an intervention to target the etiology.
  d. Search for best available synthesized evidence; if a synthesized source is unavailable, find primary evidence.
  e. Appraise the evidence source using a standardized tool to decide on applicability.
  f. Generate recommendations for implementation.
  g. Implement and gather data to evaluate outcomes.
  h. Generate further recommendations for improvement.
- Conduct "PICO" rounds:
  a. Round with nursing staff in small, brief sessions.
  b. Ask them to identify current, relevant clinical issues. If they have difficulty identifying an issue, ask them to recount the types of patients and interventions they have provided. Ask questions about how they made their clinical decisions, and solicit possible alternative decisions.
  c. Help them identify each element of the question—population, intervention, comparison, and outcome.

d. Find evidence that relates to the questions and provide short, key point summaries of synthesize evidence if it is available.

- Organize a journal club to critically appraise CPGs or systematic reviews relevant to issues identified by nursing staff.
- Participate in a product analysis team. Search for evidence related to the type of technology and gather user requirements through focus groups. Conduct a cost analysis and provide a recommendation of the product in collaboration with the team.
- Meet with nursing leaders to explore their vision for EBP and the role of CNSs in that vision.

REFERENCES

Agency for Healthcare Research and Quality (AHRQ) (n.d.). Evidence based practice centers overview. Retrieved February 11, 2014, from http://www.ahrq.gov/research/findings/evidence-based-reports/overview/index.html

Brouwers, M., Kho, M. E., Browman, G. P., Burgers, J. S., Cluzeau, F., Feder, G., & Zitzelsberger, L. for the AGREE Next Steps Consortium (2010, July 5). AGREE II: Advancing guideline development, reporting and evaluation in healthcare. *Canadian Medical Association Journal, 182*(18), E839–E842. Available online. doi:10.1503/cmaj.090449

Brown, D., & McCormack, B. (2005). Developing postoperative pain management: Utilising the promoting action on research implementation in health services (PARIHS) framework. *Worldviews on Evidence-Based Nursing, 2,* 131–141.

Cochrane Collaboration. (n.d.). *Chronology of Cochrane Collaboration.* Retrieved January 9, 2009, from http://www.cochrane.org/docs/cchronol.htm

DiCenso, A., Cullum, N., & Ciliska, D. (1998). Implementing evidence-based nursing: Some misconceptions. *Evidence Based Nursing, 1,* 38–40.

DiCenso, A., Guyatt, G., & Ciliska, D. (2005). *Evidence-based nursing: A guide to clinical nursing.* St. Louis, MO: Mosby.

Dobbins, M., Ciliska, D., Cockerill, R., Barnsley, J., & DiCenso, A. (2002). A framework for the dissemination and utilization of research for health-care policy and practice. Worldviews on evidence-based nursing presents the archives of *Online Journal of Knowledge Synthesis for Nursing, E9*: 149–160. doi: 10.1111/j.1524-475X.2002.00149.x

Doran, D. M., & Sidani, S. (2007). Outcomes-focused knowledge translation: A framework for knowledge translation and patient outcomes improvement. *Worldviews on Evidence-Based Nursing, 4,* 3–13.

Foxcroft, D. R., & Cole, N. (2006). Organisational infrastructures to promote evidence based nursing practice. *Cochrane Database of Systematic Reviews, 3.* Art. No. CD002212. doi:10.1002/14651858.CD002212.

Grimshaw, J., Eccles, M., Thomas, R., MacLennan, G., Ramsay, C., Fraser, C., & Vale, L. (2006). Toward evidence-based quality improvement: Evidence (and its limitations) of the effectiveness of guidelines dissemination and implementation strategies (1966–1998). *Journal of General Internal Medicine, 21*(Suppl. 2), S14–S20.

Harvey, G., Loftus-Hill, A., Rycroft-Malone, J., Tichen, A., McCormack, B., & Seers, K. (2002). Getting evidence into practice: The role and function of facilitation. *Journal of Advanced Nursing, 37,* 577–588.

Institute of Medicine (IOM). (2003). *Patient safety: A new standard of care.* Washington, DC: National Academies Press.

Joanna Briggs Institute (JBI). (n.d.). *About JBI.* Retrieved January 9, 2009, from http://www.joannabriggs.edu.au/pdf/about/AboutJBI.pdf

Kitson, A., Harvey, G., & McCormack, B. (1998). Enabling the implementation of evidence based practice: A conceptual framework. *Quality Health Care, 7,* 149–158.

Kitson, A., Rycroft-Malone, J., Harvey, G., McCormack, B., Seers, K., & Tichen, A. (2008). Evaluating the successful implementation of evidence into practice using the PARiHS framework: Theoretical and practical challenges. *Implementation Science, 3.* doi:10.1186/1748–5908-3–1

Ledbetter, C. A. (2000). Evidence-based best practice: The common knowledge of ethical clinical scholarship. Worldviews on evidence-based nursing presents the archives of *Online Journal of Knowledge Synthesis for Nursing, E7*: 4–9. doi: 10.1111/j.1524-475X.2000.00004.x

McCormack, B., Kitson, A., Harvey, G., Rycroft-Malone, J., Tichen, A., & Seers, K. (2002). Getting evidence into practice: The meaning of "context." *Journal of Advanced Nursing, 38,* 94–104.

McCormack, B., McCarthy, G., Wright, J., Slater, P., & Coffery, A. (2009). Development and testing of the context assessment index (CAI). *Worldviews on Evidence-Based Nursing, 6,* 27–35.

McDonald, L. (2001). Florence Nightingale and the early origins of evidence-based nursing. *Evidence Based Nursing, 4,* 68–69.

Meijers, J. M. M., Janssen, M. A. P., Cummings, G. G., Wallin, L., Estabrooks, C. A., & Halfens, R. Y. G. (2006). Assessing the relationships between contextual factors and research utilization in nursing: Systematic literature review. *Journal of Advanced Nursing, 55,* 622–635.

National Association of Clinical Nurse Specialists (NACNS). (2004). *Statement on clinical nurse specialist practice and education* (2nd ed.). Harrisburg, PA: Author.

Pearson, A., Wiechula, R., Court, A., & Lockwood, C. (2005). The JBI model of evidence-based healthcare. *International Journal of Evidence Based Healthcare, 3,* 207–215.

Pravikoff, D. S., Tanner, A. B., & Pierce, S. T. (2005). Readiness of U.S. nurses for evidence-based practice. *American Journal of Nursing, 105,* 40–51.

Rosswurm, M. A., & Larrabee, J. H. (1999). A model for change to evidence-based practice. *Image: Journal of Nursing Scholarship, 31,* 317–322.

Rycroft-Malone, J. (2004). The PARIHS framework—A framework for guiding the implementation of evidence-based practice. *Journal of Nursing Care Quality, 19,* 297–304.

Rycroft-Malone, J., & Bucknall, T. (Eds.). (2010). *Models and frameworks for implementing evidence based practice: Linking evidence to action.* West Sussex, UK: Wiley-Blackwell.

Rycroft-Malone, J., Bucknall, T., & Melnyk, B. M. (2004). Editorial. *Worldviews on Evidence-Based Nursing Practice, 1*(1), 1–2.

Rycroft-Malone, J., Seers, K., Tichen, A., Harvey, G., Kitson, A., & McCormack, B. (2004). What counts as evidence in evidence-based practice? *Journal of Advanced Nursing, 47,* 81–90.

Sackett, D. L., Rosenberg, W. M. C., Gray, J. A. M., Haynes, R. B., & Richardson, W. S. (1996). Evidence based medicine: What it is and what it isn't. *British Medical Journal, 312,* 71–72.

Stetler, C. (2001). Updating the Stetler Model of research utilization to facilitate evidence-based practice. *Nursing Outlook, 49,* 272–279.

Stetler, C. B., Damschroder, L. J., Helfrich, C. D., & Hagedorn, H. J. (2011). A guide for applying a revised version of the PARiHS framework for implementation. *Implementation Science, 6,* 99. doi:10.1186/1748–5908-6–99.

Titler, M., Kleiber, C., Steelman, V., Goode, C., Rakel, B., Barry-Walker, J.,…Buckwalter, K. (1994). Infusing research into practice to promote quality care. *Nursing Research, 43,* 307–313.

U.S. Department of Veterans Affairs. (2006). *QUERI implementation guide.* Retrieved January 9, 2009, from http://www.queri.research.va.gov/

Transformational Leadership as the Clinical Nurse Specialist's Capacity to Influence

Brenda L. Lyon

Today's demands on health care systems to improve patient care, including safety and cost effectiveness, highlight the need for the transformational leadership of clinical nurse specialists (CNSs; Institute of Medicine [IOM], 2004). CNSs are the only advanced practice registered nurses (APRNs) prepared to work in three spheres of influence: patient/client (direct care); nurses and nursing practice; and organizations/systems (NACNS, 2004). As such, CNSs are the only APRNs prepared to lead quality improvement efforts that will improve care at the unit and/or systems level (Finkleman, 2013). The transformational leadership work of the CNS is principally focused on transforming patient care by closing the gap between what is known (evidence-based practice [EBP]) and what is done in practice and by resolving systems-level problems that impede effective patient care.

Leadership is a hallmark of CNS practice in all three spheres of influence. The essence of leadership is fundamentally the capacity to influence. *Influence* is the "power of producing an effect without apparent exertion of force or direct exercise of command" (*Merriam-Webster Online Dictionary*, 2008a). Influence and, therefore, leadership is not about having position authority; it is the ability to get others to be motivated to work toward accomplishing a vision. The importance of influence as the major avenue through which CNSs positively impact both patient outcomes and cost-effectiveness is reflected in the adoption of "spheres of influence" as the framework for the National Association of Clinical Nurse Specialists (NACNS) *Statement on Clinical Nurse Specialist Practice and Education* (NACNS, 2004).

The purpose of this chapter is to present leadership as a relationship-oriented capacity to influence or motivate others to work toward shared goals in improving patient outcomes and cost-effectiveness. The *capacity* to lead is a complex quality that encompasses particular personal and relationship-focused attributes, the ability to earn and effectively use interpersonal power, and the judicious use of the principles of influence. The combination of all of these elements is necessary to enable the CNS's enactment of transformational leadership for the purpose of positively affecting others in the work of improving patient care outcomes in complex health care systems.

The chapter begins with a brief discussion of the common types of CNS work in complex systems that require leadership ability. The personal and relationship-focused attributes of effective leaders are identified. Then the concepts of interpersonal power and the principles of influence, including influence strategies, are presented as foundational to understanding the features of transformational leadership in the next section. The chapter concludes with a summary and discussion questions.

COMMON TYPES OF CNS CLINICAL WORK REQUIRING LEADERSHIP

The necessity for CNSs in health care systems is omnipresent because of the endless drive to improve patient outcomes and the cost-effectiveness of care. The high incidence of infections, skin breakdown, and falls in many hospitals, coupled with the Centers for Medicare & Medicaid Services' (CMS) initiation of value-based purchasing policies, resulting in nonpayment to hospitals for care necessitated by these and other preventable complications, simply increases organizational incentives to provide quality patient care (CMS, 2011; Rosenthal, 2007).

CNSs are well-positioned to lead change efforts within organizations to cost effectively improve patient outcomes. It is imperative that CNSs continually assess patient care outcomes to identify needs for practice improvement. Once identified, the CNS must visibly seize those leadership opportunities by working with nursing staff, other health care professionals, and administration in bringing about needed changes (see Chapter 24).

Health care facility needs for leadership to bring about nursing practice improvement may be focused in either or both the nursing sphere and the system sphere, with a wide range of foci. The nursing sphere may include, but is not limited to, needs for leadership in (a) identification of critical indicators for nurse-sensitive outcomes to enable measurement and feedback to staff regarding the effectiveness of care (Duffy, 2002); (b) bridging knowledge/skill gaps between evidence and what is done at the bedside (Dietz & Smith, 2002; Richarson & Tjoelker, 2012; Seemann, Soukup, & Adams, 2000); (c) development of evidence-based policies and procedures (Becker et al., 2012); (d) empowerment of staff to promote assertive advocacy on behalf of patients (Green & Jordan, 2004); and (e) development and implementation of innovative programs of care for patient populations (Morissette, 2004). System leadership opportunities may include, but are not limited to, (a) identification and resolution of gaps in system supports that contribute to work complexity and hazards in patient care (Ebright, Patterson, & Render, 2002; Sitterding, Froome, Everitt, & Ebright, 2012); (b) evaluation of products used in patient care (Bahr, Senica, et al., 2010); (c) identification and resolution of clinical barriers (including norms and relationships) that negatively impact patient outcomes; (d) development of critical indictor matrices for multidisciplinary quality indicators in conjunction with other disciplines (Duffy, 2002); (e) guiding multidisciplinary groups in system solutions to clinical problems (Benedict, Robinson, & Holder, 2006; Custer, 2010); and (f) boundary management between disciplines (Foggow, Solie, Tracy, & Gjere, 2005).

ATTRIBUTES OF LEADERS

To be able to positively impact changes in a health care system, the CNS must have personal and relationship-oriented attributes that give him or her the ability to be in relationship with others in a positive way so as to influence them. Several of the attributes identified in Chapter 2 as being important for CNSs to possess are consistent with attributes identified through research on transformational and authentic leaders.

Personal Attributes

Research has demonstrated that personal attributes contributing to the capacity to lead include self-confidence, proactive orientation, trustworthiness, reliability, strong sense of purpose, self-discipline, optimistic orientation, and resilience and persistence. Bass (1999) conducted a review of research on attributes of transformational leaders over a 20-year period. The two primary personal attributes necessary for a leader's ability to influence were self-confidence (a sense of security) and a proactive orientation, that is, the ability to envision a desired future and set aims. George (2003) found that authentic leaders are believable, genuine, trustworthy, and reliable. They have a strong sense of purpose, solid values, and are self-disciplined. According to George, authentic leaders possess four psychological strengths, including confidence, hope, optimism, and resiliency. Optimism is characterized by focusing on the glass as half full rather than half empty. Optimists do not take failure personally, but rather look at it as an opportunity for learning and improvement. Resiliency is an important aspect of persistence, which is the ability to deal with difficult situations with determination (George, 2003). In addition to these attributes, Spinelli (2006) and Dirks and Ferrin (2001) identified charisma as an essential personal attribute of transformational leaders.

Relationship-Oriented Attributes

In addition to person-focused attributes, there are important relationship-oriented attributes of leadership. Bass (1999) found in his study of transformational leadership that a critically important attribute was the ability to initiate and maintain positive relationships with others. The attribute is characterized by a high degree of "other-orientation" rather than narcissistic desires and is manifested by a high degree of empathy and an ability to give and contribute. Being an effective listener is one manifestation of being other-oriented. Bass also found that the ability to clearly articulate a vision that unifies values and intellectually stimulates others is very important. Consistent with Bass, Wolf et al. (2011) discuss transformational leadership qualities in the context of hospital-based Magnet initiatives, including such attributes as thoughtfulness, inclusivity, good listening skills, flexibility, resiliency, and courage.

George (2003) found that authentic leaders focus on building on people's strengths instead of focusing on weaknesses. Authentic leaders are often able to transform an organization and/or parts of an organizational system. Building self-confidence that others will see in you requires being able to see possibilities (positive visualization) and a preponderance of positive self-talk, as well as positive situational focusing (Lyon, 2001a). Positive talk can become contagious and contribute to group confidence (Avolio & Luthan, 2006). One study demonstrating the influence of authentic leadership was that of Laschinger and Smith (2013); their study of the impact of unit-leader authentic leadership on new-graduate nurses' perceptions of interprofessional collaboration yielded positive results.

Reaffirming many of the personal and relationship-oriented attributes of transformational leadership in nursing are the findings of the concept analysis conducted by Grossman and Valiga (2005) to identify the essential characteristics of leadership. The results of their analysis generated nine characteristics, including creativity, vision building, adaptability, stewardship, flexibility, risk taking, conflict management, credibility, and empowerment. These nine characteristics were used to develop The Leadership Characteristics and Skills Assessment Tool.

Importantly, all of the attributes of transformational leaders contribute to trust formation (Dirks & Ferrin, 2001; Spinelli, 2006). Basically, transformational leaders, discussed further in a later section, are able to foster a sense of trust between themselves and others and build a history of being viewed as capable of "showing the way," which is consistent with the leadership work of Kouzes and Posner (2012).

The long list of personal and relationship-oriented attributes required for leadership can seem daunting and leads some to believe that a person must be born with leadership attributes—that it is not possible to learn them. On the contrary, each of the personal and relationship-oriented attributes can be learned, developed, or enhanced over time, using targeted strategies. There is an exercise at the end of this chapter focused on helping burgeoning CNSs in the development of leadership attributes.

INTERPERSONAL POWER AND INFLUENCE

The personal and relationship-oriented attributes identified previously are fundamentally important to maximize the leader's effectiveness in influencing others. Leaders are able to envision a better way and to influence people to commit to making the vision reality. The ability to influence in a noncoercive manner is dependent on a number of factors in addition to the attributes identified previously, not the least of which is having interpersonal power (Bass, 1999; Burns, 1978; Gillespie & Mann, 2004; Kouzes & Posner, 2002). The concept of *power* is intriguing. It is often thought of as a negative attribute. When power is thought to be a bad thing, it is usually in the context of someone possessing control over others with the intent of causing harm or creating negative consequences. However, power in itself is not a bad thing and can be and often is used for positive/beneficial ends.

Interpersonal Power

Power is energy, that is, the "ability to act or produce an effect" (*Merriam-Webster Online Dictionary*, 2008b). From a physics perspective, *energy* is the capability or force to move an object. A magnet is a good analogy to explain interpersonal power. A magnet is a compound of an element (iron, nickel, cobalt, or neodymium) that has been correctly mixed together (in the right atmosphere) with a higher weight element, such as strontium, to be able to hold a charge; then the combined mixture is infused with an electrical charge to align the molecules and magnetize them. The result is a magnet that attracts, that is, draws or pulls other elements to it (How Stuff Works, 2008).

Change initiatives are more effective when they encompass "drawing to" or "pulling" strategies as opposed to "pushing" strategies (Eisenbach, Watson, & Rajinandini, 1999). The notion of "drawing to" rather than "pushing" differentiates two types of power: personal power (attributable to the person) and position power (attributable to the position). Pushing strategies are more reflective of position power. That is, persons with position or line authority, such as administrators, typically have the decisional authority to mandate direction as well as the ability to use tangible rewards and disincentives to push people in the desired direction.

Within health care organizations, CNS positions are typically salaried positions without line authority or position power. Characteristically, CNSs report directly to administrators such as the chief nursing officer (CNO) or director of advanced practice. CNSs must earn interpersonal power and purposefully use influence strategies to stimulate nursing staff and members of other health care disciplines to work toward visions focused on improving patient outcomes and cost-effectiveness.

As is evident from the previous discussion, interpersonal power and leadership are not the same constructs. Leadership is not power, per se, but is the use of power to pull others toward a goal. Power is a social construct; that is, it can only exist when two or more people are present. Although normally not incorporated into the understanding of personal power, Emerson's (1962) classic research on "dyadic resource dependence" demonstrated that when one person in a relationship has difficult-to-obtain resources that the other needs, then the person with the resources has power in that relationship. Farmer and Aquinis (2005) integrated Emerson's resource dependence theory with identity (role) theory (Ashforth, 2001) and self-verification theory (Burke, 1991) to explain power in relationships. The new theoretical postulates are applicable to any situation in which one person desires to influence another. Understanding that power is a relational concept that is in large measure affected by one person (or group) needing the resources of another person (or group) has practical implications for CNSs. It is sometimes helpful to think of it in the following manner, which is consistent with Emerson's research findings: When person or Group "A" *needs* person or Group "B" more than person or Group "B" *needs* person or Group "A," then Group "B" has more power! It is often helpful for CNSs to understand that an important derivative of their work is creating perceived *need* for their work in the organization.

The advanced nursing knowledge and skill that CNSs possess, along with expertise in their specialty area and ability to work with groups to change practice, are greatly needed by health care organizations. Therefore, there is abundant opportunity for a CNS to gain recognition as someone who is highly valued in the organization. The ability of CNSs to influence others, including staff nurses, other members of the health care team, the CNO, and the chief executive officer (CEO) is, in significant measure, dependent on the assets they bring to help meet the *organization's needs*. These assets can be categorized into the types of power discussed in the following sections, including knowledge power, charisma power, referent power, and resource power (Huber, 2000; Roberts & Vasquez, 2004).

Knowledge Power

Knowledge power is expertise. Expertise encompasses both knowledge and skill. You've often heard the phrase "knowledge is power." Knowledge is almost universally powerful in that it is needed for almost any activity; it is universal currency. Knowledge is so valuable that if protected in the form of patents or copyright or other legal means it is actually a salable commodity in the form of intellectual capital. CNSs have expert clinical knowledge and knowledge about how to advance the practice of nursing and patient care to improve patient outcomes and cost-effectiveness. As a CNS's knowledge in these areas becomes apparent in an organization, the *value* of the CNS to the organization—and, therefore, the power of the CNS in the organization—is enhanced.

Charisma Power

Charismatic power in essence is the ability to charm others. Charisma is a personal quality that is characterized by being appealing to others through a combination of factors, including pleasing appearance, enthusiasm, excellent communication skills, and the desire to be engaged with others. Charismatic people demonstrate the desire to be engaged with others by acknowledging others and remembering names and important aspects of the lives of others such as family, significant others, or pets. Being likable is important for a CNS. Different from the CNS needing to be liked by everyone, it is presenting oneself in a pleasing fashion and with an engaging demeanor. It is important to recognize that being in good relationships with others establishes social capital. Groves's (2005) research findings on charisma supported the significant positive relationship between a change agent's level of charisma and general openness to initiatives targeting organizational change.

Referent Power

While knowledge and charisma power are possessed by the person having it, referent power is network power. That is, the CNS needs to nurture and maintain good relationships with people in higher levels of position power, for example, work colleagues and professional colleagues or even friends who happen to be in positions of power. It is important that CNSs be in good relationships with key stakeholders in an organization, including the CEO, CNO, and chief financial officer (CFO).

Resource Power

While the persons you are in relationships with can be a source of referent power, the personal resources you have, including critical thinking and problem-solving ability, the ability to work with and lead groups, and other services you can provide, are a source of *resource* power. Resource power also includes tangible resources, such as money and property, but the most pertinent to CNSs is the provision of nontangible resources. A common example is the important service that CNSs provide in leading multidisciplinary group work within an organization.

The CNS can acquire considerable interpersonal power by continuing to develop knowledge/skill competencies corresponding to the needs of the organization, demonstrating charisma, attending to the development of positive relationships with those who have position authority, and being generous in the provision of services. In addition to acquiring interpersonal power, it is important to be sensitive to the basic principles of influence.

Influence

Individual effectiveness in organizations is largely dependent on the individual's ability to influence others (Cable & Judge, 2003; Kipnis & Schmidt, 1988; Yukl & Falbe, 1990). In his classic work on influence, first published in 1984 and later updated based on additional research, Cialdini (2008) identified six principles that form the foundation for the ability to influence or to get another person to say "yes." The book is a wonderful interweaving of theory and empirical evidence, and each of the principles is summarized next.

Rule of Reciprocity

The *rule of reciprocity* is based upon the norm of desiring to pay back or repay another person for something that was provided. In other words, it is common for humans to experience an obligation to repay once something is given to them. Research has demonstrated that the rule of reciprocity is very powerful and can even spur unequal exchanges, where a person feels indebted to even do a larger favor than the one received. This is another example of social capital. An example of the rule of reciprocity is helping a staff nurse with a difficult patient by demonstrating calming strategies that soothe the patient while bathing and changing the bed, and the next week the staff nurse volunteers to be on the practice improvement team focused on caring for patients experiencing confusion.

Commitment and Consistency

The principle of *commitment and consistency* is based on the human desire to be consistent in words, attitudes, and deeds. The desire to be consistent is reinforced by a society that highly values consistency.

This principle is played out by a person agreeing with or making a commitment to a stand or position, and then, based on that position, there is a greater willingness to demonstrate actions that are consistent with the prior commitment. Commitments are most effective when they are active, public, and viewed as internally motivated rather than coerced. Once a position has been taken, the person is more likely to behave in ways consistent with the stand. An example of the principle of commitment and consistency is when individuals in a multidisciplinary group agree that patient safety is a priority for their respective disciplines and then later agree to a new policy on hand washing that mandates reporting actions not consistent with the policy.

Social Proof

The principle of *social proof* is based on two human tendencies. First, when people are uncertain about what behavior is viewed as most appropriate in a group, they are more likely to view the behavior of others and accept those behaviors as correct or expected. Second, people are more inclined to follow the behavior of others who are similar to them. An example of social proof is when a CNS models asking questions about why a particular problem (symptom or functional) is being experienced by patients and then openly seeks the data/evidence to identify the etiology of the problem and what nursing care is required to prevent it. Later, a staff member, who has observed the CNS, makes it known that he or she is wondering why the patients on the orthopedic unit are experiencing breakthrough pain despite all of the analgesics being administered.

Liking

The fourth principle, *liking*, corresponds to charisma power discussed earlier. In general, people prefer to say "yes" to people that they know and like. There are several factors that affect "liking," including physical attractiveness, similarity, praise, familiarity, and association. Research has demonstrated that physical attractiveness/appearance creates an advantage in the ability to persuade and to change the attitude of others (Cialdini, 2008). Regarding similarity, we tend to like people who are like us and share common beliefs. Praise and/or the judicious use of sincere compliments can enhance liking. Repeated contact with a person can create a sense of comfort or familiarity and when we are associated with positive things or events there is often a halo effect. How a CNS dresses can promote a sense of similarity and association, and thus, CNSs should be sensitive to their audience. When working with staff nurses, many CNSs wear scrubs or a nice lab coat over comfortable everyday work clothes, but they bring business clothes for the hospital board meeting that will be attended in the evening. Further, it is essential that CNSs acknowledge, give credit, and publicly praise staff nurses and others for their contributions to accomplishing a goal and to demonstrate gratitude—to say "thank you." In this day of high-tech communications, handwritten thank-you notes stand out as something very special!

Authority

There is substantial research evidence for the principle of *authority*. There is a strong pressure in society to obey legitimate authority. Obedience to legitimate or appropriate authority is viewed as correct conduct. Research has shown that authority is demonstrated through titles (inferring knowledge), clothing, and automobiles. When a person possessed one or more of these symbols, there was more deference or obedience by those who encountered him or her (Cialdini, 2008). Examples of authority are the titles of CEO, CNO, CFO, and, increasingly, the title of CNS. Another example of authority is a classy dress suit (for women or men), interestingly often referred to as a "power" suit.

Scarcity

Scarcity is the last and sixth principle. Interestingly, people tend to assign more value to an opportunity or an object or information that is less available. For example, research has demonstrated that the act of limiting access to a message may cause people to want it more. Information that is perceived to be exclusive is more highly valued (Cialdini, 2008). This is not to say that it is a good thing to control information or resources by hoarding. It is, however, one reason why hospital CEOs and CNOs tout that their hospital has Magnet status and that they have eight CNSs! There is a national shortage of CNSs, demonstrated by the large number of open CNS positions continuously advertised by hospitals and recruiting agencies. Recognition of the fortunate position a hospital is in when there are CNSs employed by the hospital can influence administrators to be early adopters of CNS recommendations.

TRANSFORMATIONAL LEADERSHIP

Although transformational leadership has been a focus in nursing literature for the past 20 years, the importance of transformational leaders has been recognized for more than 30 years. Burns (1978), who first defined transformational leadership, asserted in his classic book on leadership that transformational leaders are able to appeal to followers' sense of values, help them see a higher vision, and encourage them to exert themselves in helping to achieve the vision. The personal attributes (including emotional intelligence, see Chapter 4) and relationship-oriented attributes, along with earned interpersonal power and the judicious use of the principles of influence covered previously, form the foundation for effective transformational leaders.

Transformational leaders motivate others to work on behalf of an organizational vision/mission and related goals. Transformational leaders inspire others to believe that the goal is both significant and attainable. They are able to intelligently articulate the rationale for and evidence undergirding the need for the goal, while inviting discussion and dialogue in refining the goal and encouraging others to be curious and to take risks. Similar to the approach advocated for leaders in the principles of complex adaptive systems is the importance of viewing difficulties as opportunities to be curious about solutions and to take risks in discovering new solutions. Taking risks is easier when members of a group share the same values because that fosters a higher level of trust (Gillespie & Mann, 2004). Transformational leaders are also able to reduce uncertainty and to reduce the experience of apathy by being visible and being positive (Bass, 1999).

Herold, Fedor, Caldwell, and Liu (2008) compared transformational leadership with change leadership in a study of 343 employees in 30 organizations representing a wide variety of industry sectors. Findings from the study demonstrated that transformational leadership and an employee's commitment to specific change projects were significantly positively related. That is, transformational leaders were able to get more commitment regardless of their ability to manage change well and regardless of the personal impact of the change on the employee's specific job situations (workload and relationships). *Commitment* was defined as encompassing both the attitude toward the change as well as the willingness to work on behalf of the successful implementation of change. This type of commitment is commonly referred to as "buy-in." Herold's findings were consistent with research on authentic leadership (George, 2003).

Transformational leadership skills are the most effective in providing clinical leadership that motivates and guides others toward practice improvements (Cook & Leathard, 2004). Thus, the development of transformational leadership skills, discussed here as *practices*, is critical to the work of CNSs.

Five Practices of Transformational Leadership

The five practices of exemplary transformational leadership were identified by Kouzes and Posner (2012). Their renowned work, initially published in 1993, was grounded in interviews of 1,100 leaders. In their study of exemplary leaders beginning in the 1980s and carried through the 2000s, they found that the attributes of leadership have not changed, but the context for leadership has changed rather dramatically. In today's world, there is a heightened degree of uncertainty and sense of chaos. Leaders must recognize (a) the reality of the speed of change as an outgrowth of new technologies; (b) the changing workforce, where trusting organizations and experiencing a sense of commitment is not necessarily commonplace; (c) the common need to search for meaning, including the desire to make a difference; (d) the connectivity of people (social capital, in that it is human networks that make the difference); and (e) the global economy requiring global understanding (Kouzes & Posner, 2012). It is imperative that CNSs be sensitive to the realities of today's world and workforce while focusing on their own self-awareness, social awareness, and interpersonal skills.

In today's context, there are many challenging opportunities for leaders in health care organizations. The leadership challenge is to mobilize others to want to do extraordinary things to turn challenges into successes. The five practices of leadership to mobilize others include modeling the way, inspiring a shared vision, challenging the process, enabling others to act, and leading with the heart (Kouzes & Posner, 2012).

Modeling the Way

In describing *modeling the way*, Kouzes and Posner (2012) make the important point that it's not titles that win you respect, it's your behavior. CNSs must model the behavior they expect from others, including talking clearly and openly about what they value, because it is important to lead from what you believe/ value. For example, "The most important people in this hospital are the patients...our primary concern must be their well-being and safety." A true leader's behavior is consistent with those values and is evidenced by spending time with those you are leading, sharing stories that make the values come alive, being there in uncertain times, and asking questions that help to focus attention on values and priorities. You can model the way by saying to staff nurses, "You are the ones on the front line—the patients need you to feel free to question and to take action to assure the quality of their care."

Inspiring a Shared Vision

Inspiring a shared vision first requires that the leader envision a desired and attractive future for the organization or service unit, such as an intensive care unit. With a "we can do it" message, that vision or dream is shared enthusiastically and in a manner and language consistent with the values and desires of those listening. In other words, CNSs must take time to listen to nursing staff to learn who they are and what they value. Tapping into those values and dreams helps to start the fire in them to take actions that will help make their hopes or dreams come alive. "You can't command commitment; you have to inspire it" (Kouzes & Posner, 2012, p. 18). Reality doesn't exist outside of us—we create it! The clear image of the future pulls the leader and others forward as a collective whole (Kouzes & Posner, 2012).

Challenging the Process

All of the leaders interviewed by Kouzes and Posner (2012) had in some way *challenged a process*—be that a new product, a rule, regulation, or legislation, or a way of doing business. In that manner, leaders are pioneers or innovators. Leaders listen. They encourage others to ask questions and challenge processes. "Why are we changing beds everyday?" "Why are we using these expensive mouth swabs—do we know that they are more effective than just good mouth care?"

It's the leader's job to sell a problem and to frame it as an opportunity to do better or to do something in a different way to produce better outcomes. Leaders also recognize that venturing into new territories carries uncertainties, potential risks, and failures. A leader always treats challenges or difficult situations as learning opportunities while acknowledging the emotions of self and others. These types of efforts are adventures—discovering what works and what doesn't and helping others feel safe while affirming that everyone is in this together (Lyon, 2001b).

Enabling Others to Act

Leaders *enable others to act*. "Leadership is a team effort" (Kouzes & Posner, 2012). Leaders manufacture hope. "Together, I know we can do this!" Hope is important in enabling change (Avolio & Luthan, 2006). Hope can be reinforced by breaking large, complex goals down into accomplishable steps and celebrating these milestones (Avolio & Luthan, 2006; Lyon, 2001a).

Good leaders foster a sense of trust and the desire for collaboration. Enabling others to act necessitates that others feel a sense of ownership and the power to take risks in trying new ways to solve problems (Lyon, 2001c). The establishment of teams that have the responsibility and authority to act on particular clinical problems, (for example, skin care or ventilator acquired pneumonia), and where members can act as consultants to other nurses or other members of the health care team is a great way to enable action.

Leading With the Heart

CNSs are commonly passionate about their specialty and the power of nursing to positively improve patient outcomes, making it easier to *lead from the heart*. It has been said that the difference between a vision and a goal is passion, that is, a vision is inspired by passion. Passion is the fire for a CNS's work. When a CNS is positively passionate about his or her work, the passion is a source of enjoyment and is evident to others. It can be contagious!

It is often helpful for CNSs to tap into the value structure of staff nurses and other members of the health care team. When a staff nurse or physician can be engaged in work that is consonant with his or her values, then it is more likely that the individual will experience satisfaction and even joy in doing the work.

Experiencing joy at work can be enhanced by being recognized and appreciated. The heart is more easily engaged when others recognize a job well done and celebrate successes. It is important for CNSs to show appreciation for individual excellence on the part of staff nurses, physicians, and other members of the team, as well as administrators.

As noted earlier, CNSs can be "hope" leaders focused on forward movement consistent with an organization's mission and the desire to improve patient outcomes. Recognizing and celebrating the achievement of patient care goals can bring joy to the work of nursing.

SUMMARY

Effective CNSs are transformational leaders in health care organizations who work to advance the practice of nursing and patient care in general to improve outcomes in a cost-effective manner. Transformational leaders have the personal and relationship-oriented attributes and the interpersonal power to effectively use influence strategies to motivate others to work toward shared goals. The interpersonal power to influence others within an organization is earned by being responsive to and appropriately meeting the needs of stakeholders, including staff nurses, other members of the health care team, and executive leadership.

The essential elements involved in the capacity to lead or influence others include particular personal and relationship-focused attributes, the ability to earn and effectively use interpersonal power, and the judicious use of the principles of influence. Each of these elements forms part of the foundation for the enactment of the five practices of transformational leadership skills: modeling the way, inspiring a shared vision, challenging, enabling others to act, and leading with the heart.

Earning the power to influence and developing transformational leadership skills requires that the CNS attend to both personal and professional development to enhance the positive attributes inherent in transformational leaders and to be cognizant of the important relationship between an organization's needs and the CNS's resources. The discussion questions and exercises that follow are designed to guide the reader in the personal development of leadership attributes.

▨ DISCUSSION QUESTIONS

- Identify and discuss the types of interpersonal power you observe in practicing CNSs. What are the common types of interpersonal power you see in the most admired CNSs within an institution? How do you know when a CNS has garnered interpersonal power?
- Identify and discuss the influence strategies that you have observed your CNS preceptors, faculty, and other leaders use to effect change.
- Discuss with practicing CNSs what they found to be the most difficult leadership challenge in effecting a practice change with staff nurses and with a multidisciplinary team.

▨ ANALYSIS AND SYNTHESIS EXERCISES

- Make a list of the personal and relationship-oriented attributes of leadership. Conduct a personal assessment of your strengths with respect to each of these attributes, and identify areas for growth. For each area of growth, identify at least one thing you can do to enhance your personal and/or relationship-oriented attributes. The list may include such things as joining "Toast Masters," taking a course in assertiveness training or conflict management, making it a priority to write thank-you notes, taking a powerful other to lunch, seeking feedback from peers, or taking a course in listening.
- Interview one transformational leader in the institution where you work, where you are having

clinical experiences, or at your school about his or her leadership experiences. Use the content in each section of the chapter to formulate your questions. Examples might be

a. "In your experiences, what have you found to be the most important personal attributes of an effective or transformational leader?"

b. "What have you found to be the most effective ways to influence others to take a desired action?"

- Discuss the questions you asked (including why you thought they were important), comparing your interviewee's responses with the content in the chapter. Identify with your classmates how your various interviewees' responses were similar or different in offering a unique perspective on leadership.

REFERENCES

Ashforth, B. E. (2001). *Role transitions in organizational life: An identity based perspective*. Mahwah, NJ: Lawrence Erlbaum Associates.

Avolio, B. J., & Luthan, F. (2006). *The high impact leader: Moments matter in accelerating authentic leadership development*. New York, NY: McGraw-Hill.

Bahr, S. J., Senica, A., Gingrae, L., & Ryan, P. (2010). Clinical nurse specialist–led evaluation of temporal artery thermometers in acute care. *Clinical Nurse Specialist, 24*(5), 238–244.

Bass, B. M. (1999). Two decades of research and development in transformational leadership. *European Journal of Work and Organizational Psychology, 8*(1), 9–32.

Becker, E., Dee, V., Gawlinski, A., Kirkpatrick, T., Lawanson-Nichols, M., Lee, B.,...Zanotti, J. (2012). Clinical nurse specialists shaping policies and procedures via an evidence-based clinical practice council. *Clinical Nurse Specialist, 26*(2), 74–86.

Benedict, L., Robinson, K., & Holder, C. (2006). Clinical nurse specialists within the acute care for elders interdisciplinary team model. *Clinical Nurse Specialist, 20*(5), 248–251.

Burke, P. J. (1991). Identify processes and social stress. *American Sociological Review, 56*, 836–849.

Burns, J. M. (1978). *Leadership*. New York, NY: Harper & Row.

Cable, D. M., & Judge, T. A. (2003). Managers' upward influence tactic strategies: The role of manager personality and supervisor leadership style. *Journal of Organizational Behavior, 24*, 197–214.

Centers for Medicare and Medicaid Services (CMS). (2011). Medicare program: Hospital inpatient value-based purchasing program. Final rule. *Federal Register, 76*(88), 26490–26547.

Cialdini, R. B. (2008). *Influence: Science and practice* (5th ed.). Boston, MA: Allyn & Bacon.

Cook, M. J., & Leathard, H. L. (2004). Learning for clinical leadership. *Journal of Nursing Management, 12*, 436–444.

Custer, M. (2010). Outcomes of clinical nurse specialist–initiated system level stardardized glucose management. *Clinical Nurse Specialist, 24*(3), 132–139.

Dietz, B., & Smith, T. T. (2002). Enhancing the accuracy of hemo-dynamic monitoring. *Journal of Nursing Care Quality, 17*(1), 27–34.

Dirks, K., & Ferrin, D. (2001). The role of trust in organizational settings. *Organizational Science, 12*(4), 450–467.

Duffy, J. R. (2002). The clinical leadership role of the CNS in the identification of nursing-sensitive and multidisciplinary quality indicator sets. *Clinical Nurse Specialist: The Journal for Advanced Nursing Practice, 16*(2), 70–76.

Ebright, P., Patterson, E. S., & Render, M. L. (2002). The "new look" approach to patient safety: A guide for clinical nurse specialist leadership. *Clinical Nurse Specialist: The Journal for Advanced Nursing Practice, 16*(5), 247–253.

Eisenbach, R., Watson, K., & Rajinandini, P. (1999). Transformational leadership in the context of organizational change. *Journal of Organizational Change, 12*(2), 80–89.

Emerson, R. M. (1962). Power-dependence relations. *American Sociological Review, 27*, 31–41.

Farmer, S. M., & Aguinis, H. (2005). Accounting for subordinate perceptions of supervisor power: An identity-dependence model. *Journal of Applied Psychology, 90*(6), 1069–1083.

Finkleman, A. (2013). The clinical nurse specialist: Leadership in quality improvement. *Clinical Nurse Specialist, 27*(1), 31–35.

Foggow, D. J., Solie, C. J., Tracy, M. F., & Gjere, N. (2005). Clinical nurse specialist leadership in computerized provider order entry design. *Clinical Nurse Specialist, 19*(4), 209–214.

Gillespie, N., & Mann, L. (2004). Transformational leadership and shared values: The building blocks of trust. *Journal of Healthcare Management, 19*(6), 588–607.

George, B. (2003). *Authentic leadership: Rediscovering the secrets to creating lasting value*. San Francisco, CA: Jossey-Bass.

Green, A., & Jordan, C. (2004). Common denominators: Shared governance and work place advocacy— Strategies for nurses to gain control over their practice. *Journal of Issues in Nursing, 9*(1).

Grossman, S. C., & Valiga, T. M. (2005). *The new leadership challenge: Creating the future of nursing* (2nd ed.). Philadelphia, PA: F. A. Davis.

Groves, K. S. (2005). Linking leader skills, follower attitudes and contextual variables via an integration of charismatic leadership. *Journal of Management, 31*, 255–277.

Herold, D. M., Fedor, D. B., Caldwell, S., & Liu, Y. (2008). The effects of transformational and change leadership on employee's commitment to a change: A multilevel study. *Journal of Applied Psychology, 93*(2), 346–357.

How Stuff Works. (2008). *Magnets*. Retrieved August 19, 2008, from http://science.howstuffworks.com/magnet.htm

Huber, D. (2000). *Power and conflict: Leadership and nursing care management*. Philadelphia, PA: WB Saunders.

Institute of Medicine (IOM). (2004). *Keeping patients safe: Transforming the work environment of nurses*. Washington, DC: National Academies Press.

Kipnis, D., & Schmidt, S. M. (1988). Upward-influence styles: Relationship with performance evaluations, salary, and stress. *Administrative Science Quarterly, 33*, 528–542.

Kouzes, J. M., & Posner, B. Z. (2012). *The leadership challenge: How to make extraordinary things happen in organizations* (5th ed). San Francisco, CA: Jossey-Bass.

Laschinger, H. K. S., & Smith, L. M. (2013). The influence of authentic leadership and empowerment on new-graduate nurses' perceptions of interprofessional collaboration. *The Journal of Nursing Administration, 43*(1), 24–29.

Lyon, B. L. (2001a). Conquering frustration: REAPing the benefits. *Reflections in Nursing Leadership, 27*(1), 38–39.

Lyon, B. L. (2001b). Positive situational focusing: Pollyanna or a powerful stress prevention strategy? *Reflections in Nursing Leadership, 27*(2), 38–39, 45.

Lyon, B. L. (2001c). Strategies to enhance positive situational focusing skills. *Reflections in Nursing Leadership, 27*(3), 36–37, 44.

Merriam-Webster Online Dictionary. (2008a). *Influence*. Retrieved July 17, 2008, from http://www.merriam-webster.com/dictionary/power

Merriam-Webster Online Dictionary. (2008b). *Power*. Retrieved July 17, 2008, from http://www.merriam-webster.com/dictionary/power

Morissette, J. (2004). Clinical nurse specialist as a leader of a bariatric program. *Clinical Nurse Specialist: The Journal for Advanced Nursing Practice, 19*(4), 209–215.

National Association of Clinical Nurse Specialists (NACNS). (2004). *Statement on clinical nurse specialist practice and education* (2nd ed.). Harrisburg, PA: Author.

National Association of Clinical Nurse Specialists (NACNS). (2012). The National Association of Clinical Nurse Specialists response to the Institute of Medicine's *The Future of Nursing* report. *Clinical Nurse Specialist, 26*(4), 222–224.

Richardson, J., & Tjoelker, R. (2012). Beyond the central line associated blood stream infection bundle: The value of the clinical nurse specialist in continuing evidence-based practice changes. *Clinical Nurse Specialist, 26*(4), 205–2011.

Roberts, D. W., & Vasquez, E. (2004). Power: An application to the nursing image and advanced practice. *AACN Clinical Issues, 15*(2), 196–204.

Rosenthal, M. B. (2007). Nonpayment for performance? Medicare's new reimbursement rule. *New England Journal of Medicine, 357*, 1573–1575.

Seemann, S., Soukup, M., & Adams, P. (2000). Hospital wide intravenous initiative. *Nursing Clinics of North America, 35*(2), 361–373.

Sitterding, M. C., Froome, M., Everitt, L., & Ebright, P. (2012). Understanding situation awareness in nursing work: A hybrid concept analysis. *Advances in Nursing Science, 35*(1), 77–92.

Spinelli, R. (2006). The applicability of Bass's model of transformational, transactional and laissez-faire leadership in the hospital administrative environment. *Hospital Topics, 84*(2), 11–18.

Wolf, G., Zimmerman, D., & Drenkard, K. (2011). Transformational leadership. In *Magnet™: The next generation. Nurses making a difference* (pp. 31–41). Silver Spring, MD: American Nurses Credentialing Center.

Yukl, G., & Falbe, C. M. (1990). Influence tactics and objective in upward, downward, and lateral influence attempts. *Journal of Applied Psychology, 77*, 525–535.

Creating a Culture of Quality

Nancy Benton

According to the National Association of Clinical Nurse Specialists' (NACNS) *Statement on Clinical Nurse Specialist Practice and Education* (NACNS, 2013), clinical nurse specialists (CNSs) "provide expert and independent care to promote health by promoting wellness, preventing illness, and providing expert assistance with disease care" (p. 55). Implied within this statement is that CNSs practice in their role with attention to the quality of care provided. Quality in health care, however, can be an elusive concept. The purpose of this chapter is to provide some insight into how quality in health care is defined, measured, and improved to create a culture of quality within the context of the practice and role of the CNS.

Historic approaches and perceptions of quality in health care are discussed, followed by contemporary approaches to ensuring health care quality. A definition for quality health care (QHC) from the nursing perspective is also discussed. Finally, the CNS's role in creating a culture of quality is explored.

BACKGROUND

To understand quality as it pertains to nursing roles, it is useful to go back to the beginning of modern nursing. Additionally, there is information and insight to be gained from reviewing the medical profession's approach to QHC.

Quality Pioneers

It could be argued that the first nurse to address quality of care was Florence Nightingale in the mid-19th century. She abhorred and fought to change the appalling conditions in which soldiers received medical care. By changing and improving the conditions in which injured soldiers were treated, mortality outcomes were improved. This could be defined as one of the first quality outcomes in health care where nursing played a key role. Florence Nightingale was the first nurse who was also a health care quality improvement specialist. Not unlike today's quality professionals, Florence Nightingale used scientific methodology to gather data and employed statistical processes to identify areas in need of improvement (Neuhauser, 2003).

Later, her aspirations to improve the quality of health care led her to open the first training academy for nurses. It could be said that modern nursing has its most fundamental beginnings in the pursuit of QHC. Florence Nightingale devoted her entire adult life to improving the quality of health care as it relates to the nursing profession. In addition to collecting data and using statistical techniques to identify improvement opportunities related to clinical practice and outcomes, she also devoted herself to improving the competence of nurses through standardized training for nurses.

In a more recent example of quality improvement in health care, a 20th-century pioneer in health care quality, Avedis Donabedian, proposed a comprehensive approach to examining quality in his landmark paper "Evaluating the Quality of Medical Care" (Donabedian, 2005). Donabedian has been called the father of quality assurance, and it is his work that is most often cited in health care quality research. Donabedian, a physician with a master of public health degree, recognized that medical care does not occur in a vacuum. The health care system and numerous health care disciplines are interwoven with each other and inextricably linked to quality outcomes. Recognizing this linkage, Donabedian proposed a structure–process–outcome model for assessing quality. *Structure* referred to the physical and organizational settings in which providers of health care practice, as well as the tools and resources they have available. *Process* referred to the manner in which health care was administered, such as patient–provider interaction, documentation of interventions, and competence of practice. Finally, *outcomes* referred to whether the desired result was achieved (Donabedian, 1980). These three dimensions of health care delivery are the framework most often used to develop methods for examining and improving the quality of health care. Measuring components of the structure, process, and outcome of health care delivery helps determine what is working well and what needs improvement.

Donabedian (2005) devoted his entire career in medicine and public health to promote better understanding of quality and methods to improve the quality of health care. In a 1996 article, he offered the following advice:

> To my mind, the most important single condition for success in quality assurance is the determination to make it work. If we are truly committed to quality, almost any reasonable method will work. If we are not, the most elegantly constructed of mechanisms will fail. (Donabedian, 1996, p. 406)

Donabedian was trying to tell us that passion for improvement is the necessary ingredient to successful quality improvement efforts.

DEFINING QUALITY

The word *quality* is used in health care frequently: for example, high-QHC, QHC organizations, improving the quality of health care, ensuring quality, quality management, and quality improvement. *Quality* as a word is easily defined, and there are many definitions. However, quality in health care is a complex concept that is not easily defined. The *American Heritage Dictionary* (2013) lists *quality* as an adjective: Having a high degree of excellence: the importance of QHC.

To be certain, quality in health care is important, but the question remains, "What is quality in health care, and how do we know it when we see it?"

The first step in understanding a complex concept such as quality in health care is to define the concept. The literature on health care quality is scant with true concept analyses as defined by Walker and Avant (1994). Nevertheless, there are some definitions available that relate to quality in health care.

In its policy statement H-450.975, the American Medical Association (AMA, 2013) defines quality of care as "the degree to which care services influence the probability of optimal patient outcomes." The Institute of Medicine (IOM, 2001, p. 52) defines quality as "the degree to which health services for individuals and populations increase the likelihood of desired health outcomes and are consistent with current professional knowledge." Both of these definitions seem to leave out key components of quality important to nursing, namely, caring and patient involvement. The American Nurses Association (ANA) states that quality is a changing concept and that, currently, quality in health care is "meeting the public's expectations in the delivery of clinically effective, efficient, and affordable health care services" (Kay, 2005, p. 75). This definition explicitly includes the patient perspective on quality. However, the concept of safety in health care is missing from this definition of quality.

Quality is a concept that is influenced by individual perceptions. Quality in health care is not necessarily a concept that demands attention when it is present in the health care experience. Indeed, quality in health care may best be noticed and described when it is missing from the health care experience. For example, the patient who waits many hours in an emergency room only to receive the wrong treatment by overworked health care professionals in an abrupt and less than caring manner is sure to recognize the lack of quality in his or her health care experience, whereas the patient who receives timely, correct treatment from health care professionals who are compassionate and caring may consider the experience routine and expected. The latter patient may not necessarily think to describe the experience as QHC.

What is quality for some may not be so for others. The indicators of quality may differ depending upon the viewpoint of the evaluator and the context in which the health care experience occurs. Patient perceptions of whether or not they have received QHC are often very different from the health care professionals' perceptions of whether QHC was delivered. Equally, the patient and professionals' perceptions may be very different from the health care system perspective of whether QHC was delivered. An all-encompassing definition of quality as it relates to health care is difficult.

PERSPECTIVES ON QUALITY

As mentioned previously, perceptions of quality in health care differ depending upon the standpoint of the observer. Patients, health care practitioners, and health care systems will all have different ideas of what represents quality.

Within the category of health care providers, nursing and medicine clearly have different definitions of quality. Most prominent in medicine's literature is outcomes of clinical care as a measure of quality (IOM, 2001). In nursing, assessment, processes, planning care delivery, and a holistic focus for QHC are evident (Attree, 1996).

In the context of the CNS's role, QHC demands that we examine the practice component as well as the patient perception of quality. Additionally, as an advanced practice nurse, an essential characteristic of the CNS is advanced expertise in "human and organizational factors that affect resource management, quality, and cost across the continuum of care" (NACNS, 2013, p. 14). The CNS must also be concerned with quality, not only as it relates to individual care but also to populations as well as health care systems.

QUALITY AND CNS SPHERES OF INFLUENCE

The conceptual model of CNS practice includes the patient/client sphere, the nurse and nursing practice sphere, and the organization/system sphere (NACNS, 2013). The concept of QHC and its relationship to the three spheres is the framework for the CNS role in creating a culture of quality.

Patient/Client Sphere

Today, most patients have some idea of the meaning of QHC; however, individual perceptions of quality may differ between patients. If there is any doubt in the patient's mind about the quality of health care he or she isreceiving, the Agency for Healthcare Research and Quality (AHRQ) has published a consumer booklet titled *Guide to Health Care Quality: How to Know It When You See It* (AHRQ, 2005). In this guide, the AHRQ places emphasis on the clinical quality of care. Did the outcome achieved match the desired outcome? There is no disagreement that outcome measures, such as whether the surgery removed all of the cancer or whether the treatment regimen improved cardiac output, are appropriate indicators of quality for patients. However, outcome measures are not the only important indicators of quality.

Age-specific quality is another consideration. A geriatric patient's view of QHC is likely different from the young adult view, which is different, yet again, from the perspective of a pediatric patient. The pediatric patient may gauge quality by whether or not the immunization injection was painful or whether the health care staff was friendly. The young adult patient may value timeliness of the appointment and waiting room times as important indicators of quality. The geriatric patient, however, may value the provider's caring attitude and willingness to take the time to listen as the most important indicator of quality. The patient viewpoint is an important measure of QHC.

Patient satisfaction reports encompass the latest research on patient perceptions, which includes domains of satisfaction related to health care provider interactions, ancillary health care staff interactions, timeliness and responsiveness of care, and whether educational needs were met. Some satisfaction surveys also include questions regarding the environment in which care was delivered, such as whether the waiting rooms and exam rooms were clean and well-appointed.

The patient as a partner in his or her own health care is also important. Most patients today are very well-informed about health care and their particular chronic disease. Being patient-centered demands that the CNS not only demonstrate a caring attitude but also be responsive to including the patient in decision making about his or her own health care. This requires the CNS to be equally well informed and well equipped to answer questions and provide the latest evidence-based information to help the patient in decision making.

The patient/client sphere of nursing practice as it relates to creating a culture of quality includes two important concepts. The first concept is patient satisfaction: Does the patient/client perceive that his or her needs were met in a manner that was competent, respectful, and caring? The second concept relates to CNS competence: Is the CNS well informed regarding the latest treatment options and alternatives, and was this information shared with the patient in a way he or she could understand and, therefore, participate in the decision making?

Nurse and Nursing Practice Sphere

Most, if not all, health care professionals enter the health care profession with the intent to ease the pain and suffering caused by illness and injury and to help to restore patients to their optimal potential functioning. The successful provision of health care is most often measured by outcome indicators. Did the patient receive a timely diagnosis? Did the surgery remove all of the cancer? Did the patient live?

CNSs advance nursing practice by setting examples and providing leadership to guide nurses in the application of evidence-based practice (EBP). There is substantial evidence in the literature with regard to improved outcomes for patients that can be directly related to the quantity and quality of nursing care (ANA, 1997). The CNS role in quality, with regard to the nurses and nursing practice sphere, is to be well versed in the measures of quality that relate to nursing practice and to facilitate optimal performance in those measures. Some examples of quality indicators for nursing care are pressure ulcer development, intravenous infiltration occurrences, and falls.

Organization/System Sphere

The health care system is also concerned with quality. Therefore, the CNS has a role in quality improvement from a systems perspective. Examples of system issues are access to the health care system in the form of access to care, waiting times for appointments, and waiting room times. These are three common indicators of quality from a system perspective. Reduction of cost, waste, and risk are other matters of quality from the health care system perspective.

The CNS role in quality from an organization/system perspective is to understand issues of quality that are important to the health care organization. The CNS can lend clinical and organizational expertise to improving performance on those indicators that have been defined by the organization.

In summary, quality in health care as it relates to the conceptual model of CNS practice and the three spheres of influence necessarily overlap. What is within the patient/client sphere and nursing and nursing practice sphere of influence overlaps into the organization/system sphere. The following case example illustrates how the three spheres of influence overlap.

CASE EXAMPLE

A 55-year-old patient is admitted to the hospital with pneumonia and chronic obstructive pulmonary disease (COPD) exacerbation. This patient has intersected the health maintenance organization (HMO) health care system six times within the past year but has not received pneumococcal or influenza immunizations. The medical team is concerned with the immediate episode of care for this patient, and immunizations have not been ordered. The CNS reviews the patient record and notices that this is his third hospital admission with pneumonia and COPD exacerbation in the past 18 months. The CNS also notices that there is no record of immunizations. The CNS approaches the patient and asks about his immunization history. The patient states that influenza and pneumococcal immunizations were offered to him once, but he refused because he does not like shots. The CNS provides information to the patient regarding recent research that indicates significantly reduced COPD exacerbations and hospitalizations for patients who have had both influenza and pneumococcal immunizations. The patient agrees to be immunized, and the CNS alerts the registered nurse (RN) assigned to that patient to administer both immunizations under a recently developed protocol (developed by the CNS) for administration of immunizations without a physician order.

After the episode with the single COPD patient, the CNS considers a system approach to immunization from an acute care perspective. The CNS gathers data on admissions of patients who could benefit from immunizations. The CNS discovers that there is no system in place to identify and administer immunizations to a particular population of patients who could benefit significantly, specifically patients with admitting diagnoses of COPD or pneumonia. This issue becomes the driver for the CNS to gather a team to explore the development of a system that identifies and vaccinates all patients with an admitting diagnosis of COPD or pneumonia.

This is an example of all three spheres of influence in CNS practice coming together to improve patient outcomes: First, the ability to recognize an opportunity to deliver evidence-based care in the form of immunizations and providing appropriate evidence-based education to the patient falls under the patient/client sphere; second, alerting the RN in charge of the care of that patient to administer the immunizations relates to the nurse and nursing practice sphere; and third, utilizing the system-level approach to identify high-risk patients who could benefit from immunizations and facilitating an organizational approach to expedient immunizations falls under the organization/system sphere.

QUALITY FRAMEWORKS

The structure, process, and outcome model of QHC proposed by Donabedian (1996) is closely aligned with the CNS spheres of influence. The organization/system sphere relates to *structure* in the Donabedian model. The nurse and nursing practice sphere relate to *process*, and the patient/client sphere relates to *outcomes*.

With the exception of Donabedian's early and enduring works, there is a dearth of conceptual models of quality in health care. Particularly lacking are conceptual models of quality as they relate to nursing practice. This reveals the nascent nature of the science of QHC within the context of nursing.

That is not to say that nursing has not been vocal about quality as it relates to nursing care. In 1995, the ANA published the Nursing Care Report Card for Acute Care in which it proposed 21 measures of nursing care purported to be linked to the quality and availability of nursing care in the acute hospital setting (ANA, 1995). In 1997, the ANA asked for proposals to develop and maintain the National Database for Nursing Quality Indicators (NDNQI). In 1998, NDNQI, which is now a registered trademark, began accepting data from hospitals and charging for the use of the system, including submission of data as well as reports from the database.

The NDNQI uses the structure, process, and outcomes (Donabedian, 1980) approach to measuring quality by identifying nurse and nursing-sensitive indicators of quality. Nursing-sensitive indicators are defined as those outcomes that improve in the presence of greater quantity (higher staffing ratios) or quality (educational levels and competence of nursing staff) of nursing care. As mentioned earlier, some examples of quality indicators for nursing care are pressure ulcer development, intravenous infiltration occurrences, and falls.

These nursing-sensitive measures help hospitals to analyze the quality and quantity of nursing care services. The national database provides benchmark performance with which the individual health care institution can compare its performance to similar hospitals across the nation.

Another quality model that incorporates a broad view of health care and seeks to define quality is the QHC model (Benton, 2010). The model contains three spheres, which encompass three domains that are most often considered important elements in

QHC. The intersection of the three spheres—that is, where the three elements exist together—encompasses the factors that define QHC (Figure 12.1).

Safe health care includes all of the processes and procedures in place to ensure that health care is delivered in a safe manner. The indicators of safety include processes such as hand-washing monitors, time-out protocols for surgery, fall reduction programs, and a *do not use* list of abbreviations, to name a few. The indicators of patient-centered health care include processes designed to measure patient satisfaction, such as emergency room waiting times and other patient-centered indicators of quality. Clinically competent health care includes education and competency of staff; adherence to clinical practice guidelines for chronic disease, such as annual retinal eye exam for diabetics who are insulin dependent; and adherence to prevention guidelines, such as screening for colorectal, breast, and cervical cancer and immunizations. The QHC model proposes that when all three elements come together for a particular patient or population, QHC is achieved.

The QHC model (Benton, 2010) differs from the Donabedian structure, process, and outcomes model. Donabedian's model proposed a framework to guide quality professionals in developing measures for quality. The QHC model is a conceptual model for defining quality in health care (Benton, 2010). The QHC model can also be used to categorize health care activities for identifying quality factors, as well as risk factors, in existing systems of health care delivery.

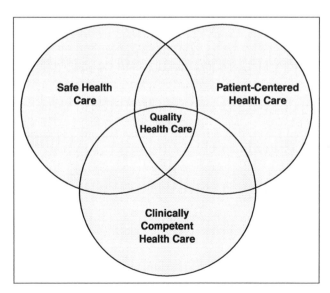

FIGURE 12.1 Quality Health Care model.

MEASURING QUALITY

Quality cannot be measured directly. Quality is measured by performance on identified indicators of quality. One indicator of quality is approval or accreditation from a quality oversight organization. Other indicators of quality encompass the domains of prevention, disease management, patient satisfaction, and patient safety.

Quality Oversight Organizations

One of the longest standing and best-known health care quality oversight organizations is The Joint Commission (TJC; formerly known as the Joint Commission on the Accreditation of Healthcare Organizations [JCAHCO]). This quality oversight organization has its roots firmly in the practice of medicine. The precursor to today's Joint Commission Standards was the Minimum Standards for Hospitals document created by the American College of Surgeons in 1917. However, it was not until 1953 that TJC first offered accreditation to hospitals and published the first Standards for Hospital Accreditation. Over the next 50 years, TJC expanded beyond hospital accreditation to nearly every venue in which health care is delivered, including inpatient and outpatient care. Today, all federally funded health care organizations and any health care organization that accepts federal payments for health care, such as Medicare, is required to maintain accreditation from TJC or an equivalent quality oversight group.

The list of accrediting agencies is long and includes organizations such as the National Council on Quality Assurance (NCQA), which has developed standards for health care plans and outpatient clinical care. The College of American Pathologists (CAP) has developed standards for the accreditation of diagnostic laboratories. The American Association of Blood Banks (AABB) has developed accreditation standards for blood and tissue banks. The Commission on the Accreditation of Rehabilitation Facilities (CARF) has developed accreditation guidelines and standards for medical rehabilitation facilities as well as behavioral health, community, child, youth, and aging services. This list is not comprehensive and accounts for only a handful of the quality oversight groups available to assess the quality of care provided by health care facilities and programs. In addition to national accreditation organizations, most states have quality oversight agencies (state inspectors) that periodically inspect health care facilities, most often in the long-term care arena of health care.

Quality Indicators

Whether an organization achieves and retains accreditation by a quality oversight group can be one indicator of quality. There are many other indicators of quality, such as adherence to clinical practice guidelines for chronic disease and population-specific prevention measures. Patient satisfaction has also become an indicator of overall quality.

Clinical Practice Guidelines

Guidelines for practice derive from research surrounding treatment of certain conditions, acute and chronic. For example, a patient with a diagnosis of insulin-dependent diabetes mellitus should receive very specific disease management elements of care, such as annual diabetic retinal examination, annual hemoglobin A1c laboratory testing, diabetic foot examination, renal function, and lipid studies, and so forth. A patient presenting to an emergency room with a chief complaint of chest pain should receive aspirin, unless contraindicated for some other reason, and an electrocardiogram within 10 minutes.

There are literally hundreds of clinical practice guidelines that are based upon the most current research. A comprehensive and searchable database of clinical practice guidelines is provided by the AHRQ under the title of National Guideline Clearinghouse (AHRQ, 2013b).

Prevention Guidelines

Although some clinical practice guidelines incorporate prevention for specific diagnoses, prevention guidelines are generally more population based. For example, colorectal cancer screening should be done for all patients older than 50 years, and a one-time pneumococcal immunization should be given to all healthy adults aged 65 and older, to name just two. The U.S. Preventive Services Task Force (USPSTF) of the AHRQ (2013a) has developed a guide to preventive services for clinicians that includes all of the recommended preventive health care services for all populations from pediatric to geriatric.

Patient Satisfaction

Another indicator of quality is patient or customer satisfaction. While the work surrounding health promotion and disease prevention was occurring in the late 1970s and early 1980s, customer satisfaction was just beginning to be explored as a potential indicator of quality (Cleary & McNeil, 1988). Until the connection between patient satisfaction and medical malpractice was made, not much attention was given to patient satisfaction in the literature. As the field of research into patient satisfaction became more active, patient satisfaction as a quality indicator emerged (Peskin, Micklitsch, Quirk, Sims, & Primack, 1995; Woodward, Ostbye, Craighead, Gold, & Wenghofer, 2000). When health care became something people sought for more than just illness or injury care, and free market principles began to affect health care organizations, a competition for patients arose, particularly in the corporate for-profit hospitals and health systems. This phenomenon helped focus attention on what the consumer of health care was looking for; thus, patient satisfaction as an indicator of quality became a popular research subject. Today, patient satisfaction is an important quality indicator in any health care organization.

Patient Safety

With all of the oversight of quality in health care by various accrediting organizations and the wealth of information to guide the health care system in delivering quality care, one might assume that high-QHC is the standard in this country. However, in 2000, the IOM published *To Err is Human*, a comprehensive look at the safety of our health care system. In this publication, the researchers estimated that between 44,000 and 98,000 deaths occur in the United States each year as a result of medical error. In other research, it was estimated that 1.3 million nonfatal medical injuries resulted in disability or lengthened hospital stay (Bates & Gawande, 2000). The cost of medical error in the form of lost income, disability, and cost to the health care system is estimated to be between $17 and $29 billion per year in hospitals nationwide (IOM, 2000). This recent information is clearly not what the consumer of health care would expect from a high-QHC system.

Just prior to the publication of the IOM's report on patient safety in 2000, the Department of Veterans Affairs (VA) instituted the National Center for Patient Safety (NCPS) in 1999. Soon after that, the AHRQ and VA collaborated to develop the Patient Safety Improvement Corps (PSIC), whose mission is to provide the knowledge and skills needed for health care organizations to improve patient safety. TJC also joined in the frenzy to improve the safety of health care by instituting the first set of National Patient Safety Goals (NPSG) in January of 2003. Then, in 2005, Congress passed the Patient Safety and Quality Improvement Act of 2005 (AHRQ, 2013c), which

was designed to analyze and aggregate patient safety information in an effort to identify system failures that could lead to improvement.

CNS Role in Quality Measurement

In order for something to be measured, it must be reduced to a numerical value. Quality oversight groups, such as TJC, issue a score or status to health care organizations. TJC has identified a cohort of universal quality measures for acute care hospitals, called ORYX measures. Acute care organizations can now measure themselves against similar organizations to determine their quality standing with regard to emergent care for acute myocardial infarction, congestive heart failure, and pneumonia care, as well as nonemergent surgical care.

Beyond TJC's ORYX measures, many health care organizations that monitor their own quality measures have adopted clinical practice guidelines based upon diagnoses, prevention guidelines based upon the populations they serve, patient satisfaction scores, and patient safety goals. For each of these categories, quality indicators are developed to determine who needs the particular intervention and whether or not the intervention occurred. This results in a performance measure for that particular indicator. Most performance measures have target levels established by the organization that are based upon national data. Approximation of the target level is then translated into quality. A scorecard is developed, and the organization sets goals for the scorecard. For example, the organization will meet or exceed the target level for at least 30 of 45 targets. For targets that are not met, the organization will institute a performance improvement project to assist in reaching the target.

In addition to occasional collection of data points for quality monitoring, the CNS role in measuring quality is to understand the organizational approach to quality. The approach of the organization may differ depending upon the business model and whether it is a for-profit, corporate-owned health care delivery system or a federal- or state-funded organization. Each organization will have unique quality goals and measures defined. The CNS should be familiar with the goals and understand the measures of quality specific to that organization.

IMPROVING QUALITY

Measuring quality is a necessary and first step to quality improvement. Before something can be improved, two things must be known: Do the data indicate a need for improvement? If so, what is the baseline upon which improvement will be determined? An improvement team cannot know that its process changes have led to improvement unless it has baseline data to which to compare the postimplementation data.

Performance Improvement Methods

The basic process in performance improvement is similar to the nursing process with which all nurses are familiar: assess, plan, implement, and evaluate. However, in performance improvement, the processes are named differently. There are numerous performance improvement methodologies, such as the Plan, Do, Study, Act (PDSA) or the Focus, Analyze, Develop, and Execute (FADE) methodologies, to name just two. What they all have in common is that they begin with identifying and analyzing the problem. This involves collecting and analyzing baseline data to determine causes and possible solutions. Based upon the analysis, a solution is identified and implemented and followup data are collected and compared to the baseline data to determine if the improvement was successful. If the desired performance level is not achieved, the process begins again and continues to repeat until the desired level of performance is achieved and sustained.

Quality Monitors

Once the improvement is accomplished, it may have to be monitored for a time to be sure the improvement efforts are sustained and that the processes put in place do not slide back into the preimprovement mode. Monitoring a new improvement is one type of quality monitor.

Another type of quality monitor is an ongoing monitor for quality, such as infection control monitoring or utilization monitoring. This type of quality monitoring is designed to continue indefinitely for the purpose of identifying problems as soon as possible. Statistical process control (SPC) techniques and control charts are often used to monitor and analyze the data for indicators of a quality problem. Details of SPC techniques are beyond the scope of this chapter; however, it is important for the CNS to know that SPC is a powerful tool that is often used in quality improvement.

The CNS Role in Improving Quality

Identifying opportunities for improvement that address or enhance patient safety issues, clinical competence and practice issues, and patient satisfaction issues is the primary role of the CNS in improving quality. The QHC model (Figure 12.1; Benton, 2010) can be used to guide the CNS in identifying areas where opportunities for improvement may exist. Once the need is identified, the CNS can facilitate the development of an improvement team to address the issue. The CNS role on the performance improvement team can be one of content expert, team leader, or team facilitator. The CNS must draw upon his or her leadership skills and often function in several roles on an improvement team in order to move the process forward.

CNS STRATEGIES FOR CREATING A CULTURE OF QUALITY

Strategies for creating a culture of quality can be aligned with the CNS core competencies. In Table 12.1, the CNS core competencies from the *Statement on Clinical Nurse Specialist Practice and Education* (NACNS, 2013) are listed on the left side of the table, and specific competencies for creating a culture of quality are provided on the right side of the table.

The CNS plays a pivotal role in identifying opportunities for improvement and in facilitating improvement in the health care organization. One of the most important skills a CNS must learn is multidisciplinary collaboration. Quality improvement opportunities rarely exist in a state where the CNS can identify the issue and improve the performance single-handedly or by collaborating only with other CNSs. Most quality issues are complex and require the input of several disciplines in identifying what must be improved to achieve the quality outcome.

Creating a culture of quality requires the CNS to understand the organizational priorities for quality. In the absence of clear organizational priorities, the CNS may use the QHC model (Figure 12.1) to explore the realm of QHC and identify areas requiring improvement. Once the opportunities for improvement are identified, the CNS can start by collecting baseline data if none exist. Armed with accurate baseline data, the CNS can then inspire others to participate in a multidisciplinary team process to brainstorm and target processes for improvement.

TABLE 12.1

CNS CORE COMPETENCIES AND QUALITY CULTURE STRATETGIES	
CNS Core Competency	**CNS Quality Culture Strategy**
1. Direct care competency: Direct interaction with patients, families, and groups of patients to promote health or well-being and improve quality of life. Characterized by a holistic perspective in the advanced nursing management of health, illness, and disease states	Using a patient-centered approach, implementing clinical practice guidelines and prevention guidelines to improve the quality of care to patients and families
2. Consultation competency: Patient, staff, or system-focused interaction between professionals in which the consultant is recognized as having specialized expertise and assists consultee with problem solving	Achieve expert understanding of prevention and clinical practice guidelines as well as patient satisfaction and patient safety to act as consultant and teacher of guidelines to other health care professionals
3. Systems leadership competency: The ability to manage change and empower others to influence clinical practice and political processes both within and across systems	Provide leadership at the institutional or community level to develop policies and procedures that support improvement on quality performance measures and adherence to clinical practice and prevention guidelines
4. Collaboration competency: Working jointly with others to optimize clinical outcomes. The CNS collaborates at an advanced level by committing to authentic engagement and constructive patient, family, system, and population-focused problem solving	Act as content expert to collaborate with multidisciplinary teams designed to improve safety and performance on quality performance measures
5. Coaching competency: Skillful guidance and teaching to advance the care of patients, families, groups of patients, and the profession of nursing	Achieve expert understanding of prevention and clinical practice guidelines as well as patient satisfaction and patient safety to act as mentor and teacher of guidelines to other nurses
6. Research competency: The work of thorough and systematic inquiry. Includes the search for, interpretation, and use of evidence in clinical practice and quality improvement as well as active participation in the conduct of research	Facilitate the research and development of additional nurse-sensitive quality indicators and competencies to address nurse-sensitive quality indicators
7. Ethical decision making, moral agency and advocacy competency: Identifying, articulating, and taking action on ethical concerns at the patient, family, health care provider, system, community, and public policy levels	Keeping the patient as the center of concern, act as an advocate for the patient's right to refuse care dictated by clinical practice guidelines when appropriate. Initiate ethical consults as appropriate

CNS, clinical nurse specialist.

■ DISCUSSION QUESTIONS

• The USPSTF (2013) recently released recommendations for HIV screening for adolescents and adults aged 15 to 65. This recommendation is discussed in the quality committee of a large HMO. A CNS is a member of the committee. The chair of the committee, the HMO's lead infectious disease physician, suggests an immediate policy change to implement the USPSTF recommendations. From a clinical as well as an ethical perspective, what considerations could be raised by the CNS?

• The CNS in surgical care has become aware of a spike in surgical site infections that appears to be limited to joint replacement surgeries. Upon closer examination of the data, it becomes clear that most of the infections are connected to one orthopedic surgeon's cases. What is the next step for the CNS?

• The CNS working in a large private hospital is rounding on the medical unit when she overhears a conversation between a staff hospitalist and one of the RN nursing staff. The hospitalist is telling the RN that he should never question the internist's process for conducting the time-out for a paracentesis. What is the next step for the CNS?

REFERENCES

Agency for Healthcare Research and Quality (AHRQ). (2005). *Guide to health care quality: How to know it when you see it.* Retrieved October 30, 2013, from http://www.ahrq.gov/legacy/consumer/guidetoq/guidetoq.pdf

Agency for Healthcare Research and Quality (AHRQ). (2013a). *Guide to clinical preventive services. Recommendations of the U.S. Preventive Services Task Force.* Retrieved September 15, 2013, from http://www.ahrq.gov/clinic/pocketgd.htm

Agency for Healthcare Research and Quality (AHRQ). (2013b). *National Guideline Clearinghouse.* Retrieved September 18, 2013, from http://www.guideline.gov

Agency for Healthcare Research and Quality (AHRQ). (2013c). *The Patient Safety and Quality Improvement Act of 2005.* Retrieved September 15, 2013, from http://www.ahrq.gov/qual/psoact.htm

American Heritage Dictionary. (2013). *Quality.* Retrieved October 28, 2013, from http://ahdictionary.com/word/search.html?q=quality

American Medical Association (AMA). (2013). *Definition of quality* (Policy No. H-450.975). Retrieved September 16, 2013, from http://www.ama-assn.org/ad-com/polfind/Hlth-Ethics.pdf

American Nurses Association (ANA). (1995). *Nursing care report card for acute care.* Washington, DC: American Nurses Publishing.

American Nurses Association (ANA). (1997). *Implementing nursing's report card: A study of RN staffing, length of stay and patient outcomes.* Washington, DC: American Nurses Publishing.

Attree, M. (1996). Towards a conceptual model of "quality care." *International Journal of Nursing Studies, 33*(1), 13–28.

Bates, D. W., & Gawande, A. A. (2000). Error in medicine: What have we learned? *Annals of Internal Medicine, 132*(9), 763–767.

Benton, N. (2010). Creating a culture of quality. In J. Fulton, B. Lyon, & K. Goudreau (Eds.), *Foundations of clinical nurse specialist practice, (p. 163).* New York, NY: Springer.

Cleary, P. D., & McNeil, B. J. (1988). Patient satisfaction as an indicator of quality care. *Inquiry, 25*(1), 25–36.

Donabedian, A. (1980). *Explorations in quality assessment and monitoring, volume 1: The definition of quality and approaches to its assessment.* Ann Arbor, MI: Health Administration Press.

Donabedian, A. (1996). The effectiveness of quality assurance. *International Journal for Quality in Health Care, 8*(4), 401–407.

Donabedian, A. (2005). Evaluating the quality of medical care 1966. *Milbank Quarterly, 83*(4), 691–729.

Institute of Medicine (IOM). (2000). *To err is human: Building a safer health system.* Washington, DC: National Academies Press.

Institute of Medicine (IOM). (2001). *Crossing the quality chasm: A new health system for the 21st century.* Washington, DC: National Academies Press.

Kay, M. (2005). Issues update. The ANA's visionary approach: Shining the light on high-quality care—one step at a time. *American Journal of Nursing, 105*(7), 73.

National Association of Clinical Nurse Specialists (NACNS). (2013). *Clinical nurse specialist core competencies, executive summary 2006–2008.* Retrieved October 28, 2013, from http://www.nacns.org/docs/CNSCoreCompetenciesBroch.pdf

Neuhauser, D. (2003). Florence Nightingale gets no respect: As a statistician that is. *Quality and Safety in Health Care, 12,* 317.

Peskin, T., Micklitsch, C., Quirk, M., Sims, H., & Primack, W. (1995). Malpractice, patient satisfaction, and physician-patient communication. *Journal of the American Medical Association, 274*(1), 22.

U.S. Preventive Services Task Force (USPSTF). (2013). *Screening for HIV.* Retrieved September 15, 2013, from http://www.uspreventiveservicestaskforce.org/uspstf/uspshivi.htm

Walker, L., & Avant, K. (1994). Concept analysis. In L. Walker & K. Avant (Eds.), *Strategies for theory construction in nursing* (3rd ed., pp. 77–102). Upper Saddle River, NJ: Prentice Hall.

Woodward, C. A., Ostbye, T., Craighead, J., Gold, G., & Wenghofer, E. F. (2000). Patient satisfaction as an indicator of quality care in independent health facilities: Developing and assessing a tool to enhance public accountability. *American Journal of Medical Quality, 15*(3), 94–105.

Patient Safety

Patricia R. Ebright

At the start of the 21st century, the health care industry made dramatic changes in its approach to patient safety. Although fundamental clinical nurse specialist (CNS) competencies outlined in the *Statement on Clinical Nurse Specialist Practice and Education* (National Association of Clinical Nurse Specialists [NACNS], 2004) equip CNSs with essential core knowledge and skills for leading and participating in a variety of program efforts, it is important that CNSs understand how these competencies complement the new approach to patient safety. Interestingly, it was through learning from other industries about the need to approach safety differently that health care inadvertently found itself aligned more than ever with nursing care theories and the advanced practice of nursing defined by CNS core competencies, which focus on the uniqueness and complexity of humans and other complex systems.

This chapter includes discussion of the events leading to the shift in patient safety focus and of subsequent legislative and regulatory developments that have had an impact on work in patient safety. Concepts and information learned from other high-risk industries about several theoretical frameworks and models underpinning the changes are explained, including the epidemiology of error, human factors, complex adaptive systems (CASs), safety culture, and characteristics of high-reliability organizations (HROs). The most recent developments in the evolving knowledge about patient safety improvement are discussed, as are ongoing and future challenges in implementation and improvement efforts. Widely used strategies and tools for assessing, improving, and evaluating safety are identified. The author outlines important organizational behaviors characteristic of

an effective patient safety program. The chapter concludes with ethical considerations for CNS work in patient safety.

HISTORY OF THE PATIENT SAFETY MOVEMENT

The nursing profession and CNSs, in particular, have always focused on the development and implementation of standards, education, and mentoring of nurses that promote patient safety and quality (Peplau, 1965/2003). Starting in the early 1980s, before the 2000 release of *To Err Is Human: Building a Safer Health System* by the Institute of Medicine (IOM) report on medical error and patient safety, a series of events drew attention to injury and deaths resulting from medical error. These events included establishment of the Anesthesia Patient Safety Foundation in 1984 for improvement of perioperative patient safety; findings reported from physician studies on the large numbers of preventable disabling injuries and deaths identified from medical records in the 1990s (e.g., Leape, 1994); 1996 regulatory and legislative activities by The Joint Commission (2013a) requiring hospital compliance with monitoring, investigation, and reporting of errors; and the creation of national organizations focused on patient safety (e.g., National Patient Safety Foundation [NPSF] in 1998 and the National Quality Forum in 1999).

Until the IOM report was released in 2000, most health care providers did not appreciate the magnitude of the medical error problem. Furthermore, those who were concerned about medical error tended to try traditional methods of approaching the problem, with little long-term success. Reading about the tens of thousands of Americans who were dying each year from errors in medical care and the hundreds of thousands who were injured, or almost injured, during their care, served as a wake-up call that more had to be done to prevent harm to patients and to improve quality of care. It became clear for many leaders in the health care industry that existing approaches to safety and quality were no longer sufficient to improve or even sustain the quality of care necessary to protect patients as recommended in subsequent IOM reports.

Authors of *Crossing the Quality Chasm: A New Health System for the 21st Century* (IOM, 2001) called for fundamental change to improve health care through six aims (Table 13.1). The aims served to broaden the scope of safety and connect it to the quality aspects of care. Health care leaders searched for solutions from industries other than health care, such as the airline, aerospace, and nuclear industries, to prevent high-stakes failures and reduce the harm resulting from error. These industries had learned long before about why errors happen, the role of human limitations in error generation, and the roles that workers and leaders play in increasing and sustaining safety (Weick & Suttcliffe, 2007).

More specifically, leaders of health care organizations began to realize that sustainable improvements in patient safety would require a switch from the traditional health care focus on individual care providers as the sole cause of error to consideration of the complex systems in which they work, and to the limited capacity within individuals themselves. This

represented a change in focus from demanding perfect individual performance in imperfect situations to understanding the imperfect situations in which imperfect performers work. This change in approach to patient safety has required swift action by health care leaders related to new learning, resources, and shifts in long-held cultural norms.

Though some health care organizations have made great progress toward the recommendations from the IOM (2001), they vary widely in sustainable achievements, demonstrating the daunting task of changing an entire industry's culture surrounding failure (Leape & Berwick, 2005; Wachter, 2010). The next section describes legislative and regulatory efforts that have affected the pace of needed change.

Legislative and Regulatory Focus on Patient Safety

Individual states continue to enact legislation to require health care organizational reporting and public disclosure of serious errors. State reporting systems vary by whether they are mandatory or voluntary; and if mandatory, the types of information reported, and what is done with the data. Two major problems with the current effectiveness of state systems are underreporting by health care organizations and lack of funding to maintain and manage the data.

Since 2003, The Joint Commission has published an annual list of Patient Safety Goals that health care organizations must achieve to receive a successful accreditation review (The Joint Commission, 2013b). The Institute for Healthcare Improvement (IHI) sponsors clinically focused improvement initiatives to challenge health care organizations toward the realization of successful patient outcomes through specific quality and safety programs (e.g., IHI, 2013). These initiatives have resulted in thousands of lives being saved. The NPSF and the Agency for Healthcare Research and Quality (AHRQ) fund research on patient safety. The following organizations have also responded to the 2000 IOM report with efforts to improve patient safety: Department of Health and Human Services (DHHS), Center for Disease Control and Prevention (CDC), Centers for Medicare & Medicaid Services (CMS), Leapfrog Group, and Healthgrades.

In early 2000, work in patient safety focused on the need to move away from the traditional focus on individuals and the so-called blame culture that enveloped error situations. We moved to more understanding of complex systems, understanding of how error occurs, and ways to redesign specific aspects of the environment based on assessments of error situations. More recent efforts in attempting to improve and sustain delivery of safe patient care have turned to building

TABLE 13.1

SIX AIMS FOR FUNDAMENTAL CHANGE IN HEALTH CARE	
Aim	**Description**
Safe	Avoid injuries to patients from the care that is intended to help them
Effective	Match care to science; avoid overuse of ineffective care and underuse of effective care
Patient-centered	Honor the individual and respect choice
Timely	Reduce waiting for both patients and those who give care
Efficient	Reduce waste
Equitable	Close racial and ethical gaps in health status

resiliency in both our health care workers and care systems to prevent error and minimize poor outcomes as much as possible. We continue to learn about why things go wrong despite best intentions and to implement interventions to reduce adverse/near-miss events. These continuing efforts require leadership.

CNSs have been leaders in their organizations for many of the new legislative and regulatory activities related to patient safety. CNSs will continue to be leaders in this work because of their educational background and unique work experience in all three spheres of health care organizations (NACNS, 2004). CNS education emphasizes problem-solving strategies at the patient, nurse, and organizational system levels based on etiology-informed interventions and evaluation. This essential aspect of their practice and education makes CNSs consumers of the new learning about error generation, human limitations, and the CASs in which care is delivered. Because of the nature of their staff versus line role position in most organizations and their influencing skills, CNSs are uniquely prepared to effect change across diverse groups of health care professionals and workers, and they are able to accommodate cultural differences and reaction to change. Most fundamental to ongoing and dramatic change in health care, CNSs are experts in illness and disease management, which is crucial to understanding the impact of design and improvement changes on patient populations and care delivery, as well as for identification of important outcomes for measurement.

NEW LEARNING ABOUT PATIENT SAFETY

Several frameworks and models provide the backdrop for new learning related to patient safety. In order to effectively lead and influence patient safety improvements, it is essential that CNSs acquire the fundamental knowledge base that supports this approach, which was introduced to health care in the late 1990s and early 2000 and continues to drive the current initiatives for improvement of patient safety and quality. The following sections cover what we have learned about CASs, evolution of error, work at the "sharp end," human limitations, safety cultures, and finally, characteristics of HROs.

Complex Adaptive Systems

In health care organizations, we have traditionally controlled the complexity inherent in situations and environments by assuming a simplistic pattern of decision making or causality. The benefit to this approach has been the appearance and feeling of control. A downside, however, is that such thinking includes

the belief that activity is consistent and continuous and that there is one best solution for multiple situations. Though nurses' basic educational preparation is grounded in a focus on the uniqueness of individual clients, maintaining this focus when providing nursing care very often competes with organizational priorities fitting with standardized, one-solution thinking. Our continuing attempts in nursing to solve problems following an error incident (e.g., wrong blood administration) with only the reeducation of nurses about the related policy or procedure demonstrates the faulty assumption that one individual is the cause of the problem.

In contrast to traditional one-solution approaches to problem solving, approaches consistent with CAS characteristics are more compatible with today's health care environments and challenges. Complex system characteristics include unpredictability, ambiguity, time-pressure and stress-laden situations, high stakes, and decision making by teams with frequently changing members (Klein, 1998). Unlike linear and more simple explanations of why things go wrong, explaining why things happen in light of CASs is very difficult. Causality is not unidirectional but most often bidirectional, involving the interaction of two or more entities. From these complex interactions emerge unpredictable behavioral patterns leading to small changes that may or may not lead to major widespread changes. Therefore, making change in complex environments requires recognition of and appreciation for the bidirectionality and unpredictability of system relationships, including human, technical, and process. The focus for CAS thinking to solve problems is not only on an ultimate end, or goal, but also on the intervening moments and processes, because it is understood that each situation holds the possibility for continuation of the same, for surprises, or for new and emerging patterns. In his book, *Diffusion of Innovations*, Rogers (2003) introduced us to findings about the realities and complexity surrounding implementation of change. In a complexity-based approach to problem solving or change, we understand we will not have complete control of situations or people in real work environments, just as we learned in nursing that we cannot control all aspects of individual client health situations.

What we in health care have learned from other high-stakes industries, such as the airlines and nuclear power plants, about the evolution of error complements the characteristics of CASs and challenges our traditional one-solution thinking approach to patient safety. Although this direction is new to health care, it is very consistent with the profession of nursing's holistic approach to care and its focus on the unique aspects of human beings for understanding illness and wellness. Demonstrated in the following sections is the natural fit of the outcomes of CNSs' advanced nursing practice, which includes the identification of etiologies as the basis for nursing care, with the focus on system etiologies for a new approach to patient safety. This new approach to patient safety requires understanding of the details of actual work within CASs and of the actual and potential contributors (etiologies) to adverse/near-miss events.

Evolution of Error

Human factors science is a science focused on human performance in varying situations and environments, often in interaction with technology. The Latent Failure Model of Complex System Failure (Woods, Dekker, Cook, Johannesen, & Sarter, 2010) is a model developed by human factors researchers based on system failure work by James Reason (1990) to explain the evolution of error or near-miss errors in health care situations. According to the model, errors are not the result of a single failure of an unreliable component (such as an individual or piece of technology), but rather the result of multiple failures in the intended defenses of a system. Developers of the Latent Failure Model suggest that improvements in patient safety can occur only when the five principles listed in Table 13.2 are appreciated by health care providers and leaders in a health care system (Woods & Cook, 1998).

Using the Latent Failure Model of Complex System Failure to Explain Failure

According to the Latent Failure Model of Complex System Failure (Woods et al., 2010) and as shown in Figure 13.1, layers of system defenses exist at all levels

TABLE 13.2

FIVE PRINCIPLES NECESSARY TO UNDERSTAND FOR IMPROVEMENT IN PATIENT SAFETY	
Principle	**Interpretation**
1. Safety is made and broken in systems, not by individuals. Adverse events result from the way work is designed and the interaction of components of the system	1. Individuals as well as the systems in which they work are complex adaptive systems (CASs) and as such reflect characteristics of complexity, including bidirectionality, relationships, and emerging and adaptive patterns
2. Progress on safety begins with understanding technical work. Our current understanding of real work is naïve and incomplete, leading to the development of performance rules that are impossible to apply in a complex, heterogeneous, and rapidly changing world. Progress in safety depends on understanding how technical and organizational factors play out in real work	2. Our tradition in health care is linear, and our tendency is to look for simple explanations. We must appreciate the delivery of health care work within complex environments to successfully implement and sustain improvements in safety. Detailed individual policies and procedures perfectly written and taught without consideration of actual work processes will not be sufficient to prevent adverse events
3. Productive discussions of safety avoid confounding failure with error. Failure results from a breakdown in systems, whereas error is usually assigned to humans and relates to a social process for attributing cause	3. The traditional culture surrounding failure and reaction to failure in health care is blame. Language following failure that reflects the traditional culture (e.g., error, blame, incident report) will lead to the same traditional reaction, or blaming, and is not a productive response in terms of improving safety
4. Safety is dynamic and not static; it is constantly renegotiated. Complex, ever-changing systems require that people change and adapt constantly. However, adaptation is often based on inadequate information and only partly successful. Understanding this dynamic is the foundation for understanding safety. Increasing complexity makes safety harder to achieve	4. Attention to improving and sustaining patient safety will require ongoing activities and continual adjustment
5. Tradeoffs are at the core of safety. Complex work environments will always be characterized by uncertainty, discontinuities, and missing information. Understanding how people cope with these challenges will increase understanding of safety	5. Understanding real work means appreciating the complexity of environments and realizing that in complex environments the resilient and most constant factor is the ability of people to adapt successfully. We need to learn how people manage in complex situations

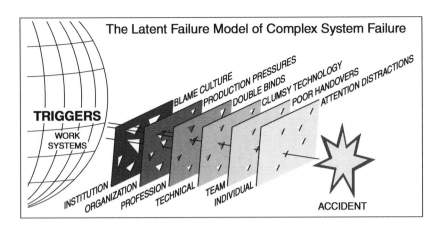

FIGURE 13.1 Complex system failure according to the Latent Failure Model. Failures in these systems require the combination of multiple factors. The system is defended against failure but these defenses have defects or "holes" that allow accidents to occur.

Source: From Woods et al. (2010).

of an organization to provide guidance and boundaries around which decisions are developed and implemented. Traditionally, health care system defenses included but were not limited to policies and procedures, standard care guidelines, chain-of-command processes for communication and decisions, budget and resource allocations, report and handoff mechanisms, competency standards, and technology. These defenses constituted important aspects of an organization's work in setting guidelines, standards, and boundaries for performance. However, in the past they have not allowed for either the situational or individual variation in naturally occurring events. They were intended for the "perfect" situation and, most often, for the experienced and knowledgeable provider.

Latent failures are discontinuities in the layers of defenses in naturally occurring, or real work, environments (Woods et al., 2010). To illustrate, a latent failure exists when a specific patient situation does not exactly fit a policy and procedure for medication administration and following the policy or procedure would not be in the best interests of the patient. A latent failure exists when there is a lack of experienced personnel on a busy unit for one specific shift, resulting in less than the needed competencies and experience required to provide care for the unit's current acuity level and number of patients.

As the previous examples demonstrate, latent failures do not represent overt failures, but they do constitute a type of latent condition that threatens the continuity of care and, when combined with latent failures enabled by a trigger event, may lead to a *near miss* (an event or situation that could have resulted in an accident, injury, or illness, but did not, either by chance or through timely intervention) or to an *adverse event* (untoward incidents, therapeutic misadventures, iatrogenic injuries, or other adverse occurrences directly associated with care or services provided within the jurisdiction of a medical center, outpatient clinic, or other facility; adverse events that may result from acts of commission or omission; VA National Center for Patient Safety, 2013).

Active failures are errors and violations caused by acts performed by workers (e.g., nurses) closest to the "sharp end" of the system (e.g., patient care), which affect system safety most directly (Reason, 2000). Reason suggested that most active failures are consequences of latent failures and not principal causes of errors. For example, using a situation discussed previously, inadequate staffing (latent failure) for a specific shift may result in a nurse who is responding to time pressures to check one, but not all, patient identifier (active failure) and then administer the wrong medication. The latent failure of inadequate staffing was a significant contributor to the error even though not checking all identifiers also contributed.

Sometimes, worker adaptation to an ongoing system latent failure becomes part of the routine work and lies dormant and unrecognized by the organization. As a consequence, implementation of new changes may unintentionally disrupt the efficacy of worker strategies to make up for latent failures, or some changes may even create new latent failures in the system. For example, a new technology or change in process may increase the time spent on a previously well-managed process and disrupt what has become a routine current flow of work. This type of disruption may cause decision *tradeoffs* (decision resolutions that involve conflicting choices between highly unlikely but highly undesirable events and more likely but less catastrophic ones). Tradeoffs are types of decisions made by nurses and other health care providers "between interacting or conflicting goals, between values or costs placed on different possible outcomes or courses of action, and between the risks of different errors" (Woods et al., 2010, p. 123) and more serious adverse patient outcomes. Using the medication error event described previously, the nurse "traded off" doing the more careful medication checks, probably relying on one or more other usually reliable cues (delivered medications to same patient earlier in shift, cared for the patient yesterday, capsules were of the same color she was accustomed to seeing, etc.) to be able to work faster and meet other organizational goals and/or patient care needs.

Leape and Berwick (2005) explained that health care lags behind other industries in safety because of its reliance on individual performance as the main key to improvement. Other industries have reduced errors by understanding that the way to be safer is to design systems so that it is difficult to make a mistake and easy to recover from mistakes that do occur (Weick & Suttcliffe, 2007).

Complexity of Work at the Sharp End Model

One of the principles stated previously for enabling progress in patient safety is about the importance of understanding actual work (Table 13.1). Woods (1988) proposed that a major barrier to making progress in safety and quality is the failure to appreciate the complexity of work. In real work situations, people anticipate, detect, and bridge gaps necessary for the delivery of safe care every day.

As Figure 13.2 (At the Sharp End of a Complex System; Woods et al., 2010) illustrates, health care workers operate at the point of care delivery (the *sharp end* and lower point of the triangle) and are involved in constantly evolving situations. Organizational resources and layers of defense from above (the *blunt end*) support, and sometimes constrain, health care workers as they continuously manage workloads using their knowledge, immediate perceptions, and own goals to handle situations. Surrounding care situations and confronting workers are multiple goal conflicts, obstacles, hazards, ambiguous and inadequate or missing data, and others'

behaviors (the system complexities on the left side of the model). Workers usually prevent things from going wrong by anticipating, reacting, accommodating, adapting, and coping (characteristics of worker resiliency on the right side of the model) with system failures. Furthermore, bridging these system failures involves constant compromise between multiple competing goals to make tradeoff decisions in the midst of a changing environment.

The cognitive, or *invisible*, work required in complex work environments is demanding and despite best efforts may result in adverse events. Four characteristic dimensions of complex environments increase cognitive problem-solving demands and difficulty (Woods, 1988): dynamism, large numbers of parts and connectedness between parts, high uncertainty, and risk. Klein (1998) identified common characteristics across different types of complex occupations and industries that influence decision making. Time pressures, high stakes, inadequate information (missing, ambiguous, or erroneous), ill-defined goals, poorly defined procedures, dynamic conditions, people working in teams, and stress contribute to complexity in work and decision making. Yet, despite these complexities, workers learn to make decisions and act, creating and actually increasing safety most of the time by using their knowledge, attending to shifts in current situational states, and balancing interacting and sometimes conflicting goals.

Human Limitations and Complexity

Human beings themselves are CASs and, despite their resilience in navigating the complexity of current

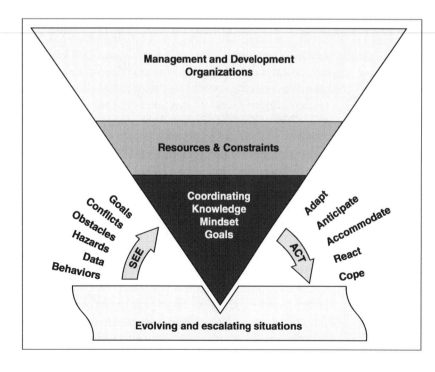

FIGURE 13.2 At the Sharp End of a Complex System: The interplay of problems–demands and practitioners' expertise at the sharp end govern the expression of expertise and error. The resources to meet problem demands are provided and constrained by the organizational context at the blunt end of the system.

Source: From Woods et al. (2010).

health care environments, we must realize that inherent human limitations may sometimes succumb to situational complexity. Human beings are not perfect. Although we can educate them about performing in complex systems and support them with system and process designs that decrease the likelihood of failure, humans are limited in the amount of information and complexity they are able to manage effectively and safely.

During situations involving multitasking, for example, human limitations may result from a variety of factors affecting "cognitive function in dynamic evolving situations, especially those involving the management of workload in time and the control of attention" (Cook & Woods, 1994, p. 270). This very type of work is crucial for ensuring safe and effective care in most situations. In addition to multitasking situations, additional human limitations have been reported relative to fatigue, negative emotions, and/or illness. For example, memory capacity, attention span, distractibility, bias, physical capability, and performance limits are human factors that are challenged during these situations. Other contributors that may affect human performance include environmental factors, such as heat, cold, noise, visual stimuli, motion, and lighting; physiologic factors, including sleep loss, alcohol, and drugs; and psychological factors, including competing activities and other emotional states (e.g., boredom).

Cook and Woods (1994) described two major human performance problems related to changes in attentional dynamics during certain situations. First, *loss of situation awareness* is the failure to maintain accurate tracking of the multiple and changing interactions between parts of processes or systems. Related to this is a lack of *mindfulness*, defined by Langer and Piper (1987) as the ability to scrutinize and refine expectations based on new information and/or contextual aspects of a situation.

Second, *fixation* is the failure to revise assessment of a situation as new information becomes available (Cook & Woods, 1994). As individuals avoid fixation, they are demonstrating *sensemaking* or reconstructing and interpreting incoming information anew in ambiguous, complex, and evolving situations (Klein, Moon, & Hoffman, 2006). Health care providers continually encounter new information in clinical care settings that requires sensemaking to make appropriate decisions about patient care.

Recognizing and appreciating the human factors that limit individual performance in complex situations, despite the best of intentions by competent and responsible care providers, are essential to initiating efforts for improving patient safety. AHRQ's *Manual on Mistake-Proofing the Design of Healthcare Processes* (Grout, 2007) provides basic information

and a guide to incorporating human factors and limitations into interventions to improve safety. The extent of our success in improving safety will always depend on our accounting for the human factors and limitations accompanying failure. Our responses to failure as well as proactive planning and design that support human performance limitations in future similar situations will create opportunities for safer care.

Hindsight Bias and Blame

Since the IOM report (2000) and as a result of learning from other industries about complex systems and human limitations, accident investigation in U.S. hospitals has begun to move from a focus on only the persons involved in an accident to more of a search for multiple potential contributors, often existing as latent failures. Before the IOM report, investigations were often influenced by the natural tendency for humans to look back from an adverse event and see only a simplified path of decision making related to the specific event (Fischoff, 1975). This tendency, which characterizes most investigations, is called *hindsight bias*. Despite ongoing education of health care providers and administrators regarding this tendency, hindsight bias remains a formidable challenge to the identification of actual contributors to an accident. Assigning blame is quick, often seems sufficient, the "fix" is viewed as simple, and formal or informal positive feedback to the person managing the aftermath by assignment of blame is frequently provided by those in charge.

What are lost through hindsight bias and swift assignment of blame are the complex human and environmental factors and the unavoidable tradeoffs that contributed to the experience of the individual(s) involved in the actual situation. Getting stuck in hindsight bias can result in the loss of important learning about (a) system failures that could be redesigned and eliminated from the organization, (b) potential system supports that might be appropriate to implement given normal human limitations that contributed to the event, and (c) opportunities for increasing individual resiliency for responding to future similar complex situations.

Organizational behaviors that are core to improving patient safety are awareness of the negative effect of hindsight bias on learning and purposeful efforts toward avoiding this bias during evaluation of contributors to near-miss and adverse events. In addition to awareness of hindsight bias, other characteristics of an effective patient safety culture and safety program that result from avoidance of hindsight bias include acknowledgment of human limitations; commitment on the part of management to, and modeling of, nonpunitive, problem-solving approaches to accident investigation; facilitation of open communication and involvement of frontline workers for learning and problem solving; design of formal systems of follow-up; and communication and training after new learning but before intended changes are developed and implemented.

The pressure on health care organizations to perform well has been increased because of the publication of patient safety "report cards," reflecting performance on patient safety goals and state medical error reporting system data where available. Compounding potential negative effects on an organization's reputation are the financial implications of reimbursement denials and regulatory penalties that involve care delivery failures related to patient safety goals and quality indicators. Many health care organizations' natural tendency will be to respond to this pressure by reverting to traditional blame and focus on individuals as the solution to improved performance. These types of responses to error usually are quickly visible and satisfying to leaders in the short run. These responses also usually involve punishment or evoke fear of punishment, but there is no evidence that they support sustained improvement in patient safety or the building of an effective patient safety culture. A major challenge for the CNS as leader for improvement in patient safety and development of an effective safety program is to influence others in the organization to implement strategies that reflect learning from other highly reliable industries that base improvement strategies on systems and human factors knowledge.

High-Reliability Organizations

Health care has learned about how to make improvements in safety from other organizations that demand high reliability because of the catastrophic nature of failure if it should occur. Key to our learning have been works by Weick and Suttcliffe (2007), who analyzed core processes for achieving high reliability across varying types of organizations. The authors identified a template of five HRO characteristics they called *mindfulness* (in contrast to the previous more general definition in "Human Limitations and Complexity"), which they proposed increase the ability to maintain reliable performance. See Table 13.3 for the five characteristics found to be common among HROs.

Patient safety researchers proposed that studying complexities and hazards at the sharp end, how providers cope with system failures, and how system failures are created or avoided through operational changes is essential for understanding human performance in complex systems (Woods et al., 2010). Before 2000, no research was found that focused on complexity of the health care system in relation to nurses' work in actual work situations. Research conducted for the purpose of understanding nursing work, including descriptions of factors characteristic of nursing work environments, factors that influence registered nurse (RN) decision making, and RN strategies to manage workflow in providing patient care during actual work situations, has increased since the IOM 2000 report (e.g., Cornell et al., 2010; Ebright, Patterson, Chalko, & Render, 2003; Potter et al., 2005; Tucker & Spear, 2006). In each of these

TABLE 13.3

CHARACTERISTICS OF HIGH-RELIABILITY ORGANIZATIONS (HROs)	
Characteristic	Example
Preoccupation with failure	Treat any lapse as a symptom that something is wrong. HROs focus on actual as well as near misses for investigation
Reluctance to simplify interpretations	Take deliberate steps to create more complete and nuanced pictures of details surrounding a failed process
Sensitivity to operations	Maintain an ongoing concern with the unexpected. HROs look for, and deal quickly with, latent failures before an event occurs
Commitment to resilience	Focus on detecting, containing, and bouncing back from adverse events. Adverse events do not disable HROs
Deference to expertise	Push decision making down to the front line and authority moves to people with the most expertise regardless of rank

studies, the researchers used methods of direct observations of nurses during actual work and/or interview strategies to elicit details of nurses' activities, thinking, and decision making while in the process of delivering care.

Reports from these studies describe latent failures confronting nurses in the midst of care delivery (e.g., missing equipment, interruptions, waiting for access to needed systems and resources, lack of time to complete interventions that were judged necessary to reach desired outcomes, and inconsistencies in how information was communicated or could be relied on for access if needed). Other results demonstrated nurse strategies for dealing with, or adapting to, the latent failures (e.g., anticipating or forward thinking, proactive monitoring of patient status to detect early warning signals, strategic delegation and handoff decisions to maintain flow of workload, individualized paper memory aids, and "stacking" management of activities to be done).

Three types of knowledge were found that affected RN decision making: knowledge about individual patients, typical patient disease profiles, and unit workflow routines (Ebright et al., 2003). Other factors affecting decision making included patterns of goal conflict or simultaneous and sometimes competing goals that, together, were difficult to reach in a timely or expected manner. Types of competing goals included maintaining patient safety, preventing getting behind schedule, avoiding increasing complexity, appearing competent and efficient to patients/families and coworkers, and maintaining patient/family satisfaction.

Moving forward with patient safety improvement efforts that fail to take into account the complexities of actual work flow and conditions will not result in increased reliability or sustained improvements. A focus only on increasing individuals' knowledge base, or fear of consequences from failure, will not result in consistent perfect performance given imperfect situations. A combined appreciation of human limitations and of system complexity is needed to reach the level of reliability achieved by HROs (Chassin & Loeb, 2011).

APPLICATION TO CNS PRACTICE

CNSs contributed to patient safety in multiple ways before the IOM report was published in 2000, and they have had a substantial impact on improvement efforts based on what we have learned since then. Health care organizations will continue to look for effective strategies to improve the quality of care and reduce error in and across settings where care is provided in light of new and evolving legislative, regulatory, and health care environment requirements.

As outlined in the *Statement on Clinical Nurse Specialist Practice and Education* (NACNS, 2004), CNSs have the educational background, including core competencies related to complex systems and leadership for implementation of change, strategic organizational positioning, and essential expert clinical knowledge, to facilitate and lead successful and sustained patient safety improvements. The CNS is in a position to influence patient safety work in five important ways: (a) role modeling behaviors of a nonpunitive safety culture, (b) facilitating and leading ongoing efforts to learn about system complexities, (c) facilitating and leading ongoing efforts to learn about health care worker resiliency, (d) proactively managing potential increases in complexity with strategic introduction of change, and (e) staying current with the evolving patient safety literature and evidence for best practice.

Providing Leadership for a Nonpunitive Safety Culture

An effective culture of safety is one in which workers are willing to share details surrounding near-miss and adverse-event situations for continuous learning about latent failures in the system. For an organization to sustain an effective culture of safety, health care workers must work in an environment that is nonpunitive, where they feel safe to speak up and where they are invited and encouraged to participate in the improvement process. Building a culture of safety requires relationships based on trust, open communication, and a belief that those closest to the work, specifically patient care, are most knowledgeable about the work itself and are needed in the improvement processes.

Successful CNS practice is dependent on nurturing and maintaining trust through relationships on a daily basis with patients and families, multidisciplinary health care personnel, and the organization's leadership. Thus, the nature of CNS practice is characterized by a unique combination of skills that includes communication strategies, relationship building, systems focus, and clinical care delivery expertise, which makes the CNS a valuable resource for others throughout the organization. Other leaders can benefit from observing the ease with which the CNS is able to blend each of these strengths to influence people and programs to achieve change across the health care continuum. Specific behaviors that the CNS should demonstrate to support and influence an effective safety culture are listed in Table 13.4.

Achieving measurable improvements in safety for patients depends on an organizational culture based on safety culture behaviors from all persons in leadership roles as well as the frontline care providers

TABLE 13.4

CNS SUPPORTIVE BEHAVIORS OF AN EFFECTIVE PATIENT SAFETY CULTURE
Behaviors
1. Open communication about, and role modeling of responses to, adverse events and near misses that reflects absence of hindsight bias
2. Commitment to and role modeling of nonpunitive, problem-solving approaches to accident investigation and follow-up interventions
3. Open communication and acknowledgment of human limitations as a contributor to adverse/near-miss events and incorporation of response interventions and systems redesigns that support and account for identified human limitations
4. Facilitation/leading and role modeling of open communication and inviting of participation of frontline workers for maximum learning and creative problem solving to reduce the risk of future events
5. Facilitating/leading the design of formal systems of adverse event/near-miss follow-up processes and dissemination of learning throughout the organization after an event
6. Role modeling timely open communication and reporting about own adverse/near-miss events and identified latent failures that could contribute to future events

CNS, clinical nurse specialist.

across the continuum of care. With their educational background and competencies used in everyday practice, CNSs can be instrumental in role modeling and leading others toward this important goal.

Outcomes of CNS practice related to development of a nonpunitive safety culture are as follows: Nurses are empowered to solve patient care problems at the point of service; nurses use resources judiciously to reduce overall costs of care and enhance quality of patient care; nurses have an effective voice in decision making about patient care; and decision makers within the institution are informed about practice problems and the significance of these problems with respect to outcomes and costs (NACNS, 2004).

Learning About System Complexities

Fundamental to improvement in patient safety is identification of the latent failures as well as active failures that contribute to complexity and hazards at the point of care (Woods et al., 2010). The CNS core competency related to differential diagnosis captures the essential critical thinking skills that allow explication of those latent failures, or etiologies, that contribute to adverse and near-miss events (NACNS, 2004, pp. 25–26). The CNS should use this core competency for direct application to specific investigations of single events or to grouped event data; lead and role model for teams of nurses and other disciplines the application of the competency to single event or grouped event data; and interpret and articulate for other leaders in the organization the process

and outcomes of differential diagnosis, including etiologies of adverse and near-miss events and the most appropriate interventions to prevent or diminish the impact of future adverse and near-miss events.

In addition, with experiential knowledge of actual work environments within which health care workers practice, the CNS brings to a variety of event investigations an informed curiosity that is essential for identification of the goals, conflicts, obstacles, hazards, data, and behaviors that contribute to the complexity surrounding care situations (Figure 13.2). Leading investigations to maintain and sustain focus on these aspects of an adverse or near-miss event provides the CNS opportunities to role model for other health care staff the acknowledgment and then the setting aside of hindsight bias, a huge barrier to safety and quality improvement. The CNS should emphasize the benefit of timely storytelling to detail the complexity surrounding adverse and near-miss event situations and for accurate identification of etiologies and potential interventions. Getting past hindsight bias and the tendency to simplify factors causing an event is paramount for learning about what is needed for improvement.

Outcomes of CNS practice related to learning about system complexities are as follows: Patient care processes reflect continuous improvements that benefit the system; change strategies are integrated throughout the system; nursing interventions target specified etiologies; and the research and scientific base for innovations is articulated, understandable, and accessible (NACNS, 2004).

Learning About Health Care Worker Resiliency

Just as important as learning what latent failures were present in adverse and near-miss event situations is learning how practitioners anticipated, accommodated, reacted, adapted, and coped with complexities to avert or decrease the impact of the adverse and near-miss events (Figure 13.2). The CNS should investigate and document during event investigations how practitioners managed to navigate the complexity of the actual work environment, how they reacted effectively or ineffectively and successfully or unsuccessfully to prevent an adverse event, or how they were able to minimize the negative outcome. Details obtained during event investigation about practitioners' cues for recognition of a problem and subsequent sequence of actions during the situation can provide excellent information for development of future interventions. Information learned from this line of investigation can be incorporated into recommended interventions for educating staff, redesigning processes and systems to support staff, or for developing new processes or designs. The CNS should facilitate the capture of event details related to coping and adaptation by probing the storyteller for the minutest information surrounding the situation that is normally lost through general questioning after an event. This detail provides less experienced staff with important knowledge that is sometimes only obtained by years of actual clinical experience.

Outcomes of CNS practice related to health care worker resiliency are as follows: Unintended consequences and errors are prevented; predicted and measurable nurse-sensitive patient outcomes are attained through evidence-based practice (EBP); collaboration with patients/clients, nursing staff, and physicians and other health care professionals occurs as appropriate; reports of new clinical phenomena and/or interventions are disseminated through presentations and publications; nurses are able to articulate their unique contributions to patient care and nurse-sensitive outcomes; nurses experience job satisfaction; nurses engage in learning experiences to advance or maintain competence; and staff comply with regulatory requirements and standards (NACNS, 2004).

Tools for Increasing Understanding of Actual Work

Health care organizations used quality management systems to manage, measure, and attempt to improve processes and outcomes before the IOM report (2000). With the new approach to patient safety, new quality management methods have been borrowed from manufacturing. These methods, some referred to as LEAN, are a particularly appropriate fit because they were processes developed to increase quality through identification of defects and inefficiencies leading to errors or failures. Henry Ford first pioneered some of the LEAN principles for workflow production in the automobile industry, and Toyota further developed the concepts (Womack, Jones, & Roos, 2007). Health care organizations continue to use LEAN principles and other strategies to guide development and improvement of systems (Toussaint & Berry, 2013). Some of the LEAN tools used by industry are useful for increasing understanding of system complexity and human limitations that contribute to adverse events. CNSs need to know about these tools to be able to use them effectively in patient safety–related projects and to understand the outcome data and implications for designing and choosing appropriate patient safety interventions. Table 13.5 lists examples of retrospective and prospective tools used in quality and patient safety work. Other methods may be called different names but are used for very similar purposes. *Retrospective* tools are useful for gathering data after an adverse or near-miss event. *Prospective* tools are very helpful in analyzing systems and processes to identify opportunities for redesign to prevent adverse events or decrease the impact of failure or to prioritize improvement efforts. Used appropriately, these tools are all about understanding details of processes, including the human component, for the purpose of learning what needs to be done to increase reliability and reduce the likelihood of failure. Like any other method or tool, inappropriate application of the methods or interpretation of outcome data will produce poor results. Appropriate use and application can result in increased and sustainable quality.

Outcomes of CNS practice related to approaches for understanding actual work are as follows: Diagnoses are accurately aligned with assessment data and etiologies; EBPs are used by nurses; clinical problems are articulated within the context of the organization/system structure, mission, culture, policies, and resources; patient care processes reflect continuous improvement that benefit the system (NACNS, 2004).

Managing the Complexity Inherent in Change

With advanced clinical knowledge, a systems orientation, and strategic positioning in the organization that is directly or closely linked to the actual clinical work environment, the CNS should be prepared to anticipate and articulate the potential contribution of planned organizational changes for creating new latent failures. As patient safety leader, consultant,

TABLE 13.5

EXAMPLES OF TOOLS FOR UNDERSTANDING WORK COMPLEXITY AND ETIOLOGIES OF FAILURE	
Tools	**Definition**
Root Cause Analysis	A process for identifying the basic or contributing causal factors that underlie variations in performance associated with adverse events or near misses (www.va.gov/ncps/glossary.html)
Event Flow Diagram	A diagram that uses graphical symbols to depict the nature and flow of events leading up to an adverse/near-miss event
Data Mining (also can be used prospectively)	The analysis of large amounts of data for relationships that have not previously been discovered and increase understanding of work complexity
Health Care Failure Mode and Effects Analysis	A prospective assessment that identifies and improves steps in a process, thereby reasonably ensuring a safe and clinically desirable outcome. A systematic approach to identify and prevent product and process problems before they occur (www.va.gov/ncps/SafetyTopics/HFMEA/HFMEA Intro.pdf)
Workflow Analysis– Process Mapping	The analysis and representation of clinical work processes from the perspective of the staff member(s)
Positive Deviance	A process whereby managers actively look for those extraordinarily successful groups and individuals and bring the isolated success strategies of those "positive deviants" into the mainstream (www.12manage.com/methods_pascale_positive_deviance.html)
Risk Resilience Assessment	Assessment of the strengths and weaknesses in the ability of an organization to manage risk (Nolan & Resar, 2008)

mentor, and change agent, the CNS should provide guidance in appreciating how new complexities may result from even well-developed and planned change efforts. Anticipating and preparing for how change might introduce new forms of latent failure and complexity in relation to the overall actual work of practitioners is also needed to maintain safe environments. The CNS should begin the design and preparation for implementing change by asking staff to answer two crucial questions designed to elicit potential consequences of the change (listed in Table 13.6). Each of these questions will result in the type of feedback not usually obtained from traditional general requests for feedback and can be very productive in identification of potential latent failures not anticipated by project planners.

Analysis of feedback from these questions allows adjustment or redesign of the change and also identifies solutions to be created and included in content for the educational rollout prior to the change. For example, when a computer software design administrator was asked 1 week before the implementation of a new computer system about what might go wrong, he identified a list of 10 possible failures. As a result, the staff was given specific directions about what to do if any of the 10 situations occurred. *Hoping* that none of the 10 identified possible failures would occur without backup planning would neither have been sufficient to prevent increased complexity for those involved in patient care nor supportive of patient safety.

Outcomes of CNS practice related to strategic planning for change are as follows: Unintended consequences and errors are prevented; desired measurable patient/client outcomes are achieved; interventions that are effective in achieving nurse-sensitive outcomes are incorporated into guidelines and policies; change strategies are integrated throughout the system; innovative models of practice are developed, piloted, evaluated, and incorporated across the continuum of care; and patient care programs are aligned with the organization's strategic imperatives, mission, vision, philosophy, and values (NACNS, 2004).

Staying Current with the Evolving Patient Safety Literature, Evidence for Best Practice, and the Changing Health Care Environment

New and emerging knowledge continues to develop about the importance of communication, teamwork, and clarifying accountabilities in this new approach to patient safety as health care organizations and patient safety researchers apply other industry models to safety improvement. CNSs should become familiar with the continuing development of innovative models

TABLE 13.6

QUESTIONS TO IDENTIFY POTENTIAL CONSEQUENCES OF CHANGE
1. Think about incorporating this new process (technology) into your actual workflow. How will this new process (or technology) in any way change the way you work, or the flow of your work?
2. As you think about incorporating this change in process (or technology) into your work, imagine that the change ends up not being successful. Why do you think that will be? What probably caused it to not be successful?

and research as the health care industry adopts and adapts other industry methods to health care work.

For example, those who have applied team development strategies for improving teamwork have had to acknowledge and adjust for the fact that health care teams often involve differing roles, numbers of members, and even differing members throughout a day. There is a shift of focus from building strong "teams" to developing "expert team member behaviors and competencies" that will transfer with members as team composition changes.

Failure in communication is the most frequently identified contributor to adverse and near-miss events. The multiple aspects of how, when, by whom, and in what situations information is communicated have been found to be very complex across a variety of complicated health care situations (Leonard, Graham, & Bonacum, 2004; Patterson & Wears, 2010). Issues related to what to standardize, how to format, or through what medium information should be disseminated by health care providers have unleashed many different models and approaches to increase accuracy and completeness. Testing and research will determine what models and critical parts of models result in successful transfer of information and in what situations.

Early learning about new approaches to patient safety included the need to create a "nonblame culture" to increase worker reporting about adverse and near-miss events. Learning about system contributors requires worker willingness to share stories about what led up to and surrounded actions resulting in failure. Health care leaders, as well as some providers, however, are uncomfortable with the term, thinking that *nonblame* reduces or eliminates workers' sense of accountability for safe decision making and actions. For some who are responsible for patient safety outcomes, it is difficult to separate the process of managing poor performance from the process of adverse and near-miss investigation. Tools such as Just Culture (The Just Culture Community, 2013) have been developed to guide managers through algorithms for determining risk behaviors in failure-related incidents and performance management actions for follow-up.

The challenge for health care organizations is to educate management on the appropriate application of these tools so that an effective culture of safety with nonblame approaches to failure investigations, separate from ongoing management of poor performance, is realized. The processes should be separated, with managing poor performance after an event only considered as a result of completed failure investigation. Some failures do not include any evidence of poor performance. Assigning blame to poor performance in the aftermath of an adverse or near-miss event but before investigations are complete may lead to biased conduct of the investigation and result in less focus on, and discovery of, system contributions. Managing poor performance continuously and separate from event aftermath helps to remove the blame from event investigation.

Recent literature focuses on approaches to patient safety and new frameworks concerning management of risk and risk resilience. Nolan and Resar (2008) proposed that once we reach a certain level of competency and consistency regarding identification of root causes and failure mode analysis, our attention should turn to evaluating and increasing the organization's risk resilience. Risk resilience is the assessment of an organization's strengths and weaknesses to adapt to variation.

Amalberti, Vincent, Auroy, and de Saint Maurice (2006) wrote about the Rasmussen/Amalberti framework for understanding violations and system migrations that occur away from standard procedures and that are sometimes necessary to maintain safety amid dynamic conditions. The authors described a continuum of safe behavior that starts with initial safe spaces of action, to creation of borderline-tolerated conditions of use, and ends with normalization of deviance and reckless individual behavior. They emphasize the need to manage risk-taking, to understand factors that influence tolerable and intolerable violations and migrations, and to understand which of these need to be supported in certain circumstances and which need to be managed.

Health care organizations' evolution toward pay-for-performance reimbursement, accountable care, and provisions of services in response to enactment of the Affordable Care Act will continue to move the focus on patient safety and quality beyond the boundaries of the acute care environment. CNSs have the knowledge and skills to lead changes in and development of new processes beyond their more prominent and past work in acute care environments.

Outcomes of CNS practice related to staying current are as follows: Predicted and measurable nurse-sensitive patient outcomes are attained through EBP; reports of new clinical phenomena and/or interventions are disseminated through presentations and publications; educational programs that advance the practice of nursing are developed, implemented, evaluated, and linked to EBP and effects on clinical and fiscal outcomes; patient care initiatives reflect knowledge of cost management and revenue enhancement strategies; and policy-making bodies are influenced to develop regulations/procedures to improve patient care and health services (NACNS, 2004).

ETHICAL CONSIDERATIONS

The CNS will continue to be involved in managing and role modeling for patient situations involving ethical aspects related to provision of safe care and the communication and decision making required. What is important and new for leadership of patient safety efforts is the commitment by the CNS to the appropriate evidence-based application of new knowledge that health care has discovered from other industries since the IOM (2000) report. It is no longer acceptable for leaders at any level to blame individuals for error and implementation of strategies that fail to explicate the system contributions to adverse events. Just as CNSs articulate the complexity of individual patient cases, they must articulate the complexity of actual work situations that leads to adverse and near-miss events, and they must provide leadership and influence for designing efforts that incorporate the new approach.

■ DISCUSSION QUESTIONS

● What was the response to the last adverse event in your organization? Was the response focused primarily on blame or details surrounding the event? How did you respond? What was your role, if any, related to event aftermath, organizational learning, or dissemination of findings after the event investigation? How could you improve on your response

to the event to have influence at each of the three spheres of your practice?
● Who is responsible for overall patient safety and quality in your organization? What is your role with patient safety and quality at each of the three sphere levels?

■ ANALYSIS AND SYNTHESIS EXERCISE

● Analyze the current patient safety efforts in your organization. Are the current activities most reflective of (a) traditional management of error; (b) developing systems and structure for error reporting, investigation, and redesign; or (c) beginning to systematically assess the organization's risk resilience ability?

■ CLINICAL APPLICATION

● Choose a change project currently in progress (may or may not be your own). Assess through sharp-end care providers and one or more prospective LEAN tools the implications of the change on total workload and systems across the continuum for patient health care outcomes (e.g., potential for new latent failure modes). Develop a response to provider input as appropriate: for example, redesign some aspects of change itself; provide helpful education for users regarding impact of change as noted by providers; and/or articulate clearly to the owner of the change initiative why new information should be considered that may alter current plans before implementation of the change.

REFERENCES

Amalberti, R., Vincent, C., Auroy, Y., & de Saint Maurice, G. (2006). Violations and migrations in health care: A framework for understanding and management. *Quality and Safety in Health Care,* *15*(Suppl. 1), 66–71.

Chassin, M. R., & Loeb, J. M. (2011). The ongoing quality improvement journey: Next stop, high reliability. *Health Affairs (Project Hope), 30*(4), 559–568.

Cook, R. I., & Woods, D. D. (1994). Operating at the sharp end: The complexity of human error. In M. E. Bogner (Ed.), *Human error in medicine* (pp. 255–310). Hillsdale, NJ: Lawrence Erlbaum Associates.

Cornell, P., Herrin-Griffith, D., Keim, C., Petschonek, S., Sanders, A. M., D'Mello, S.,…Shepherd, G. (2010). Transforming nursing workflow, part 1: The chaotic nature of nurse activities. *The Journal of Nursing Administration, 40*(9), 366–373.

Ebright, P. R., Patterson, E. S., Chalko, B. A., & Render, M. L. (2003). Understanding the complexity of registered nurse work in acute care settings. *The Journal of Nursing Administration, 33*(12), 630–638.

Fischoff, B. (1975). Hindsight does not equal foresight: The effect of outcome knowledge on judgment under uncertainty. *Journal of Experimental Psychology: Human Perception and Performance, 1,* 288–299.

Grout, J. (2007). *Mistake-proofing the design of health care processes* (Prepared under an IPA with Berry College; AHRQ Publication No. 07–0020). Rockville, MD: Agency for Healthcare Research and Quality.

Institute for Healthcare Improvement (IHI). (2013). Retrieved August 19, 2013, from http://www.ihi.org/ihi/programs

Institute of Medicine (IOM). (2000). *To err is human: Building a safer health system.* Washington, DC: National Academies Press.

Institute of Medicine, Committee on Quality of Healthcare in America. (2001). *Crossing the quality chasm: A new health system for the 21st century.* Washington, DC: National Academies Press.

The Joint Commission. (2013a). *History of The Joint Commission.* Retrieved August 19, 2013, from http://www.jointcommission.org/assets/1/6/Joint_Commission_History.pdf

The Joint Commission. (2013b). *National patient safety goals.* Retrieved August 19, 2013, from http://www.jointcommission.org/search/default.aspx?Keywords=Patient+Safety+Goals&f=sitename&sitename=Joint+Commission

The Just Culture Community. (2014). Retrieved February 16, 2014, from https://www.justculture.org/what-is-just-culture/

Klein, G. (1998). *Sources of power: How people make decisions.* Cambridge, MA: MIT Press.

Klein, G., Moon, B., & Hoffman, R. F. (2006). Making sense of sensemaking I: Alternative perspectives. *IEEE Intelligent Systems, 21*(4), 70–73.

Langer, E. J., & Piper, A. (1987). The prevention of mindlessness. *Journal of Personality and Social Psychology, 53,* 280–287.

Leape, L. L. (1994). Error in medicine. *Journal of the American Medical Association, 272*(23), 1851–1857.

Leape, L. L., & Berwick, D. M. (2005). Five years after *To Err Is Human*: What have we learned? *Journal of the American Medical Association, 293*(19), 2384–2390.

Leonard, M., Graham, S., & Bonacum, D. (2004). The human factor: The critical importance of effective teamwork and communication in providing safe care. *Quality and Safety in Health Care, 13*(Suppl. 1), 85–90.

National Association of Clinical Nurse Specialists (NACNS). (2004). *Statement on clinical nurse specialist practice and education* (2nd ed.). Harrisburg, PA: Author.

Nolan, T., & Resar, R. (2008). *Strategic system for safety.* Cambridge, MA: Institute for Healthcare Improvement.

Patterson, E., & Wears, R. (2010). Patient handoffs: Standardized and reliable measurement tools remain elusive. *The Joint Commission Journal on Quality and Patient Safety, 36*(2), 52–61.

Peplau, H. (2003). Specialization in professional nursing. *Clinical Nurse Specialist, 17*(1), 3–9. (Original work published 1965)

Potter, P., Wolf, L., Boxerman, S., Grayson, D., Sledge, J., Dunagan, C., & Evanoff, B. (2005). Understanding the cognitive work of nursing in the acute care environment. *The Journal of Nursing Administration, 35*(7–8), 327–335.

Reason, J. (1990). *Human error.* Cambridge, England:Cambridge University Press.

Reason, J. (2000). Human error: Models and management. *British Medical Journal, 320,* 768–770.

Rogers, E. M. (2003). *Diffusion of innovations* (5th ed.). New York, NY: The Free Press.

Toussaint, J. S., & Berry, L. L. (2013). The promise of LEAN in health care. *Mayo Clinic Proceedings, 88*(1), 74–82.

Tucker, A. L., & Spear, S. J. (2006). Operational failures and interruptions in hospital nursing. *Health Services Research, 41,* 643–662.

VA National Center for Patient Safety. (2013). *Glossary of patient safety terms.* Retrieved August 19, 2013, from http://www.patientsafety.va.gov/glossary.html

Wachter, R. (2010). Patient safety at ten: Unmistakable progress, troubling gaps. *Health Affairs, 29*(1), 1–9.

Weick, K. E., & Sutcliffe, K. M. (2007). *Managing the unexpected: Resilient performance in an age of uncertainty.* San Francisco, CA: John Wiley & Sons.

Womack, J. P., Jones, D. T., & Roos, D. (2007). *The machine that changed the world: The story of lean production—How Japan's secret weapon in the global auto wars will revolutionize western industry.* New York, NY: The Free Press.

Woods, D. D. (1988). Coping with complexity: The psychology of human behavior in complex systems. In L. P. Goodstein, H. B. Anderson, & S. E. Olsen (Eds.), *Tasks, errors and mental models* (pp. 128–148). London, UK: Taylor and Francis.

Woods, D. D., & Cook, R. I. (1998). *Characteristics of patient safety: Five principles that underlie productive work.* Chicago, IL: Chicago Testing Laboratory.

Woods, D. D., Dekker, S., Cook, R., Johannesen, L., & Sarter, N. (2010). *Behind human error* (2nd ed.). Burlington, VT: Ashgate.

14

Individual as Client

Janet S. Fulton and Carol L. Baird

Caring for individual persons, sick or well, is foundational to nursing practice. At the individual level, nurses provide care and comfort during acute episodes of illness, guide self-care for managing symptoms and functional problems associated with chronic illness, and offer health education, screening, and early interventions to prevent disease and maintain wellness. Today's health problems tend to be chronic, underlying, lingering pathologies prone to exacerbations and remissions and requiring anywhere from minimal to complex self-maintained treatment routines. Disease and illness are not the same thing (Larsen, 2013). Disease is pathology: a change in physical structure and function that can be quantified, measured, and described. Illness is the experience of the patient; it is what is lived in the context of cultural, social, economic, and personal worlds. Illness as lived experience is "the subjective experience of somatic discomfort, including physical discomfort, emotional discomfort, and/or a reduction in functional ability below the perceived capability level" (NACNS, 2004, p. 64). Wellness and illness are not dichotomous states where a person can pick one but not both. Nor is wellness to illness a continuum of ill to well. How would placement on such a continuum be determined? Wellness exists in disease as individuals live the experience of striving to function at maximum ability with minimal symptoms and suffering. Many people are functioning with a diagnosed chronic disease—diabetes, asthma, arthritis, and hypertension are but a few examples. Most of these individuals say they were well because they are functioning to their perceived highest level and have a good quality of life (QOL). Thus, wellness can be experienced in the presence or absence of disease. Clinical

nurse specialists' (CNSs) orientation toward advanced nursing practice is one that incorporates wellness in illness. Wellness in illness emphasizes maximizing function, promoting comfort, and relieving suffering in the lived experience of patients across disease conditions inclusive of prevention, acute and chronic. Wellness in illness presupposes nursing interventions focused on self-care, thus assisting patients to live their best lives in the presence of disease. Nursing practice incorporates knowledge of disease and its treatment with biobehavioral science, and applies this knowledge to the context of individual lives for the purpose of achieving wellness in illness. This desired outcome crosses the continuum of care settings from primary care, acute care, home care, and rehabilitation and long-term care.

Care of the individual client begins with a careful assessment. For CNSs, care begins with an advanced nursing assessment. What constitutes an advanced nursing assessment? In many care settings, the information collected for an advanced nursing assessment overlaps considerably with a medical history and physical examination. Anecdotally, when nurses are asked to explain the difference between a nursing and medical assessment they often identify the nursing assessment as more holistic. A search of the Cumulative Index to Nursing and Allied Health Literature (CINAHL) and Nursing OVID between years 2003 and 2013 identified over a thousand articles each under the term *holistic nursing* and almost 10,000 articles under *nursing assessment*. Combining these two searches—*holism/holistic nursing* and *nursing assessment*—found only a handful of articles primarily addressing focused psychosocial assessments such as spirituality, sexuality, family, culture, and

QOL. Only one article could be found that described a theoretical basis for holistic assessment (Sappington & Kelley, 1996). Using modeling and role modeling theory, Sappington and Kelley asserted that nursing care should be grounded in individual uniqueness because clients have knowledge and ability to understand what made them sick and what will make them well. A similar search for the same time period (2003–2013) identified about 200 articles when combining *nursing assessment* and *advanced nursing practice*. Physical assessment of specific symptoms, such as chest pain, shortness of breath, and depressed mood, dominated this group of articles, followed by disease-specific assessment, including asthma, diabetes, heart failure, chronic obstructive pulmonary disease, and sickle cell disease. Articles specific to critical care practice addressed using technology to monitor patients in critical care settings. Several articles address reading and interpreting laboratory tests, x-rays, scans, and other diagnostic tests.

Several empiric articles explored the content of advanced nursing assessment (Davidson, Bennet, Hamera, & Raines, 2004; Kelley, Kopac, & Rosselli, 2007). Kelley and Kopac (2001) surveyed schools of nursing about advanced health assessment courses for nurse practitioner programs and conducted a follow-up study in 2007. Consistent with the original findings, the follow-up study found the major content areas to be obtaining history and interviewing, physical assessment, health promotion, ethnic and cultural considerations, developmental assessment, and functional assessment. Pediatric and gerontological content had increased and a new content area was included: assessment strategies for persons with disabilities and special needs. In a related study, Davidson and colleagues (2004) asked nurse practitioner preceptors to rate the importance of 87 specific assessment competencies for primary care practice. Assessment competencies rated highest were in the cardiovascular, musculoskeletal, and gynecological systems and included the ability to detect and interpret abnormalities in heart rate and rhythm; determine status of circulatory, motor, and neurological systems; and conduct pelvic examinations, including collecting cervical specimens and performing and interpreting speculum and bimanual examinations. Asked about the differences between undergraduate and graduate assessment courses, faculty reported including more differential diagnosis of disease, greater focus on abnormal findings, and inclusion of testing (x-rays, EKG, wet mounts, etc.) in the graduate course. As regards conceptualizations and theoretical models used to guide assessment, faculty noted challenges in conceptualizing assessment content within nursing theory when using the medical model to establish differential diagnosis of disease

conditions (Kelley & Kopac, 2001). Among respondents indicating a theoretical basis for assessment, a holistic approach was most often reported, followed by systems theory and functional health.

Findings from the literature support the observation that advanced nursing assessment is heavily disease focused, follows the general framework of medical history and physical examination, and has a growing interest in medical testing procedures like x-rays. When the purpose of a health assessment is differential diagnosis of disease, a medical framework is appropriate and necessary. However, little evidence is available describing advanced assessment consistent with a nursing perspective (such as was described in Chapter 3). This chapter explores the importance of articulating a theoretical perspective for health assessment, offers a unique purpose of advanced nursing assessment, and suggests an assessment strategy for identifying etiologies amenable to nursing interventions consistent with a theoretical perspective.

THEORETICAL PERSPECTIVE FOR ADVANCED ASSESSMENT

The question, "What is an advanced nursing assessment?" is part of a larger unknown dealing with the nature of nursing practiced at an advanced level. What is advanced practice in nursing? What are the characteristics? What are the behaviors and outcomes? The ideas offered in this chapter about advanced assessment are *not* intended to provide *the* answer to these questions. Rather, these ideas are offered for consideration in an ongoing dialogue that is part of a quest to discover and define nursing practiced at an advanced level.

Purpose of Health Assessment

The purpose of health assessment is to collect, document, and analyze client information and to draw conclusions supported by data/information. These assessment-based conclusions direct interventions for the purpose of influencing health status. Conclusions require judgment, and conclusions made by nurses about problems amenable to nursing interventions have been called nursing diagnoses. While many judgments are made by nurses in practice, Gordon has long pointed out that the term *nursing diagnosis* is reserved for client conditions that nurses, by virtue of their education and experience, are capable and licensed to treat (Gordon, 2007).

Identifying as nursing diagnosis those conclusions made by nurses based on nursing assessment was introduced into the language of nursing in the 1970s, in part because of legislative initiatives to recognize the independent practice of nursing as distinct from medicine and to remove statutory requirements for physician supervision of nursing practice. In introducing revisions to the nurse practice act, the New York State Nurses Association included the term *nursing diagnosis* in reference to the distinctive areas in which the nurse exercised, and was expected to exercise, independent judgment (Driscoll, 1976/2007; Fulton, 2007). Scholarly work to develop nursing diagnosis can be traced to the first meeting in 1973 of the National Group for the Classification of Nursing Diagnosis, which later became the North American Nursing Diagnosis Association (NANDA). Over the years, integration of nursing diagnosis into practice has been challenging. Carpenito (1995) outlined some of the difficulties resulting from a priori application of labels to all situations in which nurses intervene, including using diagnostic terms without validation and using phrases that are little more than renamed medical diagnoses. Validation problems occur when nurses "change the data to fit the label," for example, using the label *altered nutrition* as a diagnosis for all patients being medically restricted from taking food or fluids by mouth. The renaming of medical diagnoses occurs when a nurse uses a label such as *impaired gas exchange* as a diagnosis for patients with chronic obstructive pulmonary disease, asthma, and adult respiratory distress syndrome (Carpenito, 1995). These problems aside, the need to develop nursing diagnosis is of utmost importance for communicating about our nursing conclusions, interventions, and outcomes. For purposes of this discussion, it needs to be emphasized that any statement of conclusion made by a CNS or any nurse about a patient problem, whether specified as a nursing diagnosis or not, must be logically consistent with and supported by data that were systematically collected and analyzed. Further, the conclusion should reflect a client health problem amenable to independent nursing interventions. To illustrate, the conclusion may be lower back pain related to positioning, specifically lying supine flat. Interventions are related to repositioning, such as elevating hips or moving to lateral position with knees bent. The etiology of pain, in this example, is body position supine flat. The problem is amenable to independent nursing intervention—repositioning. The specific repositioning intervention will be determined by a more in-depth assessment and understanding of the etiology of the pain problem and contextual limitations. It may be appropriate to administer prescribed medications to alleviate the pain; however, medication is a medical intervention administered based on nursing judgment within the parameters of the medical prescription and intended to alter a different etiology. Etiologies related to

position are amenable to independent nursing interventions involving repositioning.

The purpose of an advanced nursing assessment is to support an advanced judgment about a client health problem(s) amenable to independent nursing intervention. While the complexity of possible interventions varies, advanced practice is characterized by the depth and breadth of nursing judgment needed to pinpoint problems and their etiologies, not solely by the complexity of the intervention.

Theoretical Frameworks for Nursing Assessment of the Individual

Assessment concentrates heavily on collection of data about the client (Broom, 2007). The most common framework used for health assessment is the body system framework, which includes a health history and physical examination. Long used in practice, it was more formally organized in a textbook by Bates and Hoekelman (1974). It remains the dominant framework for comprehensive health assessment and is used in teaching physician and nursing students as well as students of other health professions.

The body systems framework includes a health history and a physical examination. The health history focuses on subjective data, including the client's description of symptoms and health problems and other information about the client's social background and lifestyle. Physical examination focuses on objective data determined by an examiner. The physical exam establishes a baseline, identifies normal from abnormal, and validates information obtained during the health history (Barkauskas, Baumann, & Darling-Fisher, 2002). Physical examination requires specific techniques, including inspection, palpation, percussion, and auscultation, in addition to some special positions and manipulations.

Nursing theoretical frameworks for comprehensive health assessment include Gordon's Functional Health Patterns, Unitary Person Framework, and NANDA taxonomy (Barkauskas et al., 2002). These frameworks are ways to organize information into categories and under diagnostic labels as opposed to methods for systematically collecting the data. Among the nursing frameworks, Gordon's Functional Health Patterns is the most developed.

Gordon's Functional Health Patterns framework for assessment is based on 11 areas of possible functional health problems. Health problems are determined by assessing functional patterns believed to be influenced by biological, developmental, cultural, social, and spiritual factors. The functional patterns are

1. Health perception—health management
2. Nutrition—metabolic

3. Elimination
4. Activity—exercise
5. Sleep—rest
6. Cognitive—perceptual
7. Self-perception—self-concept
8. Role—relationship
9. Sexuality—reproductive
10. Coping—stress—tolerance
11. Value—belief (Gordon, 2007)

For each functional area, a judgment of whether or not a pattern is functional or dysfunctional is made by comparing assessment data to one or more of the following: (a) individual baselines; (b) established norms for age-groups; or (c) cultural, social, or other norms. Dysfunctional patterns may occur with disease or may lead to disease. A particular pattern has to be evaluated in the context of other patterns and its contribution to optimal function of the client (Gordon, 2007). Unlike the well-established body systems assessment framework, there is no common order for collecting data, no standard questions, and no special techniques of physical examination.

PHILOSOPHICAL UNDERPINNINGS OF ASSESSMENT

Assessment involves combining general knowledge from theory and research with particular knowledge about a client for the purpose of clinical decision making. To explain the paradox of knowledge that is both general (from theory and research) and specific (to a client), Gadow (1995) used a dialectic framework (a method of inquiry in philosophy) to explore the process by which clinical assessment in nursing resolves the opposite positions of general and particular knowledge. The dialectic method was selected because it supports arriving at the most complete understanding of a process. Understanding the overall process, not the outcome, is the goal of this method. Knowledge generated by the dialectic method is considered complete when it incorporates—not eliminates—the opposing elements into the process (Gadow, 1995).

Gadow's (1995) inquiry identified five levels to the assessment process: vulnerability, disengagement, reduction, holism, and engagement, summarized in Table 14.1. The vulnerable level is focused on the

TABLE 14.1

LEVELS OF NURSING ASSESSMENT DERIVED FROM DIALECTIC INQUIRY	
Level of Assessment	**Characteristics**
1. Vulnerability	Level of greatest immediacy Focus on subjectivity (experience) of symptoms Urgent symptoms receive attention, etiology not addressed
2. Disengagement	Symptoms are objectified Experience is framed in general terms; no longer personal Objectified experiences are moved to abstract categories for explanation
3. Reduction	Objectively identifiable elements are the basis for diagnostic certainty Search for etiology underlying the symptom Identify a wealth of possible etiologies Multiple competing etiologies generate greater complexity
4. Holism	Knowledge about all competing elements is incorporated Comprehensive view of patient experience in context with no single type of data being more important Patient viewed as an object assembled by data analysis, not as a person encountered by another person
5. Engagement	Patient engaged as "author" of experience rather than object of assessment Patient interprets the data to create internal coherence Patient and nurse become coauthors of a relational narrative, reconstructing the situation as meaning Situation becomes unified, existentially, as a lived situation

Source: Gadow (1995).

patient's immediate experience and is marked by the patient's vulnerability. The patient is experiencing an urgent and distressing symptom, such as pain or dyspnea. At this level, the patient's experience is the reason for beginning the assessment and the focus of assessment is entirely on the patient's subjective report. No attention is given to exploring the etiology of the problem at this time. At the second level, disengagement, the symptom becomes objectified. The patient's experience of the symptom is reframed in more general terms for the purpose of finding an explanation or etiology. Individual patient distress or suffering associated with the symptom is ignored, and the objectified symptom is moved to an abstract category. At the third level, reduction, the objectified symptom becomes the basis for determining an etiology—the "thing" that explains the symptom. Pain, for example, may be explained by orthopedic fracture, local tissue inflammation, or many other causes. For some symptoms, there may be more than one "thing" that explains the symptom. For example, psychosocial problems may have multiple competing etiologies, such as loss, grief, and anger related to situations past or recent events. Orthopedic fracture may cause pain; however, posture, movement, and other etiologies can explain pain intensity in the presence of fracture. At the fourth level, holism, multiple competing elements, or explanations are viewed simultaneously as the focus shifts back to the individual in context. No one data type is more important. Creating a holistic perspective allows the "tangled web" of cause and effect to emerge (Maher & Hemming, 2005). However, while the holistic level provides a comprehensive view of patient experience, the patient is still viewed as an object assembled by the nurse's data analysis, not as a person encountered by another person.

At the last level of assessment, engagement, the patient is engaged as the author of the experience rather than the object of assessment. Internal coherence is created when the patient interprets the data and assigns meaning. Engagement is complete when intersubjectivity is established between the nurse and the patient. The nurse and patient become coauthors of the narrative and reconstruct the situation as meaning. The narrative is no longer objective; it becomes existential as a lived situation.

A UNIQUE PURPOSE FOR ADVANCED NURSING ASSESSMENT

Multiple theoretical perspectives and theories are used in nursing practice to explain phenomena and provide supportive scientific evidence for interventions. Gordon (2007) noted that there is no consensus around a single conceptual focus of nursing and, thus, no consensus on the focus of nursing diagnosis. In medicine, the focus of the assessment is singularly on diagnosis of physical disease. In nursing, depending on the theoretical perspective used to guide practice, nursing diagnoses may be focused on self-care agency, dysfunctional health patterns, or other. Plurality of purpose for assessment within the profession is acceptable; what is not acceptable is a lack of logical consistency between the theoretical perspective/theory and procedures (questions, techniques, data sources, etc.) and subsequent conclusions about problems in a nursing assessment–diagnosis process.

Nursing's definition of health and health-related problems has evolved to reflect more than body system pathology and biological function. However, labeling nursing as *holistic* does not provide clarity for assessment purposes. Holism as a theoretical perspective has many interpretations, including *adding together different parts to construct a whole* and a more Gestalt notion of *the whole is greater than the sum of parts*. Based on the nursing assessment literature, it appears that holistic assessment means adding one or more focused assessments to a body system assessment, such as a focused assessment on sexuality or spirituality. Focused assessments, individually or in addition to physical assessment of body systems, provide additional information, but conclusions based in a focused assessment are no more holistic than the traditional physical examination of body systems—the conclusions reflect a circumscribed area of interest.

Gadow's finding that the theoretical perspective of the nurse, holistic or otherwise, helps shape a patient's experience suggests that nursing should actively address the theoretical underpinnings of assessment. No one theoretical perspective is absolute or best; however, it is important to have a defined theoretical perspective (or theory) underpinning the assessment process. Being clear and defining a theoretical perspective for assessment is important for several reasons. First, a theoretical perspective defines what counts as data, including necessary data to be collected, and boundaries around a complete data set. Second, a theoretical perspective guides data analysis and interpretation by logically aligning data with conclusions consistent with the theory. Third, conclusions should align with interventions and outcomes consistent with the theory. This logical flow from data collection, analysis, conclusions, interventions, and outcomes is evident when the traditional body systems medical examination framework is used. Using a medical framework to assess body systems for pathological states leads to conclusions about disease, interventions focused on disease treatment, and goals for disease cure or stability. In nursing practice, this logical flow often breaks down because of nursing's espoused beliefs about holistic perspective, and the conclusions nurses draw about patient problems are often disconnected. Greater attention is needed to clarify the multiple theoretical perspectives underpinning nursing assessment. The theoretical basis of focused assessments should be articulated to clarify the rationale for selection of data to be collected, to guide the interpretation and selection of interventions, and to identify targeted outcomes.

In a complex multidisciplinary health care environment where team collaboration is paramount, our challenge is to identify a theoretical perspective supporting nursing's unique contributions to patient/client health outcomes. Self-care, a theoretical perspective that views patients and families engaging in purposeful actions directed at maintaining or improving their health, has been proposed as a theoretical perspective underlying much of nursing practice and distinguishing nursing from other disciplines. Sidani (2003) noted that self-care is a framework that underpins the design of health-promotion interventions and guides nursing practice across the continuum of care. Table 14.2 summarizes Sidani's arguments supporting self-care as a philosophical orientation underlying and distinguishing nursing as a discipline. Considering assessment is a process composed of levels that culminate in a patient–nurse narrative, the self-care framework could be used to shape the intersubjective patient–nurse narrative. A self-care framework would provide a directed purpose for the nurse–patient relationship and would guide the assessment process, drive nursing interventions, and frame target outcomes. Self-care is consistent with nursing's ontology and enjoys considerable empiric evidence.

SELF-CARE PERSPECTIVE FOR ADVANCED NURSING ASSESSMENT

Self-care is defined as decisions and actions taken by individuals to cope with a health problem and to improve or maintain health status. The notion of self-care has also been referred to as self-management, self-care agency, self-efficacy, and other related terms. While similar in meaning, nuances are present, as individual authors use different definitions of similar concepts. For the purpose of the perspective presented here, self-care is considered a broad umbrella term for a philosophical orientation that views patients and families engaging in purposeful actions directed at maintaining or improving their health. The self-care perspective assumes that (a) the purpose of nurse–patient engagement is to support the patient in managing his or her own health; (b) engagement is intersubjective, whereby patient and nurse become coauthors of a relational narrative, reconstructing the situation as meaning; and (c) self-care is central to meaning in the nurse–patient narrative.

The goal of self-care is an individual's experience of wellness, which is manifest and measured as perceived satisfaction with functional status and QOL. Individual wellness is derived from ongoing interaction of life processes—the combination of biological and psychosocial processes of an individual. The processes are ever present and together are reflected in the total functioning of a human being (Nguyen, Donesky-Cuenco, & Carrieri-Kohlman, 2008). Changes in biological or psychosocial processes are threats to wellness. The purpose of the nursing assessment is to identify threats to wellness (functional status and QOL) and determine etiologies of those

TABLE 14.2

SUMMARY OF ARGUMENTS SUPPORTING SELF-CARE AS A PHILOSOPHICAL ORIENTATION THAT UNDERLIES AND DISTINGUISHES NURSING AS A DISCIPLINE
1. Self-care serves as a framework that underpins health promotion interventions
2. Self-care guides practice across the continuum of care in multiple care settings
3. Self-care provides theoretical foundation for psychoeducational, cognitive, behavioral, and symptom management interventions that focus on 　a. Self-monitoring, perceiving, and identifying changes in functioning 　b. Judging the meaning and severity of these changes 　c. Assessing options for actions to manage these changes 　d. Selecting and performing appropriate actions
4. Self-care is viewed as an outcome of nursing care where patients are expected to select and perform actions to maintain life, healthy functioning, and well-being

Source: Sidani (2003).

threats. Nursing interventions are actions to facilitate self-care and to alter etiologies, thereby alleviating or minimizing threats. Self-care actions initiated by patients/clients at the direction of the nurse alter problem etiologies, thus alleviating or minimizing threats and improving perceived functioning and QOL. Threats to wellness and desired self-care outcomes are coconstructed between patient and nurse in the relational narrative of assessment. Figure 14.1 depicts the elements of a self-care theoretical perspective.

Overview of Self-Care Perspective

Self-Care. *Self-care* is purposeful actions by patients or their family members directed at maintaining or improving health. Self-care is a complex construct, and definitions may vary based on the *purpose* of the actions and on the *ability* of the individual or family/caregivers. Self-care differs depending on whether the purpose is maintenance of current health status by preventive measures or maintenance/management of a chronic disease state. For example, self-care of older adults may have the purpose of maintaining or improving functionality, responsibility, integrity, and/or growth (Hoy, Wagner, & Hall, 2007). Self-care of adults newly diagnosed with epilepsy may have the purposes of management of medications and treatments, safety, seizures, and life issues (Unger & Buelow, 2009). These purposes, however, are dependent upon *abilities*, the patient's emotional status, and physical comfort and functioning. A debate that surrounds the discussion about self-care is whether the concept is appropriate if the individual is unable to perform, that is, paralyzed or comatose.

Orem (as cited in Sidani, 2003, p. 67) considered self-care to be both self-care agency and self-care

behavior, although her perspective was rather medical (Koch, Jenkins, & Kralik, 2004). Self-care agency is the capability of the individual to carry out necessary tasks to maintain, improve, or manage health. This agency comprises multiple domains, including cognitive (knowledge of health status and behaviors needed), physical (ability to perform needed task), emotional and psychosocial (motivation, desire, environmental, and family support), and performance (the ability to carry out the self-care tasks; Sidani, 2003). Self-care behaviors are the processes that individuals or caregivers take in order to maintain or improve health status or manage a health problem. Self-care capability and self-care processes are mutually reinforcing concepts, not separate entities (Hoy et al., 2007). Examples of behaviors are self-monitoring of health, communicating with health care providers and caregivers, coping with and preventing stress, taking medication or following other treatment regimens, changing ways of doing in order to maintain independence, preventing injury, maintaining safety in maneuvering about home and community (including transportation), and learning about health and illness.

Wellness. Wellness is experience; consistent with the nature of experience, wellness is subjective. Wellness is often characterized by pleasant sensations and a perception of comfort (Fakouri & Lyon, 2005; National Association of Clinical Nurse Specialists [NACNS], 2004). As an experience, wellness imbeds individual values, culture, past experiences, and future expectations (DiLalla, Hull, & Dorsey, 2004). Wellness represents balance between the biological strengths and needs and the psychosocial strengths and needs. Wellness can exist in the presence of disease (McMahon & Fleury, 2012). From a nursing perspective, wellness can exist in the presence of disease because wellness is an experience through which individuals, with support as necessary, maximize potential for satisfactory functional status and QOL (Uno & Ruthman, 2004).

Functional Status. Functional status is the perceived ability to perform necessary and valued behaviors for the purpose of meeting basic physiologic needs, fulfilling social roles, and maintaining psychosocial well-being (Wang, 2004; Whitcomb, 2011). The adequacy of functional status is determined by an individual based on whatever the individual thinks is adequate or satisfactory for desired activities.

Current level of function should be distinguished from functional capacity and functional reserve (Doran, 2003). Current functioning is defined as performance dependent on functional *capability*. For example, walking in the community depends on an individual having muscular strength, adequate range of motion of lower extremities, balance, and

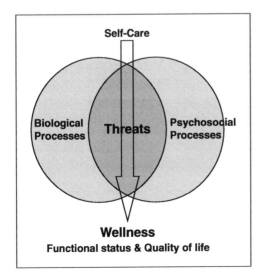

FIGURE 14.1 Model describing relationships of concepts in a self-care theoretical perspective.

cardiopulmonary stamina, as well as the motivation to walk that far. Biological processes may limit strength through muscle wasting. Psychosocial processes, such as fear of falling, may limit motivation to walk. An individual with chronic problems of biological processes may have less functional capability. Capability may be improved through interventions, such as exercise. *Functional capacity* is the maximum potential to perform activities. *Functional reserve* is the difference between the current performance and the capacity to perform. Most people have a large reserve that is not tapped in usual or basic needs performance.

Perceived function is associated with well-being (Mazanec, Daly, Douglas, & Lipson, 2010), effective coping (Ostwald, Swank, & Khan, 2008), adaptation to changes in health status, environment, or work status (Sandqvist, Scheja, & Eklund, 2008), further disablement (Harrison & Stuifbergen, 2001), self-efficacy for learning new skills (Swor et al., 2003), and perceived cognitive function and neuropsychological performance (Vardy et al., 2008). In addition to the association with well-being, low levels of functioning may predict increased dependency in activities of daily living, increased use of health care services, increased admission to nursing homes, and increased mortality (de Rekeneire et al., 2003).

Perceived functional status may or may not be the same as objective or viewed functioning. Perceived functional status is assessed as a verbal self-report from the individual and is therefore subjective. Verbally reported data may be augmented by objective findings from physical exam or clinical testing. For example, subjective and objective cognitive status in neurological disorders may be poorly correlated (Schultze-Lutter et al., 2007). Subjective visual effect from cataracts may not be strongly associated with actual objective measure of cataract (Hakim-Banan, n.d.). Younger dialysis patients with high levels of physical performance reported significantly higher strength, mobility, and balance than could be demonstrated using objective measures, suggesting that early impaired sensory nerve function disability may not be realized by patients (Blake & O'Meara, 2004). Safety may become a consideration when perceived function is not well supported by objective measures as patients over- or underestimate abilities to engage in functional tasks.

QOL. Functional status is closely associated with QOL; however, QOL is not the same as functional status. QOL is the perception of being able to enjoy life and is influenced by but independent of functional status. QOL is also associated with, but not the same as, wellness. An individual may report having satisfactory QOL with poor levels of wellness.

QOL is a broad and complex concept that includes an array of physical and psychosocial characteristics that, if limited or threatened, may affect the individual's ability to derive satisfaction in/from life (Kroenke, Kubzansky, Adler, & Kawachi, 2008). QOL can be influenced by biologic and physiological factors such as symptoms and functional status (Lin, Chen, Yang, & Zhou, 2013), attachments, and perceived role value, security, and personal control (Grewal & Porter, 2007). Importantly for this discussion, enhanced self-care is associated with greater QOL (Bounthavong & Law, 2008). QOL is independent of physical and social functioning (Lau & McKenna, 2002). In fact, medical therapies to stabilize disease and improve physical function, including pharmacologic agents, have been associated with poorer QOL (Smith, Olin, & Madsen, 2006).

Life Processes

Biological Processes. Biological processes are the micro- (chemical, hormonal, cellular) and macro- (movement, digestion, respiration, etc.) mechanisms that support life, physiologic functioning, and adaptation. These biological processes may be normal and abnormal variations, or they may be pathological. Pathophysiological phenomena may cause alterations in naturally occurring life processes (Carrieri-Kohlman, Lindsey, & West, 2003), as can compensatory physiological mechanisms.

Biological processes may be affected by psychosocial processes. Carrieri-Kohlman et al. (2003) divide life processes into five broad areas: regulation, cognition, sensation, protection, and motion. Disruptions to life processes in any of these five areas can threaten an individual's functioning. Disruption in any one area of life processes will cause disruption in others, so interactions of the areas are mutual and may be additive and/or synergistic, involving one or more of the broad areas. The resulting disruption in functioning results in threats to wellness.

The typical pattern of disruption of life processes tends to vary between specialty populations more greatly than within populations. For example, the pattern of symptoms experienced by persons with head and neck cancer treated with radiation therapy are similar and different from the pattern of symptoms experienced by persons with heart failure. Persons with heart failure share a similar within-group pattern of symptoms that are different from the pattern of symptoms experienced by persons with Alzheimer's disease. Patients with multiple health problems change the symptom pattern even more.

As specialists, CNSs focus on self-care around life processes alterations common within the specialty population; therefore, a comprehensive body system assessment is not often useful. The challenge for

CNSs is to develop assessment guidelines for common disruptions in life processes for specialty populations.

Psychosocial Processes. Psychosocial processes are the other half of the life processes and are intimately associated with health and wellness. Disruptions in psychosocial processes may be both etiologic factors associated with a health disruption or consequences of dealing with a health disruption. Psychosocial processes include all of the mental processes necessary for protection, interaction, learning, creation, aesthetics, and valuing. Because health and wellness are not simply a biological phenomenon but the interaction of the individual's perception within a social constructed environment, there are many examples of the interaction of psychosocial processes and health.

Psychosocial processes encompass cognition and emotions. Cognitive processes include orientation, learning ability, perception, beliefs, and negative thinking and may mediate health status through beliefs such as control, learned helplessness, attribution, locus of control, optimism/pessimism, problem solving, and emotion (Harttman-Maeir, Harel, & Katz, 2009). Research on learning ability indicates that ability, even controlling for age and education level, has a major role in inadequate health literacy; inadequate health literacy is associated with health outcomes (Levinthal, Morrow, Wanzhu, Jingwei, & Murray, 2008). *Emotions* are responses to events determined by cognition and perception, causing physiological changes, and usually altered behavior. Pleasure and self-realization are also psychosocial processes; threats to both may lead to threats to wellness. Another psychosocial process often associated with self-care is motivation (Gore-Felton & Koopman, 2008).

Individuals should be considered in context of a social environment. Interpersonal relationship may be considered a psychosocial process; however, relationships are often identified as a social factor necessity for health and wellness. The social part of psychosocial processes of health and wellness include interpersonal and intergroup relationships. Other social factors that are associated with health and wellness are income, employment, education and literacy, gender and gender issues, culture, and environment. For example, increased real and perceived social support is related to improved outcomes after hip fracture (Mortimore et al., 2008). Psychosocial relationships maintain functioning, wellness, and QOL.

Emotions are responses to events determined by cognition and perception, causing physiological changes and usually altered behavior. There are multiple examples of the interaction between emotion and health. For example, evidence suggests that depression is associated with heart disease (Lichtman et al., 2008), negative feelings are related to sleep disturbances (Steptoe, O'Donnell, Marmot, & Wardle, 2008), and anxiety may predict decreased functional status (Ostwald et al., 2008).

QOL is defined by psychosocial and social aspects as well as physical aspects. Therefore, psychosocial processes directly affect the perception of wellness (Blane, Netuveli, & Montgomery, 2008; Buenaver, Edwards, Smith, Gramling, & Haythornthwaite, 2008; Davis, 2007; Muslimovic, Post, Speelman, Schmand, & de Haan, 2008). Social factors associated with wellness are often affected by geopolitical issues. Income inequalities, environmental safety, and discrimination certainly affect health, but also QOL. For example, racial/ethnicity disparities in total knee replacement are evident, particularly in black men with no supplemental insurance to Medicare (Hanchate, Zhang, Felson, & Ash, 2008).

Threats to Wellness

Threats to wellness arise from changes in biological and psychosocial processes. Changes in biological processes may lead to physiologic compensatory mechanisms such as inflammatory processes resulting in pain or pathophysiological alterations resulting in organ-focused disease. Changes in psychosocial processes may result in decreased sensation or perception, decreases in cognition and changes in affect, difficulty with activities of daily living, and alterations in role performance, social relationships, and social support networks (Lindqvist, Widmark, & Rasmussen, 2006).

Threats to function have multiple etiologies that may overlap both biological and psychosocial processes. For example, the ability to provide for personal hygiene requires perception (touch, vision, and hearing), cognition, motivation, and central and peripheral neurophysiologic mechanisms (strength, range of motion). In addition, a suitable environment to allow for hygiene, adaptive equipment, or support from others may also be necessary. Threats to personal hygiene may include interruption in any or part of any of these biological or psychosocial processes.

Threats to QOL are biological and psychosocial. Biological threats to QOL include developmental issues (aging, pregnancy), acute illnesses or injuries, and poorly controlled chronic diseases (Bounthavong & Law, 2008; Chen, Chen, Lee, Cho, & Weng, 2008). Psychosocial threats to QOL include education (Bounthavong & Law, 2008), socioeconomic status, employment/occupation (Mountain, Mozley, Craig, & Ball, 2008), and environment (Collier & Truman, 2008). The multidimensional nature of QOL requires skilled assessment to identify complex etiologies. For example, a patient may report limited enjoyment in life. An advanced assessment with relational narrative discovers that the Asian refugee patient is worrying about breast cancer recurrence, compounded by fatigue with difficulty sleeping and lack of appetite plus minimal social network and limited social support from family and friends. The complexity of etiologies requires ongoing, in-depth assessment.

CONDUCTING AN ADVANCED SPECIALTY HEALTH ASSESSMENT

This chapter opened by asking, *What constitutes an advanced nursing health assessment?* Thus far, in consideration of the question, we explored the philosophical basis of assessment, discussed the importance of articulating theoretical perspective and a purpose and proposed self-care as a theoretical perspective closely aligned with nursing's unique contribution to patient/client outcomes. Now we need to bring some of these discussion points forward and consider the conduct of assessment.

From philosophy we learned that assessment is a process of nurse and patient coauthoring a relational narrative. Through narrative a situation becomes unified, not objectively, but as a lived situation. An assessment should include generous opportunity for inclusion of patient experience and interpretation of health-related problems along with the CNS's expertise, which also becomes part of the relational narrative. The purpose of assessment should always be clear. Any and all assessment data should be collected with the endpoint in mind. For this chapter, we are proposing an endpoint of individual assessment as altering the experience by engaging the nurse and patient in self-care within the specialty domain to maintain wellness by improving functional status and of life. Self-care is well supported in the nursing literature as a philosophical orientation unique to nursing. Sidani (2003) noted that QOL. Self-care underpins health-promotion interventions; guides practice across the continuum of care in multiple care settings; provides theoretical foundation for psychoeducational, cognitive, behavioral, and symptom management interventions; and is viewed as an outcome of nursing care where patients are expected to select and perform actions to maintain life, healthy functioning, and well-being.

Wellness as experience is therefore subjective and characterized by pleasant sensations and a perception of comfort, and it imbeds individual values, meanings, culture, past experiences, and future expectations. Wellness represents balance between the biological

life process and psychosocial life processes and is manifested as functional status and QOL. Self-care is directed at eliminating or minimizing biological and psychosocial threats to wellness, thereby maximizing functional status and QOL. Advanced nursing assessment involves understanding a patient's meaning of wellness, identifying the gap between a patient's perceived and desired wellness and ability to achieve desired wellness, and drawing conclusions about etiologies of problems preventing closure of the gap. Using a traditional body systems framework, advanced practice nurses have concentrated on gathering a comprehensive medical and surgical history along with a complete system review and physical examination for the purpose of determining a differential disease diagnosis, useful in the practice of primary care and other settings, but not directed at an endpoint of self-care. Within a self-care perspective, the purpose of assessment is to determine gaps between perceived wellness (functional status and QOL), desired wellness, and patient self-care abilities (knowledge, skills, and resources) for achieving desired wellness. Nursing interventions are designed to address the causes (etiologies) of the gaps and assist patients in self-care to achieve desired wellness. Assessment shifts to greater focus on the patient's perspective. Patient perspective of wellness is foreground, with traditional elements of medical and surgical history, habits, lifestyle, and physical examination of the nurse/provider-focused assessment as background. CNS practice expertise shapes nursing interventions to address gaps between perceived and desired wellness. Nursing interventions minimize threats and maximize self-care. The outcome of CNS interventions can be measured as improved perception of wellness (functional status and QOL).

CNSs, while prepared broadly in a population, also specialize in a delimited area of practice, which may be focused on a problem (e.g., pain, wound management), setting (e.g., critical care unit, operating room, community clinic), or disease/pathology (e.g., diabetes, oncology). CNSs have mastery in the application of scientific knowledge to specialty practice. CNSs in specialty practice areas can use a self-care theoretical perspective to design assessment guidelines for determining gaps and self-care interventions for specialty patient populations. Assessment, for a specialist, should be consistent with the distinctive problems and concerns of patients within the specialty scope for purpose of altering the patient's experience. For example, a CNS specializing in diabetes would engage in patient assessment for the purpose of altering the patient's experience of having diabetes. For persons living with diabetes, there are biological threats and psychological threats to well-being, and while there are individual variations, there are also commonalities among problems that allow a diabetes specialist to assess and conclude (diagnose) with much more depth and nuance than a nonspecialist.

A growing body of scientific evidence is shedding light on the dimensions of the wellness experience for specialty populations. For example, older women with multiple chronic diseases described a core of similar problems (Roberto, Gigliotti, & Husser, 2005). For these women, disease faded into the background, while problems related to functional status and QOL (pain, falls, sleep disturbances, reduced energy, worrying, financial strain, medication side effects, and functional limitations) became foreground concerns for daily living. The women in this study described self-care strategies for managing the problems. Here is the place for advanced nursing assessment—to see common problems as threats to wellness, to assess the patient's perception of his or her experience, and to use a CNS's expertise to cocreate interventions that will reduce threats and improve functional status and QOL. Thorne, Patterson, and Russell (2003) noted that individuals with chronic disease are experts in self-care with priorities and principles different from textbook recommendations and provider prescriptions.

A SELF-CARE ASSESSMENT FORMAT

What follows is a suggested template or guide for incorporating the patient's perspective of wellness into an advanced nursing health assessment. CNSs are encouraged to develop assessment templates for specialty populations, addressing common threats and gaps across specialty, to consider the patient as the expert in determining wellness, and to become coauthor in eliminating or minimizing biological and psychosocial threats.

Wellness (Experiential) Data

- Describe your general state of health
- Describe any health-related problems or concerns
- What does it mean to you to have these problems or concerns?
- How does any one problem or concern aggravate or cause other problems?
- How do you think nurses or other health care providers can help with any problems or concerns that interfere with your functioning and enjoying life?

Functional Status

- Do you function at the level you think you should?
- Are there any problems or concerns that interfere with your ability to function at your maximum level?

- How much and in what way do problems or concerns interfere with your ability to take care of your personal needs such as bathing and dressing?
- How much and in what way do problems or concerns interfere with your ability to do necessary things such as shopping, cooking, or paying bills?

Quality of Life

- Do you enjoy life as much as you want?
- Any there any problems or concerns that interfere with your satisfaction with life or enjoying life as much as you think you can?
- How much and in what way does the symptom or problem affect your feelings, such as feeling sad, worried, or nervous?
- How much and in what way does this symptom or problem interfere with relationships with family and friends?
- What would you like to do that you find you cannot do? What might help you with doing what you want?

Psychosocial Processes

Patient's Understanding of Problem or Disease and Cause
- What is your understanding of the problem/disease?
- What do you think caused the problem?

History of Present Problem or Disease
- Describe the history of your current problem from the time it first started until present. Include how it interfered with things you wanted to do, how it has made you feel, and how it has caused you to change the way you live your life.

Past History of Problem or Disease
- Have you ever had the same or similar problems at another time? If so, when?
- What do you think caused that problem?
- Do you think that past problems are related to current problems? If so, how?
- How did you manage the problem in the past? What did you do?

Patient's Suggestions for Relieving Problem or Disease
- What do you think would help the current problem?
- What do you see as obstacles to getting the help you need?

Family Diseases
- Describe any health problems that family members have had that are similar to your problem
- How did they manage their problem?
- What happened to these family members?

Family and Social Support

- Who helps you with problems?
- Are you satisfied with the help you get?
- Who could help you but is not? Why not?
- How could you tell this person(s) you need more or different help?

Biologic Processes

Review of preventative health practices/risk factors (data obtained from medical record/patient interview):

- Immunizations
- Screenings (hearing, vision)
- Disease (diagnosed pathologies)
- Allergies to medicine, food, plants, other
- Caffeine/tobacco/alcohol/recreational drug use
- Dental health
  - Do you have a dentist?
  - When was your last dental checkup?
  - Do you have any current problems with your teeth or mouth?
- Exercise
  - Do you exercise regularly? Describe regular exercise routine.
  - What motivates or interferes with exercise?
- Nutrition
  - How would you describe your daily diet/foods you eat?
  - What foods do you like?
  - What foods do you not like or avoid?
  - Do you have problems buying food?

Patient's Perception of the Relationship Between Lifestyle and Health

- What do you think is the relationship between your lifestyle and your general state of health?
- Is there anything you think you should do to improve your health?

Medications and Medical Therapies

- Current prescribed medications
  - What medications are you currently taking?
  - What are the effects of taking these medications?
  - If you skip the medications, do you feel better, worse, or no difference?
  - What kinds of concerns do you have about obtaining the medications, such as cost, delivery, or problems getting refills?
- What medications have you taken that were not prescribed for you, such as medications prescribed for a family member with a similar problem?
- What, if any, medications do you think might help that you are not taking, or would help if you stopped taking?
- Over-the-counter medications or supplements
  - What over-the-counter medications are you taking?
  - What are the effects of taking these medications?
  - What vitamin, mineral, or other nutritional supplements are you taking?
  - What are the effects of taking these supplements?
  - Where did you learn about these over-the-counter medications and supplements?

Physical Alterations

- The physical examination for advanced nursing assessment varies and is generally a focused assessment based on the specialty patient population and/or the health-related problem. For example, where risk of falling is identified, the physical examination should be tailored to include assessment of parameters involving gait, balance, and muscle strength. Physical examination techniques including inspection, palpitation, percussion, and auscultation in addition to special tests should be used.

ANALYZING DATA AND DRAWING CONCLUSIONS

From the assessment data, a CNS draws conclusions about the patient's desired wellness and threats to wellness, both biological and psychosocial. Problems represent gaps between desired wellness and patient abilities (knowledge, abilities, and resources). The etiologies (causes) of problems are determined and interventions are designed to alter etiologies and promote self-care for the purpose of wellness.

Begin analysis of assessment data by first framing the patient situation in a context. Summarize the patient's physical, emotional, social, functional abilities and resources. Identify the patient's strengths. Cues to the patient's strengths are often imbedded in descriptions of the patient's past experiences, level of functioning, and family and social support. Strengths focus on what is going well. In promoting self-care, a CNS will need to mobilize and develop the patient's strengths (Gottlieb, 2013).

After constructing a contextual frame for the patient, the following steps will assist in the data analysis process.

1. What key issues emerged?
2. What are the problems amenable to nursing interventions?
3. How are nursing problems linked/related to each other and to disease problems?
4. What are the self-care demands?
   a. What are/will be the patient requirements for self-care?
   b. Is there a gap between self-care agency and self-care demands?

5. What are the desired outcomes?
   a. What are the gaps between desired outcomes and present state?
   b. What are the clinical indicators that outcomes are achieved?
6. What are the patient's strengths? How can strengths be framed to support self-care demands?

Identify key problems by listing all the concerns and problems identified by the patient and any nursing observations. Include data from the medical record, including diseases and documented alterations in physiology. At this point, all problems have equal weight; don't exclude a problem because it seems minor.

Explore how problems are related to each other. Look for one or two key problems that are central to others. Example: A patient being treated with chemotherapy for breast cancer is experiencing sleep disturbance, hot flashes, fatigue, and agitation. Which, if any, problem is central? Will improving the quality of sleep help ameliorate hot flashes, fatigue, and agitation, or are the hot flashes an etiology of the sleep disturbances and improving sleep will lead to reduced fatigue and agitation? Thinking in terms of key problems reduces chances for a piecemeal approach to care and gives equal weight to patient experiences, such as symptoms, and disease-based pathophysiology. The goal is to find those central problems that can result in improvement of related problems. In this example, making changes to control or minimize the effects of hot flashes can lead to better quality sleep, thus reducing fatigue and agitation. Hot flashes, while difficult to eliminate, are sometimes managed with pharmacologic agents; however, their effects can be minimized by nursing interventions directed at environmental manipulation such as keeping the room cool, wearing light sleepwear, and wearing sleepwear that wicks moisture. In this example, the problem is amenable to nursing interventions, the interventions are managed by the patient as self-care, and the self-care fills the gap between the desired quality sleep and current poor quality sleep.

Analysis of the assessment data results in conclusions about the key problem(s) and their relationships to one another. The next step is to consider interventions to enable patients to fill the gap between desired and actual level of functioning and QOL.

1. What are recommended nursing interventions?
2. Who will deliver the intervention(s)?
3. How will the intervention(s) delivery be monitored?
4. How will the intervention(s) be evaluated?
5. How does the intervention address the patient's strengths?
6. What referrals to/consultations with other health care providers should be obtained?
7. Resources considerations: How will the patient obtain the necessary resources for the recommended interventions?

Well-written interventions clearly delineate the dose (intensity), frequency, and any delivery procedures or considerations. Interventions should be delivered as intended; validate that the patient can follow through on the intervention. Check the patient's level of understanding and provide written instructions as appropriate. Where psychomotor skills are involved, validate that the patient can manipulate equipment or perform procedures. Include follow-up plans by noting when the nurse should evaluate the outcome of the intervention.

SUMMARY

Nurses provide care and comfort to individuals during acute episodes of illness and guide self-care for managing symptoms and functional problems associated with chronic illness. Problems related to chronic illness are due to underlying, lingering pathologies prone to exacerbations and remissions and requiring anywhere from minimal to complex self-maintained treatment. Advanced nursing assessment should articulate a theoretical perspective, which will facilitate a logical link between data collection, data analysis, and intended clinical outcomes. Promoting self-care has been identified as the unique contribution of nursing to health care of individuals. A model discusses the relationship between biological and psychosocial threats to wellness, measured as functional status and QOL. The assessment framework explored in this chapter is focused on self-care. A template for assessment is presented; it can be adapted for specialty populations. CNSs need to provide leadership in advancing nursing care of individuals across the life span and to assure self-care ability for maximum function and QOL.

■ DISCUSSION QUESTIONS

- What constitutes an advanced nursing assessment? Discuss the importance of addressing this question.
- How does theory guide an advanced nursing assessment? Give an example of how the purpose of an advanced nursing assessment would shift based on the theory guiding the assessment.
- Discuss the concepts in the self-care perspective presented in this chapter. How would you apply these concepts to your specialty population?

ANALYSIS AND SYNTHESIS EXERCISES

- Advanced nursing assessment involves coauthoring a narrative with the patient. An emerging body of scientific work is providing insight into the patient's perspective. Review a qualitative research study describing experience with a health-related problem or chronic illness. Based on the findings, what assessment data should be included in assessing patients with similar problems or illnesses?
- Conduct a case study and identify the biological and psychosocial threats experienced by the patient

CLINICAL APPLICATION CONSIDERATIONS

- Consider the information on the suggested assessment guide and use it to help develop a specialty-focused advanced nursing assessment that targets a selected specialty patient population. Focus on information that will lead to conclusions about problems that are amenable to nursing interventions. The final assessment format may be in a design or configuration of your choosing (e.g., order of information, questions asked, etc.) that best facilitates a coauthored narrative in the context of common threats to wellness, involving biological and psychosocial processes evidenced in the specialty population.
- Conduct a health assessment of a patient using your specialty assessment format. Revise the format as needed after piloting.

REFERENCES

Barkauskas, V. H., Baumann, L. C., & Darling-Fisher, C. S. (2002). *Health and physical assessment.* St. Louis, MO: Mosby.

Bates, B., & Hoekelman, R. A. (1974). *A guide to physical examination.* Philadelphia, PA: Lippincott.

Blake, C., & O'Meara, Y. M. (2004). Subjective and objective physical limitations in high-functioning renal dialysis patients. *Nephrology Dialysis Transplantation, 19,* 3124–3129.

Blane, D., Netuveli, G., & Montgomery, S. M. (2008). Quality of life, health and physiological status and change at older ages. *Social Science & Medicine, 66*(7), 1579–1587.

Bounthavong, M., & Law, A. V. (2008). Identifying health-related quality of life (HRQL) domains for multiple chronic conditions (diabetes, hypertension and dyslipidemia): Patient and provider perspectives. *Journal of Evaluation in Clinical Practice, 14*(6), 1002–1011.

Broom, M. (2007). Exploring the assessment process. *Paediatric Nursing, 19*(4), 22–25.

Buenaver, L. F., Edwards, R. R., Smith, M. T., Gramling, S. E., & Haythornthwaite, J. A. (2008). Catastrophizing and pain-coping in young adults: Associations with depressive symptoms and headache pain. *Journal of Pain, 9*(4), 311–319.

Carpenito, L. J. (1995). *Nursing care plans and documentation: Nursing diagnosis and collaborative problems.* Philadelphia, PA: Lippincott.

Carrieri-Kohlman, V., Lindsey, A. M., & West, C. (2003). The conceptual approach. In V. Carrieri-Kohlman, A. M. Lindsey, & C. West (Eds.), *Pathophysiological phenomena in nursing: Human responses to illness* (pp. 1–12). St. Louis, MO: Saunders.

Chen, K., Chen, M., Lee, S., Cho, H., & Weng, L. (2008). Self-management behaviours for patients with chronic obstructive pulmonary disease: A qualitative study. *Journal of Advanced Nursing, 64*(6), 595–604.

Collier, L., & Truman, J. (2008). Exploring the multi-sensory environment as a leisure resource for people with complex neurological disabilities. *NeuroRehabilitation, 23*(4), 361–367.

Davidson, L. J., Bennett, S. E., Hamera, E. K., & Raines, B. K. (2004). What constitutes advanced assessment? *Journal of Nursing Education, 43*(9), 421–425.

Davis, L. A. (2007). Quality of life issues related to dysphagia. *Topics in Geriatric Rehabilitation, 23*(4), 352–365.

de Rekeneire, N., Visser, M., Peila, R., Nevitt, M. C., Cauley, J. A., Tylavsky, F. A., . . . Harris, T. B. (2003). Is a fall just a fall: Correlates of falling in healthy older persons. The Health, Aging and Body Composition Study. *Journal of the American Geriatrics Society, 51*(6), 841–846.

DiLalla, L. F., Hull, S. K., & Dorsey, J. K. (2004). Effect of gender, age, and relevant course work on attitudes toward empathy, patient spirituality, and physician wellness. *Teaching and Learning in Medicine, 16*(2), 165–170.

Doran, D. M. (2003). Functional status. In D. M. Doran (Ed.), *Nursing sensitive outcomes* (pp. 27–64). Boston, MA: Jones & Bartlett.

Driscoll, V. M. (1976/2007). The movement to secure statutory definition of the unique and independent practice of nursing. *Clinical Nurse Specialist, 21*(1), 7–12.

Fakouri, C., & Lyon, B. (2005). Perceived health and life satisfaction among older adults. The effects of worry and personal variables. *Journal of Gerontological Nursing, 31*(10), 17–24.

Fulton, J. S. (2007). The unique and independent practice of nursing. *Clinical Nurse Specialist, 21*(1), 5–6.

Gadow, S. (1995). Clinical epistemology: A dialectic of nursing assessment. *Canadian Journal of Nursing Research, 27*(2), 25–34.

Gordon, M. (2007). *Manual of nursing diagnosis.* Boston, MA: Jones & Bartlett.

Gore-Felton, C., & Koopman, C. (2008). Behavioral mediation of the relationship between psychosocial factors and HIV disease progression. *Psychosomatic Medicine, 70,* 569–574.

Gottlieb, L. N. (2013). *Strengths-based nursing care: Health and healing for person and family.* New York, NY: Springer.

Grewal, P. K., & Porter, J. E. (2007). Hope theory: A framework for understanding suicidal action. *Death Studies, 31*(2), 131–154.

Hakim-Banan, N. (n.d.). *Association between subjective visual function and both low contrast visual acuity and contrast sensitivity in cataract.* City University London. Retrieved January 21, 2009, from http://www.city.ac.uk/optometry/research/eyenet/projects/cataract.html

Hanchate, A. D., Zhang, Y., Felson, D.T., & Ash, A. S. (2008). Exploring the determinants of racial and ethnic disparities in total knee arthroplasty: Health insurance, income, and assets. *Medical Care, 46*(5), 481–488.

Harrison, T., & Stuifbergen, A. (2001). Barriers that further disablement: A study of survivors of polio. *Journal of Neuroscience Nursing, 33*(3), 160–166.

Harttman-Maeir, A., Harel, H., & Katz, N. (2009). Kettle test—A brief measure of cognitive functional performance. Reliability and validity in stroke rehabilitation. *American Journal of Occupational Therapy, 63*(5), 592–599.

Hoy, B., Wagner, L., & Hall, E. O. C. (2007). Self-care as a health resource of elders: An integrative review of the concept. *Journal of Caring Sciences, 21*(4), 456–466.

Kelley, F. J., & Kopac, C. A., (2001). Advanced health assessment in nurse practitioner programs. *Journal of Professional Nursing, 17*(5), 218–225.

Kelley, F. J., Kopac, C. A. & Rosselli, J. (2007). Advanced health assessment in nurse practitioner programs: Follow-up study. *Journal of Professional Nursing, 23*(3), 137–143.

Koch, T., Jenkin, P., & Kralik, D. (2004). Chronic illness self-management: Locating the "self." *Journal of Advanced Nursing, 48*(5), 484–492.

Kroenke, C. H., Kubzansky, L. D., Adler, N., & Kawachi, I. (2008). Prospective change in health-related quality of life and subsequent mortality among middle-aged and older women. *American Journal of Public Health, 98*(11), 2085–2091.

Larsen, P. D. (2013). Chronicity. In I. M. Lubkin & P. D. Larsen (Eds.), *Chronic illness: Impact and intervention.* Boston, MA: Jones & Bartlett.

Lau, A., & McKenna, K. (2002). Perception of quality of life by Chinese elderly persons with stroke. *Disability and Rehabilitation, 24*(4), 203–218.

Levinthal, B. R., Morrow, D. G., Wanzhu, T., Jingwei, W., & Murray, M. D. (2008). Cognition and health literacy in patients with hypertension. *Journal of General Internal Medicine, 23*(8). Retrieved January 21, 2009, from http://www.springerlink.com/content/yg110886517k6863/

Lichtman, J. H., Bigger, J. T. Jr., Blumenthal, J. A., Frasure-Smith, N., Kaufmann, P. G., Lespérance, F.,…Froelicher, E. S; American Heart Association Prevention Committee of the Council on Cardiovascular Nursing; American Heart Association Council on Clinical Cardiology; American Heart Association Council on Epidemiology and Prevention; American Heart Association Interdisciplinary Council on Quality of Care and Outcomes Research; American Psychiatric Association. (2008). Depression and coronary heart disease: Recommendations for screening, referral, and treatment: A science advisory from the American Heart Association Prevention Committee of the Council on Cardiovascular Nursing, Council on Clinical Cardiology, Council on Epidemiology and Prevention, and Interdisciplinary Council on Quality of Care and Outcomes Research: Endorsed by the American Psychiatric Association. *Circulation, 118*(17), 1768–1775.

Lin, S., Chen, Y., Yang, L., & Zhou, J. (2013). Pain, fatigue, disturbed sleep and distress comprised a symptom cluster that related to quality of life and functional status of lung cancer patients. *Journal of Clinical Nursing, 22*(9), 1281–1290.

Lindqvist, O., Widmark, A., & Rasmussen, B. H. (2006). Reclaiming wellness—Living with bodily problems, as narrated by men with advanced prostate cancer. *Cancer Nursing, 29*(4), 327–333.

Maher, D., & Hemming, L. (2005). Understanding patient and family: Holistic assessment in palliative care. *British Journal of Community Nursing, 10*(7), 318–322.

McMahon, S., & Fleury, J. (2012). Wellness in older adults: A concept analysis. *Database Nursing Forum, 47*(1), 39–51.

Mortimore, E., Haselow, D., Dolan, M., Hawkes, W. G., Langenberg, P., Zimmerman, S., & Magaziner, J. (2008). Amount of social contact and hip fracture mortality. *Journal of the American Geriatrics Society, 56*(6), 1069–1074.

Mountain, G., Mozley, C., Craig, C., & Ball, L. (2008). Occupational therapy led health promotion for older people: Feasibility of the Lifestyle Matters programme. *British Journal of Occupational Therapy, 71*(10), 406–413.

Muslimovic, D., Post, B., Speelman, J. D., Schmand, B., & de Haan, R. J. (2008). Determinants of disability and quality of life in mild to moderate Parkinson disease. *Neurology, 70*(23), 2241–2247.

National Association of Clinical Nurse Specialists (NACNS). (2004). *Statement on clinical nurse specialist practice and education* (2nd ed.). Harrisburg, PA: Author.

Nguyen, H. Q., Donesky-Cuenco, D., & Carrieri-Kohlman, V. (2008). Associations between symptoms, functioning, and perceptions of mastery with global self-rated health in patients with COPD: A cross-sectional study. *International Journal of Nursing Studies, 45*(9), 1355–1365.

Ostwald, S. K., Swank, P. R., & Khan, M. M. (2008). Predictors of functional independence and stress level of stroke survivors at discharge from inpatient rehabilitation. *Journal of Cardiovascular Nursing, 23*(4), 371–377.

Roberto, K. A., Gigliotti, C. M., & Husser, E. K. (2005). Older women's experiences with multiple health conditions: Daily challenges and care practices. *Health Care for Women International, 26,* 672–692.

Sandqvist, G., Scheja, A., & Eklund, M. (2008). Working ability in relation to disease severity, everyday occupations and well-being in women with limited systemic sclerosis. *Rheumatology, 47,* 1708–1711.

Sappington, J., & Kelley, J. H. (1996). Modeling and role-modeling theory. *Journal of Holistic Nursing, 14*(2), 130–141.

Schultze-Lutter, F., Ruhrmann, S., Picker, H., von Reventlow, H. G., Daumann, B., Brockhaus-Dumke, A.,…Pukrop, R. (2007). Relationship between subjective and objective cognitive function in the early and late prodrome. *British Journal of Psychiatry, 191*(Suppl. 51), s43–s51.

Sidani, S. (2003). Self-care. In D. M. Doran (Ed.), *Nursing-sensitive outcomes* (pp. 65–113). Boston, MA: Jones & Bartlett.

Smith, R. E., Olin, B. R., & Madsen, J. W. (2006). Spitting into the wind: The irony of treating chronic disease. *Journal of the American Pharmaceutical Association, 46*(3), 379–400.

Steptoe, A., O'Donnell, K., Marmot, M., & Wardle, J. (2008). Positive affect, psychological well-being, and good sleep. *Journal of Psychosomatic Research, 64*(4), 409–415.

Swor, R., Compton, S., Farr, L., Kokko, S., Vining, F., Pascual, R.,...Jackson, R. E. (2003). Perceived self-efficacy in performing and willingness to learn cardiopulmonary resuscitation in an elderly population in a suburban community. *American Journal of Critical Care, 12*(1), 65–70.

Thorne, S., Paterson, B., & Russell, C. (2003). The structure of everyday self-care decision making in chronic illness. *Qualitative Health Research, 13*(10), 1337–1352.

Unger, W. R., & Buelow, J. M. (2009). Hybrid concept analysis of self-management in adults newly diagnosed with epilepsy. *Epilepsy & Behavior, 14,* 89–95.

Uno, K., & Ruthman, J. L. (2004). Wellness as a self-care philosophy for nurses and their leaders. *Holistic Nursing Practice, 20*(1), 3–4.

Vardy, J. L., Xu, W., Booth, C. M., Park, A., Dodd, A., Rourke, S.,...Tannock, I. F. (2008). Relation between perceived cognitive function and neuropsychological performance in survivors of breast and colorectal cancer (ASCO Annual Meeting Proceedings, Post-Meeting Edition). *Journal of Clinical Oncology, 261,* 15(S), 6016.

Wang, T. J. (2004). Concept analysis of functional status. *Journal of Nursing Studies, 41*(4), 457–462.

Whitcomb, J. J. (2011). Functional status versus quality of life: Where does the evidence lead us? *Advance in Nursing Science, 34*(2), 97–102.

Family as Client

Barbara S. O'Brien, Ginette G. Ferszt, Cheryl L. Crisp, and Desiree Hensel

Modern providers have come to understand that improving safety and health care outcomes requires looking at patients as full partners and the source of control in their care (Cronenwett et al., 2009). Consistent with family systems theory, whenever children are involved, the patient is the family and the family is defined by the patient. The advanced practice registered nurse (APRN) consensus model recognizes six patient populations (National Council of State Boards of Nursing [NCSBN], 2008). Of those six, family across the life span, pediatric, and neonatal populations have a clear family focus. Women's health, psychiatric health, and adult/gerontology health populations will also involve effective adjustment and adaptation of the entire family unit to achieve desired outcomes. Family-centered care is an approach to health care incorporating active participation of families in the planning, delivery, and evaluation of health care. When the family is the client, a clinical nurse specialist (CNS) considers all members and the family as a whole when interventions are designed. The family is recognized as a full partner with health care providers and included in decision making based on their level of comfort and ability. When working with the family as a unit, assessment and interventions strategies are highly complex. Regardless of the nature of family interventions designed by the CNS, family inclusion in nursing care and patient decision making is increasingly recognized as an essential component of care.

Dynamic shifts in health care today reflect continued efforts to effectively involve families in patient care. Challenges created by a fast-paced delivery system—including shortened length of hospital stay,

technologically driven diagnostics that yield rapid results, the need for prompt decision making, and greater acuity of patients cared for in the home—increasingly press nurses to develop trust with family members in abbreviated periods of time. At the forefront of this movement, family-centered care and family as client have emerged as essential nursing care concepts and philosophies. Families are an integral part of the continuum of care, and their effective involvement with the patient and providers can profoundly influence patient outcomes. As informed consumers, families are no longer content to take backseat positions to professionals. They are demanding more information and greater participation in issues related to the care of a loved one. The Institute of Medicine (IOM) supported patient-centered health care systems where treatment recommendations and decision making included patients' (and family) preferences (IOM, 2001). In addition, today's focus on cost containment has generated a resurgence of home care provisions, so inclusion and support of families becomes increasingly salient in accomplishing safe, optimal recovery for the vast majority of patients. Facilitating transitions is becoming particularly important, both the traditional process of transitioning from inpatient to outpatient settings and newer challenges of transitioning children living with chronic conditions from pediatric to adult care settings, made possible by advances in care for conditions that children had previously died from before reaching adulthood.

Families vary greatly in their capacity to respond to health-related stressors. In many cases, staff nurses adeptly manage the family education, support, health coaching, and resource needs required to facilitate continuing care. However, it is important to recognize that the specific nature of the challenge and the abilities of the family will impact adjustment and adaptation. The CNS has the educational preparation to analyze barriers to an individual's active involvement in his or her care and to create strategies to empower families. For families with established, functional systems who are experiencing alterations that fall within their capacity to respond, the staff nurse is generally able to provide the support that sufficiently responds to family needs. Staff nurses may not have the time, knowledge, and/or skills to respond to complex family needs, especially in light of the increasing nursing workloads combined with high patient acuity and shortened lengths of hospital stays. Consequently, home care issues may surface that escalate the risk of poor patient outcomes or increase recidivism rates, all contributing to the escalating cost of health care. Additionally, the risk of resulting low patient satisfaction ratings and conflict situations escalate when family needs are neglected.

The CNS is the ideal resource to respond to the increasing needs of today's complex families. This chapter addresses CNS interventions for the family unit, focusing on the family as client and the family as the context of care. Strategic interventions in advocating for and role modeling of family-centered care are discussed. Within the CNS spheres of practice framework described by the National Association of Clinical Nurse Specialists (NACNS, 2004), CNSs must be competent in addressing family needs. This practice includes assessing family needs and designing interventions for families experiencing the stress of illness/injury, as well as providing support and education to staff while establishing system changes that address family needs and focus on positive patient care outcomes.

BACKGROUND

The literature is rich in descriptions of CNS practice involving families. CNSs intervene to help families in acute care, outpatient, private practice, and community-based settings and in numerous specialties, including but not limited to community health, critical care, gerontology, medical-surgical (MS), neurology, pediatrics, maternal child health, psychiatric mental health, and rehabilitation. The following discussion provides a few examples that illustrate the scope of CNS practice.

CNS practice has been shown to improve pediatric outcomes in a wide variety of clinical settings. As a leader in advancing clinical care, CNSs support the adoption of evidence-based practices (EBPs) at the bedside (Gurzick & Kesten, 2010). Canam (2005) described CNS- provided health care for children with complex needs and their families across the continuum of care. In addition to focusing on individual children and their families, the 16 CNSs who were studied were found to contribute to high-quality, cost-effective care at the population level. In home care, CNSs have provided essential follow-up for low-birth-weight babies in the transition from hospital to home (Brooten et al., 2002). In-home and telephone support for 4 months for these infants and their families resulted in an increase in the mother's confidence in providing care for her infant and a decreased use of emergency departments and pediatrician offices (Lasby, Newton, & Von Platen, 2004). CNSs' participation in a multidisciplinary community effort to improve oral health among school-aged children on Medicare resulted in an increase in preventative services and decrease in restorative services after 2 years (Melvin, 2006).

CNS-led outpatient follow-up services have been shown to be an effective way to manage various pediatric health problems. In a randomized controlled trial, Burnett, Juszczak, and Sullivan (2004) compared clinical outcomes of CNS-managed clinics with pediatric gastroenterology (GI) clinics in 102 pediatric patients with functional constipation and found that children treated in the CNS clinics were more likely to be cured (hazard ratio 1.33), and this cure happened more rapidly at a mean time of 18 months versus 23 months at the GI clinics. Traumatic brain injuries, including concussions, are significant sources of pediatric morbidity. Falk (2013) examined the effects of CNS follow-up services for pediatric patients with head injuries in Sweden. The follow-up was conducted 2 to 3 weeks after the initial injury and was tailored to the child's specific injury and symptoms. Of 149 patients who received follow-up service, 91% reported late symptoms including headache. Eight percent of the children required several visits to assure that symptoms were resolved. Falk concluded that the advanced practice nursing services helped minimize the complications and long-term impact of head injuries. In critical care, CNSs have made significant contributions, intervening to promote communication between the patient, family, and health care staff in these stressful care settings. Notable success has been reported in decreasing length of stay in intensive care units (ICUs) as a result of improved communication between patients, families, and staff facilitated by CNSs teamed with the medical director (Ahrens, Yancey, & Kollef, 2003; Coyle, 2000). Coyle described the benefit of the CNS in assuming a primary supportive role for families by providing information and answering very difficult questions related to health care decisions about a family member with suspected brain stem death.

Gerontological CNSs continue to be in high demand because the current population of Americans older than 65 years is 36 million, or 12% of the population. By 2030, the number is expected to rise to 20%, or 71.5 million (Burbank, 2007). Despite this growing need, attracting enough CNSs to serve the health care requirements of this rapidly growing population is a persistent challenge (Thornlow, Auerhahn, & Stanley, 2006). Gerontological CNSs practice in a wide variety of settings, including acute care, long-term care facilities, outpatient practices, senior housing facilities, and in the community. A decrease in the amount of total hospital days and health care costs and therefore decreased stress for the patient and family was presented by Barnes et al. (2012). Decreased hospital readmissions along with prolonged stabilization of the patient's mental status resulted in decreased family distress. Austrom et al. (2006) described the benefits of providing care to Alzheimer's patients and their families in the primary care setting by multidisciplinary teams coordinated by a geriatric advanced practice nurse. Furthermore, positive patient outcomes for elders receiving institutional or home care may depend on successful integration of family resources and coping abilities. The CNS is uniquely positioned to provide this support.

Oncology CNSs have provided psychosocial support and education for families in diverse settings. CNSs in community oncology and palliative care programs have enhanced communication across the continuum of care and improved patients' and families' abilities to successfully navigate complex systems (Vooght & Richardson, 1996; Wittenberg-Lyles, Goldsmith, & Ragan, 2010). Oncology CNSs in a perioperative nurse liaison program intervened with a designated family point person for families experiencing high degrees of distress and were able to demonstrate decreased patient and family anxiety while improving communication (Cunningham, Hanson-Heath, & Agre, 2003). CNSs have also been identified as having an important role in providing support and education for patients receiving chemotherapy for colorectal cancer and their families (Wright & Myint, 2003).

Palliative care CNSs help families to navigate the often difficult practice of caring for their loved ones with life-limiting illness in both inpatient and outpatient settings. The CNSs help families care for their loved ones in a location chosen by the patient and families, allowing the families to have precious time with their loved ones in a safe, comfortable environment. Quinn and Bailey (2011) describe how the use of CNS-directed palliative care teams in Ireland have helped families to negotiate and receive the care needed to keep their children with life-limiting illness at home, a more satisfying option for both the children and their families. Wittenberg-Lyles, Goldsmith, and Ragan (2010) described a communication system known as the COMFORT initiative as a way for families to have a greater understanding of the information they receive regarding their loved ones' diagnoses, care, and progression through the palliative care process. Treating the family in addition to the patient provides greater satisfaction by engaging family members in planning sessions to establish goals of care and to define realistic expectations regarding the patient's condition.

These selective examples illustrate the importance of CNS practice focusing on family involvement. A long and rich history of the beneficial impact of CNS intervention with family is documented in the literature.

CARING FOR FAMILIES: CNS FOCUS

Important challenges confront families when a member develops an acute or chronic health problem. The response of the family to this altered state will depend on many variables and warrants a systematic analysis. Nurses expect families to be responsive to their suggestions and teaching. Typically, busy bedside nurses expect that families will be amenable to their suggestions, instructions, and any limitations imposed by the health care system. Although the majority of families acquiesce to these system conditions, such as limited visiting hours, a dilemma arises for the family whose response fails to conform to expectations. For these families, significant conflict can arise between family members and health care providers. When conflict with family members occurs, staff nurses frequently consult a CNS. Valuing shared decision making and empowering families, even when conflicts occur, is a competency of graduate nursing education the CNS should possess (Cronenwett et al., 2009). While a CNS may be able to negotiate a resolution to the conflict, future crises may be averted by mentoring and coaching staff nurses in providing early attention to family issues and building on family strengths.

CNSs work with families in multiple care settings. Family management issues may present different challenges depending on the setting and CNS specialty practice area. CNSs are commonly involved with management of family responses specific to identified health care issues. In these circumstances, the goal of family assessment is evaluation of the effectiveness of family activities and coping strategies needed for immediate and/or ongoing management of an impaired member. When available, it is recommended that CNSs working in other health care areas take advantage of consultation from psychiatric/mental health care provider colleagues to assist with families exhibiting behavioral pattern challenges or a history of psychiatric problems. In most instances, the CNS can have tremendous impact on family adaptation when armed with a systematic approach for assessment and intervention.

Positive patient outcomes often require a team approach when addressing family concerns and needs. Internalized personal attitudes, biases about families, and what constitutes an appropriate response to the needs and care of an ill member can affect the actions of health care providers. Premature judgment of family reactions can be devastating to therapeutic relationships. Therefore, the CNS needs to recognize and examine personal values as well as those of collaborating staff to avoid compromising care outcomes. Actions and responses that are appropriate for one family may be completely unrealistic or unacceptable for another. Family composition and coping strategies are dependent on many factors. Therefore, it is important for the CNS to obtain a comprehensive understanding of the family system, family members' perceptions of the situation, and response patterns.

SPHERES OF INFLUENCE

Nurses often make valiant efforts to work with families experiencing illness stressors. Unfortunately, absence of a systematic approach to assessment coupled with time constraints may result in ineffective actions. When the situation is compounded by direct conflicts between staff and family, the task is even more daunting and neglected. Early attention to family issues and the use of family strengths to avert the development of a crisis are important strategies that the CNS can incorporate into clinical practice. Operating in the three spheres of influence, the CNS can make great strides to improve patient and family outcomes, educate staff to work effectively with families, and effect organizational and policy-level changes to advocate for family care across all settings. Effective management of family issues necessitates the use of all three spheres of influence of the CNS (NACNS, 2004):

1. Patient/client: use of specific knowledge of assessment of family stress and adaptation as well as the use of therapeutic family intervention strategies.
2. Nurses and nursing practice: focus on prevention strategies targeting implementation of staff education programs as well as role modeling of appropriate interventions needed to work effectively with families in crisis.
3. Organization/system: apply research and leadership skills designed to create a hospitable environment of care that will incorporate family needs.

Sphere I: Family Focus

Family Assessment and Intervention. CNSs prepared in the specialties of pediatrics or family therapy have typically incorporated practice competencies for assessing and intervening with family units. Because a family is a dynamic system, intervention requires specialized practice competencies. All CNSs can benefit by improved understanding of the family as an integrated unit.

It is often difficult to predict how different families will respond when confronted with the same health care problem. A framework that continues to be used by the CNS in family assessment and intervention to describe family stress and coping is the Resiliency Model of Family Stress, Adjustment, and Adaptation. This model helps to identify stressors and suggests ways to assist the family in adjustment strategies and adaptation. Since its inception, this model has continued to evolve and to be used by nursing and other disciplines from the social sciences in a variety of clinical settings.

Application of this model is consistent with the first sphere of influence related to the practice of CNSs: patient/client. The model relates important variables specific to the assessment of family stress and adaptation and provides a guide for developing therapeutic family intervention strategies.

The Resiliency Model can be used for working with families throughout the illness trajectory. It has been applied to a variety of health care challenges for families in various stages of development and across socioeconomic boundaries (Danielson, Hamel-Bissell, & Winstead-Fry, 1993; Pozo, Sarriá, & Brioso, 2013). The model identifies interacting factors that influence family adaptation. Numerous valid and reliable assessment instruments are available to obtain systematic, objective data useful in designing effective interventions for each unique situation. Use of the model can serve as a foundation to guide the CNS to a greater understanding of issues involved in providing family care. The Resiliency Model is an expansion and compilation of the work of Hill (1949), the Double ABCX Model of Family Stress (McCubbin & Patterson, 1981), and the Typology Model of Family Adjustment and Adaptation (McCubbin & McCubbin, 1987). These theories take into consideration available family resources, family perception of the stressor, and established family coping patterns and problem-solving skills. The Resiliency Model reframes these multiple factors and expands the model for the purpose of explaining family adaptation (Danielson et al., 1993).

The Resiliency Model has practical application for CNSs working in inpatient settings as well as in community care areas. Because health issues may precipitate family stress/crisis, having a model to guide understanding of a family's response patterns can facilitate designing effective, individualized nursing interventions. The Resiliency Model focuses on identifying and building on family strengths. Families may be in either the initial (adjustment) or long-term (adaptation) phases of response to illness.

The *adjustment phase* of the model is initiated when a new illness stressor places a demand on the family system. The adjustment phase begins when the family becomes aware of an illness or injury that provokes more than a limited and contained response. Such stressors include accidents, traumatic injuries, or any illness diagnosis. Health concerns evoke a cascade of effects that influence family actions, reactions, and functions. Severity of illness will impact family response: The more severe the illness (stressor), the greater the impact on the family system. For example, a planned elective surgery for hip replacement for an older adult member is unlikely to demand major, long-term changes for the family and could be expected to be far less distressing than an unanticipated accident resulting in a spinal cord injury for a young adult.

Family vulnerability highlights the importance of other factors that may impact the stress experience. The existence of concurrent, multiple stressors increases a family's vulnerability to effective management of a new demand. If the illness represents the single stressor requiring adjustment, it will be easier to focus on needed activities required to meet the illness demands. Conversely, a family grappling with multiple changes will be highly vulnerable. Events such as the recent death of a family member, relocation of a family member (e.g., sending a child to college), financial difficulties (e.g., loss of wages), and marital friction may all increase family vulnerability. The additional stressors often tax the family's capacity to manage the illness situation and may be enough to adversely affect the ability to respond to the transitions and strains produced by the illness. The model uses the term *pileup* to label this phenomenon. Multiple stressors compound in a synergistic manner and can alter interpersonal relationships and threaten stability of the family system. In these circumstances, members may become overwhelmed, have difficulty coping, or be plummeted into a crisis mode if buffering factors are inadequate to manage the situation.

To appropriately evaluate the impact of vulnerability, one must consider other factors that may influence family adjustment. Family types, the existing established patterns of functioning for a family, provides information about the ability of the family to deal with the illness event. It is important to determine how the family usually operates and behaves. The range of family types and established behavior

patterns can be extensive. In general, the most resilient families are described as cohesive but flexible. A cohesive family remains emotionally, if not physically, close and supportive despite changes in circumstances. A flexible family is able to realign priorities and relationships in order to accomplish mutual goals. These families are highly adaptive and have clear open communication patterns. Family roles can change to accommodate the needs of the ill family member. Families with characteristics of cohesion and flexibility are better able to effectively problem solve and manage stressors. Families that are disorganized, loosely bonded, and inflexible should be considered at-risk. For example, a disorganized family may have difficulty communicating among themselves and, subsequently, bombard the nurses with questions and complaints. Ineffective communication often leads to confusion for both the family and the health care team. These families often have difficulty collaborating, problem solving, and making health care decisions. Chaotic activity is evidenced in the care setting where disagreements, control issues, hostility, and displaced priorities are commonly exhibited.

Family resistance resources is a variable in the model that considers the strengths and capabilities of the family system that are useful in managing the stressful situation. Resistance factors provide the family with the ability to avert a crisis or major family disruption. For example, in a flexible family system, the ability and willingness of members to assume roles previously held by the ill member provides a smooth transition for recovery within the family system. Assessing resistance factors facilitates identifying interventions to support those strengths that are useful in promoting effective adjustment. Appropriate assessments might include evaluation of economic stability, cohesiveness, flexibility, hardiness, shared spiritual beliefs, traditions, celebrations, routines, and organization (McCubbin & McCubbin, 1993).

Though extremely significant, the family's view of their situation is often ignored. If perception is everything, then family appraisal of the stressor demands priority attention. Problems may be created when health care providers inadvertently act on their own beliefs regarding the meaning of the illness and its expected impact on the family system. It is most important to acknowledge that individual appraisal of any event is personal and, therefore, variable and subjective. Avoidance of imposing external beliefs in the situation is imperative. In order to help a family adjust to a member's illness, nurses need to understand the family's perspective of the situation. If viewed as a catastrophic, uncontrollable event, adjustment will require interventions aimed at providing education and realistic expectations to avert further deterioration. On the other hand, a family viewing the situation as a challenge will benefit from support in their efforts to rally an effective defense.

The last factor, problem solving and coping, takes into account the abilities that exist within a family to confront new or distressing situations. Problem-solving skills require the family to identify the problem, break it into manageable parts, and take action to resolve it. Some families do not communicate openly, directly, and effectively; therefore, communication within the family must be assessed. Distressed communication between family members frequently evokes difficulties and creates conflicts among the family members and in the health care environment. For example, a family member may infer that nursing care is inadequate when the real issue is anxiety about the family's ability to manage the affected individual at home.

Techniques to reinforce problem-solving skills include support of previously effective strategies and keeping the focus on the problem and not the family members. Clarifying decisions and strategies may avert competitive or even hostile reactions over power and control issues. Undoubtedly, most nurses have confronted difficulties in this area when decisions related to life-support measures, comfort measures, or nursing home placement were being considered.

These elements of typology, appraisal, problem-solving skills, and availability of resources interact as the family strives to manage the illness-related stressor. Eventually, the response culminates in some level of adjustment for the family. The model predicts that if all factors are in balance and function to reduce the level of tension in the family, there will be a *bonadjustment*, an optimistic and constructive ability to manage the situation. Illness places a major strain on the family system because there are often burdensome demands that occur in all of the components of the model. Yet, many families are capable of making this adjustment with little or no assistance. When demands are too high, *maladaptation* may result. Demands can include shifting roles within the family, changing goals (or even values), new rules or priorities, boundary changes, and alterations in patterns of functioning (McCubbin & McCubbin, 1993). When demands exceed mediating factors, maladjustment occurs and a resulting crisis may loom. Too frequently, it is only at this juncture that the CNS is consulted. Problems in the health care setting escalate as families in crisis exhibit disorganization and disruptive behaviors. Nurses and other care providers describe the situation as out-of-control and express fear of negative patient and family outcomes. McCubbin and McCubbin caution against labeling these families as dysfunctional. It is the experience of crisis that initiates the adaptation phase. When things are very painful, humans tend to seek assistance

in reducing suffering. Therefore, the CNS should approach these situations armed with the knowledge that with supportive care these families are likely to be amenable to interventions and strategies that enable them to better manage their situation.

When illness recovery has a distinct resolution, interventions targeting adjustment may be enough. Once the illness resolves, the family is likely to reestablish itself at a previous or higher level of functioning. Conversely, if the family has maladjusted to the stressor or the changing situation adversely impacts adjustment, a crisis may occur. If emotional stability is at risk, additional assistance may be indicated, such as a referral for family counseling. However, the CNS should anticipate entry into the next phase of the model when working with families dealing with chronic illness. Chronic conditions will create periodic additional or ongoing demands for the family.

The adaptation phase of the Resiliency Model explains the interacting factors that affect family response in this stage. While the factors are similarly labeled, the duration of the stressor requires major and enduring change within the family—adaptation as opposed to adjustment. *Adjustment* involves immediate and often temporary changes in managing an illness, whereas *adaptation* infers acceptance of more durable and long-lasting alterations. Family survival may depend on the acceptability of these changes within the family group. Successful adaptation is defined as the existence of a balance between meeting individual member needs and the well-being of the family as a whole (Danielson et al., 1993). No single strategy can be prescribed in any of the components and, as in the adjustment phase, the interactions between the variables will change the approach. Also, effective adaptation to chronic illness will require integration with the larger community, including the health care system. This mutual relationship facilitates identification of appropriate care, support, and essential education provided to families, while the families reciprocate by following through on the plan of care.

As a family strives to manage a chronic illness, challenges to their prior adjustment will be inevitable. The CNS should anticipate and monitor the occurrence of pileup over time. Families will become increasingly vulnerable to crisis when demands related to the chronic illness mount or when factors required in managing the situation are compounded by other stressors, strains, and transitions of family life. When pileup of stressors is suspected, the CNS needs to identify impending or actual stressors impacting the family. Assessment of life changes, hardships, concurrent competing demands, prior strains, situational demands, efforts to cope, ambiguities, and normal life cycle transitions experienced by the family need to be explored. A clinical interview and assessment is important in identifying issues in this area and in affirming rapport with the family. Additionally, the CNS might elect to use a structured assessment instrument designed to measure family stress (Table 15.1).

When stressors are overwhelming, a family crisis situation may ensue. Again, family strengths and resources are rallied in an attempt to manage the situation. Many components of family response must be reassessed in an effort to obtain currently valid data to guide future interventions to assist with adaptation. It is important for the CNS to identify the family types and newly instituted patterns of functioning, as multiple family types exist. In general, families with greater breadth and depth in their patterns of functioning will be better equipped to support family integrity, unity, flexibility, and predictability when struggling to manage an illness and its long-term impact. To supplement the clinical interview, instruments are available to the CNS to assist in determining family types; two of these are provided in Table 15.1.

Additionally, it is important to reassess the adaptive strategies being used by the family. Historically established patterns may be inadequate in the face of new demands imposed by the illness. However, the adoption of new methods may be problematic as well. For example, a mother may seek employment outside the home to decrease the burden of financial stress resulting from the illness, or a family may move closer to health services for the ill member. Such changes may evoke a chain reaction because needs, desires, and roles of other family members can be dramatically impacted. In assessing this component, the clinical interview should focus on the family's values, priorities, expectations, goals, and rules over time as well as on any change in patterns of family functioning and their impact on the system. Effective patterns will be congruent with family functioning and positively correlated with the ease and level of adaptation to the illness. Assessment of family patterns provides insight into functioning and elucidates important family strengths and valued resources.

Efforts to adapt will be affected by available family resources. Effective assessment in this area should include review of resources of the individual

TABLE 15.1

ASSESSMENT INSTRUMENTS FOR FAMILY ASSESSMENT/FUNCTIONING		
Instrument	**Primary Reference**	**Focus of Measure**
Family Inventory of Life Event and Changes (FILE)	McCubbin & Thompson (1991)	Evaluates stressors present in family at one point in time
Family Hardiness Index	McCubbin & Thompson (1991)	Identifies stress resistance and adaptation resources, mitigating stressors, and demands
Family Time and Routines Scale	McCubbin & Thompson (1991)	Family integration and stability
Family Inventory of Resources for Management (FIRM)	McCubbin & Thompson (1991)	Measures family social, psychological, community, and family income resources
Social Support Index	McCubbin, Patterson, & Glynn, (1996)	Measures type and availability of social support for family
Family Problem Solving and Communication	McCubbin, Thompson, & McCubbin (1996)	Explores type of problem-solving methods used by family and primary communication patterns existing within the system
Coping Health Inventory for Parents (CHIP)	McCubbin & Thompson (1991)	Measures coping skills of families where a child has a health condition; greater repertoire of coping skills predicts improved family management
Family Crisis-Oriented Personal Evaluation Scale	McCubbin & Thompson (1991)	Identifies problem-solving and behavioral strategies used in difficult or problem situations
Family's Sense of Coherence Index (FSOC)	McCubbin, Thompson, & McCubbin (1996)	Evaluates degree of connection and loyalty within family unit
Family Index of Resiliency and Adaptation (FIRA-G)	McCubbin & Thompson (1991)	Evaluates flexibility for use of various problem-solving strategies

Source: McCubbin, Thompson, & McCubbin (2003).

family members, the family working as a unit, and the community. Resources may be tangible (having a home that is appropriately modified for a person with a disability) or intangible (such as personality attributes of family members). Desirable and abundant resources facilitate adaptation. The CNS needs to assess existing resources while planning interventions for the acquisition and maintenance of ongoing support needs. Case managers and social workers can be valuable in identifying and procuring resources, such as assistive devices, financial relief, and community support systems. Intangible resources are more difficult to identify but may have significant influence on the level of adaptation. For example, a caregiver who is depressed is likely to have a diminished capacity to meet the demands of the situation regardless of past performance. There are myriad family resource considerations, and the unique constellation of these factors can affect family hardiness and the ability to adapt at any point in time. Family interviews often reveal resources that are operational and those that are lacking in a specific situation. To assist in this process, the Family Inventory of Resources for Management (FIRM) can be useful (Table 15.1).

Social support is an important and powerful interpersonal resource for family adaptation. Broadly defined, it includes all persons and agencies that may assist the family in coping with the illness. Extended family, personal friends, health care providers, and even government policies can serve as affirming sources of support to families coping with illness conditions. Recent attention and policy statements at the national and international level have legitimized attention to effective pain management for many. A broad network of effective social support promotes family adaptation by enhancing a sense of respect and efficacy on the part of the family as well a sense of being valued in the larger community. Families may openly share social support resources with providers on interview, but additional assessment can be accomplished through administration of specific assessment instruments (Table 15.1).

The Resiliency Model describes three levels of family appraisal that impact family adaptation. Level 1 occurs in the adjustment phase and refers to the family's definition of the stressor and its impact—how they view the illness. Level 2, the situational level, requires an assessment of the family's appraisal of their capacity to cope with the challenge—their ability to balance the demands with the strengths and capabilities of the family. These appraisals must be reevaluated over time and can vacillate from positive to negative depending on the circumstances at the time. Many factors affect the family's assessment of the situation and are capable of altering perceptions. For example,

when a family member is initially diagnosed with a myocardial infarction, families may panic, fearing the worst. With successful treatment, family fears may be substantially allayed and optimism (realistic or not) may result. If treatment fails or the member develops heart failure, this appraisal will shift again as the family must adjust to new circumstances and arrive at a revised interpretation of the meaning, demands, and suspected outcomes of the situation. It must be noted that the family's appraisal of the situation may differ significantly among the members and from that of health care providers. Evaluation should focus on the impact of the perception on effective adaptation and what strategies should be employed to reduce adverse outcomes. Positive appraisals of an illness and the family's ability to manage it will support effective problem solving, coping, and use of resources directed at adaptation. The CNS needs to encourage families to share their thoughts and feelings about the illness and its impact on the family, thus obtaining data useful in designing interventions to support realistic and constructive appraisals. Even for families dealing with terminal illness, a positive outlook is possible by focusing on interventions such as spending quality time with the member or facilitating a "good death."

Level 3, family schema appraisal—family meaning, requires insight into the meaning the family attaches to the illness and the subsequent family changes. Arriving at a shared family meaning of the illness and its impact on the family system is a complex endeavor requiring time and effort on the part of the family. Most providers have heard families report that the presence of an unexpected stressful event, such as the birth of a child who is medically fragile or has a disability, "brought the family together." It may even be stated that such cohesiveness would not have otherwise occurred. Accomplishments in this area involve a reappraisal of family values, goals, priorities, rules, and expectations and a realignment of the perception of the family, its meaning to the members, and even its patterns of functioning resulting from the illness situation. The family's ethnic, religious, and sociocultural background will influence how the family appraises and makes meaning of the situation that they are confronting. The new meaning involves the intense work of altering expectations, reframing previously held views, and arriving at a family schema that is accepted by all members. The CNS is challenged to elicit data from the family that reveal their shared meaning and understanding of their situation. Cultural factors must be accounted for in this process. Data about the family's meaning and understanding of the situation can be used to support development of a positive and constructive view that is congruent with the changed family situation.

The last variable of the model that interacts to influence family adaptation is problem solving and coping. Coping behaviors are defined as efforts of a family member or the family as a whole to reduce or manage a demand on the system. While problem solving is frequently viewed on the individual level, it can operate as a coordinated effort across the family system. A plan can be established so that various members assume complementary functions to accomplish a desired outcome. In a family with a child with a disability, older siblings may assume more household tasks to enable the parents to have quality time with each other and other children in the family. Danielson et al. (1993) noted that coping and problem solving may be directed at (a) reducing or eliminating stresses and hardships, (b) acquiring additional resources, (c) managing family system tension, and (d) shaping the appraisal at both the situational and the schema level. Having a broad array of problem-solving and coping strategies combined with an open, honest, and effective communication style establishes a positive environment for adaptation. As an adjunct to the clinical interview, the CNS may select an instrument developed to measure family problem-solving and coping skills (Table 15.1).

The components of the model interact to predict the effect on adaptation outcomes for families managing an illness situation. In *bonadaptation*, family coherence is demonstrated through alignment of family schema and patterns of functioning, appropriate growth and development of members, maintenance of family integrity, and the existence of mutually supportive relationships with the community. For families dealing with chronic illness, this process is ongoing and requires revision as the illness or family situation undergo change. The continuing nature of the adjustment requires the CNS to be vigilant in systematically reevaluating and addressing emergent family needs. Assessment of the family related to all factors that influence adaptation is imperative. Again, instruments specifically designed to assess family adaptation can be useful (Table 15.1).

The CNS must anticipate the life transition and family adaptation as adolescents move from dependent to independent managers of their health care needs. Decisional conflict is likely to occur as part of the letting-go process for both the parent and emerging adult. Maternal and Child Health Bureau identifies a core quality measure assuring that youth with special needs receive the services they need to transition to adult life (U.S. Department of Health and Human Services, 2008). Yet, one national survey found only 15% of these youth were meeting the transition outcome (Lotstein, McPherson, Strickland, & Newacheck, 2005). The CNS can play a key role in facilitating this transition, in part by assessing adolescents' readiness to assume greater responsibility for their own care. An overview of tools that may be useful in such an assessment are listed in Table 15.2. Assessment findings then can help the family in the decision-making process as they plan for the next phases of chronic illness management.

TABLE 15.2

TOOLS TO MEASURE TRANSITION READINESS IN ADOLESCENTS WITH CHRONIC ILLNESS		
Tool	**Primary Reference**	**Focus**
TRAQ—Transition Readiness Assessment Questionnaire	Sawicki et al. (2011)	Based on transtheoretical model, the 29-item Likert-type scale measures self-advocacy and self-management skills in special health care needs of patients 16 to 26 years of age
Transition Readiness Survey Adolescent/Young Adult Version (TRS:A/YA) and Transition Readiness Survey: Parent Report (TRS:P)	Fredericks et al. (2010)	The TRS:A/YA version is a 38-item 3-point scale that measures self-management, regimen knowledge, demonstrated skills, and psychosocial adjustment in liver transplant patients from 11 to 20 years of age. The TRS:P contains 36 items
The Readiness for Transition Questionnaire (RTQ-teen; RTQ-parent)	Gilleland, Amaral, Mee, & Blount (2012)	Designed for use in kidney transplant patients ages 15 to 21; parallel tool versions rate adolescent involvement and parent involvement in 10 behaviors on a 4-point scale
UNC TR(x)ANSITION Scale	Ferris et al. (2012)	Designed for use in patients with chronic illness from ages 12 to 20 years, the 33-item scale assesses 10 domains: *T*ype of illness, *Rx*, medications, *A*dherence, *N*utrition, *S*elf-management, *I*nformed reproduction, *T*rade/school, *I*nsurance, *O*ngoing support, and *N*ew health providers

The Resiliency Model integrates a multitude of factors that influence family response to illness events. This explanation is useful in assessing family adjustment and/or adaptation and in designing effective interventions needed to provide assistance to families in their struggle to manage stress and garner appropriate support. Left unaddressed, illness stressors can result in harmful outcomes for patients and their families.

Sphere II: Nursing and Nursing Practice

Formal and informal educational programs for nurses and other health care professionals must be built into the fabric of our health care systems to meet the needs of today's diverse families. Formal, ongoing educational programs must include topics such as cultural and religious influences on family responses to a patient's illness, cultural and spiritual needs or concerns of families, family coping styles, the family developmental life cycle, preparing children for visiting their loved one, the prevention and management of crisis, and assessing families for anxiety, depression, and posttraumatic stress disorder (Ferguson, Ward, Card, Sheppard, & McMurtry, 2013; Hughes, Bryan, & Robbins, 2005; Jones et al., 2004). CNSs can provide updates and ongoing attention to these issues for nursing care personnel and students.

CNSs can facilitate staff participation in the development of informational materials for patients and families in hospital or community settings. Print and digital materials can assist families with understanding the dimensions of an illness or treatment and provide a realistic perspective upon which to shape their response. In one hospital, a digital recording illustrating a realistic portrayal of a code was made available to families struggling with a resuscitation decision. The CNS viewed the digital recording with family members and facilitated a question-and-answer discussion. This intervention often paved the way for families to engage in decisions with an improved understanding of the implications for the patient.

Children are curious, and in many families it is appropriate for children to visit members in the acute care setting. It is important to prepare children for what they will see and hear in an effort to avoid misinterpretations that may result in enduring traumatic experiences. In preparing children for visiting their loved one, particularly in a critical or ICU, the CNS can provide age-appropriate educational programs. These programs, designed to reduce the fear and anxiety experienced by children, may be one-on-one play sessions, digital recordings, storybooks, or other formats familiar to children. Staff may need to be reminded of the importance of child visitation and

also supported with strategies to assist in making it a satisfactory experience for all.

Attitudes toward health, illness, and health care providers are strongly influenced by cultural and ethnic factors (Campinha-Bacote, 2003; Herz, 1987; Ravindran & Myers, 2012). When individuals respond to an illness in a manner that is similar to a member of the health care subculture, they are most often labeled *normal* (Herz, 1987). Given the changing demographics in our country, nurses are caring for individuals and families from a broad spectrum of ethnic backgrounds who often respond differently than the expected norm. It has long been known that emotional expressiveness in minority cultures is less valued by the dominant culture (Boiger & Mesquita, 2012) and families who respond with a great deal of emotion may be judged in a negative way or misunderstood by health care providers. The judgment of health care personnel influences the health care agency's attitude. CNSs can facilitate effective response to families in stressful situations by encouraging an attitude of respect for diversity.

CNSs can assume a pivotal role in interacting with families and educating nursing staff. Cultural bias can blind one to another's reaction to illness (Baider, 2012). Because our cultural values and assumptions are usually outside of our awareness and we see the world through our own knowledge, beliefs, and cultural lens, assisting the staff, in a gentle way, to explore their own values, beliefs, and assumptions is often a first step. Providing consultation to nurses and educating them about different cultures must be a priority in today's health care systems.

Given the high level of stress that nurses experience at various times during their career, support services for staff must also be an integral part of health care systems today. Staff support is needed to decompress and confront feelings about family members, their reactions and behaviors, or patient care outcomes. In the past, support groups for nurses have often come under the purview of psychiatric CNSs. However, CNSs in other specialties can also provide support for nurses in a variety of ways. For instance, one of the authors developed a creative approach for supporting and empowering nurses in clinical situations where they had provided care for a patient who was hospitalized for a long period of time. In one situation, the patient's pain and related distress were unable to be totally relieved. Often, the nurses felt inadequate in their inability to provide comfort for this patient. When the patient died, nurses, residents, unit secretaries, family members, nursing assistants, and clergy were brought together around the patient's bed. The purpose of this ritual was not only to remember the patient but also to provide the opportunity for health care professionals and other staff members to acknowledge each other and all of their efforts. Gathered together over the patient, the surgical resident recalled a time when he had chastised one young nurse for intrusion on his time by calling him in the middle of the night. However, in reflection, the resident was able to acknowledge the importance of the nurse advocating for the patient. This intervention facilitated the grieving process of staff and enabled them to reflect positively on their efforts to provide appropriate care. Perhaps more importantly, this intervention made it possible for the team to reframe the staffs' efforts by acknowledging and validating their actions despite the outcome of death of the patient.

Another avenue for role modeling and educating nursing staff about family needs, as well as designing family interventions, is regular interprofessional patient care conferences. These conferences provide an opportunity for establishing honest, accurate, and understandable information to be communicated to families. Questions and concerns raised by family members can also be addressed individually and collectively. An intervention study conducted in a neonatal ICU reported that using a shared decision-making model in scheduled meetings between health care professionals and patients resulted in less conflict, more accurate knowledge, more realistic parent expectations, and improved provider relationships with families (Penticuff & Arheart, 2005).

The CNS can play an integral role in working with staff to provide knowledge, competence, and confidence for integrating families in patient care to promote quality outcomes. CNSs can also serve the nursing staff by providing expert knowledge and skills for managing difficult and challenging family situations, whether through role modeling, education, or personal support. Clearly, this resource function serves to promote job satisfaction and staff retention. These factors further highlight the value-added service of the CNS in the practice setting.

Sphere III: Organization/System

The CNS must work to advocate for inclusion of the family as a partner in multidisciplinary decision making and care. To accomplish this goal, attention must be focused on broader organizational and societal policies that appropriately incorporate a family focus in health care. Research and leadership skills of the CNS are useful in promoting an environment of care that fosters family involvement and emphasizes family-centered care.

Improving the environment of care for families may necessitate challenges to existing practices. The CNS must become actively involved in evaluating the needs of families and the practices of nurses and other health care providers in working with families. The

conduct and dissemination of nursing research on family care is needed to substantiate best practices. Long-standing disputes over access to patients in the institutional setting is a classic exemplar. Notably, restrictive policies related to flexibility in visiting hours, visitation by young children, and even pet visitation policies are being reviewed in many facilities. These practices should be challenged and revised based on the best evidence to ensure care that promotes quality patient/family outcomes.

Institutional environments need to consider the needs of families as well. Becoming involved in the creation or redesign of a facility affords the CNS an opportunity to promote areas where families feel welcome and not external to the care setting. While attractive lounge areas are important, providing a private, quiet, and safe space for visitors; ensuring comfortable sitting or sleep accommodations; and access to staff care providers represent more enduring needs. For the most part, these needs have not been adequately addressed and may create artificial barriers to family involvement in care procedures. The CNS is prepared to explore family environmental needs and to implement cost analysis profiles measuring the impact on patient response.

Challenging long-established policies and embedded beliefs may lead to dramatic changes in health care practice. For example, while many health care providers may resist the movement, evidence is mounting that family presence at resuscitation procedures is beneficial. Not only are patients and families expressing not just a desire, but a right to be present (Hung & Pang, 2011), but also studies have indicated that with appropriate preparation and support during the event, families reported that witnesses felt comforted that everything was done to save the loved one and that they experienced no greater stress than a control group (Duran et al., 2007; Leung & Chow, 2012, Thacker & Long, 2010). As families are invited to observe care processes, a reduction in legal actions may be an additional benefit. The CNS needs to be active in pursuing evidence to advocate for best-practice agency policy changes that will increase responsiveness to family needs and outcomes and that are supported by financial efficacy.

As the population continues to age, provisions for palliative care are an increasingly relevant concern. Recently, Clinical Practice Guidelines for Quality Care were developed (National Consensus Project for Quality Palliative Care, 2004). Families need to know that their loved one is being treated with respect and that suffering is kept at a minimum. Additionally, families need emotional support and timely, honest information about what to expect in the dying process (Quinn & Bailey, 2011; Wittenberg-Lyles, Goldsmith, & Ragan, 2010). The growing need for and evidence guiding the provision of palliative care will impel greater CNS involvement in this important area of practice. Organizations need to be presented with accurate facts that support implementation of conscientious, cost-effective decisions regarding palliative care services.

Finally, nurses are being called upon to influence the development of health policy on the local, state, and federal levels (Buerhaus et al., 2012; Richter et al., 2013) and CNSs need to provide leadership in this area. CNSs should also advocate for improved agency-to-agency communication. Policies affecting timely patient/family information that protects confidentiality when moving across the system, such as transfer to another facility or discharge to the home setting, must be established, monitored, and evaluated to ensure continuity of quality care. The ethical use of electronic medical record and its availability to all needed health care providers is also required. Public policy impinging on the access to care or stigmatization of patients returning to communities demands attention. HIV/AIDS, escalating antibiotic-resistant infections, attention to effective pain management, and potential public health crises, such as the threat of a flu epidemic or a bioterrorism attack, are examples of contemporary issues where public education, assistance, and policy decisions have been impacted by the actions of nurses. Additionally, CNSs need to be involved in the development of comprehensive, evidence-based standards of care. Nurses are capable of viewing practice from a variety of perspectives. The CNS can take the lead in representing family inclusion in standards wherever relevant.

To accomplish outcomes in this area, CNSs may choose to serve on hospital committees, community boards, and local, state, or national committees. The ability to conduct or support research studies and to analyze and logically apply research findings to practice is a process where CNSs must use their expertise to advocate for patient/family care. Exercising leadership skills, expert interpersonal communications, and advanced knowledge are essential in influencing policies directed at meeting the needs of patients and families in the face of dynamic changes in the health care system.

SUMMARY

The integration of family care into nursing practice continues to evolve. While other models and theories of family may be equally relevant, the Resiliency Model was selected to provide the CNS with a systematic approach for assessment and development of intervention strategies for families confronting a health care challenge. Examples of methods and instruments useful in obtaining comprehensive assessment leading to effective therapeutic interventions were presented. Provisions for family care across the three spheres of influence of CNS practice were highlighted. The need for CNS leadership in family care requires a continued focus on the development of this practice component.

■ DISCUSSION QUESTIONS

- In your professional life, how would the elements of the Resiliency Model have been helpful in preventing personal bias about family responses that might affect nursing care?
- How would you incorporate the issues related to power and family structure into the Resiliency Model?
- How would you incorporate issues involving transitions in your own practice?
- What family stressors have you confronted in your own practice?
- What interventions have you employed when working with a challenging family situation? How might a theoretical model help you to design effective new methods?
- How can the CNS promote collaboration with the total health care team in meeting the challenge of family care in your setting?
- What EBP project would be relevant to the enhancement of family care in your nursing specialty?
- What policy changes can you identify that would promote family involvement and *bonadaptation*?

■ REFLECTION

- Reflect on your past clinical experiences with a challenging family that stands out in your mind. Identify possible reasons for the difficulty you experienced in delivering family-centered care. Refer to the Resiliency Model, and consider other interventions that you might use in the future with this type of family that might be more successful.
- Reflect on a current challenge in a family clinical situation. Apply the three levels of influence to analyze how you might have been effective in all three spheres of influence.

■ ANALYSIS AND SYNTHESIS EXERCISES

Select a movie with a family focus, for example, *My Big Fat Greek Wedding, Away From Her, The Other Sister, Our Family Wedding, The Big Wedding, Follow the Stars Home.*

Points to Consider: Observe your responses to different family members as you watch this movie. Identify which family member(s) you would have the most difficulty communicating with and discuss possible reasons for your responses. Discuss methods or interventions you could employ to improve the situation.

■ CLINICAL APPLICATION

The face of the family is evolving. Nurses have long maintained that "pain" is a subjective experience defined by the individual. The CNS should recognize that what constitutes a "family" is also defined by the patient. Strict definitions of family that do not allow for patient preferences may result in inadequate patient support and conflicts with the health care team. Review your institution's policies related to family visitation within the context of the three spheres of influence. Consider how these policies evolved? Were they created with patient input? Are they evidence based? Are they difficult to enforce? Do they improve patient safety? Do they improve the quality of care? Create a plan to share your findings with recommendations for next steps.

REFERENCES

Ahrens, T., Yancey, V., & Kollef, M. (2003). Improving family communication at the end of life: Implications for length of stay in the intensive care unit and resource use. *American Journal of Critical Care, 12*(4), 317–323.

Austrom, M. G., Hartwell, C., Moore, P., Perkins, A., Damush, T., Unverzgagt, F. W.,...Christopher, M. (2006). An integrated model of comprehensive care for people with Alzheimer's disease and their caregivers in a primary setting. *Dementia: The International Journal of Social Research and Practice, 5*(3), 339–352.

Baider, L. (2012). Cultural diversity: Family path through terminal illness. *Annals of Oncology, 23*(Suppl. 3), 62–65. doi:10.1093/annonc/mds090

Barnes, D. E., Palmer, R. M., Kresevic, D. M., Fortinsky, R. H., Kowal, J., Chren, M.-M., & Landefeld, C. S. (2012). Acute care for elders units produced shorter hospital stays at lower cost while maintaining patients' functional status. *Health Affairs, 31*(6), 1227–1236. doi:10.1377/hlthaff.2012.0142

Boiger, M., & Mesquita, B. (2012). The construction of emotion in interactions, relationships, and cultures. *Emotion Review, 4*(3), 221–229. doi:10.1077/1754073912439765er.sagepub.com

Brooten, D., Genaro, S., Knapp, H., Jovene, N., Brown, L., & York, R. (2002). Classic article: Functions of the CNS in early discharge and home follow up of very low birthweight infants. *Clinical Nurse Specialist: The Journal for Advanced Practice Nursing Practice, 16*(2), 85–90.

Buerhaus, P., DesRoches, C., Applebaum, S., Hess, R., Norman. L. D., & Donelan, K. (2012). Are nurses ready for health care reform? A decade of survey research. *Nursing Economics, 30*(6).

Burbank, P. (2007). Introduction. In P. Burbank (Ed.), *Vulnerable older adults. Health care needs and interventions* (pp. xviii–xxiv). New York, NY: Springer.

Burnett, C. A., Juszczak, E., & Sullivan, P. B. (2004). Nurse management of intractable functional constipation: A randomized controlled trial. *Archives of Disease in Childhood, 89*(8), 717–722.

Campinha-Bacote, J. (2003). Guest editorial: Cultural desire: The key to unlocking cultural competence. *Journal of Nursing Education, 42*(6), 239–240.

Canam, C. (2005). Illuminating the clinical nurse specialist role of advanced practice nursing: A qualitative study. *Canadian Journal of Nursing Leadership, 18*(4), 70–89.

Coyle, M. A. (2000). Meeting the needs of the family: The role of the specialist nurse in the management of brain death. *Intensive and Critical Care Nursing, 16*(1), 45–50.

Cronenwett, L., Sherwood, G., Pohl, J., Barnsteiner, J., Moore, S., Sullivan, D.,...Warren, J. (2009). Quality and safety education for advanced nursing practice. *Nursing Outlook, 57*(6), 338–348.

Cunningham, M. F., Hanson-Health, C., & Agre, P. (2003). A perioperative nurse liaison program: CNS interventions for cancer patients and their families. *Journal of Nursing Care Quality, 18*(1), 16–21.

Danielson, C. B., Hamel-Bissell, B., & Winstead-Fry, P. (1993). *Families, health, and illness.* St. Louis, MO: Mosby.

Duran, C. R., Oman, K. S., Abel, J. J., Koziel, V. M., & Symanski, D. (2007). Attitudes toward and beliefs about family presence: A survey of healthcare providers, patients' families and patients. *American Journal of Critical Care, 16*(3), 270–279.

Falk, A. C. (2013). A nurse-led paediatric head injury follow-up service. *Scandinavian Journal of Caring Sciences, 27*(1), 51–56.

Ferris, M. E., Harward, D. H., Bickford, K., Layton, J. B., Ferris, M. T., Hogan, S. L.,...Hooper, S. R. (2012). A clinical tool to measure the components of health-care transition from pediatric care to adult care: The UNC TRxANSITION Scale. *Renal Failure, 34*(6), 744–753.

Ferguson, L. M., Ward, H., Card, S., Sheppard, S., & McMurtry, J. (2013). Putting the "patient" back into patient-centered care: An education perspective. *Nurse Education in Practice, 13*(4), 283–287.

Fredericks, E. M., Dore-Stites, D., Well, A., Magee, J. C., Freed, G. L., Shieck, V., & James Lopez, M. (2010). Assessment of transition readiness skills and adherence in pediatric liver transplant recipients. *Pediatric Transplantation, 14*(8), 944–953.

Gilleland, J., Amaral, S., Mee, L., & Blount, R. (2012). Getting ready to leave: Transition readiness in adolescent kidney transplant recipients. *Journal of Pediatric Psychology, 37*(1), 85–96.

Gurzick, M., & Kesten, K. S. (2010). The impact of clinical nurse specialists on clinical pathways in the application of evidence-based practice. *Journal of Professional Nursing, 12*(1), 42–48. doi:10.1016/j.profnurs.2009.04.03

Herz, F. B. (1987). Ethnicity, families and life-threatening illness. In M. Leahey & L. Wright (Eds.), *Families and life-threatening illness* (pp. 232–233). Springhouse, PA: Springhouse.

Hill, R. (1949). *Families under stress.* New York, NY: Harper & Row.

Hughes, F., Bryan, K., & Robbins, I. (2005). Relatives' experiences of critical care. *Nursing in Critical Care, 10*(1), 23–30.

Hung, M., & Pang, S. (2011). Family presence when patients are receiving resuscitation in an accident and emergency department. *Journal of Advanced Nursing, 67,* 56–67.

Institute of Medicine (IOM). (2001). *Crossing the quality chasm: A new health system for the 21st century.* Washington, DC: National Academies Press.

Jones, C., Skirrow, P., Griffiths, R. D., Humphris, G., Ingleby, S., Eddleston, J.,…Gager, M. (2004). Post-traumatic stress disorder-related symptoms in relatives of patients following intensive care. *Intensive Care Medicine, 30,* 456–460.

Lasby, K., Newton, S., & Von Platen, A. (2004). Neonatal transitional care. *Canadian Nurse, 100*(8), 18–23.

Leung, N. Y., & Chow, S. K. Y. (2012). Attitudes of healthcare staff and patients' family members towards family presence during resuscitation in adult critical care units. *Journal of Clinical Nursing, 21,* 2083–2093. doi:10.1111/j.1365–2702.2011.04013x

Lotstein, D. S., McPherson, M., Strickland, B., & Newacheck, P. W. (2005). Transition planning for youth with special health care needs: Results from the National Survey of Children with Special Health Care Needs. *Pediatrics, 115*(6), 1562–1568.

McCubbin, H. I., & Patterson, J. M. (Eds.). (1981). *Systematic assessment of family stress, resources and coping: Tools for research, education and clinical intervention.* St. Paul, MN: Family Social Stress.

McCubbin, H. I., Patterson, J. M., & Glynn, A. (1996). Social support index. In H. McCubbin, A. Thompson, & M. McCubbin (Eds.), *Family assessment: Resiliency, coping, and adaptation—Inventories for research and practice.* Madison, WI: University of Wisconsin.

McCubbin, H. I., & Thompson, A. (1991). *Family assessment inventories for research and practice* (2nd ed.). Madison, WI: University of Wisconsin.

McCubbin, H. I., Thompson, A., & McCubbin, M. (Eds.). (1996). *Family assessment: Resiliency, coping and adaptation—Inventories for research and practice.* Madison, WI: University of Wisconsin.

McCubbin, H. I., Thompson, A., & McCubbin, M. (2003). *Family measures: Stress, coping and resiliency (CD-ROM).* Madison, WI: University of Wisconsin.

McCubbin, M., & McCubbin, H. I. (1987). Families coping with illness: The resiliency model of family stress, adjustment and adaptation. In H. McCubbin & A. Thompson (Eds.), *Family assessment inventories for research and practice* (2nd ed., pp. 3–232). Madison, WI: University of Wisconsin.

McCubbin, M., & McCubbin, H. I. (1993). Family coping with illness: The resiliency model of family stress, adjustment and adaptation. In C. Danielson, B. Hamel-Bissell, & P. Windstead-Fry (Eds.), *Families, health, and illness* (pp. 21–63). St. Louis, MO: Mosby.

Melvin, C. S. (2006). A collaborative community-based oral care program for school-age children. *Clinical Nurse Specialist, 20*(1), 18–22.

National Association of Clinical Nurse Specialists (NACNS). (2004). *Statement on clinical nurse specialist practice and education* (2nd ed.). Harrisburg, PA: Author.

National Consensus Project for Quality Palliative Care: Clinical practice guidelines for quality palliative care, executive summary (2004). *Journal of Palliative Care Medicine, 7*(5), 611–627.

National Council of State Boards of Nursing (NCSBN). (2008). Consensus model for APPN regulation: Licensure, accreditation, certification, and education. Chicago, IL: APPN Consensus Work Group and the APPN Joint Dialogue Group. Retrieved from http://www.nursingworld.org/consensusmodeltoolkit

Penticuff, J. H., & Arheart, K. L. (2005). Effectiveness of an intervention to improve parent-professional collaboration in neonatal intensive care. *Journal of Perinatal Neonatal Nursing, 19,* 187–202.

Pozo, P., Sarriá, E., & Brioso, A. (2013). Family quality of life and psychological well-being in parents of children with autism spectrum disorders: A Double ABCX Model. *Journal of Intellectual Disability Research.* Advance online publication. doi:10.1011/jir.12042

Quinn, C., & Bailey, M. E. (2011). Caring for children and families in the community: Experiences of Irish palliative care clinical nurse specialists. *International Journal of Palliative Care, 17*(11), 561–567.

Ravindran, N., & Myers, B. J. (2012). Cultural influences of health, illness, and disability: A review and focus on autism. *Journal of Child and Family Studies, 21*(2), 311–319. doi:10.1007/s10826–011-9477–9

Richter, M. S., Mill, J., Muller, C. E., Kahwa., E., Etowa, J., Dawkins, P., & Hepburn, C. (2013). Nurses' engagement in AIDS policy development. *International Nursing Review, 60*(1), 52–58. doi:10.1111/j1466–7657.2012.01010.x

Sawicki, G. S., Lukens-Bull, K., Yin, X., Demars, N., Huang, I. C., Livingood, W.,… & Wood, D. (2011). Measuring the transition readiness of youth with special healthcare needs: Validation of the TRAQ—Transition Readiness Assessment Questionnaire. *Journal of Pediatric Psychology, 36*(2), 160–171.

Thacker, K., & Long, J. (2010). Presence in final moments: A precious gift. *Journal of Christian Nursing, 27,* 38–42.

Thornlow, D. K., Auerhahn, C., & Stanley, J. (2006). A necessity not a luxury: Preparing advanced practice nurses to care for older adults. *Journal of Professional Nursing, 22*(2), 116–122.

U.S. Department of Health and Human Services, Health Resources and Services Administration, Maternal and Child Health Bureau. (2008). *The National Survey of Children with Special Health Care Needs chartbook 2005–2006.* Rockville, MD: U.S. Department of Health and Human Services.

Vooght, S., & Richardson, A. (1996). Community oncology. A study to explore the role of a community oncology nurse specialist. *European Journal of Cancer Care, 5*(4), 217–224.

Wittenberg-Lyles, E., Goldsmith, J., & Ragan, S. L. (2010). The COMFORT Initiative: Palliative nursing and the centrality of communication. *Journal of Hospice and Palliative Nursing, 12*(5), 282–292. doi:10.1097/NJH.0b013e3181ebb45e

Wright, K., & Myint, A. S. (2003). The colorectal cancer clinical nurse specialist in chemotherapy. *Hospital Medicine, 64*(6), 333–336.

Community as Client: Clinical Nurse Specialist Role

Naomi E. Ervin

The specialty of *community health nursing* was titled *public health nursing* until the late 1960s (Freeman, 1970; Sullivan, 1984). Recently, members of the specialty are encouraging a return to this original title to better reflect the focus of the specialty on the community or population. Defined as a synthesis of knowledge from nursing and social and public health sciences (American Public Health Association [APHA], 1996), public health nursing may be practiced in any setting. The hallmark of the practice is prevention of illness and injury toward improvement of the health of communities or populations.

In early public health nursing textbooks, the emphasis was on the community (Freeman, 1950). In a later book, Freeman (1970) stated, "The purpose of community health nursing is to further community health through the selective application of nursing and public health measures within the framework of the total community health effort" (p. 31). The focus on the community has been expanded and refined over the decades but remains essentially true to the original focus. This chapter provides an overview of the historical, theoretical, conceptual, and ethical background and foundations of advanced public/community health nursing practice. In particular, the chapter focuses on the public health/community health clinical nurse specialist (CNS) role in working with the community as client, offering extensions/interpretations of the NACNS (2004) competencies when the community is the client rather than an individual.

HISTORICAL BACKGROUND

In 1948, Esther Lucile Brown issued a report calling for the incorporation of public health nursing and related sciences into collegiate undergraduate curriculums (Brown, 1948). This recommendation was implemented in 1965, making public health nursing a required component of all undergraduate baccalaureate nursing programs. The implementation of this requirement for providing public/community health nursing programs resulted from the 1967 publication of a Western Interstate Council on Higher Education in Nursing (WICHEN) monograph series, one of which was about community health nursing. These documents provided a theoretical basis for practice through a conceptual framework based on key concepts from theories and practice (Sullivan, 1984).

Early in the development of the specialist level of public health nursing, master's programs were housed in schools of public health long before 1967. The trend to offer master's programs in schools of nursing began in the 1970s with phasing out of public health nursing master's level study in most schools of public health (Ervin, 2007). Because the first programs to prepare CNSs began in the 1950s in schools of nursing (National League for Nursing, 1958), public health nursing differed from the larger nursing profession at the inception of the specialty.

During the late 1970s and early 1980s, when public health nurse leaders were concerned about the focus of the specialty, a conference was planned to address the definition and title of the specialty. The Consensus Conference on the Essentials of Public Health Nursing Practice and Education was held in 1984 to define public health nursing and community health nursing and to identify education needed for generalist and specialist practice. The term *community health nurse* was referred to in the consensus document as an umbrella term for any nurse working in the community. A *community health nurse specialist* was defined as "a nurse with at least a master's degree in any area of nursing, such as maternal-child health, psychiatric-mental health or medical-surgical nursing or some sub-specialty of any clinical area" (U.S. Department of Health and Human Services, Consensus Conference, 1985, p. 4). A *public health nurse specialist* is prepared at the graduate level with a focus in the public health sciences. One recommendation from the Consensus Conference was that a certification examination be developed.

The differentiation between community health nursing and public health nursing has not been clearly identified by the profession. The title of the specialty continues to be in flux, as indicated in the introduction. A useful rubric for differentiating the specialty from practice in the community is to use the term *community-based nursing* as nursing in the community and *public/community health nursing* to refer to the specialty. In this chapter, the author uses the term *public/community health nursing* as the title of the specialty that focuses on care of the community or population.

Another step toward realization of a certification examination came with the development of standards of practice. The 1986 American Nurses Association's (ANA) *Standards of Community Health Nursing Practice* delineated differences between the generalist and the specialist. These standards identified the specialist's practice as care of the community. The certification examination for the clinical specialist in public/community health nursing was developed by a committee with representatives from both the ANA and the Public Health Nursing Section of the APHA. The examination was offered for the first time in October 1990. The original content areas of the certification examination closely approximated the essential content areas identified in the authoritative documents at that time, for example, epidemiology, biostatistics, community assessment and diagnosis, nursing theory, management theory, and research (ANA, 1986; U.S. Department of Health and Human Services, Consensus Conference, 1985; Selby, Riportella-Muller, Quade, Legault, & Salmon, 1990). The committee that developed the original certification examination was chaired by the author of this chapter.

The original standards of practice were revised by representatives of the Quad Council of Public Health Nursing Organizations, which is composed of the ANA, the Association of Community Health Nursing Educators (ACHNE), the Association of State and Territorial Directors of Nursing (now titled the APHN), and the Public Health Nursing Section of the APHA (Quad Council of Public Health Nursing Organizations, 1999). The 1999 document was deliberately titled public health nursing to more accurately reflect the definition of the specialty that was widely accepted at that time. Review of the 1999 scope and standards document was begun in 2004 with representation from the four member organizations of the Quad Council. The revised standards were published in 2007 (ANA, 2007). The revised scope and standards statement contains measurement criteria, which are indicators of competent practice, for both generalist and specialist roles. The scope and standards were revised again during the period 2010 to 2012 and published in 2013 (ANA, 2013).

The latest phase of the evolution of public/community health nursing is the changes in certification, which went into effect in January 2014. The certification examination for the CNS in public health nursing was retired at the end of 2013. Certification renewal will be available if the nurse meets the recertification requirements as listed in the certification booklet. ANCC will continue to offer certification of advanced public health nurses as a specialty, but only by a portfolio method after the end of 2013 (American Nurses Credentialing Center, 2013).

Public/community health nursing has almost always been defined as care of individuals, families, and communities (ANA, 1986; Freeman, 1950; Gardner, 1926). Care at the population level is paramount in advanced practice. Direct care of individuals and families is included in the scope of practice of the public/community health nurse generalist and specialist (ANA, 2013; Quad Council of Public Health Nursing Organizations, 1999).

THEORETICAL AND CONCEPTUAL BACKGROUND

The foundations of advanced practice are in the categories of philosophical, conceptual, and knowledge. A major philosophical framework for practice of the public/community health nurse specialist is social justice (Ervin, 2002a). Complementary to social justice is the field of environmental justice, which focuses on fair treatment of populations under laws, policies, and regulations about the environment (Institute of

Medicine [IOM], 1999). Among the major concepts included in advanced community health nursing practice are nursing, public health, primary prevention, health promotion, population focus, community, autonomy, and interprofessional practice (Ervin, 2002a). The public health sciences particularly include biostatistics, epidemiology, and environmental health. Theoretical foundations are found in the areas of, but not limited to, health behavior, health promotion, disease and injury prevention, health education, demography, and ecology.

Several models of practice at the advanced level have been developed and are described in the literature. The most prevalent models are community as client (Anderson & McFarlane, 1988), community as partner (Anderson & McFarlane, 2010), Helvie's energy theory (1998), and the Integrative Model for Holistic Community Health Nursing (Laffrey & Kulbok, 1999).

The focus of care is the community or population for the clinical specialist in public/community health nursing. The core processes used at the advanced practice level are community assessment, program planning, program implementation, and program evaluation (Ervin, 2002a).

The Core Competencies for Public Health Nursing (Quad Council of Public Health Nursing Organizations, 2012), based on the public health competencies developed by the Council on Linkages (Council on Linkages between Academia and Public Health Practice, 2010), provided added clarification for the specialist role. The public health competencies are general and apply to all categories of public health workers. A task group of representatives of the Quad Council (2012) used the public health competencies to delineate competencies at three levels or tiers: basic or generalist level (Tier 1), specialist or midlevel (Tier 2), and executive and/or multisystems level (Tier 2). The document spells out the competencies expected of the CNS in public/community health nursing, which fits within the Tier 2 level of practice.

The title *clinical specialist* in public/community health nursing has not been widely adopted by practice settings. An informal review of local health department websites revealed little use of the title. Position titles listed were director, consultant, supervisor, coordinator, and public health nurse. More striking is that the term *community health nurse* is used instead of *public health nurse* in some state and local health departments (Ervin, 2007).

Whatever model is employed by advanced practice public/community health nurses, the paradigm of multiple determinants of health remains a constant. Health and disease are outcomes of complex factors referred to as multiple determinants of health (Evans, Barer, & Marmor, 1994). This paradigm is becoming more accepted as scientists discover causes of health and disease previously unknown or understood differently. New knowledge has helped us to understand that the physical environment has a much greater effect on health and disease than we believed in previous centuries. The evidence about the physical environment and its relationship to the human condition is also becoming more accepted (IOM, 1995, 1999).

APPLICATION TO CNS PRACTICE

The National Association of Clinical Nurse Specialists' (NACNS) *Statement on CNS Practice and Education* (2004) is not a natural fit with all aspects of advanced public/community health nursing practice. On the one hand, the competencies are worded to be directed primarily at care of individuals, but this section provides interpretation of the patient/client sphere of influence that fits with the community as client. On the other hand, the statement on CNS practice does not contain all aspects of CNS practice that are key to competent advanced public/community health nursing practice. Broad areas that have been omitted are included in this section. Components related to systems and staff education are universally compatible with all specialties of CNS practice.

Patient/Client Sphere of Influence

The major goals of public/community health nursing are to prevent disease and injury and to promote health of communities and populations. These goals contrast with the goal of CNSs in other specialties: "to decrease or prevent symptoms/suffering and improve functioning" (NACNS, 2004, p. 18). CNS services may also be sought by patients or clients to maintain or improve health by modifying risk behaviors and increasing health-promoting lifestyles. One major difference between the goals of public/community health clinical nurse specialists (P/CHCNSs) and CNSs in other specialties is the client: the community vs. the individual or family.

As emphasized elsewhere in this chapter, the patient/client of the P/CHCNS is the community or population under the jurisdiction of a P/CHCNS's responsibility. For example, in a local health department, the P/CHCNS may be responsible for the residents of a specific county, which could contain a few thousand to a few million residents. The ability to "take care" of thousands of individuals has been questioned. The P/CHCNS does not take care of each individual, but organizes programs, services, collaboratives, and/ or partnerships to meet protection, prevention, and health promotion gaps in services not provided by other sectors of the community (IOM, 1988).

Services made available to a community through an agency with P/CHCNSs are not just in a community but are part of that community. This means that the P/CHCNS develops outreach activities to take services to people and does not wait until people come to a facility. For example, a community nursing center may hold an immunization day at a local elementary school or Women, Infants, and Children (WIC) program site. WIC is a federal program that provides grants to states for supplemental foods, health care, referrals, and nutrition education for low-income pregnant, breast-feeding, and non-breast-feeding postpartum women and to infants and children up to age 5 who are at nutritional risk (Food & Nutrition Service, U.S. Department of Agriculture [USDA], n.d.).

The first core competency listed in the NACNS statement is "Use knowledge of differential illness diagnoses and treatments in comprehensive, holistic assessments of patients within the context of disease, diagnoses, and treatments" (NACNS, 2004, p. 25). The language of disease and treatments is not a good match with the words used to define competencies of P/CHCNSs. For competent community practice, advanced practice nurses need knowledge of community diagnoses and interventions, which may equate to treatments, at the community and/or population levels; nevertheless, the term *treatments* conveys more of a connotation to care of ill individuals.

The basis for developing programs and services is a community assessment. The outcome of such an activity is comparable to the assessment done on an individual patient: a diagnosis. In public/community health nursing, the diagnosis is at the community or population level and is labeled community diagnosis or community health diagnosis (Ervin, 2002a; Muecke, 1984; Neufeld & Harrison, 1990). Diagnoses serve the same purpose at the individual or community level: to provide the focus for identifying the intervention or potential interventions to address the diagnosis or problem.

As with a diagnosis about an individual, identifying the cause of the community diagnosis is a necessary step in order for an appropriate intervention to be determined or developed. Evidence-based interventions are a necessary component of the P/CHCNS's practice for effectiveness and for achieving desired outcomes. Causes of problems or conditions at the community level are numerous. The evidence to determine what is the cause or causes of a specific diagnosis must be obtained after the community assessment process is completed, if not collected during the process. Infant mortality is one example of a problem that has multiple causes, for

example, sudden infant death syndrome (SIDS), low birth weight, birth injury, and congenital anomalies. With the details about the factors related to infant mortality in a specific community, the P/CHCNS can explore the research about specific interventions to decrease infant mortality. For example, if the leading cause of infant mortality in a specific community is low birth weight, then the risk factors for low birth weight have to be explored. Low birth weight due to poor maternal nutrition may require a much different intervention than low birth weight related to young maternal age.

For P/CHCNS practice, interventions are embedded in programs or services delivered to an aggregate or community in need of such actions (Ervin, 2002a). For example, if statistics demonstrate a low rate of immunization among specific members of a population or community, the intervention of immunizations must be delivered in a program designed to reach children and adults in need of immunizations. The outreach program must be tailored to reach such members of a community in order to protect not only the specific individuals but also the total community against outbreaks of preventable diseases. Immunizations for adults also decrease costs to society and prevent deaths from preventable illnesses such as pneumonia among adults older than 65 years.

Interventions applied to ameliorate community diagnoses may be policy development and enforcement (Public Health Nursing Section, 2001). P/CHCNSs practice in an interprofessional mode in many practice settings, but they may also work with professional organizations to bring about policy changes. Policy development may be at a local, state, or national level. One example in which public health nurses have been involved for many years is legislation to prohibit smoking in public places. Other policy areas that require continued attention are access to health care, safety in the community, and surveillance.

Public/community health nursing practice is based on evidence (NACNS, 2004), but evidence-based interventions are not abundant. In a survey of local health departments, a large majority of agencies reported using evidence in practice, but most guidelines were from other public health agencies and not specific to nursing (Ervin, Bell, & Bickes, 2009). The most frequently used model for implementing evidence-based practice (EBP) in public/community health nursing is the Minnesota model (Public Health Nursing Section, 2001). The model, informally titled the "intervention wheel," integrates three components: the population basis of interventions, three levels of practice (community, systems, individual/family), and 17 public health interventions. *Interventions* are defined as "actions taken by public health nurses on behalf of individuals, families, systems, and communities to improve or protect health status" (Public Health Nursing Section, 2001, p. 1). Each intervention is described, and documentation is provided for the evidence base in the publication.

One example of an intervention employed by advanced practice public/community health nurses is coalition building. The intervention is aimed at promoting and developing alliances among organizations for a common purpose. Through this intervention, linkages are built, problems are solved, and local leadership is enhanced to address health concerns. Steps for coalition building include recruiting members, developing preliminary objectives and activities, convening the coalition, estimating needed resources, selecting a coalition structure, maintaining the coalition, and conducting continuous process and outcome evaluation (Public Health Nursing Section, 2001).

Nurses and Nursing Practice Sphere of Influence

Although the title of clinical specialist is not often used in public/community health nursing practice, the role of nurses with advanced preparation is often directed toward the sphere of influence of nurses and nursing practice. The titles *supervisor, director, coordinator,* and *inservice educator* have position descriptions with components related to this sphere of influence. Assisting public/community health nurses to become more effective is a major part of any public/community health nurse in an advanced role.

A preferred approach to developing the competencies of staff nurses is through the process of coaching (Ervin, 2005). Building on baccalaureate education, the P/CHCNS provides regular guidance for each nurse to emphasize strengths and focus on improving areas of less strength. The first activity for implementing a clinical coaching process is an assessment of the nurse's strengths and weaknesses. This assessment may be conducted in several ways, but a self-assessment should be part of the process. The P/CHCNS then schedules regular appointments with the nurse to discuss the assessment and develop objectives and a plan for achieving the objectives.

In public/community health nursing practice, most staff nurses have some preparation regarding care of the community, but the P/CHCNS can make great strides for team strength by working with each nurse individually as well as in group activities. For example, the basis of program planning is a community assessment. Most advanced practice public/community health nurses do not conduct community assessments by themselves; a group effort is generally needed to accomplish this task in a timely manner.

Furthermore, most staff nurses do not have time in their assignments to gather data and information unless they are given some direction about how to do so efficiently. The P/CHCNS plans the community assessment with the knowledge of team assignments, strengths, and time constraints for team members.

The evidence base for public/community health nursing comes from a variety of fields, such as epidemiology, health behavior, and health promotion. Many studies have identified effective interventions for various aggregates of the population. Agencies that base practice on evidence generally have policies, procedures, protocols, and guidelines for nurses' use (Ervin et al., 2009). The organizational approach to EBP is appropriate because each nurse could not possibly review research and other evidence and develop interventions to meet community needs (Ervin, 2002b).

Several resources are available for nurses to use in practicing from an evidence base. Among those already mentioned is the "intervention wheel" (Public Health Nursing Section, 2001). Also available for nurses' use are books on EBP (e.g., Brownson, Baker, Leet, & Gillespie, 2003; Melnyk & Fineout-Overholt, 2010), data-based articles about research findings, and research syntheses (e.g., Rice & Stead, 2004). Over 20 years of research supports the effectiveness of home visiting to pregnant, low-income women and their children (Olds, Henderson, Tatelbaum, & Chamberlin, 1986; Olds & Kitzman, 1990; Olds et al., 1997). P/CHCNSs locate resources about EBP so that the evidence base for practice is readily available in each agency.

In addition to the evidence base for practice in specific agencies, P/CHCNSs engage in lifelong learning to maintain and enhance competence (NACNS, 2004). Membership in professional organizations is one approach for accomplishing this goal. Several organizations provide opportunities for learning as well as leadership involvement. In addition to the NACNS and the ANA, associations specific to public/community health nursing are the Public Health Nursing Section of the APHA, the ACHNE, and the APHNs. Most states also have a public health association with a public health nursing section to address continuing education needs of public health nurses in the specific state.

Organization/System Sphere of Influence

Advanced practice public/community health nurses often hold positions that require them to have influence and control of organization or system activities, such as director of a community nursing center or director of public health nursing. Such positions of authority permit nurses to have more control over practice as well as the development of policies that support quality community care. However, many official agencies, such as local and state health departments, function within structures and policies determined outside the influence of the nursing department or service area (Turnock, 2011). For example, state regulations may dictate the perimeters of health department functions as well as the qualifications of directors of public/community health nursing at the local level. Some states require that local health departments meet accreditation criteria that may have been developed without nursing representation. In public health, advanced practice nurses may gain more influence in the organization/system sphere by serving on state boards of health, holding policy positions in the offices of state legislators and national congresspersons, and gaining appointment to state regulatory agencies.

One of the greatest constraints for practice in public official agencies often is the lack of funding for activities to benefit the community-at-large. Because most funding for official public health agencies comes from taxes, local voters often decide the fate of funding. Funding for local official agencies is also derived from state and federal funding, both of which are, in turn, derived from taxes. Advanced public/community health nurses are also involved in writing grants to generate funding.

For community nursing centers, the issue of sustainability is paramount as a focus for the P/CHCNS who establishes and practices in such a center (Glick & Kulbok, 2002; Krothe, 2002; Murphy, 1995). Revenue generated from third-party reimbursement is the second largest stream of revenue for P/CHCNS services. Because much of the focus for these services is prevention, reimbursement may not be abundantly available. Often, too, the population that needs prevention services is not insured or is underinsured.

EVALUATION

The basis for evaluation of the effectiveness of interventions by the P/CHCNS is the evaluation plan, which is developed as part of the program planning process. The evaluation plan puts forth explicit measurable outcomes. Some of the outcomes may be at the individual, family, group, aggregate, or community level. At times, outcomes may be identified at more than one level because of the type of intervention. For example, a smoking cessation program for pregnant women, may track not only the smoking cessation level in specific sessions attended by the women but also the percentage of women who reported smoking during pregnancy, by reviewing birth certificates. Each outcome measure is important to monitor the success of a long-term community program.

In evaluating the impact of interventions of the CNS in public/community health nursing, the ideal measures are those at the community or population level. Some common measures of population health include mortality, morbidity, infant mortality, and immunization levels (Valanis, 1999). However, these indicators of health at the community level are difficult to attribute to the actions of P/CHCNSs or to any one organization in the community, such as the local health department.

Program planning by the P/CHCNS provides a mechanism for the specialist to develop realistic measures of success for specific programs. The programs may be provided through local health departments or any other community-focused organization, such as a community nursing center, visiting nurse association, or community health center. Rather than measure outcomes for the total community, the P/CHCNS must develop outcome measures for the target population or community segment identified as in need of the service or intervention.

To determine if an intervention had an effect, the P/CHCNS must gather baseline data about the target population before the intervention is implemented. For example, the immunization level of 2-year-olds in a specific targeted geographical community was identified at 29% by the local health department. The P/CHCNS identified that the immunization level of 2-year-old children attending the community nursing center was also 29%. If resources allow for a program to reach all 2-year-old children in the community, the follow-up evaluation would have to survey all children in that community. The resources to conduct this type of intervention and evaluation are rarely available to community nursing centers. However, through chart audits, the nursing staff could identify the immunization levels of children who attended the nursing center. If children did not return to complete an immunization series, the P/CHCNS would need to include a portion of the intervention that called for follow-up by phone, e-mail, mailed reminder notices, home visits, or a combination of these methods for reaching parents.

One example of a project to improve outcomes was coordinated by the author working with a home health care agency. The program focused on improving outcomes for patients with heart failure. Patients who had home visits after the inservice education program for the nursing staff improved in several outcomes, including fewer hospitalizations, improved medication adherence, and more exercise (Ervin, Scrivener, & Simons, 2004).

Working with low-income communities is often the focus of P/CHCNSs. Examples of the outcomes focused upon in these communities are increasing the immunization levels of targeted groups such as homeless children, prevention and early detection and treatment of lead poisoning, and preventing low-birth-weight infants (Ervin, Nelson, & Sheaff, 1999). Other examples of improvements in a community's health can be seen in the work done by community nursing centers to provide care in low-income communities in various parts of the country. Numerous examples demonstrate that advanced practice nurses are among the vanguards in recognizing that barriers to health care create inequities that will not be solved by the government anytime soon (IOM, 2003; Murphy, 1995).

ADVANCED NURSING PRACTICE

Focus on the population or community for public/community health nursing practice is applicable at both the generalist and specialist levels. However, the specialist level encompasses the total spectrum of practice activities in providing leadership to nurses who practice at the generalist level. Knowledge and skills required to fulfill the specialist role are acquired at the master's or doctoral level. Baccalaureate nursing education provides the foundation for graduate study.

Interventions to address community or population issues are based on a broad array of knowledge about biostatistics, epidemiology, demography, health behavior, environmental health, and health policy as well as advanced nursing knowledge. The P/CHCNS is qualified to develop or adapt interventions and plan programs needed to implement the interventions. Generalist public/community health nurses are members of teams to implement the interventions. The scope and standards of practice delineate the criteria for both the generalist and specialist levels of practice (ANA, 2013).

Although the scope of practice for the generalist and specialist is a continuum, the public/community health nursing generalist in some agencies may provide care to individuals and families more than to total communities and populations. In order to maintain or enhance the health of a community, often interventions are carried out at the individual level, such as immunizations. Care at the individual level is not a negation of the community focus but part of the total scope of practice needed to achieve healthy communities.

ETHICAL CONSIDERATIONS

Advanced practice public/community health nurses embrace the Code of Ethics that applies to all nurses. The Code of Ethics makes reference to individuals as patients and specifically lists the community as a patient in the second edition (ANA, 2001). As outlined earlier, a major philosophical foundation and ethical orientation for advanced public/community health nursing practice is social justice. The original focus of public health nursing was care of indigent families, especially in the major cities of the United States (Sullivan, 1984). Even though public health nursing services were expanded to the total population in the early 20th century, the ethical ideals of the specialty have persisted.

Social justice calls for equal entitlement of all persons to basic aspects of a healthy life, such as health protection and minimum standards of income. This approach requires that the total society protect the public's health vs. the idea that the individual's lifestyle needs remediation (Beauchamp, 1999; Fry, 1985). Societal protection of health is mandatory if societies are to prosper because individuals cannot provide the infrastructure to support small and large communities with items such as clean air and water.

The greatest advancements in health have been made through public health measures such as control of communicable diseases and regulation of air, water, sewage treatment, and food quality. These and other public health measures have contributed greatly to the 30-year increase in the life span seen in the 20th century (Brownson et al., 2003). Without an investment in the public health approach that the public's right to safe water, air, food, and environment is greater than the market approach (Shi & Singh, 2008), the United States would not have as high a standard of living as it now enjoys. If individuals purchased what each could afford, millions of individuals and families would live in squalor. The U.S. society is not without inequities (Ervin & Bell, 2004), but society has made strides toward improving the environment and standard of living for millions of citizens and residents.

Advanced public/community health nurses are committed to achieving the *Healthy People 2020* objectives, which are focused on four overarching goals: (1) "attain high quality, longer lives free of preventable disease, disability, injury, and premature death"; (2) "achieve health equity, eliminate health disparities, and improve the health of all groups"; (3) "create social and physical environments that promote health for all"; and (4) "promote quality of life, healthy development, and healthy behaviors across all life stages" (U.S. Department of Health and Human Services, 2010, n.p.). Achieving the *Healthy People 2020* goals and objectives is in part dependent upon access to health services. P/CHCNSs work toward improving access to services through various interventions, for example, developing community nursing centers, promoting equity in access to services, and improving health care coverage through legislation. Assessing access to health services includes ethical questions about who has access and why (Bambas & Casas, 2003).

Research over the past several decades has demonstrated that medical care is not the most important factor in improving health and length of life. Improving social and environmental determinants of health is necessary in order to see appreciable improvements in health, well-being, and length of life. Most notable of the social determinants of health are income and education (Evans et al., 1994; Lantz, Golberstein, House, & Morenoff, 2010; Lantz & Pritchard, 2010).

■ DISCUSSION QUESTIONS

- What advanced public/community health nursing practice conceptual frameworks are commonly found in the literature? Describe one of them.
- How has society influenced the development of advanced public/community health nursing practice?
- How do public/community health nursing and community-based nursing differ?
- What place does social justice have in advanced public/community health nursing practice?
- How does the Code of Ethics for nurses compare with the social justice orientation?

■ ANALYSIS AND SYNTHESIS EXERCISES

- For a specific geographical community, locate vital statistics about the population and compare and contrast with the state and national vital statistics for the same time period.
- Gather data about the leading causes of death for a specific geographical community, and formulate one community diagnosis. Use comparisons with the state and U.S. statistics.
- Locate environmental standards for air and water quality. Analyze the data about air and water quality for a specific community using the standards.
- Identify the location of toxic sites in a specific geographical community. Compare morbidity and mortality data for the populations who live near these sites with state and national morbidity and mortality data for selected conditions, for example, asthma, cancer, or premature births.

■ CLINICAL APPLICATIONS

- Interview three key leaders of a specific community to gain their perspectives on the leading community problems.
- Identify the three leading health problems or potential problems in a given community.
- Compare the three leading health problems identified for a specific community with the focus of the major health care providers in the community.

REFERENCES

American Nurses Association (ANA). (2001). *Code of ethics for nurses with interpretive statements.* Washington, DC: American Nurses Publishing.

American Nurses Association (ANA). (2007). *Public health nursing: Scope and standards of practice.* Silver Spring, MD: Author.

American Nurses Association (ANA). (2013). *Public health nursing: Scope and standards of practice* (2nd ed.). Silver Spring, MD: Nursesbooks org.

American Nurses Association (ANA), Council of Community Health Nurses. (1986). *Standards of community health nursing practice.* Kansas City, MO: Author.

American Nurses Credentialing Center. (2013). *2013 certification renewal requirements.* Retrieved from www.nursecredentialing.org/RenewalRequirements.aspx

American Public Health Association (APHA), Public Health Nursing Section. (2013). *Definition and practice of public health nursing.* Retrieved from http://www.apha.org/membergroups/sections/aphasections/phn/

Anderson, E. T., & McFarlane, J. M. (1988). *Community as client: Application of the nursing process.* Philadelphia, PA: Lippincott.

Anderson, E. T., & McFarlane, J. M. (2010). *Community as partner: Theory and practice in nursing* (6th ed.). Philadelphia, PA: Lippincott Williams & Wilkins.

Bambas, A., & Casas, J. A. (2003). Assessing equity in health: Conceptual criteria. In R. Hofrichter (Ed.), *Health and social justice: Politics, ideology, and inequity in the distribution of disease* (pp. 321–334). San Francisco, CA: Jossey-Bass.

Beauchamp, D. E. (1999). Public health as social justice. In D. E. Beauchamp & B. Steinbock (Eds.), *New ethics for the public's health* (pp. 101–109). New York, NY: Oxford University Press.

Brown, E. L. (1948). *Nursing for the future.* New York, NY: Russell Sage Foundation.

Brownson, R. C., Baker, E. A., Leet, T. L., & Gillespie, K. N. (2003). *Evidence-based public health.* New York, NY: Oxford University Press.

Council on Linkages Between Academia and Public Health Practice. (2010). *Core competencies for public health professionals.* Retrieved from http://www.phf.org/programs/corecompetencies

Ervin, N. E. (2002a). *Advanced community health nursing practice: Population-focused care.* Upper Saddle River, NJ: Prentice Hall.

Ervin, N. E. (2002b). Evidence-based nursing practice: Are we there yet? *Journal of the New York State Nurses Association, 33*(2), 11–16.

Ervin, N. E. (2005). Clinical coaching: A strategy for enhancing evidence-based nursing practice. *Clinical Nurse Specialist, 19*(6), 296–301.

Ervin, N. E. (2007). Clinical specialist in community health nursing: Advanced practice fit or misfit? *Public Health Nursing, 24*(5), 458–464.

Ervin, N. E., & Bell, S. E. (2004). Social justice issues related to uneven distribution of resources. *Journal of the New York State Nurses Association, 35*(1), 8–13.

Ervin, N. E., Bell, S. E., & Bickes, J. T. (2009). Evidence-based nursing practice in local public health. *Michigan Journal of Public Health, 3*(1), 33–46.

Ervin, N. E., Nelson, L. L., & Sheaff, L. (1999). Preventing adverse outcomes: A population focus. *Journal of Nursing Care Quality, 13*(6), 25–31.

Ervin, N. E., Scrivener, K., & Simons, T. (2004). Using the linkage model for integrating evidence into nursing practice. *Home Healthcare Nurse, 22*(9), 606–611.

Evans, R. G., Barer, M. L., & Marmor, T. R. (Eds.). (1994). *Why are some people healthy and others not?* New York, NY: Aldine de Gruyter.

Freeman, R. B. (1950). *Public health nursing.* Philadelphia, PA: Saunders.

Freeman, R. B. (1970). *Community health nursing practice.* Philadelphia, PA: Saunders.

Fry, S. T. (1985). Individual vs. aggregate good: Ethical tension in nursing practice. *International Journal of Nursing Studies, 22*(4), 303–310.

Gardner, M. S. (1926). *Public health nursing* (2nd ed.). New York, NY: Macmillan.

Glick, D. F., & Kulbok, P. A. (2002). Revising programs. In N. E. Ervin, *Advanced community health nursing practice: Population-focused care* (pp. 451–462). Upper Saddle River, NJ: Prentice Hall.

Helvie, C. O. (1998). *Advanced practice nursing in the community.* Thousand Oaks, CA: Sage.

Institute of Medicine (IOM). (1988). *The future of public health.* Washington, DC: National Academies Press.

Institute of Medicine (IOM). (1995). *Nursing, health, & the environment.* Washington, DC: National Academies Press.

Institute of Medicine (IOM). (1999). *Toward environmental justice.* Washington, DC: National Academies Press.

Institute of Medicine (IOM). (2003). *Unequal treatment: Confronting racial and ethnic disparities in healthcare.* Washington, DC: National Academies Press.

Krothe, J. S. (2002). Monitoring program implementation. In N. E. Ervin, *Advanced community health nursing practice: Population-focused care* (pp. 349–369). Upper Saddle River, NJ: Prentice Hall.

Laffrey, S. C., & Kulbok, P. A. (1999). An integrative model for holistic community health nursing. *Journal of Holistic Nursing, 17*(1), 88–103.

Lantz, P. M., Golberstein, E., House, J., & Morenoff, J. (2010). Socioeconomic and behavioral risk factors for mortality in a national 19-year prospective study of U.S. adults. *Social Sciences and Medicine, 70*(10), 1558–1566.

Lantz, P. M., & Pritchard, A. (2010). Socioeconomic indicators that matter for population health. *Preventing Chronic Disease, 7*(4), A74. Retrieved from http://www.cdc.gov/pcd/issues/2010/jul/09 0246.htm

Melnyk, B. M., & Fineout-Overholt, E. (2010). *Evidence-based practice in nursing & healthcare: A guide to best practice* (2nd ed.). Philadelphia, PA: Lippincott Williams & Wilkins.

Muecke, M. A. (1984). Community health diagnoses in nursing. *Public Health Nursing, 1*(1), 23–25.

Murphy, M. (Ed.). (1995). *Nursing centers: The time is now.* New York, NY: National League for Nursing Press.

National Association of Clinical Nurse Specialists (NACNS). (2004). *Statement on clinical nurse specialist practice and education* (2nd ed.). Harrisburg, PA: Author.

National League for Nursing. (1958). *The educational preparation of the clinical nurse specialist in psychiatric nursing.* New York, NY: Author.

Neufeld, A., & Harrison, M. J. (1990). The development of nursing diagnoses for aggregates and groups. *Public Health Nursing, 7*, 251–255.

Olds, D. L., Eckenrode, J., Henderson, C. R., Jr., Kitzman, H., Powers, J., Cole, R., et al. (1997). Long-term effects of home visitation on maternal life course and child abuse and neglect. Fifteen-year follow-up of a randomized trial. *Journal of the American Medical Association, 278*(8), 637–643.

Olds, D. L., Henderson, C. R., Jr., Tatelbaum, R., & Chamberlin, R. (1986). Improving the delivery of prenatal care and outcomes of pregnancy: A randomized trial of nurse home visitation. *Pediatrics, 77*(1), 16–28.

Olds, D. L., & Kitzman, H. (1990). Can home visitation improve the health of women and children at environmental risk? *Pediatrics, 86*(1), 108–116.

Public Health Nursing Section. (2001). *Public health interventions: Applications for public health nursing practice.* St. Paul: Minnesota Department of Health.

Quad Council of Public Health Nursing Organizations. (1999). *Scope and standards of public health nursing practice.* Washington, DC: American Nurses Publishing.

Quad Council of Public Health Nursing Organizations. (2012). *Core competencies for public health nursing.* Retrieved from http://www.achne.org/Quad%20Council/QuadCouncilCompetenciesforPublicHealthNurses.pdf

Rice, V. H., & Stead, L. F. (2004). Nursing interventions for smoking cessation. *Cochrane Database Systematic Reviews, 1*, CD001188.

Selby, M. L., Riportella-Muller, R., Quade, D., Legault, C., & Salmon, M. E. (1990). Core curriculum for master's community health nursing education: A comparison of the views of leaders in service and education. *Public Health Nursing, 7*(3), 150–160.

Shi, L., & Singh, D. A. (2008). *Delivering health care in America* (4th ed.). Sudbury, MA: Jones & Bartlett.

Sullivan, J. A. (Ed.). (1984). *Directions in community health nursing.* Boston, MA: Blackwell.

Turnock, B. J. (2011). *Public health: What it is and how it works* (5th ed.). Sudbury, MA: Jones & Bartlett.

U.S. Department of Agriculture (USDA), Food & Nutrition Service. (n.d.). *Women, infants, and children.* Retrieved from www.fns.usda.gov/wic

U.S. Department of Health and Human Services. (1985). *Consensus conference on essentials of public health and nursing practice and education.* Rockville, MD: U.S. Department of Health and Human Services, Bureau of Health Professions, Division of Nursing.

U.S. Department of Health and Human Services. (2010). *Healthy people 2020: Improving the health of Americans.* Retrieved from www.healthypeople.gov/2020/default.aspx

Valanis, B. (1999). *Epidemiology in health care* (3rd ed.). Stamford, CT: Appleton & Lange.

Population-Based Data Analysis

Ann L. Cupp Curley

There is increasing awareness among health care professionals of the importance of population-based care. Problems are defined (diagnoses) and solutions proposed (interventions) for defined populations or subpopulations. While clinical decision making related to individual patients is important, it has little impact on overall health outcomes for populations. Conversely, population strategies have the potential to impact the health and the health care–related activities of large groups of people. Clinical nurse specialists (CNSs) are educated to provide evidence-based care to specialty populations. These populations may be defined by the demographic characteristics of the population, the setting or environment, the type of care required, or the diagnosis (National Association of Clinical Nurse Specialists [NACNS], 2004). The focus of population-based care is on populations at risk, comparison groups, and demographic factors. It is concerned with the patterns of delivery of care and outcomes measurement at the population or subpopulation level.

How can we improve the quality of care for our patients by taking a population-based care approach? If we altered how we define our population, how would the care we provide differ, and who would benefit from this difference? What would be the cost benefit of changing how we provide individual care based on a deeper understanding of population health needs? These are questions that the CNS encounters in everyday practice. Successful CNS practice depends on the ability to recognize the difference between the individual and population approaches to

the collection and use of data and the ability to assess needs and evaluate outcomes at the population level. This chapter provides the CNS with the tools to be able to follow a critical chain of evidence and avoid the pitfalls of faulty inference in population analysis.

BACKGROUND

The historical evolution of epidemiology and public health provides a background for an understanding of the population approach to patient care. The publication of Farr's "Vital statistics" in J. R. McCullach's *A Statistical Account of the British Empire* in 1837 laid the foundation for the use of vital statistics in public health. Up until the 19th century, appeals for public health reform were based on subjective information and were dependent on emotional appeal. Vital statistics supplied public health reformers with objective data and the ability to support their requests for reform with facts and figures. For example, using information that he gathered on cholera victims, Snow compared the incidence rates for cholera in one water district with those in another to support his hypothesis that cholera resulted from the contamination of water supplies. Perhaps one of the earliest documented examples of evidence-based practice (EBP) occurred in 1854 when the handle of the contaminated well in London was removed, resulting in a sharp decrease in the incidence rate for cholera and the end of an epidemic.

Florence Nightingale was educated in arithmetic, geometry, and algebra. During the Crimean War, she used statistical analysis to plot the incidence of preventable deaths among British soldiers. She created a diagram to dramatize the unnecessary deaths caused by unsanitary conditions and the need for reform. After the Crimean War, Nightingale worked with Farr to standardize data collection and classification in hospitals. This work led to the development of her Model Hospital Forms. She used the standardized data to support her crusade for hospital reform, especially improvements in sanitation (Dossey, 2000). With her analysis, Florence Nightingale revolutionized the idea that social phenomena could be objectively measured and subjected to mathematical analysis. She was one of the earliest health care practitioners to collect and analyze data in order to persuade people of the need for change. Her work in medical statistics led to her election in 1858 to the Statistical Society of England (Dossey, 2000; Lipsey, 1993).

Since Farr and Nightingale, the use of statistics in public health has expanded and become more sophisticated. Statistics are now used to explain the linkages between many different variables and health and disease. The Framingham Heart Study is one of the most important population studies ever carried out in the United States and provides an example of how the methods pioneered by early practitioners such as Farr and Nightingale can be effectively employed. In 1948, researchers recruited the original cohort of 5,209 men and women between the ages of 30 and 62 from the town of Framingham, Massachusetts. It was through the monitoring over time of these participants that the variables associated with cardiovascular disease were identified. The idea that individuals could modify *risk factors* (a term coined by the study) tied to heart disease, stroke, and other diseases originated with the Framingham Heart Study. Still in operation, a fourth cohort of participants was enrolled in 2003. The study has generated more than 1,000 scientific papers to date (National Heart, Lung and Blood Institute [NHLBI] & Boston University, 2013).

The Nurses Health Study was established in 1976 with funding from the National Institutes of Health (NIH). The primary goal was to investigate the potential long-term consequences of the use of oral contraceptives, but the goal has since expanded to include the investigation of other diseases and conditions. Every 2 years cohort members receive a questionnaire about diseases and health-related topics, including smoking, hormone use, and menopausal status. It has also expanded to include investigations into the risk factors for major chronic diseases in women. The Nurses Health Study has made many contributions to the understanding of women's health. It was through this study that it was discovered that women who used estrogen plus testosterone to reduce postmenopausal symptoms were about twice as likely to develop breast cancer as women who had never used postmenopausal hormones. A point of interest is that nurses were originally chosen for the study because investigators believed that nurses would be highly likely to respond to the surveys and not drop out of the study. This has proven true, as response rates have been consistently high and the mortality rate due to participant dropout is low (Harvard Medical School, 2013).

The work of Farr, Snow, Nightingale, and others laid the foundation of today's studies; however, statistics must be used with caution. Health is a multidimensional variable—factors that affect health, and that interact to affect health, are numerous. Many relationships are possible. There are problems inherent in the use of statistics to explain differences between groups. Although statistics can *describe* disparities, they cannot *explain* them. It is left to the researchers to explain the *differences*. In addition to the problem of using statistics to explain differences, one must also be aware of the validity and reliability of the data. There are problems associated with the categorizing and gathering of statistics during the research process that can have an effect on how the data should be interpreted. In order to formulate change, one must do more than just collect data; one must look at the theoretical issues associated with explaining the relationship between the variables. Practice must clearly indicate a commitment to high standards for research, with an emphasis placed on adherence to careful and thorough procedure and ethical practice.

ISSUES IN POPULATION-BASED ANALYSIS

Population strategies are used to identify populations at risk and to evaluate interventions at the population level. When evaluating data at the population level, it is important to avoid ecologic fallacy. An ecologic fallacy occurs when an observed association in a population is assumed to exist on an individual level. For example, higher rates of falls are seen in elderly populations than in younger populations. Polypharmacy also occurs at higher rates in elderly populations, so we might be tempted to believe that polypharmacy is responsible for the higher rates of falls. However, we cannot conclude that whenever an elderly individual falls it is due to polypharmacy. Population-based evaluation and planning depend on understanding the many and varied factors that influence health and disease. Statistics alone cannot explain relationships between variables or differences among groups. The

CNS should make use of the sound investigative principles and a broad theoretical perspective to interpret the results. When a clinical problem is identified, one of the next steps is a systematic review of the literature to discover what is already known about the issue.

Another potential difficulty in population research is that indirect associations can appear causal. An indirect relationship occurs when a factor and an attribute seem to be related only because of some underlying common condition. A classic example occurred when Farr detected an inverse relationship between cholera and altitude. This finding seemed to support the then commonly held belief that cholera was caused by bad air or *miasmas*. In fact, cholera deaths occurred more frequently at low-lying altitudes because the water was less pure in these areas. When a factor appears to be causally linked to a health problem, additional studies and further scrutiny are warranted in order to rule out alternative explanations.

PRINCIPLES OF POPULATION-BASED ANALYSIS

The five basic principles of the population approach to care described by Ibrahim, Savitz, Carey, and Wagner (2001) provide a framework for the CNS in the area of population-based evaluation. These principles include the following: a community perspective, a clinical epidemiology perspective, EBP, an emphasis on prevention, and an emphasis on outcomes.

The *community perspective* refers to the collection of data related to the frequency of disease, disability, and death in a population and the number of people in the population of interest. This information allows the CNS to calculate rates. The evaluation of outcome measures in populations begins with an identification of the totality of health problems, the needs of defined populations, and the differences among groups. The rates calculated from these numbers can help the CNS target populations at risk and supply the evidence for changes in clinical practice.

The *clinical epidemiology perspective* refers to the need to manage all patients with similar needs or problems—congestive heart failure patients, for example, or dependent elderly people being cared for at home. The care of specialized groups is the core of CNS practice.

EBP is a principle of population-based health care and one of the core competencies of CNS and basic nursing practice (American Nurses Association [ANA], 2010; NACNS, 2004). EBP is "a problem-solving approach to the delivery of health care that integrates the best evidence from studies and patient care data with clinician expertise and patient preferences and values" (Gallagher-Ford, Fineout-Overholt, Melnyk, & Stillwell, 2011, p. 54). Quality and cost-effectiveness are also important considerations in EBP. The basic sciences of public health (particularly epidemiology and biostatistics) provide tools for the CNS working with specialized populations to provide evidence for effective interventions.

Prevention can also best be carried out at the population level. For example, a falls prevention program within a hospital can lead to decreased injuries and related costs. Interventions that are appropriate at the individual level and applied at the population level can result in widespread change.

Outcomes measurement refers to collecting and analyzing data using predetermined outcomes indicators for the purposes of making decisions about health care (National Database of Nursing Quality Indicators [NDNQI], 2013). Outcomes research in CNS practice is research that focuses on the effectiveness of nursing interventions. Outcomes measurement in population-based care begins with the identification of the population and the problem, followed by the generation of a clinical question related to outcomes. An outcomes measure should be clearly quantifiable, relatively easy to define and diagnose, and lend itself to standardization.

In outcomes measurement, the CNS is ultimately concerned with whether or not a population benefits from an intervention (care). The CNS also needs to be concerned with the question of efficacy (does the intervention work under ideal conditions?) and effectiveness (does it work under real life situations?). Other important considerations are efficiency (cost–benefit), affordability, accessibility, and acceptability. The identification of outcomes is an important first step in planning interventions, and comparing outcomes before and after an intervention is an excellent way to evaluate effectiveness. Data obtained through outcomes measurement can provide evidence for needed change at local, regional, state, or national levels by identifying areas for improvement in practice (Oppewal, 2012).

POPULATION-BASED ANALYSIS FOR CNS PRACTICE

Methods derived from epidemiology can be used to identify the etiology or the cause of a disease and the risk factors, identify the impact of risk factors in a population, determine the extent of a disease and/or adverse events found in a population, evaluate both existing and new preventative and therapeutic measures and modes of health care delivery, and provide the foundation for developing public policy and making regulatory decisions.

Descriptive Epidemiology

Descriptive epidemiology is used to describe the distribution of disease and other health-related states and events in terms of personal characteristics, geographical distribution, and time. There are four types of descriptive studies: case reports, case series, correlation studies, and cross-sectional surveys. This chapter will focus on the use of correlation studies and cross-sectional surveys in population analyses. The data used in descriptive studies are often readily available—from hospital records, census data, or vital statistics records.

Correlation Studies

Correlation studies are also referred to as ecologic studies. Ecologic studies are used to conduct studies of group or population characteristics. In ecologic studies, rates are calculated for characteristics that describe populations and used to compare frequencies between different groups at the same time or the same group at different times. They are useful for identifying long-term trends, seasonal patterns, and event-related clusters. Because data are collected on populations instead of individuals, an event cannot be linked to an exposure in individuals, and the investigator cannot control for the effect of other variables (confounders). A confounder is a variable that is linked to both a causative factor and the outcome. A good example of a potential confounder is socioeconomic status. Low-income individuals may avoid treatments or choose suboptimal, inexpensive treatments because of cost. They may also experience poor outcomes due to stress or poor nutrition. A failure to account for socioeconomic status may therefore skew study results (Hoffman & Podgurski, 2013).

A study by Babones (2008) provides an illustration of a correlational study. The author used data from the *World Institute for Development Economics Research* to investigate the relationship between inequality and three population health outcomes (life expectancy, infant mortality, and murder rate) in more than 100 countries. The results of these analyses indicate that income inequality correlates negatively with population health. That is, populations in poorer countries experience poorer health, and populations in wealthier countries experience better health. The author points out that "the existence of a correlation between income inequality and population health does not, in itself, imply a causal relationship between the two variables" (p. 1623). These data indicate a relationship between the variables—but not a causal one. There are many possible explanations for the relationship, including (but not exclusively) cultural and social differences among the countries. Correlational studies can provide researchers with insight into a problem, as this one does, but it requires further study to understand why such a relationship exists.

Cross-Sectional Studies

In cross-sectional studies, both exposure to a factor and an outcome are determined simultaneously. They provide a "snapshot" at one point in time. One problem with cross-sectional studies is that the investigator is studying prevalent cases only—not new cases—and the cases may not be representative. They exclude people who have died, and temporal relationships are difficult to determine. Cross-sectional studies can be used to suggest possible risk factors and to identify prevalence rates, but they are not useful for evaluating interventions.

Scott (2013) conducted a cross-sectional study to identify the prevalence of risk factors for type 2 diabetes among school-age children (Grades 1 through 5) and to determine eligibility for type 2 diabetes screening. The 2010 American Diabetes Association guidelines were used to determine the percentage of students eligible for screening. The medical records of children enrolled in school-based health clinics in Kentucky public schools were reviewed for several variables associated with risk for developing type 2 diabetes, such as body mass index (BMI), family history of diabetes, and the presence of acanthosis nigricans. Of the students 10 years of age or older enrolled in this study, 39.3% were eligible for further screening for type 2 diabetes.

This study serves to illustrate both the advantages and the disadvantages of cross-sectional studies. There are problems inherent in using medical records for data collection, such as accuracy of information (measurement errors) and missing information. In this study, students with evidence of insulin resistance (such as hypertension or hyperlipidemia), while eligible for further type 2 diabetes screening, may have been missed because these measurements were not part of the required, school-based health screenings in Kentucky schools at the time of the study. On the other hand, a cross-sectional study is fairly quick and can be used to identify prevalence rates for specified populations, as this one did.

Rates

Knowledge of the distribution of illness and injury within a population can provide valuable information on etiology and can lay the foundation for the introduction of new interventions. Rates are a useful method of measuring attributes, illness, and injury in a specific population, and they can also be used to evaluate outcomes. Both low and high rates can provide useful information for the CNS.

The *Morbidity and Mortality Weekly Report (MMWR)* published by the Centers for Disease Control and Prevention (CDC) provides an example of how rates can be used to identify trends and provide policy makers with information for designating resources. The CDC surveys the incidence and prevalence of many diseases and conditions. These figures provide health care workers and policy makers with information on the risks and burden of various diseases and conditions. For example, the *MMWR* published in July of 2013 reveals that in 2010 the rate of deaths among women attributed to a drug overdose occurred at a rate of 9.8 per 100,000. Deaths from opioid pain relievers (OPRs) were five times higher in 2010 than in 1999 for women. During the same time period OPR deaths among men increased 3.6 times. Emergency department (ED) visits related to the misuse or abuse of OPR among women more than doubled between 2004 and 2010. The highest ED visit rates were for cocaine or heroin (147.2 per 100,000 population), benzodiazepines (134.6), and OPR (129.6). An important fact highlighted in this report is that "More women have died each year from drug overdoses than from motor vehicle–related injuries since 2007" (CDC, 2013b, July 5, p. 537). In addition to the usefulness mentioned earlier, these rates provide health care workers with important information to guide prescribing, alerts them to the need for the screening of patients' conditions that may lead to drug abuse, and highlights the need to use states' prescription drug monitoring programs.

In rates, the numerator is the number of events that occur during a specified period of time, and the denominator is the average population of interest during that time period. The numerator is divided by the denominator, then this number is multiplied by a constant: 100, 1,000, 10,000, or 100,000 and is expressed as per that number. Simply put, the rate is calculated as follows:

Rate = Numerator/Denominator × Constant Multiplier

In order to calculate rates, the CNS must first have a clear and explicit definition of the patient population and of the event. For a rate to make sense, anyone represented in the denominator must have the potential to enter the group in the numerator.

Rates can be either crude or specific. Crude rates apply to an entire population without any reference to any characteristics of the individuals in it. Crude mortality rate is an example. To calculate crude mortality, the numerator is all deaths during a specific period of time. The denominator is the number of people in the population of interest. Typically, the population number that is used is the population at midyear.

Specific rates can also be calculated. Specific rates are calculated after a population has been categorized into groups. Let us suppose that a CNS wants to calculate the yearly fall rate for patients 65 years of age and older who are on a particular unit. The formula would be as follows:

Total number of falls of patients 65 years of age and older during the specified year (numerator) divided by total number of patient days of patients 65 years of age and older for that unit during the year (denominator) × 100 = rate per 100

In order to compare rates in two or more groups, the events in the numerator must be defined in the same way, the time intervals must be the same, and the constant multiplier must be the same. Rates can be used to compare two different groups or one group during two different time periods. Returning to the example about falls, the fall rates could be compared on the same floor but at two different times, for instance, before and after implementation of a planned intervention.

Formulas for the rates discussed in this chapter, as well as many other useful examples, can be found in Table 17.1.

Incidence rates describe the occurrence of new events in a population over a period of time relative to the size of the population at risk. Prevalence rates are the number of all cases of a specific disease or attribute in a population at a given point in time relative to the size of the population at risk. Incidence provides information about the rate at which new cases occur. It is a measure of risk. The formula for the incidence rate for type 2 diabetes in a community is as follows:

Total number of people diagnosed with type 2 diabetes in a population during the year (numerator) divided by population at midyear (denominator) × 1,000 = rate per 1,000

Prevalence measures the amount of an existing problem during a specific time and is a measure of burden. The formula for the prevalence rate for type 2 diabetes during 1 year in a community is as follows:

Total number of people with type 2 diabetes in a population during the year (numerator) divided by population at midyear (denominator) × 1,000 = rate per 1,000

In the previous formula, all newly diagnosed cases for the year plus existing cases are included. It

TABLE 17.1

CALCULATING RATES		
Type	**Description**	
Incidence rates	Describe the occurrence of *new* disease cases in a community over a period of time relative to the size of the population at risk. *RISK* $\text{Incidence rate} = \dfrac{\text{Number of new cases during a specified period}}{\text{Population at risk during the same period}}$	× constant multiplier
Prevalence rates	Are the number of *all* cases of a specific disease in a population *at a given point in time* relative to the population at risk. *BURDEN* $\text{Prevalence rate} = \dfrac{\text{Number of existing cases at a specified time}}{\text{Population at risk at the same specific time}}$	× constant multiplier
Crude rates	Summarize the occurrence of births (crude birth rate) or deaths (crude death rate); the numerator is the number of events, and the denominator is the average population size. $\text{Crude death rate} = \dfrac{\text{Number of deaths in a population during a specified time}}{\text{Average population estimate during the specified time}}$	× constant multiplier
Specific rates	Used to overcome some of the biases seen with crude rates; used to control for variables such as age, race, gender, and disease. $\text{Age-specific death rate} = \dfrac{\text{Number of deaths for a specified age group during a specified time}}{\text{Population estimate for the specified age group}}$	× constant multiplier
Case fatality rates	Used to measure the percentage of people who die after diagnosis with a certain disease and within a certain time after diagnosis. $\dfrac{\text{Number of individuals dying during a specified period of time after disease onset or dx}}{\text{Population estimate for the specified age group}}$	× constant multiplier
Proportionate mortality ratio	Useful for determining the leading causes of death $\dfrac{\text{Number of deaths from a specified cause in the United States during specified time period}}{\text{Total deaths in the United States during the specified time}}$	× 100
Years of potential life lost (YPLL)	Used for setting health priorities; predetermined standard age at death in United States is 65 years. $\dfrac{65 - \text{age at death from a specific cause} = X}{\text{Add the years of life lost for each individual for specific cause of death} = \text{YPLL}}$	
Sensitivity	The ability of a screening test to identify accurately those persons with the disease $= TP/(TP + FN)$	
Specificity	Reflects the extent to which it excludes the persons who do not have the disease $= TN/(TN + FP)$	
Positive predictive value	$= TP/(TP + FP)$	
Negative predictive value	$= TN/(TN + FN)$	

FN, false negatives; FP, false positives; TN, true negatives; TP, true positives.

is important to note that undiagnosed cases are not captured in either prevalence rates or incidence rates.

The *National Health Interview Survey (NHIS)*, which is conducted annually by the U.S. Census Bureau, provides data with which to track the achievement of national health objectives. The 2011 report shows that the prevalence of diagnosed diabetes in the U.S. population has increased from 2.5 per 100 in 1980 to 6.9 per 100 in 2011, an increase of 175% (CDC, 2013a). Information on the rising incidence and prevalence of diabetes in the United States has led to increased attention to factors that cause diabetes (especially lifestyles) and programs targeted at primary prevention.

Incidence rates provide us with a direct measure of how often new cases occur within a particular population and provide some basis on which to assess risk. By comparing incidence rates among population groups who vary in one or more factor, the CNS can begin to get some idea of the association between a factor and risk. For example, taking the example on falls one step further, if the CNS compares the fall rates on two different floors and discovers that they are significantly different, the characteristics of the two floors can be compared and the etiology can be hypothesized.

The case fatality rate is often used to determine when to use a screening test and for evaluating acute, infectious diseases. It is a measure of the probability of death among diagnosed cases. Its usefulness for chronic diseases is limited because the length of time from diagnosis to death can be a long one. The formula is as follows:

The number of deaths due to the disease in a specified period of time divided by the number of cases of the disease in the same period of time × 100

The case fatality rate can provide health care professionals with information on how deadly a disease is.

Standardization of crude rates is an important consideration in ecologic studies. Standardization is used to control for the effects of age and other characteristics in order to make valid comparisons of rates. Age adjustment is an example of rate standardization and perhaps the most important one. No other factor has a bigger effect on health outcomes than age. Consider the problem of comparing two communities with very different age distributions. One community has a much higher mortality rate for cancer than the other one, leading investigators to consider a possible environmental hazard in that community, when in fact that community's aging population is the factor most responsible for the higher rate. Age adjustment allows a researcher to eliminate the problem of age differential and, thus, compare rates for health events across population groups or to assess changes in rates over time.

There are two methods of age adjustment: direct and indirect. The direct method applies observed age-specific rates to a standard population. The indirect method applies the age-specific rates of a standard population to the age distribution of an observed population.

As mentioned previously, rates can be used to describe the distribution of disease and other health-related states and events, but sometimes the CNS may be more concerned with knowing how data can be used to describe the relevancy of clinical practice. Health impact assessment is the assessment of the potential health effects, positive or negative, of a particular intervention on a population. The number needed to treat (NNT) statistic, the disease impact number (DIN), and the population impact number (PIN) are formulas that are used in health impact assessment. NNT is the number of patients needed to receive a treatment to prevent one bad outcome. DIN is the number of those with the disease in question among whom one event will be prevented by the intervention. PIN is the number of those in the whole population among whom one event will be prevented by the intervention. Years of potential life lost (YPLL) measures premature mortality, the productive years that are lost related to early death (Gordis, 2008).

More extensive information on health impact assessment formulas and standardization can be found in most advanced epidemiology texts. It is important for the CNS involved in population-based evaluation to be aware of these concepts.

Analytic Epidemiology

Analytic epidemiology looks at the origins and causal factors of diseases and other health-related events. These analyses are often carried out to test hypotheses formulated from a descriptive study. The goal of analytic epidemiology is to identify factors that increase or decrease risk. *Risk* is the probability that an event will occur. For example, a patient who smokes might ask the CNS, "What is the likelihood that I will get lung cancer if I continue to smoke?"

Although descriptive studies allow a basis for comparison and can provide the CNS with data to identify etiology and differences among groups, further studies must be carried out to determine the significance of a factor. To do this, the CNS can use comparison of exposed and nonexposed groups; comparison is an essential component of population studies. One design is the case–control study.

Case–Control Studies

In a case–control study, the CNS must first identify a group of individuals with the attribute of interest (cases). A second group is identified without the attribute of interest (controls). The proportion of those *cases* who were exposed to the suspected causal factor are then compared to the proportion of the cases who were not exposed, and the proportion of the *controls* who were exposed are compared to the proportion of the controls who were not exposed. The measure of the effect of exposure is expressed as an odds ratio (OR), which is the ratio of the odds of having been exposed if you are a case to the odds of having been exposed if you are a noncase. If the exposure is not related to the attribute, the OR will equal 1. If the exposure is related to the attribute, the OR will be less than 1.

In a case–control study, if there is an association of an exposure with an attribute, the prevalence of history of exposure should be higher in persons who have the attribute in cases than in controls. It is important to keep in mind that only a subset of the population will be at risk from a particular exposure—in other words, only a proportion of those exposed will become a case as a result of their exposure. The fact that an elderly individual is overmedicated may put that person at risk for a fall, but it does not mean that that person *will* fall. The calculation of the OR can tell the CNS something about the risk of exposure in becoming a case, but it does not calculate certainty.

There are some problems with case–control studies that the investigator must keep in mind. People in the groups are not randomly assigned; association may be the result of exposure to another, unknown, variable. The problem with randomization in case–control studies is that the investigator cannot always assign exposure to a variable randomly for ethical reasons.

Case–control studies can be used to study the effects of a practice or pattern of behavior that is not under the control of the researcher.

Selection of the sample is an important step in case–control studies. Definite criteria should be used so that there is no ambiguity about how to distinguish between a case and a control. Exposure is not always all or nothing. Controls should resemble the cases as closely as possible except for exposure to the factor under study. If the cases are drawn from a particular clinic, then ideally the controls should be drawn from the same clinic population. Matching is one method that can be used to select a sample so that potential confounders are distributed equally between the cases and controls. A good example would be if a CNS planned to evaluate the odds of falling if a patient is taking a certain class of drugs. It is known that some patients have a higher risk of falling than others. In general, for example, people who have problems with their eyesight, such as macular degeneration or cataracts, are at higher risk of falling than those who do not have those conditions. By matching for physical disabilities that may contribute to a fall, the CNS can eliminate potentially confounding variables. The problem with matching is that the investigator is not always aware of all of the potentially confounding factors, and it can be expensive and time consuming to match for multiple variables and to match each subject in a study.

Recall bias is also an important consideration in case–control studies. This can happen when people who experience an adverse outcome think over and remember the events leading up to the outcome. It makes it more likely that they will recall details that people who did not experience the adverse outcome will not. A woman who gives birth to a child with birth defects is more likely to remember every event leading up to and including birth than a woman who gives birth to a normal baby. This can lead to a false association between an event (such as a fall) and a birth defect.

Table 17.2 can be used to calculate an OR in a case–control study.

Cohort Studies

Cohort designs can be either prospective or retrospective. In a *prospective* cohort design, the investigator

TABLE 17.2

CALCULATION OF ODDS RATIO		
	CASES	**CONTROLS**
Exposure	a	b
No exposure	c	d
Totals	a + c	b + d
	Proportion of cases exposed = a/a + c	Proportion of controls exposed = b/b + d
Odds Ratio = ad/bc		

selects a group of individuals who were exposed to a factor and a group of nonexposed individuals and follows both groups to compare the incidence of an attribute (more than two groups can be compared in this design). In a *retrospective* cohort design, exposure is ascertained from past records and outcome is ascertained at the time the study begins. If an association exists between the exposure and the outcome, then the proportion of the incidence rate of the exposed group will be greater than the incidence in the nonexposed group. The ratio of these is the relative risk (RR), which is the incidence rate in the exposed divided by the incidence rate in the nonexposed. RR is the measure of the strength of an association between an exposure and a disease.

If the RR is equal to 1 (numerator equals the denominator), then the risk to the two groups is equal. If the RR is greater than 1 (numerator is greater than the denominator), the risk in the exposed groups is greater than the risk in the nonexposed group. If the RR is less than 1 (denominator is greater than the numerator), the risk in the exposed group is less than the risk in the nonexposed group.

Cohort studies are carried out when the investigator has good evidence that links an attribute to an outcome, when the time interval between exposure and the attribute is short, and when the outcome occurs relatively often.

A cohort study was carried out to ascertain the risks associated with hospitalization and delirium in people with Alzheimer disease (Fong et al., 2012). The study took place from January 1, 1991, to December 31, 2006. People diagnosed with Alzheimer disease who were hospitalized during this time period were compared to a cohort of people with the disease who were not hospitalized. A significant finding in this study was that those people who were hospitalized and who did not have delirium had an increased risk for death (adjusted RR, 4.7; 95% confidence interval [CI], [1.9, 11.6]) and institutionalization (adjusted RR, 6.9; CI, [4.0, 11.7]). With delirium, risk for death (adjusted RR, 5.4; CI, [2.3, 12.5]) and institutionalization (adjusted RR, 9.3; CI, [5.5, 15.7]) increased. The results provide health care providers with important information on the care of people with Alzheimer disease, particularly the importance of taking steps to prevent delirium in such patients.

One of the major problems with cohort studies is that they can be time consuming and expensive if the sample must be followed for any length of time. The longer the time period that people are followed, the more likely it is that participants will be lost for follow-up. This can lead to problems with calculating incidence rates. Recall that in the Nurses Health Study one reason for choosing nurses was because of the belief that they would have a low dropout rate. Cohort studies are not feasible if there is difficulty involved in identifying exposed versus nonexposed populations or when data for the subjects is incomplete or lacking. Table 17.3 can be used to calculate the RR in a cohort study.

Case–Control and Cohort Studies

It is important to understand that the difference between case–control and cohort studies is not a function of calendar time. In case–control studies the investigator begins with people who have the attribute of interest and those who do not. In cohort studies the investigator begins with exposed and nonexposed individuals. Case–control and cohort studies are used to establish etiologic relationships. If associations are found, further studies are necessary to determine causal links and to prevent false inferences (ecologic fallacy). When examining the results of case–control and cohort studies, it is important for the CNS to consider whether or not all other explanations for an identified association have been eliminated. No single epidemiological study can satisfy all criteria for causality. The CNS needs to look at the accumulation of evidence as well as the strength of individual studies.

TABLE 17.3

CALCULATION OF RELATIVE RISK				
	Disease	No Disease	Totals	
Exposure	a	b	a + b	Incidence in Exposed a/a + b
No exposure	c	d	c + d	Incidence in Nonexposed c/c + d
Relative Risk (RR) = incidence in the exposed/incidence in the nonexposed				

Risk

RR and the OR are measures of the association between a factor and an outcome. They can be used to derive causal inference, but they do not provide any information regarding the actual change in magnitude of a risk related to a factor. *Risk* is the probability of an event occurring. *Attributable risk* (AR) is an estimate of the amount of risk that is attributable to a particular risk factor and is calculated in cohort studies. The formula for the AR is as follows:

AR = (risk in exposed) − (risk in nonexposed)

If an exposure is harmful, the AR will be greater than 0. If an exposure is protective, the AR will be less than 0. If a study determines that the likelihood of dying in middle age is 0.2 for someone who is normal weight and 0.4 for someone who is morbidly obese, then the AR for being obese is 0.4 − 0.2 = 0.2.

Population attributable risk is important to policy makers. For the previous example, the question becomes, "Among the general population, how much of the total risk for death in middle age is due to morbid obesity?" This decade, the question about how much risk is accrued by people who are overweight has become a concern for health care professionals and policy makers alike.

Randomized Trials

Randomized trials are useful for evaluating treatments (including technology) and for assessing new ways of organizing and delivering health services. In population-based studies, the issue is often health promotion and disease prevention, rather than treatment of an existing disease. The intervention is undertaken on a large scale, with the target involving defined populations rather than individuals, and often involves educational, program, or policy interventions. When carefully designed, randomized trials can provide the strongest evidence for a cause-and-effect relationship.

The basic design of a clinical trial is to assign the sample randomly to either receive the new treatment or not to receive the new treatment. The difference between a randomized trial and a cohort study is that in a randomized trial, the subjects are randomly selected to be exposed or not be exposed. Inclusion and exclusion criteria for the participants must be precise and spelled out in advance. Like cohort studies, more than two groups can be compared using this design. Analysis is carried out to determine how many people in the new treatment group (or groups) improve and how many people in the current treatment group improve.

A clinical trial design was used to evaluate the effects of a pedometer intervention for low-active adolescent girls (Schofield, Mummery, & Schofield, 2005). The purpose of the study was to compare the effectiveness of daily step count targets with time-based prescription (the more traditional method) for increasing the health-related physical activity of low-active adolescent girls. The study was carried out over a 12-week period. The participants were assigned to a control group, a pedometer group, or a minutes group. The pedometer group set daily step count targets, while the time group set time-based goals for physical activity. The authors used analysis of variance (ANOVA) to analyze the differences among the groups. There was a significant difference in activity between the pedometer group and the time group, suggesting that this piece of technology has the potential to change the activity behavior of low-active adolescent girls in the short term. The investigators state that more research is needed. This study illustrates how useful the clinical trial design is for testing a new intervention on a specialized population.

Sample Size

Sample selection and sample size determination is a critical step in the research process. The sample size is an important factor in determining whether or not the investigator has ample resources to carry out the study and what size sample is required in order to identify true differences and associations. Power analysis is used to determine sample size. There are several factors that influence the size of the sample that is needed: power, effect size, and significance.

Significance is the probability that an observed difference or relationship exists. Power is the capacity of the study to detect differences or relationships that actually exist in the population. It is the capacity to correctly reject a null hypothesis, that is, prevent a Type II error. The larger the power required, the larger the necessary sample size. The smaller the sample size, the smaller the power of the study. Effect size is the actual differences between groups and treatments. It can be determined by reviewing previous studies or by conducting a pilot study. The smaller the effect size is, the larger the necessary sample size. The more stringent the significance level, the greater the necessary sample size.

Power analysis can be conducted using computer programs. There are many free software programs available on the Internet to assist with power analysis. Typing sample size calculation in a search engine such as Yahoo! or Google will lead the investigator to many sites. Power analysis allows the CNS to use resources efficiently and to provide data that are meaningful (Kellar & Kelvin, 2013).

Screening

Screening is used to describe programs that deliver a testing mechanism to detect disease in groups of asymptomatic individuals. It is a method used in secondary prevention for early detection in order to improve prognosis. There are several concepts that are important to understand about screening.

Screening is neither available nor appropriate for all diseases. In order for a screening program to be effective, certain criteria should be met: (a) the target population should be identifiable and accessible, (b) the disease should affect a sufficient number of people to make screening cost-effective, (c) the disease should be relatively serious, (d) an effective treatment is available for the disease, and (e) the preclinical period should be sufficient to allow treatment before symptoms appear so that early diagnosis and treatment make a difference in terms of outcome. To be effective, it is necessary for the screening test to be sensitive enough to detect most cases of the disease and to be specific enough to exclude most other causes of positive results. Screening tests should also be relatively inexpensive, easy to administer, and have minimal side effects (Gordis, 2008).

The validity of a screening test refers to its ability to accurately identify those who have the disease. Sensitivity and specificity are measures of a screening test's validity. *Sensitivity* is a measure of a screening test's ability to accurately identify disease when it is present. *Specificity* is the probability of a negative test when the disease is absent. The *positive predictive value* is a measure of the probability of a positive test result when the disease is present. The *negative predictive value* of a test is a measure of the probability that the disease is absent when there is a negative test. The higher the prevalence of a condition in a population, the higher the predictive value is. The formulas for these values can be found in Table 17.1.

The CNS can evaluate the success of screening programs by determining whether or not there is a reduction in overall mortality, a reduction of the case fatality rate in screened individuals, an increase in the percentage of cases detected at earlier stages, a reduction in complications, and improvement of quality of life in screened individuals.

ETHICAL CONSIDERATIONS IN POPULATION-BASED EVALUATION

Population-based evaluation provides the CNS with information for EBP. There is no reason to assume that a new intervention or therapy will have only positive effects; research can detect evidence of harm as well as benefit. The question is not whether studies should be conducted, it is *how*. Ethics is as important as a sound methodology in population research. Population-based interventions should relate to a well-understood disease etiology, be feasible, and entail an appropriate trade off of rights of the individual against benefit that is accrued to the population. Population-based research can have direct and often immediate societal relevance, and although this research involves human subjects, individuals may derive no personal benefits from the results of a study.

One of the best examples of population research that violated the principle of "do no harm" was the Tuskegee Study. The U.S. Public Health Service, working with the Tuskegee Institute, began the study in 1932. Nearly 400 low-income black men with syphilis were enrolled in the study. They were never told they had syphilis, and they were never treated. At the start of the study, there was no proven treatment for syphilis. After penicillin became a standard cure in 1947, the medicine was withheld from the men. The Tuskegee scientists wanted to continue to study how the disease spreads and kills. The experiment lasted four decades, until public health workers leaked the story to the media. Many family members also became infected and died as a result. The *New York Times* exposed the study in 1972, 40 years after the study began and after many articles on the study had been printed in professional journals (National Public Radio, 2002).

In 1978, the National Commission for the Protection of Human Subjects of Biomedical and Behavioral Research created *The Belmont Report: Ethical Principles and Guidelines for the Protection of Human Subjects of Research*. *The Belmont Report* sets forth the basic ethical principles required for research involving human subjects. Autonomy (the right of self-governance), beneficence (prevent evil or harm to others), and justice (balance between the benefits of participating in a study and the burden) are the three core principles of *The Belmont Report*.

The CNS should be aware of some special considerations in population-based research. A randomized trial can provide strong evidence for adopting a new intervention, but not all interventions are appropriate for study. A randomized trial is considered unethical if the current intervention is believed to be the best available, whether or not that fact has been established scientifically by well-designed studies. A good example would be a study to determine whether or not legislation to prevent people from talking on handheld cell phones while driving decreases motor vehicle accidents. It would be unethical to undertake a clinical trial where some people would be randomly selected to talk on a cell phone while driving.

Group comparison is a basic method in population-based research, and a related issue is the use of race and ethnicity as a grouping variable. Genetic research has been unable to find a clear genetic break between races, and biological differences are poorly understood. Using race to identify subgroups is of questionable validity. Ethnicity may be a better category, but if it is used the researcher should have a justifiable reason for the use of ethnicity as a variable, and it should be clearly defined. No variable should be used routinely, and there should be a clear and justifiable reason for the use of every variable.

There are also special ethical concerns related to screening programs. Individuals in a well population take part in screening programs, and health care professionals need to show that the benefits of screening outweigh the costs. Screening programs should be safe and free of side effects. Errors in results can cause concerns. False positive results create both extra costs for diagnostic procedures and anxiety for the individual. False negative results are equally problematic because they can place individuals at ease and make them less likely to seek help when they have early symptoms of a disease.

The CNS who is involved with population-based research has an obligation to protect and consider the interests of the populations studied. Population-based research should be concerned with the larger systemic effects that new information generates. Recent proposals to restrict the size of soda servings, reduce the amount of sodium in foods, and to display calorie counts for restaurant foods represent efforts to improve population health based on what is now known about added sugar, salt, and calories. These proposals, which are similar to other measures that have been taken to protect public health, such as helmet laws, regulations for the fluoridation of water supplies, and vaccination policies, have been met with mixed (and at times harshly critical) reactions. It is important to keep in mind that policies are associated with costs. There are the financial costs to public institutions such as those related to enforcement, the personal costs (buying a helmet, for example), and the costs of the loss of personal freedom (Frieden, 2013). Health care policies should be created by duly authorized bodies on the basis of valid evidence or data and both group need and group demand should be the strongest determinants. Finally, they should be designed to prevent premature death and injury, and over the long haul, reduce costs in health care and increase productivity. When a CNS is making decisions related to population-based evaluation, the decisions have to be based on a sound methodological framework that includes ethical considerations of the effect of the research on the population as a whole.

CONCLUSION

Two nurse practitioners enrolled in a doctorate in nursing practice program investigated the fall rate in a long-term care/subacute rehabilitation (SAR) setting (Rosner & Sirkin, 2007). They found that the facility was near the 50th percentile for falls when compared to similar institutions and that there was a need for an improved fall prevention program, particularly in the SAR setting. Following an in-depth literature review to gain a better understanding of the known contributors to falls and a careful evaluation of the existing fall prevention program, a comprehensive, interprofessional fall prevention program was initiated in the SAR. The program was evaluated using a cohort design, with fall rates calculated for the SAR population before and after the intervention. The fall rate decreased from 19 falls per 1,000 patient days before the intervention to 9 falls per 1,000 patient days after the intervention with an RR of 0.4, demonstrating a decreased risk of falling after the intervention.

This project provides an example of how population methods can be used to identify a problem, design and implement an intervention, and evaluate the intervention to improve patient care.

SUMMARY

Population-based analysis is a complex practice area, and the challenges for the CNS are diverse. Interventions at the population level can have a more far-reaching effect than interventions at the individual level. A falls intervention program based on carefully researched evidence, for example, will have a bigger impact on fall rates in a hospital than an uncoordinated, individual approach. The CNS requires skills in EPB, comprehensive assessment, and evaluation of interventions at the population level. Population-based data can assist the CNS to target at-risk populations, identify risk factors, evaluate interventions, and make decisions to improve the health of populations. This chapter outlines the basic principles and processes of population-based analysis. The CNS can use this information in practice and also to explore the issues related to population health further.

▪ DISCUSSION QUESTIONS

- During 1996, 215 new cases of AIDS were reported in Williamson, a city of 500,000. This brought the total number of active cases of AIDS to 2,280. During this time there were 105 deaths attributable to the disease.

a. What was the incidence rate per 100,000 for AIDS during 1996?
b. What was the prevalence rate of AIDS per 100,000?
c. What is the cause-specific death rate of AIDS?

• Let us hypothesize that BMI is associated with type 2 diabetes. Using health records, ascertain the BMIs of adolescents at your clinic who have not been diagnosed with diabetes. Classify every individual as either obese or not obese, and then follow each one over time. Classify each adolescent who is diagnosed with diabetes as a case and each one who is not as a control. Match cases and controls in your study for age and gender. Out of 20 adolescents who are obese, 17 are diagnosed with diabetes. Four out of 20 adolescents who are not obese are diagnosed with diabetes[1] (see Exhibit 17.1).
a. What is the study design?
b. What is the appropriate statistic for testing the hypothesis?
c. Carry out the calculations.
d. Why use other clinic patients for the control group?

3. Use Exhibit 17.2 to answer the following questions:
a. What is the sensitivity of the test?
b. What is the specificity of the test?
c. What is the positive predictive value?
d. What is the negative predictive value?
e. What effect do you get from lowering the screening cutoff point in terms of false positives and false negatives ?

4. Go to www.cdc.gov/nccdphp/burdenbook2004 / toc.htm; research the state that you live in or work in
a. What is the burden of chronic diseases in this state?
b. How do the leading causes of death in the state compare to U.S. figures?

EXHIBIT 17.1

Summary of Clinic Information

	Cases	Controls
Obese	17	4
Not obese	3	16
Total	20	20

---

[1] These data are not based on a real case and were created solely for use in this exercise.

EXHIBIT 17.2

Screening Information

Screening Test Results	Population		
	Disease	No Disease	Total
Positive	TP 66	FP 98	164
Negative	FN 84	TN 9,752	9,836
Total	150	9,850	10,000

c. Identify five important risk factors that should be targeted in the state
d. Identify vulnerable groups. To whom should targeted services be provided?

Answers to Discussion Questions

1. a. $215/500,000 \times 100,000$
   = 43 cases per 100,000
   b. $2,280/500,000 \times 100,000$
   = 456 cases per 100,000
   c. $105/500,000 \times 100,000$
   = 21 deaths per 100,000

2. a. This is a cohort design.
   b. RR
   c. $RR = \dfrac{17/17 + 4}{3/3 + 16} = 0.81/0.16$

   RR = 5.06 risk is greater in exposed than non-exposed group
   d. Matching is one method that can be used to select a sample so that potential confounders are distributed equally between the cases and controls. Controls should resemble the cases as closely as possible except for exposure to the factor under study.

3. a. TP/(TP + FN) 66/(66 + 84) = 0.44 or 44%
   b. TN/(TN + FP) 9,752/(9,752 + 98) = 0.99 or 99%
   c. TP/(TP + FP) 66/(66 + 98) = 0.402 or 40%
   d. TN/(TN + FN) 9,752/(9,752 + 84) = 0.991 or 99%
   e. Lowering the screening cutoff level that distinguishes between diseased and nondiseased populations will increase the false positives and decrease false negatives. Sensitivity will be increased and specificity will be decreased.

REFERENCES

American Nurses Association (ANA). (2010). *Nursing: Scope and standards of practice* (2nd ed.). Washington, DC: Author.

Babones, S. J. (2008). Income inequality and population health: Correlation and causality. *Social Science & Medicine, 66,* 1614–1626.

Centers for Disease Control and Prevention (CDC). (2013a). *Diabetes data and trends.* Retrieved August 1, 2013, from http://www.cdc.gov/diabetes/statistics/prev/national/figage.htm

Centers for Disease Control and Prevention (CDC). (2013b, July 5). Vital signs: Overdoses of prescription opioid pain relievers and other drugs among women—United States, 1999–2010. *MMWR. Morbidity and Mortality Weekly Reports.* Retrieved August 1, 2013, from http://www.cdc.gov/mmwr

Dossey, B. (2000). *Florence Nightingale: Mystic, visionary, healer.* Springhouse, PA: Springhouse.

Fong, T. G., Jones, R. N., Marcantonio, E. R., Tommet, D., Gross, A. L., Habtemariam, D.,...Inouye, S. K. (2012). Adverse outcomes after hospitalization and delirium in persons with Alzheimer disease. *Annals of Internal Medicine, 156,* 848–856.

Frieden, T. (2013, June 14). Government's role in protecting health and safety. *The New England Journal of Medicine, 368*(20), 1857–1859.

Gallagher-Ford, L., Fineout-Overholt, E., Melnyk, B. M., & Stillwell, S. B. (2011). Implementing an evidence-based practice change: Beginning the transformation from an idea to reality. *American Journal of Nursing, 111*(3), 54–60.

Gordis, L. (2008). *Epidemiology* (4th ed.). Philadelphia, PA: Elsevier Saunders.

Harvard Medical School. (2013). *Nurses' health study.* Retrieved August 28, 2013, from http://www.channing.harvard.edu/nhs/?page_id=70

Hoffman, S., & Podgurski, A. (2013). Big bad data: Law, public health, and biomedical databases. *Journal of Law, 41*(Suppl. 1), 156–160.

Ibrahim, M., Savitz, L., Carey, T., & Wagner, E. (2001). Population-based health principles in medical and public health practice. *Journal of Public Health Management Practice, 7*(3), 75–81.

Kellar, S., & Kelvin, E. A. (2013). *Munro's statistical methods for health care research* (6th ed. Kindle Edition). New York, NY: Wolters Kluwer/Lippincott Williams & Wilkins.

Lipsey, S. (1993). *Mathematical education in the life of Florence Nightingale.* Retrieved August 31, 2013, from http://www.agnesscott.edu/lriddle/women/night_educ.htm

National Association of Clinical Nurse Specialists (NACNS). (2004). *Statement on clinical nurse specialist practice and education* (2nd ed.). Harrisburg, PA: Author.

National Database of Nursing Quality Indicators (NDNQI). (2013). *FAQS.* Retrieved August 5, 2013, from http://www.nursingquality.org/FAQs

National Heart, Lung and Blood Institute (NHLBI) & Boston University. (2013). *History of the Framingham study.* Retrieved August 28, 2013, from http://www.framinghamheartstudy.org/about/history.html

National Public Radio, Inc. (2002). *Remembering Tuskegee.* Retrieved August 31, 2013, from http://www.npr.org/templates/story/story.php?storyId=1147234

Oppewal, S. (2012). Identifying outcomes. In A. L. Cupp Curley & P. A. Vitale (Eds.), *Population-based nursing: Concepts and competencies for advanced practice* (pp. 19–46). New York, NY: Springer.

Rosner, N., & Sirkin, A. (2007). *A multifaceted falls reduction strategy in a sub-acute rehabilitation setting* (Unpublished doctoral capstone project). University of Medicine and Dentistry of New Jersey, School of Nursing, Newark.

Schofield, L., Mummery, W., & Schofield, G. (2005). Effects of a controlled pedometer-intervention trial for low-active adolescent girls. *Medicine & Science in Sports and Exercise, 37*(8), 1414–1420.

Scott, L. K. (2013). Presence of type 2 diabetes risk factors in children. *Pediatric Nursing, 39*(4), 190–196.

Client-Focused Teaching and Coaching: The Clinical Nurse Specialist Role

Kelly A. Goudreau

Learn about a pine tree from a pine tree and about a bamboo plant from a bamboo plant. *(Matsuo Basho, 1644–1694)*

Client-focused teaching and coaching has undergone many name changes over the years. Names for the process are varied and include patient education, patient-centered education, coaching, and client-focused education. Each of these variations reflects a need to clearly define the process of providing needed information to the individual who is experiencing a health challenge of some kind. The health challenge may be either short- or long-term/chronic in nature. Today, the focus from many organizations, such as The Joint Commission (TJC, 2011) and the Institute for Healthcare Improvement (IHI, 2013) in collaboration with the Institute of Medicine (IOM, 2001), is on empowering or activating patients to manage their own care more effectively. Issues around providing education to patients and focusing on the needs of the patients as they seek specific information are many. One of the issues is frustration on the part of both the patient/client and the health care provider due to the plethora of conflicting information now available to patients/clients. Additional frustrations on the part of the health care provider include whether or not the patient/client is ready to listen and use the information presented (readiness to learn), how best to

get the information to the patient/client in an understandable manner (health literacy), and, finally, how best to assess whether or not the information has had a positive effect on the patient/client (assessment of learning outcomes).

What role does the clinical nurse specialist (CNS) play in this ongoing dance between the patient/client and the health care provider working to inform the patient/client? A concentration on client-focused teaching and coaching or patient education is specifically reflected in the outcomes of CNS practice articulated by the National Association of Clinical Nurse Specialists (NACNS) *Statement on Practice and Education* (2004) and in the more recent definition of the core CNS competencies (NACNS, 2010). In the statement, NACNS identifies that two of the expected outcomes of CNS care and function are (a) development of innovative educational programs for patients, families, and groups that are then implemented and evaluated; and (b) expertise in diagnosis and treatment to prevent and remediate, or alleviate illness and promote health with a defined specialty population (NACNS, 2004, pp. 25–26). Within the core CNS competencies, the direct care competency includes statements pertaining to being patient centered in approaching care (NACNS, 2010, p. 19). This chapter relates patient education concepts and offers evidence-based interventions to support critical elements of CNS practice. Client-focused teaching is an important function of nursing practice and critical to the role of the CNS. This chapter addresses

1. The current practice of client-focused teaching and coaching in the clinical environment
2. The changing role of client-focused teaching and coaching in health care delivery
3. Evidence-based strategies that the CNS can use to support nursing staff and other health care providers to effectively educate patients/clients from a patient-centered approach

BACKGROUND

Staff nurses within a hospital system, home care, or long-term care environment must demonstrate how their practice meets certain standards of care established by TJC (2011), the major accrediting agency for most health care facilities. A focus on patient education is a component of the delivery, design, and testing of nursing interventions related to preventing, lessening, or alleviating the illness experience. Educating patients in the management of their own care is integral across the health care continuum, in health promotion and disease prevention, and in the diagnosis, treatment, and self-management of acute and chronic diseases. The CNS provides support for both the staff nurse and the patients as they attempt to meet the educational needs of the patients/clients regardless of the setting (home, inpatient, rehabilitation, ambulatory care, or long-term care).

In addition to the role in CNS practice and outcomes (NACNS, 2004, 2010), patient education is also mandated by TJC (2011). CNSs typically play a key role in ensuring that strategies are put in place to meet or exceed TJC standards. In the past, there was a separate section in TJC standards that addressed patient education. With the recent revisions, however, the expectations for patient education are now dispersed across almost all of the standards. Specific Joint Commission standards that refer to patient education include the following: assessment of patients' learning needs, infection control, national patient safety goals, medication management and reconciliation, transfer and follow-up care, participation in decisions about care, receiving information in an understandable manner, how to seek assistance if the patient's condition changes, and informed consent (TJC, 2011). Further, the focus is now on being patient centered in response to the IOM report first shared in 2001, which focused on the quality "chasm" and how health care providers are not listening to the needs of the patient but instead are focused on the needs of the system.

The role of the CNS expands beyond meeting the needs of nursing staff and accrediting agencies and addresses the needs of patient care directly. CNSs care for patients with both acute and chronic disease within a specialty population (NACNS, 2010). Of note is the fact that the chronic disease burden in the United States will continue to increase as the population ages (Ward & Schiller, 2013). The CNS's role in this area must be especially evident. To effectively self-manage chronic disease, patients must first think that they need to manage their disease. After the acknowledgment that they have a disease that has to be managed, they then need to understand their condition(s) and the disease process. They must also be able to self-monitor, record, and track self-monitoring data; know what, when, and how to report changes in their condition; problem solve; modify their medications, diet, and physical activity as appropriate; enlist the support and involvement of family members and their social support systems; and cope on a day-to-day basis (Holy Cross Hospital, 2012; Lorig, 2001; Wagner et al., 2005). This activity is no longer termed patient education because it is so much more than that. The CNS educates patients with chronic disease regarding the information and skills needed to accomplish these critical tasks. As an advanced practice nurse, the CNS may also be the patient's point of contact regarding the self-monitoring data and offer guidance about needed changes in the treatment plan. The CNS also offers advice and suggestions to help patients solve self-management problems. The process of coaching the patient to care for his or her own chronic disease is so much more than that and involves more than just the patient sphere of influence. The nurse/nursing sphere is heavily impacted by the need to know how best to approach the patient and whether or not he or she is ready to approach self-care of the chronic illness. The systems sphere is also heavily influenced, as the CNS must identify and create tools and find resources for the nursing staff to use when providing support to the patient who is beginning to grapple with the fact that he or she has a chronic illness that will have to be managed. All of these come into play as the CNS works with the population. The CNS plays a key role in the development and use of evidence-based interventions to provide in-depth education, coaching, and counseling to patients and family members, nursing staff, and administrators who need to provide the resources for patient-centered care of chronic illness.

Like health care delivery and the role of the CNS, patient education has evolved. In the 1970s, patient education was frequently viewed as offering patients print materials or audiovisuals to provide information about their conditions and the diagnostic or surgical procedures they were about to undergo. The educational content frequently focused solely on anatomy and pathophysiology, emulating the medical model of teaching. Clinicians truly believed that providing information in this way would motivate patients to comply with the treatment plan and make the recommended health behavior changes. This approach was frequently unsuccessful in accomplishing either education or compliance with treatment plans.

There are several reasons for this lack of success. The first reason for this failure was the misconception that information alone, especially about anatomy and pathophysiology, was sufficient to cause people to change health behaviors. Another reason for lack of success was the common use of fear messages. Clinicians believed that if they informed patients about the negative consequences of noncompliance, patients would certainly follow the treatment plan and make the recommended lifestyle changes. There is ample evidence to suggest that fear messages are ineffective (Wagner et al., 2005). Fear elicits anxiety. Most people who experience anxiety try to avoid the situation that is making them anxious, which in turn makes it very difficult to positively influence a patient's willingness to adhere to treatment plans and make the desired health behavior changes (Nolte, Elsworth, Sinclair, & Osborne, 2007). The patient education materials of this era were designed to foster compliance. Patients who appeared in these materials and audiovisuals were usually depicted as White. Little, if any, attempt was made to tailor and personalize patient education materials to age, race, gender, or ethnicity of the specific target audience for whom they were intended.

The field of patient-centered care has evolved both conceptually and as a field of practice since the 1970s. In particular, a shift occurred in 2001 with the release of the landmark document from the IOM, *Crossing the Quality Chasm* (2001), when the words "patient-centered care" were first put into the public forum for health care leaders to implement.

An ample body of research currently exists on evidence-based interventions drawing from the health education, nursing, clinical psychology, and health care communications literature (Wagner et al., 2005). The evolution of patient education parallels changes in society, health care delivery, and the patient's role. In the 1970s, the relationship between patients, physicians, and health care team members was significantly different than it is today. Physicians were considered to be solely responsible for designing treatment plans and the subsequent regimens, and there was little opportunity for other members of the health care team, much less the patient, to contribute to the design of the treatment plan. The patient was held responsible and accountable for carrying out the treatment plan as designed by the physician, but there were few attempts to solicit patient input in order to create a tailored, individualized treatment plan that accommodated the patient's goals and lifestyle. We now know that the better a treatment plan is tailored to accommodate the patient's goals, perceptions of health, and lifestyle, the more likely it is to be followed (Bruce, Lorig, & Laurent, 2007; Holy Cross Hospital, 2012).

The Current Practice of Client-Focused Teaching/Coaching in the Clinical Environment

Two key differences between the 1970s and the clinical practice of patient-centered care and coaching today are first, the client is expected to be a full partner and the key decision maker in how his or her health will be managed (Turner, Thomas, Wagner, & Moseley, 2008). Second, to be the key decision maker, the client must clearly understand the health care issues, and health literacy is key to that understanding (U.S. Department of Health and Human Services [USDHHS], 2013a, 2013b). Patients are now recognized as key active participants in the process of health care. An informed and empowered patient is active and participatory in his or her own care and also takes greater responsibility for his or her own health care outcomes. This active participation is necessary to achieve the desired clinical outcomes. The Chronic Care Model presented by the Institute for Chronic Care (2013) displays in graphic form how the patient who is activated and understands the need to be participatory with the health care team has better outcomes than the patient who is not engaged and proactive. Their activated and empowered participation also impacts the economics of health care delivery (Ament, 2008; Goudreau et al., 2008; Kennedy et al., 2007; Mayer & Villaire, 2004). Patients need information and skills to:

1. Access health care services. Patients must not only be able to access the needed health care services in a timely manner, but they must also have the skills needed to navigate complex health care delivery systems and interface with insurers
2. Adopt a healthy lifestyle to promote health, prevent disease, and enhance their quality of life
3. Prepare for diagnostic tests and procedures
4. Participate as active partners in all aspects of their care
5. Self-manage acute and chronic diseases and conditions
6. Obtain optimal benefits from rehabilitation
7. Engage the needed support from family members and friends

8. Employ the needed coping skills
9. Communicate effectively with their providers and members of the health care team

The kind of communication required to do this is fostered by a true partnership between patients and their providers and health care team members (Institute for Chronic Care, 2013; Schwartzenberg, Cowett, Van Geest, & Wolf, 2007).

CNSs are able to lay a foundation for this therapeutic relationship and, depending on the clinical practice environment and the population they work with, they can maintain it over time. This is especially important for patients with chronic diseases. The role of the CNS in inpatient care allows for standardization, assessment of appropriate materials, and the introduction of patient education through a variety of methods and techniques. Methods include such processes as print media, verbal instruction, computer-based instruction, and return demonstration (London, 1997). The CNS role in outpatient environments ensures that the initial work done by the inpatient nursing staff can be maintained or modified to better meet the patient/client needs. The nursing staff in the outpatient environment can be instructed on the use of Motivational Interviewing (MI; Rollnick, Miller, & Butler, 2008) and the Stanford Living Well (Holy Cross Hospital, 2012) program for coaching and support of patients and their caregivers in the battle on chronic illness. The patients/clients are seen more than just in the hospital or in a clinic visit and can now be maintained on an ongoing basis.

To be a full partner in his or her own health care, the patient/client must be able to communicate effectively with his or her provider. Communication must be reciprocal and must include ways to contact the provider or team when questions arise and answers are needed. The changing era of the information age has seen increased expectations for communication between patients and their providers. As patients become more technology savvy and increasingly competent, they are seeking greater amounts of information from both their provider and other sources such as the Internet. They are also demanding immediate opportunities to communicate with their providers. As a result, use of secure e-mail between patients and members of the health care team is now possible and increasing (Lorig, Ritter, Laurent, & Plant, 2006; B. Don Burman, personal communication, September 2, 2013). To make this an effective environment for learning and support of client-focused education, patients need to be comfortable with and understand the process and the "business" rules for both how and what is appropriate for this method of communication. Just as there is an expectation of behavior in a personal interaction, there are also behavioral expectations in an online environment.

When a patient is admitted to an inpatient area, a rehabilitation unit, or is simply seeing a provider in a time-limited clinic interaction, there is a need to clearly and effectively communicate and understand. A health partnership, or medical home model of care (National Conference of State Legislatures [NCSL], 2012) cannot be established if there is a lack of understanding of the topics at hand. Health literacy in combination with MI and the concept of a medical home or patient-centered care model are key elements in ensuring that patients/clients understand the content being presented or discussed.

Health care providers are not always good at creating materials or presenting content that truly meets the needs of the patients/clients they are intended to serve. Content is not clear or simply is too complex to assist comprehension (Schwartzenberg et al., 2007; Seligman et al., 2007). These poor efforts at provision of health information that is inappropriate to the patient/client needs only serve as bad examples of how to accommodate low health literacy.

Health literacy was identified as a major issue in the U.S. Department of Health document *Healthy People 2020* (USDHHS, 2013a) and continues to be an issue on the rise. In *Healthy People 2020* (USDHHS, 2013a), health literacy is defined as "the degree to which individuals have the capacity to obtain, process, and understand basic health information and services needed to make appropriate health decisions" (p. vi). All people need health literacy skills to find their way to the right place in a hospital, self-monitor and self-manage chronic and acute conditions, safely take prescribed medications, fill out medical and insurance forms, and communicate with members of the health care team.

A national survey of adults in the United States found that a significant number of Americans have low-level general literacy skills that hamper their participation in the economy and society (Kirsch, Jungeblut, Jenkins, & Kolstad, 1993; National Center for Education Statistics, 2006). Upwards of 90 million Americans

> were much less likely to respond correctly to the more challenging literacy tasks in the assessment—those requiring higher level reading and problem-solving skills. In particular, they were apt to experience considerable difficulty in performing tasks that required them to integrate or synthesize information from complex or lengthy texts. (Kirsch et al., 1993, p. xvii)

These difficulties with general literacy are only compounded when one considers the complexity of health care information and the added stressors of learning about a health condition not previously known.

People from all ages, races, incomes, and education levels are challenged by health literacy. Individuals with limited health literacy incur medical expenses that are up to four times greater than patients with adequate literacy skills, costing the health care system billions of dollars every year in unnecessary doctor visits and hospital stays (Nielsen-Bohlman, Panzer, & Kindig, 2004; IHI, 2013; IOM, 2001). The health literacy problem is compounded by the fact that most patients hide their confusion because they are too ashamed and intimidated to ask for help.

Effective communication between health care providers and their patients is hindered when patients or family members have limited health literacy. Difficulties in communication can cause medical errors, delay in care, treatment mishaps, and other costly, unwanted consequences that are sometimes fatal (Nielsen-Bohlman, Panzer, & Kindig, 2004). Issues surrounding health literacy are also recognized by TJC (2011). TJC mandates patients' right to receive information in a manner that they can understand. Elements of this standard deal with information specifically tailored to the patient's age, language, and ability to understand and accommodation of physical and cognitive impairments.

Patient and environmental health literacy relate to the CNS's core competencies in the client direct care, nursing practice, and organizations and systems spheres of practice. The CNS impacts the patient/client directly by ensuring that he or she understands the content presented by the provider or other health care staff. The CNS impacts the care provided by the nurse through defining the issues surrounding patient/client-focused education and providing support and education to the nursing staff. Specifically, the CNS educates the nursing and support staff about how to empower patients/clients and how to create materials that are within the boundaries of health literacy guidelines. The CNS impacts the health care system by putting in place policies and programs that allow for and encourage an active and participatory patient/client. Additionally, the fact that these policies and programs are based on the best available evidence adds to the value the CNS brings to the clinical environment. The final system-level impact of the CNS is the standardization of patient/client educational materials and processes at an appropriate grade level and with a culturally appropriate focus. Each of these influences at the patient/client level, the nursing staff level, and the systems level will lead to improved patient/client outcomes.

Most health education materials should be written at the sixth-grade reading level to accommodate current health literacy levels in the United States (National Center for Education Statistics, 2006). Using materials that incorporate the appropriate reading level and a clear graphical layout can make a big difference in promoting patients' comprehension, because appropriate graphics and pictures reinforce the written text. Many options are available for evaluating the reading level of written materials. Most focus on sentence length, complexity of words used, numbers of words in a phrase, and number of syllables in the words. The Fleisch-Kincaid test is often built into current software programs' readability indices and can be used to assess a document's reading level.

CNSs can also decrease the demands on patient literacy through effective patient–clinician communication. Most patients want and need to have effective relationships with their physicians and health care team members. Providing patients with pamphlets, directing patients to a website, or having patients watch a video can supplement but never replace face-to-face interactions. Successful discussions with patients about health behavior change and self-management are founded on trust and a therapeutic relationship. Effective relationships help patients take a more active role in their health care. The CNS can extend the invitation for patients to participate in different ways at different times. The goal is to keep the dialogue flowing.

Two issues must be taken into consideration when looking at any health education and client-focused interventions related to acute or chronic illnesses: (a) the client is expected to be a full participant in the health care process, and (b) health literacy is potentially compromised. The CNS is an essential element in the assessment of the client/patient and his or her ability to fully participate. Methods to approach clients/patients must be based in evidence-based practice (EBP) and firmly founded in theoretical constructs that provide strength to the interventions and provide methods to evaluate the outcomes. Many theories and processes have been proposed, and many of those are currently being researched. The impact of patient participation and ability to understand the content are key to whichever method/theoretical model is used.

Conceptual and/or Theoretical Support: Evidence-Based Patient Education Interventions

There are many different theoretical constructs for patient/client-focused educational interventions. TJC (2011), *Healthy People 2020* (USDHHS, 2013a), and the IOM (2001), Nielsen-Bohlman, Panzer, & Kindig (2004) have all pointed to the need for activated, empowered, and informed patients/clients; therefore, research is underway to find the best methods to achieve improved patient outcomes. Evidence-based patient education can be integrated into all aspects of CNS practice through a variety of methods and techniques. Due to the current time constraints in health care (Ament, 2008; London, 1995), many of the evidence-based methodologies discussed in this section are those that can be easily accomplished in time-limited clinical encounters. Others are longer term but are supportive of the overall concepts of empowerment and activation of the patient/client in his or her own care.

TJC (2011) mandates that patient education be based on each patient's needs and ability to understand. This requires assessing the preferred learning modality of the patient and documenting the stated educational needs, including any physical, cognitive, and social barriers that may impact the patient's ability to learn the needed information and skills. Identification of the patient's needs and concerns facilitates the integration of the clinical and patient priorities. These patient-centered or client-focused needs assessment techniques use active involvement of the patient because they focus on the patient's ownership of the problem, identification of the issues, and problem solving.

Some of the theories that can be used to provide a foundation for the educational intervention that follows the assessment include the Salient Belief Model (Miller, 1957), the Health Belief Model (Rosenstock, Strecher, & Becker, 1994), and the Stages of Change Model (Prochaska & DiClemente, 1983). A more recent midlevel theory and application focuses on how to address and empower patients/clients who have chronic diseases and assists in long-term management of the chronic disease. The Chronic Disease Self-Management Program (CDSMP; Holy Cross Hospital, 2012; Lorig, 2001) offers some hope for positive long-term outcomes of care.

Salient Belief Model

One of the quickest and most effective strategies to elicit patient concerns is based on the work of Miller (1957). Miller's Salient Belief Model is based on research demonstrating that people have a limited number of strong beliefs about any topic. Miller identified that the number of strong beliefs an individual can have can be as many as seven (±2). If you can determine what those beliefs are, you can design your teaching to address those beliefs and concerns.

The term *salient* is derived from the Latin word *salire,* to leap or jump. Synonyms for salient include apparent, obvious, self-evident, first, or significant. A clinician can use the Salient Belief Model as an assessment strategy in a one-on-one situation with a patient. To identify the patient's salient beliefs, ask, "When you think of ____, what do you think of?" Here's an example that's not related to health:

"When you think of Thanksgiving, what do you think of?" People may respond with family gatherings, turkey, football, or the beginning of the holiday shopping season. Although asked the same question, the responses demonstrate the diversity of strong beliefs on Thanksgiving. If a CNS needed to effectively educate an individual about Thanksgiving, the topic would be framed around its relationship to the person's response to the salient belief question. A CNS questioning two patients who are not taking their antihypertensive medications might discover that one worked swing shifts and found it difficult to follow the regimen due to differences in work schedule. Another might express concern regarding loss of sexual function. The CNS can then approach these two patients with very different counseling strategies. CNSs can use the Salient Belief Model to identify patient concerns and then to frame their education to those specific needs and concerns. These are tools that the CNS can use in difficult situations where the staff nurse and other clinicians have not had success.

The Health Belief Model

The Health Belief Model (Rosenstock, Strecher, & Becker, 1994) was first described by U.S. Public Health officials in the 1950s in an effort to define the process of change and how best to motivate an individual to change existing health behaviors. The model specifies that for a change to occur in an individual's health behaviors, there must be some motivating factors. These factors initiate the change in behavior and assist in sustaining the change until it becomes a habit. The model contains perceived threat: There must be a perceived threat to the individual in order for a change to be initiated. The threat consists of two parts: (a) perceived susceptibility and (b) perceived severity of a health condition. Perceived susceptibility is the individual's subjective perception of the risk of contracting a health condition. If they do not perceive that they are susceptible, then no change will be made to the health behaviors that are likely to lead to the health condition. Perceived severity is feelings concerning the seriousness of contracting an illness or of leaving it untreated and is based on the evaluations of both medical and possible social consequences. This particular belief falls clearly into the 1970s perspective of health education and could be used to generate fear in the individual in order to motivate action on his or her part. Although the Health Belief Model can still be used today, the provider needs to be aware of the tendency toward potential use of scare tactics. In an environment that is attempting to empower a new generation of learners, this tendency must be taken into consideration and used carefully.

The second part of the Health Belief Model relates to perceived benefits to participating in the prescribed treatment plans. The empowered and activated patient will likely see this as the most palatable component of the model, and it includes the individual belief about the effectiveness of strategies designed to reduce the threat of illness. There are, however, also perceived barriers that would prevent the individual from participating. These barriers include the potential negative consequences that may result from taking particular health actions, including physical, psychological, and financial demands. In today's health care environment, where many individuals do not have sufficient health care plans to provide support for long-term maintenance of chronic illnesses, this can be a defining factor in the success of the planned change.

Cues to action, the final element in the Health Belief Model, include events, either bodily (e.g., physical symptoms of a health condition) or environmental (e.g., media publicity), that motivate people to take action. However, this area of the Health Belief Model has not been systematically studied.

Other variables also articulated in the model include the impact of (a) indirect, diverse demographic, psychosocial, and structural variables that affect an individual's perceptions of his or her ability to change; and (b) the belief of the individual that he or she is able to be successful, or self-efficacy (Bandura, 1977).

Stages of Change Model

An additional perspective on how an individual can be approached regarding health behaviors and how he or she is impacting activities of daily living is the Stages of Change Model, first articulated by Prochaska and DiClemente (1983). The stages of change are experienced by each individual and can be used to assess whether an individual is ready to make changes in his or her life and whether or not those changes are likely to be maintained over time. Stage 1 is *precontemplation*. When in this stage, the individual has the health problem (whether he or she recognizes it or not) and has no intention of changing. Stage 2 is *contemplation*. In contemplation, the individual recognizes that there is a health problem and is seriously thinking about changing. He or she has not yet made any plans to change at this time. The third stage of change is *preparation for action*. When preparing for action, the individual recognizes the problem and intends to change the behavior within the next month. At this time, some behavior change efforts may be reported, but whatever has been defined as the successful behavior change criterion has not yet been reached. The fourth stage of change is *action*. In this stage, the

individual has enacted consistent behavior change for less than 6 months. Without positive reinforcement of the change, he or she may revert to the contemplative or precontemplative stage. Use of both overt and covert reinforcements is appropriate at this stage, in addition to social support and avoiding high-risk cues. The final stage is *maintenance*. In order to reach this stage, the individual must maintain the new behavior for at least 6 months.

Another theory or model of care that is increasing in use and has shown successful outcomes is the mid-level theory of chronic disease self-management (Holy Cross Hospital, 2012; Lorig, 2001). The CDSMP is clearly evidence based, with more than 20 years of research supporting the findings that patients feel empowered and activated and make changes in their lives that are manageable and maintained over time (Kennedy et al., 2007; Lorig, 2001). The program consists of a combination of self-directed change that is supported by a peer group and that is sustained over a period of 6 weeks. Although this is not a program that can be managed quickly in a short interaction with a client, it is one that can be managed by the CNS with his or her client/patient population. The CDSMP model brings the best of patient empowerment, peer support, health literacy, and ongoing positive interaction with the health care system together into a single program.

Application to CNS Practice. There are several evidence-based strategies to help patients change their health behaviors. In the process of learning how to improve delivery of patient education services, it is important to understand the factors that help a person gain control over specific health behaviors.

Each of the theories identified has specific elements that can be applied directly to CNS practice. Although conceptual, each of the models previously identified can be used by the CNS as he or she addresses specific patient/client education needs.

The first action by the CNS as he or she addresses the individual patient/client is to assess the educational needs. Next is to identify how best to address the needs in collaboration with the patient/client and the health care team. Each of the models previously identified indicates a need to assess the patient/client, the preferred method of learning, and whether or not he or she is ready to make the behavioral changes required to attain improved health outcomes.

Self-efficacy theory (Bandura, 1977), a component of both the Stages of Change (Prochaska & DiClemente, 1983) and the CDSMP (Lorig, 2001) models, can be used in two ways: first with the health care providers as they are releasing control of the management of the patient's/client's health plan, and again when assisting the patient to feel more self-assured as he or she assumes the management of his or her own care. It is important to remember that self-efficacy relates to a person's belief about his or her ability to do some future activity. It is predictable and related to a specific activity. It is not a personality trait.

Self-efficacy involves:

1. Behavior choices—Which activities people will choose to attempt and which they will avoid. People will not attempt behaviors that they believe are impossible even if they have the needed skills to complete the task.
2. Effort—How much effort people will expend and how long they will persist in the face of obstacles. Some people will persevere longer, trying to complete a task despite obstacles and failures.
3. Amount of anxiety tolerated—How much anxiety or distress people experience during their efforts.

A CNS can use self-efficacy theory to help patients change health behaviors. When suggesting a change in the treatment that requires a new health behavior, ask the patient, "On a scale from 1 (*being totally unsure*) to 10 (*being totally sure*), how certain are you that you will be able to (identify the behavior)?" The numerical score is important. People who give themselves scores of 7 or higher are much more likely to be able to perform the behavior. Scores of less than 7 indicate the need to go back and problem solve. People have very different reasons regarding why they feel they cannot perform a behavior. By working with a patient to identify his or her specific concerns, you can effectively problem solve with the patient to facilitate the needed health behavior change (Lorig, 2001).

In dealing with patients/clients, it is important to discuss options and specifically ask the patient/client what behavior he or she wants to change. Assist the patient/client to select one behavior that he or she feels he or she can realistically change within the period of time that he or she identifies. Typically, small increments of time are more achievable and realistic. Assist the patient to make a plan that will help him or her to achieve the goal. It is important for the patient/client to identify previous activity related to this behavior that will help him or her to be successful in this attempt.

The CNS can do this by asking what problems the patient/client expects to encounter. Once difficulties have been identified, the CNS can ask him or her to identify strategies that could overcome the issues, then re-ask the self-efficacy question. Plan to follow up with the patient as needed or appropriate. At the point of follow-up, congratulate the patient if he or she was successful; problem solve if the patient experienced difficulty or was not successful.

There are several ways to enhance patients' self-efficacy. Modeling is one technique. Modeling is also called imitation learning. This technique is effective for learning new behaviors and strengthening previously learned behaviors that are slipping. When dealing with any patient/client, offer him or her models or examples of others similar to the patient/client (i.e., condition, age, educational background, job, social support system) who have successfully dealt with similar problems related to self-management or coping strategies. Your patient may develop a stronger belief in his or her own capabilities if the person is similar in age, sex, social status, situation, and type of problem. By using multiple events or models, the patient will be more likely to identify with one of the subjects or situations. It is also important to offer an example of a person who had to cope with problems and work out solutions in order to attain mastery.

The modeling technique can also be used in patient education classes or groups. In a group teaching session, when one participant poses a problem, an effective group leader will not offer the solution. The CNS should facilitate group problem solving by asking, "Does anyone have a suggestion for solving this problem?" The CNS can write down the ideas on a flip chart or dry erase board and probe the group for additional suggestions. After several suggestions have been made, turn to the person who posed the problem or question and ask, "Does this offer you a few hints you can use?" After group members have offered suggestions, the CNS may contribute a few more. In using this process, the group members become models for the group. The process generates creative solutions and, because group members have helped each other, enhances their self-efficacy.

MI is another technique that the CNS can use to assist patients/clients in the process of change (Hall & Finegood, 2006; Miller & Rollnick, 2002; Rollnick, Miller, & Butler, 2008). Often described in conjunction with Prochaska and DiClemente's (1983) Stages of Change, MI is a process of assisting the patient/client to more clearly define reasons why change has not been successful in the past. Of utmost importance is recognition that the patient/client is in complete control of the decision to make a change. The health care provider must always remember and respect the patient's/client's right to refuse to change.

The first component of MI is to establish rapport. Rapport is an essential element if the relationship is to develop into the therapeutic discussion that will assist patients/clients to change. As an advanced practice nurse, the CNS is in the best position to assist patients/clients to change. There are four core MI skills:

1. Express empathy—acknowledge that there are issues that must be addressed.

2. Roll with resistance—resistance is normal and must be acknowledged as a component of the change process.
3. Develop discrepancy—create "cognitive dissonance" or the acknowledgment of the difference between where the individual is at the present and where he or she would like to be once his or her goal is accomplished.
4. Promote self-efficacy and change—encourage successful outcomes and assist the patient/client with reaffirmation of his or her success (Hall & Finegood, 2006).

Use of MI permits the CNS to demonstrate respect for the patient's values, preferences, and needs, while at the same time encouraging the change that the patient/client is seeking. MI helps identify patients' concerns and needs by asking open questions, for example, "What's concerning you most right now?" CNSs can use patients' responses to tailor treatment plans to their specific concerns, goals, and lifestyles. Open questions also help identify behaviors that patients would like to change by focusing on the patient's motivation, willingness, and ability to change specific behaviors.

Conversations about behavior change optimally occur when patients and CNSs view each other as partners, an important component of the spirit of MI. Patient–CNS partnership also maintains the relationship even if the patient is not ready to take action. The CNS can ask,

As your CNS, I am concerned about you and your health. I recognize (reflective listening) that you have said that, for now, you are not interested in *(insert health behavior change),* but out of my concern for you, may I have your permission to ask about it in the future?

MI also encourages CNSs to express empathy. When patients share their concerns or fears, CNSs can offer emotional support, another dimension of patient-centered care. Understanding the patient's feelings and perspectives without judging or blaming does not need to imply agreement. Acceptance is possible without agreement or endorsement. The CNS may differ with a patient's views and respectfully express the divergence. However, it is extremely important to listen to patients to understand their perspectives. Listening, accepting, and respecting patients' perspectives builds the therapeutic, patient-centered relationship.

Setting the agenda is the next component of MI. Setting the agenda permits the CNS to identify and respect the patient's values, preferences, and expressed needs, the first component of patient-centered care. CNSs can effectively use this information

to create a treatment plan specifically tailored to each patient, increase adherence, and engage the patient in health behavior change. It also opens the door to discussion about possible health behavior changes. Permitting patients to identify behaviors they would like to change immediately increases buy-in to the change process. Patient engagement is another attribute of patient-centered care.

CNSs can assess importance to patients by affirming patients' past successful behavior changes or coping strategies. This enhances patient confidence to make new health behavior changes. For example, "Remember when you started walking more, and you started by just walking to the mailbox, then worked your way up gradually to walking for 30 minutes a day?" or "Remember when we added two new medicines to the ones you were already taking? You did a great job juggling times you take your medicines, even though one of the new ones could not be taken close to mealtimes."

MI also includes assessing readiness. It can be done using the self-efficacy needs assessment technique ("People can differ a lot when it comes to how ready they are to [*insert health behavior change*]. How ready do you think you are?") or using numerical scale ("If 0 was *totally unprepared* and 10 was *absolutely sure you will be able to* [*insert health behavior change*], what number would you give yourself?"). If the patient responds less than 7, it alerts the CNS to the likelihood that the patient will not be able to succeed with the behavior change.

Additional probing may identify specific barriers that the patient would need to overcome, and the CNS may be able to help the patient find ways to resolve those problems. The CNS can also ask the patient what it would take to achieve a higher number. Then, the CNS can specifically deal with the issues the patient identifies.

Negotiation is a critical component of the partnership, the therapeutic relationship, and patient-centeredness. It permits clinicians to use their clinical expertise, and it allows patients to use their knowledge of their goals and lifestyle experiences to achieve the desired clinical outcomes while keeping patients in control. Asking open questions, affirming, reflective listening, and summarizing help clinicians and patients discuss possibilities for behavior change. These core skills help patients make changes that are important to them and lead to enhanced health outcomes.

MI is an effective way to enhance patient–clinician communication and facilitate health behavior change. Its effects are more powerful than active listening or simple reflection used alone. MI also helps clinicians build therapeutic relationships. It creates rapport and engages patients in discussions about their needs, priorities, and health behavior change. To counsel patients most effectively, it is important for clinicians to use a variety of approaches (Miller & Rollnick, 2002), self-efficacy, and modeling, along with MI. These strategies complement MI. They permit clinicians to work with each patient as an individual and use evidence-based counseling techniques to gain important information to create the most effective treatment plan, engage the patient, and support health behavior change.

Health literacy is an issue that cannot be forgotten as you deal with the issue of change and informing patients/clients of their options. Keeping in mind that health literacy is an issue for approximately two-thirds of the American population, Chew, Bradley, and Boyko (2004) identified a series of questions that allow fast screening of patients who may have low health literacy. These questions focus on how often an individual must ask for assistance, confidence levels, and admitting difficulty with understanding written materials. Unfortunately, they rely on the individuals being able to admit they have difficulty understanding information. CNSs can easily and quickly assess health literacy by asking the patient to repeat information that has been shared with them in their own words (London, 1997).

It is important to remember that print materials are most effectively used as an adjunct to support, complement, augment, and remind patients of what is important for maintaining or improving their health. They can also use print materials to share information about their condition and treatment plan with family members. By using the following communication techniques, CNSs can effectively counsel patients and family members who have limited health literacy skills:

1. Ask open-ended questions to ascertain patients' comprehension
2. Use everyday language to explain terms
3. Build on what the patient knows
4. Be alert for nonverbal behavior that indicates misunderstanding
5. Provide opportunities for patients to report on what they have understood
6. Provide names and numbers for staff that can be called for questions

The "teach-back" technique is recommended to nonjudgmentally permit patients to report what they have learned in a patient education session. The CNS can use questions such as

1. "So I can make sure that I was clear, please tell me what you think we have discussed during this visit," or
2. "Please tell me what you will tell your wife/husband about the changes we have made in your treatment plan at today's visit."

The emphasis is a check on the clarity of the CNS, not a test of the patient.

All of the methods described in this section are active ways in which a CNS can implement elements of the models described in the previous section. By using these tools, the CNS can have a significant impact on the patients/clients and the health care team. Ultimately, the goal is to provide examples, models, and behaviors that will increase the likelihood of success in patient health outcomes. The CNS also has a role to play in the system.

Systems-Level Health Literacy. Because of the leadership role of CNSs, they can also impact the health literacy of the care environment. Patients must navigate the physical grounds and buildings of health care facilities, read signs and informational postings, complete forms, find the correct departments, and correctly check in for services. CNSs can assume a leadership role in assessing their health care environments and clinical settings. In addition to information on health literacy and strategies to effectively educate patients and families with limited health literacy, the Harvard School of Public Health's Health Literacy Program provides information on how to conduct an environmental health literacy assessment. One of the valuable resources on the Harvard Health Literacy Program's website is the text of the seminal work on health literacy written by Doak, Doak, and Root (1985). Upon their retirement, the team of Doak, Doak, and Root offered the text of their book to the Harvard School of Public Health Literacy Program with permission to make it freely available to all disciplines to promote health literacy in hospitals and other health care organizations. This book provides CNSs with very specific strategies to educate patients and family members with low health literacy.

Evaluation of Patient/Client-Centered Teaching and Coaching. Patient/client-centered teaching and coaching focus on the use of interpersonal relations skills as well as the use of print materials that are tailored to the needs of the patients/clients. Evaluation of the interpersonal relationship is not easily measured. Assessment of clinical outcomes resulting from the interaction and adherence to the treatment plan agreed to by the patient/client in collaboration with the health care provider is perhaps the best measure. These must be measured on a one-on-one basis, however, and are difficult to quantify. Measurements of an established criterion, such as ability to stay within evidence-based boundaries of care (e.g., performance measures for hemoglobin A1c for diabetic patients), may be an indirect measure of the success of patient/client-centered teaching. To use these measures as a potential direct measurement of success is difficult and biased at best.

Evaluation of materials is much easier to accomplish. The use of the Simple Measure of Gobbledygook (SMOG) scale provides a process to evaluate printed materials (McLaughlin, 1996). The SMOG scale, in collaboration with the Fleish-Kincaid analysis of grade level, also provides a means to measure the health literacy levels of various educational materials provided to the patient/client as a supplement to any other educational process. As mentioned previously, it is important to maintain reading levels between the sixth and eighth grade levels in order to reach the majority of the U.S. population.

Ethical Considerations

There is a potential for breach of ethics in any circumstance where a health care provider has access to a patient/client's personal feelings related to his or her self-efficacy to make change. Each and every CNS should be vigilant to the potential abuses of patients/clients in their vulnerable state.

CONCLUSION

The roles and responsibilities of CNSs offer important opportunities at the direct client care through the health system levels to impact patients' quality of life and clinical outcomes. They can also serve as role models and mentors to nurses and other clinical disciplines in promoting use of evidence-based patient education and counseling techniques. Their role in effectively educating patients and family members and positively impacting the health care environment promotes care that is patient-centered.

Through the use of techniques and tools that support the patient/client as he or she makes changes in his or her lifestyle and health, the CNS can impact the patient, the nursing staff, and the system. Through these actions on the three spheres of influence, the care of patients/clients will be improved.

A focus on empowerment, activation, and inclusion of the patient in a manner that he or she can understand can only result in improved cost-effectiveness and increased access for patients/clients everywhere. The time has come for patient/client-focused education that increases the ability of the individual to make decisions regarding his or her care. The CNS can and does play a significant role in making it possible.

■ DISCUSSION QUESTIONS

- If you were to ask a group of CNSs (barring unforeseen events) to rate on a scale from 10 (*being absolutely certain*) to 1 (*being absolutely uncertain*), how likely it is that they will successfully get dressed tomorrow morning, most will respond "10." Ask the same group of CNSs how likely it is that they could successfully scale Mount Everest tomorrow, and their responses may be very different. Discuss how you have seen this same kind of situation play out with patients in the clinical area. How would you apply self-efficacy theory to assist patients to perhaps see themselves doing something that they may consider impossible?

- According to Hall and Finegood (2006), 40% of the population is in precontemplative stage of change, 40% are in contemplative, and only 20% of the population is engaged in active change processes. Does this number surprise you? Why or why not?

- What types of patient education material does your facility have? Are there any gaps in the information available and the information that your patients need? Are standardized patient/client education materials available, or does each unit use something different?

■ ANALYSIS AND SYNTHESIS EXERCISES

- Think of an individual that you have worked with, or who may be a part of your circle of family or friends, who has successfully managed to change his or her health behaviors and has sustained the change over a year or more. What was it that assisted him or her to make the change? If you do not know of anyone who has successfully changed health behaviors, think of someone who has attempted change. Why do you think he or she was not successful?

- Interview leaders of a CDSMP (you can often find one by doing a search online for leaders in your area). Ask them about their background. Are they a health care provider or a lay person? Ask them about the program and why they chose to become a leader. What role do you see the CNS having in support of a CDSMP group?

- Look at the patient/client education materials in your facility. Do a SMOG analysis and a Fleish-Kincaid analysis of the grade level of the materials. Do your materials meet the standard? What would have to be done to make them meet the standard?

REFERENCES

Ament, L. (2008). Getting patients to follow treatment plans is challenging, costly. *Hospitals and Health Networks*, April. Retrieved February 11, 2009, from http://www.hhnmag.com/hhnmag_app/jsp/articledisplay.jsp?dcrpath=HHNMAG/Article/data/04APR2008/0804HHN_InBox_DisMgt&domain= HHNMAG

Bandura, A. (1977). Self-efficacy: Toward a unifying theory of behavior change. *Psychology Review, 84,* 191–215.

Bruce, B., Lorig, K., & Laurent, D. (2007). Participation in patient self-management programs. *Arthritis and Rheumatism, 57*(5), 851–854.

Chew, L. D., Bradley, K. A., & Boyko, E. J. (2004). Brief questions to identify patients with inadequate health literacy. *Family Medicine, 36*(8), 588–594.

Doak, C. C., Doak, L. G., & Root, J. H. (1985). *Teaching patients with low literacy skills.* Philadelphia, PA: J. B. Lippincott.

Goudreau, K. A., Geiselman, J., Sutterer, W., Tarvin, L., Toothaker, A., Pincock, L.,…Henry, P. (2008). Economics of standardized patient education materials with veteran patients. *Nursing Economics, 2*(26), 111–115, 121.

Hall, D., & Finegood, K. (2006). *Motivational interviewing: Enhancing readiness to change.* Retrieved December 29, 2008, from http://www.nadcp.org/preconference/Pre-Conf_ Motivational_ Interviewing.pdf

Holy Cross Hospital. (2012). *Living well: Chronic disease self-management—A toolkit for hospitals.* Retrieved September 14, 2013, from http://www.ncoa.org/improve-health/center-for-healthy-aging/content-library/Hospital-Toolkit-MD-2012.pdf

Institute for Chronic Care. (2013). *The Chronic Care Model.* Retrieved September 15, 2013, from http://www.improvingchroniccare.org/index.php?p=The_Chronic_Care_Model&s=2

Institute for Healthcare Improvement (IHI). (2013). *The patient experience: Improving safety, efficiency and CAHPS through patient-centered care.* Retrieved September 14, 2013, from http://www.ihi.org/offerings/Training/ThePatientExperience/Pages/default.aspx

Institute of Medicine (IOM). (2001). *Crossing the quality chasm.* Washington, DC: Author.

The Joint Commission (TJC). (2011). *R3 Report: Patient centered communication standards for hospitals.* Retrieved September 14, 2013, from http://www.jointcommission.org/assets/1/18/R3%20Report%20Issue%201%2020111.PDF

Kennedy, A., Reeves, D., Bower, P., Lee, V., Middleton, E., Richardson, G.,…Rogers, A. (2007). The effectiveness and cost effectiveness of a national lay-led self care support programme for patients with long-term conditions: A pragmatic randomised controlled trial. *Journal of Epidemiology and Community Health, 61*(3), 254–261.

Kirsch, I., Jungeblut, A., Jenkins, L., & Kolstad, A. (1993). *Adult literacy in America: A first look at the findings of the National Adult Literacy Survey* (Publication No. 9375). Washington, DC: National Center for Education Statistics, U.S. Department of Education.

London, F. (1995, August). Teach your patients faster and better. *Nursing, 95,* 68, 70.

London, F. (1997, February). Return demonstrations: How to validate patient education. *Nursing, 97,* 32j.

Lorig, K. R. (2001). *Patient education: A practical approach* (3rd ed.). Thousand Oaks, CA: Sage.

Lorig, K. R., Ritter, P. L., Laurent, D. D., & Plant, K. (2006). Internet-based chronic disease self-management: A randomized trial. *Medical Care, 44*(11), 964–971.

Mayer, G., & Villaire, M. (2004). Low health literacy and its effectives on patient care. *Journal of Nursing Administration, 34*(10), 440–442.

McLaughlin, G. (1996). SMOG grading—A new readability formula. *Journal of Reading, 12*(8), 639–646.

Miller, G. (1957). The magical number seven, plus or minus two: Some limits on our capacity for processing information. *Psychological Review, 63,* 81–97.

Miller, W. R., & Rollnick, S. (2002). *Motivational interviewing: Preparing people for change* (pp. 201–216). New York, NY: Guilford Press.

National Association of Clinical Nurse Specialists (NACNS). (2004). *Statement on clinical nurse specialist practice and education* (2nd ed.). Harrisburg, PA: Author.

National Association of Clinical Nurse Specialists (NACNS). (2010). *Clinical nurse specialist core competencies: Executive summary 2006–2008.* Retrieved September 14, 2013, from http://www.nacns.org/docs/CNSCoreCompetenciesBroch.pdf

National Center for Education Statistics. (2006). *National survey of adult literacy.* Retrieved September 8, 2013, from http://nces.ed.gov/pubsearch/pubsinfo.asp?pubid=2007469

National Conference of State Legislatures (NCSL). (2012). *The medical home model of care.* Retrieved September 5, 2013, from http://www.ncsl.org/issues-research/health/the-medical-home-model-of-care.aspx

Nielsen-Bohlman, L., Panzer, A. M., & Kindig, D. A. (Eds.). (2004). *Institute of Medicine Committee on health literacy.* Washington, DC: National Academies Press.

Nolte, S., Elsworth, G. R., Sinclair, A. J., & Osborne, R. H. (2007). The extent and breadth of benefits from participating in chronic disease self-management courses: A national patient-reported outcomes survey. *Patient Education and Counseling, 65*(3), 351–360.

Prochaska, J. O., & DiClemente, C. C. (1983). Stages and processes of self-change of smoking: Toward an integrative model of change. *Journal of Consulting and Clinical Psychology, 51*(3), 390–395.

Rollnick, S. R., Miller, W. R., & Butler, C. C. (2008). *Motivational interviewing in health care: Helping patients change behavior.* New York, NY: Guilford Press.

Rosenstock I., Strecher, V., & Becker, M. (1994). The Health Belief Model and HIV risk behavior change. In R. J. DiClemente & J. L. Peterson (Eds.), *Preventing AIDS: Theories and methods of behavioral interventions* (pp. 5–24). New York, NY: Plenum Press.

Schwartzenberg, J. G., Cowett, A., Van Geest, J., & Wolf, M. S. (2007). Communication techniques for patients with low health literacy: A survey of physicians, nurses and pharmacists. *American Journal of Health Behavior, 31*(Suppl. 1), S96–S104.

Seligman, H. K., Wallace, A. S., DeWalt, D. A., Schillinger, D., Arnold, C. L., Shilliday, B. B.,...Davis, T. C. (2007). Facilitating behavior change with low literacy patient education materials. *American Journal of Health Behavior, 31*(Suppl. 1), S69–S78.

Turner, S. L., Thomas, A. M., Wagner, P. J., & Moseley, G. C. (2008). A collaborative approach to wellness: Diet, exercise and education to impact behavior change. *Journal of the American Academy of Nurse Practitioners, 20,* 339–344.

U.S. Department of Health and Human Services (USDHHS). (2013a). *Healthy People 2020: Understanding and improving health.* Retrieved September 14, 2013, from http://www.healthypeople. gov/2020/topicsobjectives2020/default.aspx

U.S. Department of Health and Human Services (USDHHS). (2013b). *Health literacy.* Retrieved September 14, 2013, from http://www.health.gov/ communication/literacy/

Wagner, E. H., Bennett, S. M., Austin, B. T., Greene, S. M., Schaefer, J. K., & Vonkorff, M. (2005). Finding common ground: Patient centeredness and evidence based chronic illness care. *The Journal of Alternative and Complementary Medicine, 11*(Suppl. 1), S7–S15.

Ward, B. W., & Schiller, J. S. (2013). Prevalence of multiple chronic conditions among US adults: Estimates from the National Health Interview Survey, 2010. *Prevention of Chronic Diseases, 10,* E65.

19

Consultation in the Clinical Nurse Specialist Role

Geraldine S. Pearson

Consultation has been a central component of the clinical nurse specialist (CNS) role since the role was first identified in the 1950s and implemented as part of specialty role designation. It is prominently identified in the newest competencies proposed for CNSs by the National Association of Clinical Nurse Specialists (NACNS). In this document, *consultation* is defined as "patient, staff, or system-focused interaction between professionals in which the consultant is recognized as having specialized expertise and assists consultee with problem solving" (NACNS, 2010, p. 14).

Historically, nurses prepared at the master's level as specialists in clinical nursing were seen as part of a movement to improve care. Peplau (1965), Reiter (1966), and Smoyak (1976) all wrote about specialized clinical preparation as an additional educational component of traditional nursing education. Consultation was an integral part of this expanded nursing role and remains one of the core competencies of the CNS role. Defined as the indirect provision of care through helping others implement change, the process of CNS consultation has reflected the tumultuous fiscal and professional pressures that nursing in general has faced. These pressures include managed care and reimbursement issues, funding streams, erosion of the value placed on the CNS role, and the inherent difficulty capturing the essence of the CNS role, especially with regard to consultative activities and outcome measures. For CNSs the purpose of consultation is to implement a unit of change that will result, either directly or indirectly, in improved health care. The CNS consultant may deal with various systems, including educational, health care, and corporate environments. Consultation may be case specific to an individual, group specific to staff or patients, or system specific. Consultation is often integrated into direct care roles and occurs in all specialties of advanced practice nursing. Some aspect of consultation is usually central to the functioning of a CNS regardless of the nursing practice specialty.

Many theorists, both in nursing and in other disciplines, have identified the structure and process of consultation with distinct boundaries and rules. In reality, consultation activities, like much of the CNS role, have evolved and changed, often to fit the CNS practice situation. Currently, consultation competency is a required skill in a clinical specialist role and, as already defined by the NACNS (2010), involves focused interaction among professionals in which the consultant has specialized expertise and assists with problem solving. More specifically, Berragan (1998) noted that consultation in nursing appears to follow two trends: "external or independent consultancy where the incumbents focus purely upon this role as their 'job,' and internal consultation where consultancy is seen as an integral part of their role and is a subrole of the advanced practitioner" (p. 139). These two trends are applicable to the consultation roles taken by CNSs in the current health care system. Barron and White (2009) advocate differentiating clinical consultation from other CNS roles involving comanagement, referral, and supervision.

Their algorithmic model carefully details the process of consultation from request to consultative intervention and assessment.

It is impossible to underestimate the influence of third-party reimbursement and fiscal restraints on the CNS consultation role, at least as it was originally conceptualized. The fiscal constraints on the CNS role, including the need for direct third-party reimbursement, have had a significant impact on role continuation and development. Many CNSs have compromised with the fiscal pressures or the systems where they practice and incorporate the consultative process into other aspects of their work that are more likely to result in third-party reimbursement.

In spite of the financial complexities of continuing to do consultation as the predominant part of a CNS's job, most nurses in a CNS role would cite consultation as the arena where they have the most impact on a changing health care system. It is the area of work where all the skills possessed by a CNS are called into play and actively used as part of a consultation process.

The CNS role requires knowledge, expertise, and experience in an area of specialty practice. Consultation evolves out of the evidenced expert knowledge base of a CNS who knows how to practice and how to improve situations through indirect application of expertise. This chapter reviews the historical development of consultation in CNS practice, conceptual models of consultation, and outcome measures pertaining to efficacy of the consultative role.

HISTORICAL PERSPECTIVE

The role of consultant is rooted in specialty practice, which, in turn, has been the hallmark of the CNS role. The 1960s saw an increase in graduate nursing programs that trained nurses in specialty fields. This trend continued into the 1970s and was influenced dramatically by the federal funding available to nurses who went on to graduate study (Hoeffer & Murphy, 1984). By 1980, the American Nurses Association (ANA) had issued a social policy statement that defined specialization in nursing for its nursing members and community constituents (ANA, 1980). From here developed the Council of Clinical Nurse Specialists, which first met in 1983 and became a forum for CNSs, their developing role, and their evolution within specialty practice. The entry level for CNS practice is a graduate nursing degree originally defined with key components of educational content in theory, clinical practice, and research (Field, 1983). Course content around the consultation role was generally embedded in the clinical practice aspect of educational preparation.

Barron (1989) noted that consultation has historically been an essential part of the CNS role. The key types of consultation are divided into expert, resource, and process consultation. The expert is seen as having unique skills necessary to prescribe specific solutions to problems in specific situations. In contrast is the resource consultant, who provides relevant information allowing the consultee to choose alternative solutions (Sparacino & Cooper, 1990). The third type of consultation, involving process, initiates changes in situations that allow the consultee to make decisions applicable to this situation and ones in the future (Kohnke, 1978).

Historically, Berragan (1998) suggested that nurses, in the early years of the CNS role, were reluctant to take on the role of consultant. She suggested that this was rooted in a lack of suitable role models and nurses' questionable need for consultation. Chinn and Wheeler (1985) suggested that consultation models in nursing were impeded because of the perceived inferiority of nursing when compared to medicine. It was also suggested that the consultation role development was rooted in the development of nursing knowledge within the framework of womens' positions within a largely patriarchal medical system (Hagell, 1989).

In the 1970s and 1980s, the consultation role in nursing was promoted in the United States, specifically for advanced practice nurses and CNSs (Blake, 1977; Lareau, 1980). In Britain, Wright and Pearson (in Marr, 1993) began the nurse consultant role in the 1980s in nursing development units. Wright (1991) and Marr (1993) began the work in Britain at the same time that Braddock and Sawyer (1985) were defining nurse consultation in the United States, and Keane (1989) was describing similar role development in Australia.

Fenton (1985, p. 33) further developed Benner's model of expert nursing practice (1984) by defining the consulting role as a specific domain of CNS practice. She noted that this aspect of the CNS role included

- Providing patient care consultation to the nursing staff through direct patient intervention and follow-up;
- Interpreting the role of nursing in specific clinical patient care situations to nursing and other professional staff; and
- Providing patient advocacy by sensitizing staff to the dilemmas faced by patients and families seeking health care.

Fenton's early descriptors of the consultation aspect of the CNS role are one of the few that directly identify advocacy as an important component to consultation. As such, the provision of improved patient care is the goal of a consultative process, whether through direct or indirect means.

Currently, consultation is one of the core competencies for CNSs (NACNS, 2004) and is prominently noted to be part of revised competencies. Consultation is accomplished within three spheres of influence, including patient/family, nursing personnel, and organizational systems (NACNS, 2004). The CNS is both a resource and a process consultant (Klein, 2007).

As a resource consultant, the CNS provides relevant information that enables the staff nurse and others to make decisions based on alternatives. As a process consultant, the CNS facilitates change so that decisions can be made in specific and future situations. "CNS consultation can be measured by outcome achievement and documentation of specific process activities" (Klein, 2007, p. 13).

Klein notes that consultation can be both internal (within the institution) or external (outside the institution). External consultation can involve specialty organizations, other health care providers, or other health care systems (Klein, 2007).

In current practice, the consultation provided by a CNS of any specialty is complex, complicated, elegant, astute, and powerfully effective in transitioning systems of care. Most often integrated into a broader CNS role, consultation continues to be a hallmark of CNS practice with the ultimate aim of improving patient care.

CONCEPTUAL MODELS OF CONSULTATION

Hamric and Spross (1989) defined *consultation* as an interactional process occurring between two professionals trying to solve a problem. Most consultation is based on a problem-solving approach. Lippitt and Lippitt (1978) note that "the ultimate goal of consultation is learning, change, and growth" (p. 130).

Certainly one of the first nursing theorists to touch on the consultative practice of the CNS, at least indirectly, was Patricia Benner (1984). Her research on clinical expertise identified seven domains of practice defining the process of clinical judgment. These include the helping role, administering and monitoring therapeutic interventions and regimens, effective management of rapidly changing situations, the diagnostic and monitoring functions, the teaching–coaching function, monitoring and ensuring the quality of health care practices, and organizational and work role competencies. The process of consultation is embedded in each domain. Inherent in a consultation practice is clinically expert knowledge about a particular disease entity or population of people (Spross & Baggerly, 1989). Benner would likely view nurses at the expert level of practice as embodying the characteristics necessary to be a nurse consultant.

Barron and White (2009) defined the distinct differences between the processes of consultation, collaboration, comanagement, and referral. Consultation is distinguished by the degree to which the nurse assumes direct responsibility for clinical management. Consultants are generally not responsible for direct management of the clinical dilemma on which they are consulting. If they become responsible for the direct clinical intervention, then the process moves away from consultation and into comanagement or supervision. The consultee assumes responsibility for the clinical outcomes and is free to use or not use the advice offered by the consultant.

Approaches to consultation are varied and may be based on specific or multiple theoretical structures. Also, in the current practice arena for CNSs, consultation is less likely to be bounded by strict rules and structures and more apt to ebb and flow with the clinical work inherent in the CNS role. This is influenced by utilization of resources, reimbursement for services, and workforce needs. Few health care systems have the luxury of employing a CNS who does only consultation. Most CNSs integrate consultation into other core competencies of the role.

Gerald Caplan is best known for his model of mental health consultation rooted in his work in Israel in 1949 when, as a child psychiatrist, he was faced with the mental health needs of 16,000 immigrant children. He believed that a traditional model of referral, diagnosis, and psychotherapy of individual children was not possible. As a response, he developed an indirect service model of consultation with colleagues caring for groups of children. Eventually his model was used by nurses and clergy, and it has become the framework for mental health consultation used by many disciplines (Caplan, Caplan, & Erchul, 1995).

Caplan (1970) defined consultation as a process in which a specialist's help is sought to identify ways of system or work problems. He advocated for the following principles:

- Guide the development of consultation by understanding its ecological field
- Explicate all consultation contracts
- Keep the consultant relationship noncoercive
- Promote consultee-centered consultation
- Avoid uncovering types of psychotherapy
- Use the displacement object
- Foster orderly reflection
- Widen frames of reference
- Train those who consult to be consultants (Caplan et al., 1995, pp. 25–26)

Caplan and Caplan (1993) also conceptualized four models for consultation. These included client-centered case consultation, consultee-centered case consultation, program-centered administrative consultation, and consultee-centered administrative approach. Differences in individual or system define the specific consultation model.

While Caplan's model has been used widely in school environments, many CNSs, especially those working in psychiatric settings, use his principles to guide their consultation work. Caplan et al. (1995) emphasized that consultation is only one part of a "larger conceptual framework designed to prevent mental illness and promote mental health in the population at large" (p. 30). His model also tends to be more structured in terms of consultative role and behavior than the roles taken by CNSs. Caplan's major premise has great applicability to nursing practice. He maintains that consultation is only one piece of a larger conceptual framework aimed at preventing mental illness and promoting mental health. Similarly, CNSs involved with nonpsychiatric specialty areas are likely to see consultation as one part of their role.

In the early decades of the CNS role, there was much debate about whether the consultative role was a primary or subrole for CNSs. It was argued that consultation was the foundation for the educator, researcher, and clinician roles that make up the CNS components of functioning (Noll, 1987). Currently, most would agree that the process and function of consultation is integrated into all aspects of the CNS role.

Alvarez (1990) described developmental stages of consultative relationships of psychiatric CNSs in nonacute settings. They were seen as testing via crisis referrals, referrals by a few psychologically minded staff, widening islands of staff support, regular in services and increasing visibility, regular referrals and active working relationships, and skilled staff using the consultant as a source of education and support for staff-generated interventions.

Blake and Mouton (1983) proposed an organizational consultative model used by many nurses. It involved a definition of four focal issues (power/authority, morale/cohesion, norms/standards, and goals/objectives) and their interdependence. Defining change in one focal issue influences functioning in the other issues. Interventions were planned accordingly and included the following categories: acceptant, catalytic, confrontation, prescription, and theories and principles.

The most evolved descriptions of the CNS consultation role have come from Barron (1989) and Barron and White (2009). They wrote about the CNS as consultant and outlined the steps needed to facilitate this process. Modeled along the nursing assessment, they included assessment, planning the intervention, the intervention, and evaluation/closure. Barron advocated for an organizational assessment whenever a CNS consultant entered a system. She also identified establishing relationships and negotiating roles with administrators, physicians, and other professionals as essential to the process. Establishment of credibility involves fostering effective mutual relationships with consultees that ultimately allows the CNS "to offer practical, theoretically sound, successful problem-solving strategies and clinical expertise" (p. 137). Barron and White (2009) defined an ecological model of CNS consultation that considered characteristics of the nurse consultant, characteristics of the consultee, patient and family factors, and situational factors. Formal and informal consultation and various consultation situations can include CNS to CNS, CNS to physician, and CNS to staff nurse consultations.

SPECIALTY DIFFERENCES IN CNS CONSULTATION

Many specialty areas of nursing have developed strong CNS components and role development. These include pediatrics, oncology, cardiology, internal medicine, community health, and psychiatry.

The specialty of psychiatric nursing has been cited as the first to develop curriculum-specific education around the consultation role. In 1946, with the passage of the National Mental Health Act, research and training funds were given to the core mental health disciplines (Hamric, 1989). The designation of psychiatric nursing as one of these core disciplines furthered the scope of psychiatric nursing education and practice and likely fostered the early development of the CNS role specifically aimed at psychiatric consultation liaison nursing (PCLN).

PCLNs often serve as system consultants in their work settings, using systems theory to assess feelings, motivations, and interactions with others. The goals are often to resolve interpersonal difficulties and conflicts among staff and to facilitate change. The ultimate goals are improved outcomes and better patient care (Robinette, 1996).

The PCLN role is well defined in the literature as a role taken by nurses who have both psychiatric/mental health and medical-surgical (MS) experience. They practice mostly in MS inpatient or outpatient settings and long-term care facilities (Happell & Sharrock, 2001; Minarik & Neese, 2002).

Similarly, the child and adolescent psychiatric clinical specialist traditionally undertakes case-based consultation activities with community agencies, schools, and pediatricians. Pediatric populations tend to be more involved in multiple systems as compared to their adult counterparts, and providing comprehensive care demands consultation to involved individuals and organizations.

OUTCOME EVALUATION OF CNS CONSULTATION

Because the consultation role of the CNS is often integrated into other work tasks and is sometimes difficult to quantify, many have struggled with measuring outcome. In spite of these difficulties, it is essential that the aspects of CNS practice that result in change be measurable and quantifiable to illustrate their value to the individuals and organizations that fund the practice. Prevost (2002) noted that CNSs can demonstrate cost-effectiveness by understanding the data elements that define changes. These can include admission rates, average lengths of stay, rates of complication, numbers of educational consultation requests, employee turnover rates, and rates of infection. Measuring the outcome means understanding exactly what is to be measured to gauge change or improvement.

Oermann and Floyd (2002) identified a comprehensive outcome model that included clinical, functional, costs, and satisfaction. They see outcome studies as complementary to evidence-based practice (EBP). Findings are integrated into practice and subsequent outcome studies "validate the effectiveness of those interventions and confirm whether they continue to work over time" (p. 142). Prevost (2002) emphasized the need to quantify clinical expertise and to justify the CNS role by measuring, communicating, and marketing effectiveness, impact, or outcome.

The concept of outcome has become increasingly important in this fiscally driven health care environment. Consultation activities of the CNS are especially subject to scrutiny because many of these clinical activities are difficult to quantify or measure. Consultation is a specialized nursing intervention with focus on various systems. Yakimo (2006) has written about measuring outcomes in PCLN, noting that little attention has been paid to outcomes in this area of specialization. This is likely true in other subspecialties of CNS.

Yakimo, Kurlowicz, and Murray (2004) reviewed PCLN studies that illustrated effective interventions by CNSs acting in a consultative role. These included reduction of demanding patients' requests of staff nurses' time (Mallory, Lyons, Scherubel, & Reichelt, 1993), decreasing length of stay associated with untreated mental health issues (Ragaisis, 1996), and identifying and treating delirium and depression in the elderly (Kurlowicz, 2001).

Yakimo (2006) has advocated for a broader emphasis on comprehensive outcome dimensions relating to the patient and family, the provider, and the institution. The Donabedian model of health care delivery suggests that there are three sources of evidence from which quality can be determined: structure, process, and outcome (Donabedian, 1966, 1980). Yakimo and others (2004) advocate using a systematic model to evaluate the outcome of consultative activities. Types of outcome include clinical, psychosocial, functional, fiscal, and satisfaction. Oermann and Floyd (2002) note that advanced practice nurses are in the best position to conduct the outcome studies demonstrating the effectiveness of their practice.

Brooten and Naylor (1995) have questioned whether or not traditionally measured outcomes are sensitive enough to evaluate nursing actions. This has particular implications for nurse consultation activities, which are often integrated into other aspects of nursing practice and thus difficult to quantify and measure.

This issue is applicable to more recent literature. Fairley and Closs (2006), in their study evaluating a nurse consultant's clinical activities and the effect on patient outcomes, note that clinical activities were complex processes involving clinical judgment and decision making. They found it difficult to pinpoint the exact activities that resulted in their definition of patient care success: "a state free from risk or harm that optimizes rehabilitation" (p. 1113).

Becker (2013) notes the measurable positive outcomes of implementing a clinical specialist role on a night shift. The goal was CNS availability for improved patient outcomes, communication, education, and cost-effectiveness. This role was rooted in a model in which the night-shift CNS was available to every area of the hospital for consultation and clinical assistance. The measured outcomes included a decrease in medical errors, a reduction in overtime, and consistent education through the night shift. In general, the morale and quality of nursing practice improved and this was attributable to the CNS on the night shift.

SUMMARY

The consultation aspect of the CNS role has evolved and grown into a well-accepted, essential part of advanced nursing practice. The nursing literature is filled with descriptive papers and anecdotes about successful nursing consultations at all subspecialties of CNS practice. It is more difficult to find research-based evidence about the efficacy of the role, probably because it is very difficult to measure the outcome of consultation.

Nearly all CNSs engage in some process of consultation as part of their nursing role. The groups and individuals who have benefited from the process of consultation do not question the utility of CNS consultation. The complexity of the consultation role assumed by CNSs has evolved in direct proportion to the development of the total role. CNSs in a variety of specialty practice arenas use consultation as part of their daily work. Most engage in consultation as part of their more multidimensional CNS role.

There is increasing pressure on nurses who provide consultation to identify and measure the direct impact of the intervention, especially as it relates to reducing health care costs. It is essential that nurses engaged in consultation begin systematically measuring the effect of this intervention. At no other time in the history of the consultative role has this been more essential. By illustrating the value of the activity in measurable terms, nurses will ensure that they can continue offering the creative, dynamic, and thoughtful consultative activities that directly and indirectly improve and enhance patient care.

DISCUSSION QUESTIONS

- What role does consultation have in current CNS practice?
- Can a CNS practice without incorporating consultation in his or her role?
- How does consultation differ across specialties of CNS roles?
- What is the advantage of adhering strictly to a theoretical model of consultation vs. developing a version that fits the practice, situation, and needs of the consultee?
- When, after receiving nursing education, is a CNS able to provide effective consultation? What factors influence this?
- What are the pitfalls of offering consultation?
- How does a CNS integrate the other aspects of functioning, such as direct care or teaching, with a consultation role? Identify the positives and negatives of this when all parts of the role are integrated in the same setting.
- How does the CNS build in the research component to his or her consultative practice that builds an EBP and justifies the consultation?
- What administrative and clinical supports are required by a CNS in order to offer consultation?

ANALYSIS AND SYNTHESIS EXERCISES

- Choose one description of a CNS consultation in literature from the past three years. Evaluate the paper from the perspective of use of a theoretical model, role description, and incorporation of evaluation that is measurable and determines effectiveness.

- Evaluate the clinical practices of five CNSs. Query them about the role of consultation in their work and the ways they measure their effectiveness.

CLINICAL APPLICATIONS

- Observe a consultation conducted by a CNS. Note the following:
  - How did the consultation begin? Did it have a discrete beginning, or was it integrated into the CNS role?
  - What was the predominant question from the consultee?
  - What theoretical model did the CNS use while conducting the consultation?
  - How did the consultation fit into the CNS role and the setting?
- Develop a consultation project in a clinical setting where you are practicing. Include the following:
  - Identify the individuals requesting the consultation (consultees).
  - Listen to the request for consultation. Is it related to an educational need, a clinical problem, a staffing problem, or another issue influencing care?
  - Develop a plan for providing the consultation, including the consultee in the process.
  - Ascertain how the consultation will be evaluated, identifying measurable goals and objectives while quantifying whether or not the consultation accomplished original goals of the process.

STEPS TO CNS CONSULTATION

- Request for consultation is received
  a. Define the type of consultation requested (consultee-centered, patient-centered, program-centered)
  b. Define the role of the individuals requesting the consultation
  c. Assess the issues involved
  d. Decide whether or not consultation can be provided
- CNS agrees to conduct the consultation
  a. Define the question and the issues
  b. Define the recipients of the consultation
  c. Define the intervention that could potentially come from the consultation
- Consultation is provided
  a. Document process and progress
  b. Determine need for follow-up
- Evaluate outcome of consultation
  Adapted from Barron and White (2009).

CASE STUDY OF THE CONSULTATION PROCESS FOR A CHILD AND ADOLESCENT PSYCHIATRIC CNS

Jane is a CNS working on an inpatient child unit in a large metropolitan hospital. The average length of stay on the unit is 7 days, and the average age of the child patients is 10 years. The head nurse for the unit, Tim, requests a consultation about a particular staff person with whom he is "struggling." Jane determines that this is a consultation to the head nurse about a program-(staff-) centered issue. The head nurse will be using Jane's consultation to better provide supervision to the staff nurse. Jane will have no role in any formal intervention with the staff person.

After establishing the process of the consultation and their roles, the consultation begins. Tim begins to define his difficulties with the staff nurse and the way this individual interacts with very young children on the unit. As he talks about his observations, he also shares his self-doubts and his concerns that he is overreacting to what he is observing.

Jane asked Tim to define the role expectations for the staff nurse and to think about the ways this staff person was meeting these expectations. She also asked Tim to think about why he was hesitant to confront this particular staff. He shared that the individual's age and long experience was in direct contrast to his relative newness to the head nurse role. Jane and Tim looked at what he brought to the role and discussed ways of supervising the staff so she would have more positive interactions with the younger patients on the unit.

One week later, when Jane and Tim spoke again, he indicated that the supervision process had gone "much better" with this person and that the consultation helped him. Jane documented the consultation and filed it. She made sure Tim knew he could use her consultative expertise in the future with other unit issues.

REFERENCES

Alvarez, C. A. (1990). The psychiatric clinical nurse specialist in the non-acute setting. In P. S. A. Sparacino, D. M. Cooper, & P. A. Minarik (Eds.), *The clinical nurse specialist: Implementation and impact* (pp. 145–162). East Norwalk, CT: Appleton & Lange.

American Nurses Association (ANA). (1980). *Nursing: A social policy statement.* Kansas City, MO: Author.

Barron, A. M. (1989). The CNS as consultant. In A. B. Hamric & J. A. Spross (Eds.), *The clinical nurse specialist in theory and practice* (2nd ed., pp. 125–146). Philadelphia, PA: W. B. Saunders.

Barron, A. M., & White, P. A. (2009). Consultation. In A. B. Hamric, J. A. Spross, & C. M. Hanson, (Eds.), *Advanced practice nursing: An integrative approach* (4th ed., pp. 191–216). St. Louis, MO: Elsevier.

Becker, D. M. (2013). Implementing a night-shift clinical nurse specialist. *Clinical Nurse Specialist, 25,* 26–30.

Benner, P. (1984). *From novice to expert: Excellence and power in clinical nursing practice.* Upper Saddle River, NJ: Prentice Hall.

Berragan, L. (1998). Nursing practice draws upon several different ways of knowing. *Journal of Clinical Nursing, 7*(3), 209–217.

Blake, P. (1977). The clinical specialist as nurse consultant. *Journal of Nursing Administration, 7*(10), 33–36.

Blake, R. R., & Mouton, J. S. (1983). *Consultation: A handbook for individual and organizational development* (2nd ed.). Reading, MA: Addison Wesley.

Braddock, B., & Sawyer, D. (1985). Becoming an independent consultant. *Nursing Economics, 3*(6), 332–335.

Brooten, D., & Naylor, M. (1995). Nurses' effect on changing patient outcomes. *Image, 27,* 95–99.

Caplan, G. (1970). *The theory and practice of mental health consultation.* New York, NY: Basic.

Caplan, G., & Caplan, R. B. (1993). *Mental health consultation and collaboration.* San Francisco, CA: Jossey-Bass.

Caplan, G., Caplan, R. B., & Erchul, W. P. (1995). A contemporary view of mental health consultation: Comments on "Types of Mental Health Consultation" by Gerald Caplan (1963). *Journal of Educational and Psychological Consultation, 6,* 23–30.

Chinn, P. L., & Wheeler, C. E. (1985). Feminism and nursing. *Nursing Outlook, 33*(2), 74–77.

Donabedian, A. (1966). Evaluating the quality of medical care. *Milbank Member Fund Quarterly, 44*(Suppl. 3), 166–206.

Donabedian, A. (1980). Methods for deriving criteria for assessing the quality of medical care. *Medical Care Research and Review, 37*(7), 653–698.

Fairley, D., & Closs, S. J. (2006). Evaluation of a nurse consultant's clinical activities and the search for patient outcomes in critical care. *Journal of Clinical Nursing, 15,* 1106–1114.

Fenton, M. V. (1985). Identifying competencies of clinical nurse specialists. *Journal of Nursing Administration, 15,* 31–37.

Field, L. (1983). Current trends in education and implications for the future. In A. B. Hamric & J. Spross (Eds.), *The clinical nurse specialist in theory and practice.* New York, NY: Grune & Stratton.

Hagell, E. I. (1989). Nursing knowledge: Women's knowledge. A sociological perspective. *Journal of Advanced Nursing, 14*(3), 226–233.

Hamric, A. (1989). History and overview of the CNS role. In A. Hamric & J. Spross (Eds.), *The clinical specialist in theory and practice* (pp. 3–18). Orlando, FL: Grune & Stratton.

Hamric, A. B., & Spross, J. A. (1989). *The clinical nurse specialist in theory and practice* (2nd ed.). Philadelphia, PA: W. B. Saunders.

Happell, B., & Sharrock, J. (2001). The psychiatric consultation-liaison nurse: Towards articulating a model for practice. *Journal of Psychiatric and Mental Health Nursing, 8,* 411–417.

Hoeffer, B., & Murphy, S. A. (1984). *Specialization in nursing practice.* Kansas City, MO: American Nurses Association.

Keane L. (1989). Independent nurse consultant: The lateral leap. In: R. Pratt & G. Gray (Eds.). Issues in Australian Nursing, 2nd ed. Edenburgh: Churchill Livingstone.

Klein, D. G. (2007). From novice to expert. In M. G. McKinley (Ed.), *Acute and critical care clinical nurse specialists: Synergy for best practices* (pp. 11–28). St. Louis, MO: Saunders.

Kohnke, M. (1978). *Case for consultation in nursing: Designs for professional practice.* New York, NY: Wiley.

Kurlowicz, L. H. (2001). Benefits of psychiatric consultation-liaison nurse interventions for older hospitalized patients and their nurses. *Archives of Psychiatric Nursing, 15*(2), 53–61.

Lareau, S. C. (1980). The nurse as clinical consultant. *Topics in Clinical Nursing, 2*(3), 79–84.

Lippitt, G., & Lippitt, R. (1978). *The consulting process in action.* San Diego, CA: University Associates.

Mallory, G. A., Lyons, J. S., Scherubel, J. C., & Reichelt, P. A. (1993). Nursing care hours of patients receiving varying amounts and types of consultation/liaison services. *Archives of Psychiatric Nursing, 7*(6), 353–360.

Marr, J. F. (1993). Consultant nurse. *Surgical Nurse, 6,* 25–26.

Minarik, P. A., & Neese, J. B. (2002). Essential educational content for advanced practice in psychiatric consultation liaison nursing. *Archives of Psychiatric Nursing, 16*(1), 3–15.

National Association of Clinical Nurse Specialists (NACNS). (2010). *Clinical nurse specialist core competencies: Executive summary 2006–2008.* Harrisburg, PA: Author.

Noll, M. (1987). Internal consultation as a framework for clinical nurse specialist practice. *Clinical Nurse Specialist, 1,* 46–50.

Oermann, M. H., & Floyd, J. A. (2002). Outcomes research: An essential component of the advanced practice nurse role. *Clinical Nurse Specialist, 16*(3), 140–144.

Peplau, H. E. (1965). The nurse in the community mental health program. *Nursing Outlook, 13*(11), 68–70.

Prevost, S. S. (2002). Clinical nurse specialist outcomes: Vision, voice, and value. *Clinical Nurse Specialist, 16*(3), 119–124.

Ragaisis, K. M. (1996). The psychiatric consultation-liaison nurse and medical family therapy. *Clinical Nurse Specialist, 10*(1), 50–56.

Reiter, F. (1966). The nurse-clinician. *American Journal of Nursing, 66*(2), 274–280.

Robinette, A. L. (1996). PCLNs: Who are they? How can they help you? *American Journal of Nursing, 96*(7), 48–50.

Smoyak, S. A. (1976). Specialization in nursing: From then to now. *Nursing Outlook, 24*(11), 676–681.

Sparacino, P. S. A., & Cooper, D. M. (1990). The role components. In P. S. A. Sparacino, D. M. Coooper, & P. A. Minarik (Eds.), *The clinical nurse specialist: Implementation and impact* (pp. 11–40). East Norwalk, CT: Appleton & Lange.

Spross, J. A., & Baggerly, J. (1989). Models of advanced nursing practice. In A. B. Hamric & J. A. Spross (Eds.), *The clinical nurse specialist in theory and practice* (2nd ed., pp. 19–40). Philadelphia, PA: W. B. Saunders.

Wright, S. (1991). The nurse as consultant. *Nursing Standard, 5,* 31–34.

Yakimo, R. (2006). Outcomes in psychiatric consultation-liaison nursing. *Perspectives in Psychiatric Care, 42*(1), 59–62.

Yakimo, R., Kurlowicz, L. H., & Murray, R. B. (2004). Evaluation of outcomes in psychiatric consultation-liaison nursing practice. *Archives of Psychiatric Nursing, 18*(6), 215–227.

Mentoring

Kelly A. Goudreau

You take people as far as they will go, not as far as you would like them to go. (*Jeannette Rankin, 1880–1973*)

The art of mentoring is a complex interchange of give, take, readiness to learn, sensing of readiness to learn, and integration of the learner's needs as perceived by both the learner and the mentor. This dynamic dance typically takes place within the context of a one-on-one relationship established between two people: a mentor and his or her protégé. There are other models of mentorship that are described in the literature (Goran, 2001; Grossman, 2007; Rhodes et al., 2009), but the key concept is one of sharing of knowledge and information from one who is more experienced or expert with one who seeks to learn from the expert (Busen & Engebretson, 1999; Yoder, 1990). The definition of mentoring or mentorship is more than just sharing knowledge and teaching skills, however. It also includes career counseling, guidance, advice, and enhanced opportunities for career advancement as a result of the networks that the mentor has established that assist the protégé. The role of the clinical nurse specialist (CNS) as the expert clinician, guide, and mentor to the experienced and inexperienced nursing staff embodies the concept of mentorship.

Although the concept of mentoring has been in existence for centuries, there continues to be little research-based literature on the topic. The enculturation of the concept as an expectation, however, has occurred in relatively recent history. Over the past 30 years, mentoring was integrated into the stream of consciousness in the business world and has also become a construct of the CNS's world. Mentoring is both provided and received by the CNS as he or she develops and grows. The expectation is to return the gift of knowledge and expertise gained through experience that was provided by a mentor through mentoring the next generation of staff nurses and CNSs as they grow and develop.

The intent of this chapter is to provide an overview of the current state of the literature on mentoring and mentorship, define conceptual models of mentoring and mentorship currently in use, apply these models to CNS practice in a variety of settings, and discuss the current cultural expectation for mentoring and mentorship. Examples of how and why to implement the concept in practical terms is provided.

MENTORSHIP: WHERE DID IT COME FROM?

The concept of mentoring and mentorship is actually derived from ancient Greek mythology. In the *Odyssey*, the story purportedly written by Homer (Bell & Goldsmith, 2013; Fitzgerald, 1961), Odysseus (Ulysses) left his young son, Telemachus, in the hands of Mentor, who guided him into becoming a loved and trusted leader in his father's absence. The story brings in elements of Greek mythology through the introduction of the concept that it was not actually a man named Mentor who guided and taught young Telemachus but was in fact the goddess Athena in disguise. The principle is that a more experienced person can provide counsel and guidance to the less experienced person who is learning and growing under the watchful eye of his or her mentor. The element of the goddess Athena brings in a matronly perspective as well and suggests some aspects of the parent–child, mother–son relationship. According to Peddy (2001), although it has not changed significantly, a more contemporary description of a mentor is "a friend and role model, an able advisor, a person who lends support in many different ways to one pursuing specific goals" (p. 28).

The Roman Catholic Church saw mentoring as an important means of succession planning. The church leaders identified that in order for the church to ensure its continued success, not only did they have to draw in new members but there also needed to be a sense of community. In an effort to achieve that sense of community they established formal mentoring relationships between clergy and community youth. Mentoring was identified as a professional responsibility of all the members of the church. Mentoring young members of the church to become devout practitioners and take the place of the aging clergy provided continued growth and development of the church. Not only was growth achieved but also an increased diversification in the ranks of parishioners was attracted to the church as the young of the various populations became church leaders. The church increased its ability to reach out to the widening array of cultures it was attempting to convert.

The concept of mentoring became embedded in the business world for the same reasons articulated by the church. Success of any business rests on planning and growth of the potential pool of candidates for leadership. Succession planning in the face of a shrinking pool of employable personnel is a strong driver of the rationale for mentoring. The same reasons exist currently in nursing.

In 2010, the most current statistics in nursing indicated that by the year 2020 there would be a shortfall of 340,000 available nurses (Hart, 2007; Health Resources and Services Administration, 2006). The downturn in the economy changed the perspective slightly, as many of the Baby Boomer generation chose not to retire immediately, meaning they have stayed in the workforce longer than they perhaps intended. That has had some interesting effects on the workforce, in that those young nurses who graduated from nursing programs between 2009 and now (2013) have had few opportunities to practice. Many of them have either chosen or been forced to leave nursing as a result. The downstream effect is twofold: (a) there have been fewer young nurses in the workforce to mentor, and (b) the departure of the young nurses from the discipline will only serve to enhance the pending shortage. The numbers have not been "crunched" at this point in time so the perceptions are anecdotal at best. The difficulty becomes that this

unknown effect and impact is the creation of a false sense of a nursing "glut" in the workforce. At no time have the concepts of mentoring and mentorship been more important to nursing. Mentoring and mentorship are primary components in keeping nursing a viable profession for the same key reasons that the church identified:

- Succession planning in a time of shortage
- Increasing diversity in both culture and age variation in the workplace
- The need for a sense of community and professional responsibility

A variety of so-called mentoring programs have gained popularity in recent years. A number of facilities that hire nurses have developed residency or internship programs with the focused goal of both attracting and retaining new nurses graduating from schools of nursing (American Association of Colleges of Nursing [AACN], 2013; Bally, 2007; Hayes & Scott, 2007; Hunnerkopf, 2007; Poynton, Madden, Bowers, & Keefe, 2007). Key to these programs is the relationship that is established between the new graduate and his or her preceptor/mentor. Expectations for these preceptors do not often extend beyond the relationship with the new graduate and assessment of his or her competence to provide minimally safe patient care. These skills do not often move beyond the skills of a staff nurse. The preceptors are not mentors in the truest sense of the meaning found in the literature (Grossman, 2007; Yoder, 1990). According to Dracup and Bryan-Brown (2004), "mentors do more than teach skills; they facilitate new learning experiences, help new nurses make career decisions, and introduce them to networks of colleagues who can provide new professional challenges and opportunities" (p. 450). The overall intent of the residency is to decrease the numbers leaving the profession through development of current registered nurses (RNs) as preceptors or mentors, provision of support to new RNs, and increasing overall satisfaction with the profession through opportunities for growth, development, and collegial relationships for both the mentor and the protégée. The role of the CNS clearly fulfills all of these expectations.

LITERATURE REVIEW

A clear definition of *mentorship* versus *preceptorship* has been the primary confusion within the literature. The concept of mentoring and mentorship as described in this chapter has been clearly defined and articulated by only a few authors (Angelini, 1995;

Grossman, 2007; Murray, 2001; Shea, 2001; Stewart & Kreuger, 1996; Yoder, 1990; Yonge, Billay, Myric, & Luhanga, 2007). Most authors on the topic assume that the reader has the same understanding of the concept, and they proceed to describe the relationship as one that is focused on skills attainment. Typically, in United States and Canadian literature the relationship focused on skills attainment is called preceptorship rather than mentorship (Grossman, 2007; Yonge et al., 2007). Mentoring and mentorship is most accurately defined as follows:

> Mentoring in nursing encompasses a guided experience, formally or informally assigned, over a mutually agreed-on period, that empowers the mentor and mentee to develop personally and professionally within the auspices of a caring, collaborative, culturally competent, and respectful environment. (Grossman, 2007, p. 28)

There has been tremendous international interest in mentoring recently. This interest, however, has only served to perpetuate the confusion and lack of clarity surrounding the terms *preceptorship* and *mentorship*. The work surrounding the initiation of Project 2000 in the United Kingdom has generated tremendous interest in the process and outcomes of what is being called mentoring and mentorship (Andrews & Wallis, 1999; Hyatt, Brown, & Lipp, 2008; Moseley & Davies, 2008; Nettleton & Bray, 2008; Webb & Shakespeare, 2008). An additional international discussion on mentoring and mentorship is the Leonardo da Vinci project undertaken in the European Union (Fulton et al., 2007). On closer examination of the articles, however, it is clearly evident that in both instances the articles describe support of the nursing students who are entering the workplace in greater numbers now that the educational institutions are responding to the call for increased enrollment. The articles describe mentorship as a supportive educational environment that links the student with a particular individual who will assess his or her clinical competency. In the United States, these relationships are more often called preceptorships rather than mentoring relationships.

Although the concept of mentoring and mentorship has existed for literally generations, there has been very little actual research on the topic. Perhaps this is due to the current state of confusion regarding the extent to which the support is provided and the duration of the support. Articles in both the business and nursing literature are most likely to be anecdotal in nature and discuss the "how to" of mentoring rather than assessing research-driven benefits of mentoring (Cahill & Payne, 2006; Tuohig, 2007). In many research-focused articles the concept of mentoring has not been defined clearly, so it is difficult to determine if the research was conducted on mentoring or preceptoring as the concept; there continues to be confusion about the terms (Dyer, 2008; Fulton et al., 2007; Hyatt et al., 2008; Moseley & Davies, 2008; Myall, Levett-Jones, & Lathlean, 2008; Nettleton & Bray, 2008; Webb & Shakespeare, 2008; Yoder, 1990). Rhodes et al. (2009) did conduct evidence-based analyses of the concept of mentoring of young adults and defined six standards that address six critical dimensions of mentoring program operations: (a) recruitment; (b) screening; (c) training; (d) matching; (e) monitoring and support; and (f) closure (p. 3). These standards are not, however, definitive to the creation of the mentored relationship but again outline the "how to" in reference to establishing a mentoring operation. Additionally, a literature review by Pompa (2012) found that there are several positive impacts from the mentoring relationship, for both the mentee and the mentor. As part of the literature review, Pompa (2012) found in more than 100 studies that the following were the most regularly quoted benefits for mentees:

> improved performance and productivity; improved knowledge and skills; greater confidence, empowerment and well-being; improved job satisfaction and motivation; faster learning and enhanced decision-making skills; improved understanding of the business; improved creativity and innovation; encouragement of positive risk-taking; development of leadership abilities. (p. 9)

Benefits to the system that used a mentor/mentee relationship to develop staff included "strategic change, facilitation of partnerships, innovation and change, problem solving and better project management" (p. 9).

On the other hand, Noe (1998) argues for caution in assessing the impact of mentoring. He found that mentors tend to overestimate the value and impact of their support, and attributed a greater proportion of the business success to the mentoring than protégés did.

For purposes of the research review, and application within the advanced practice role, mentoring continues to be defined much as Yoder (1990) and later Grossman (2007) and Yonge and colleagues (2007) defined it and includes a component whereby the mentor specifically works with the protégée to develop a long-term plan for specific personal development in addition to skills development. Areas that need growth are collaboratively identified by both the mentor and the protégé and, in turn, are developed, explored, and expanded. Unfortunately, there is little research examining this definition and the outcomes of same.

The research that has been done with the broader definition in mind has been structured around the implications of the relationship between the mentor and the protégé and, subsequently, the behaviors that are most conducive to establishing and maintaining the mentoring relationship (Allen, Eby, & Lentz, 2006; Nedd, Nash, Galindo-Ciocon, & Belgrave, 2006; Nickle, 2007). The focus on individual development has been identified as a means to increase personal and professional satisfaction for both the mentor and the protégé (Finley, Ivanitskaya, & Kennedy, 2007). By clearly identifying opportunities for improvement and opportunities for personal development, the mentor and the protégé are collaborative partners, and both have stated they experience personal satisfaction with both the growth and the relationship that develops (Shea, 2001). Although not research-based, Shea blends the concepts of preceptoring and mentoring but distinctly separates them in terms of time and structure. He describes various stages of the relationship on a continuum ranging from highly structured, short-term relationships (preceptorships) to informal, long-term friendships that are intermittent in nature but are sustained relationships that last from 3 years to a lifetime (mentorships).

Research conducted includes both qualitative and quantitative work (Angelini, 1995; Benner, 1984; Dyer, 2008; Dracup & Bryan-Brown, 2004; Nedd et al., 2006; Nickle, 2007; Schweibert, 2000; Stewart & Kreuger, 1996). Unfortunately, most of the work is survey or self-report in nature and has little academic or scientific rigor. Additionally, little has been done in terms of evaluation of the outcomes of a mentoring relationship (Grossman, 2007; Rhodes et al., 2009).

The work done to date supports the anecdotal perceptions that there is value in the relationship that is largely of an intangible nature but is reported as positive for both the mentor and the protégé (Allen et al., 2006; McKinley, 2004; McWeeny, 2002; Morse, 2006; Robert Wood Johnson Foundation, 2004; Zucker et al., 2006). Further, the relationship that holds the most promise of sustained and positive outcomes are the informal long-term friendships described by Shea (2001; Allen et al., 2006).

CONCEPTUAL AND/OR THEORETICAL SUPPORT FOR MENTORING

The rigorous research that has been conducted has been based on one of three conceptual frameworks or theories. Within nursing, Benner (1984) is the most frequently cited work that supports the perception

that an individual can move from being a novice to being an expert under the watchful eye of a guide, or through self-reflection and experiential growth (Nedd et al., 2006). Although this theory provides some strength to the concept of mentoring, it is not specifically focused on the relationships of the novice with the experts in his or her environment and provides only tangential support for the premise that mentoring will strengthen and ensure overall satisfaction with the new role.

The issue of a lack of strong theoretical constructs to support research and researchable outcomes of mentoring and mentorship are also found outside of nursing. Strong theory development was undertaken in the field of psychology, however, and theoretical constructs around mentoring relationships by Kram (1985) suggest that mutual interpersonal appreciation is key to being able to initiate and maintain a mentoring relationship. Kanter's (1977) work on organizational development and individual development also provides theoretical structure to mentoring relationships in the workplace similar to that posited by Kram. These theories are rarely seen within nursing, however.

Finally, the strongest theoretical construct that directly relates to mentoring is that presented by Collins, Brown, and Holum (1991) in their discussion of the theories of a Russian educator, Lev Vygotsky (Nickle, 2007). Collins et al. describe the theory of constructivism as defined by Vygotsky. Vygotsky was a contemporary of Piaget's, but neither man knew of each other due to the fact that the Iron Curtain separated their research during their lifetimes. What Vygotsky, and later Collins et al. (1991), described is a process where by a mentor/teacher/guide assesses the learner's abilities with lower and upper thresholds of comfort. That comfort zone is called the zone of proximal development, and it is the job of the guide and mentor to push the learner to move along the continuum of learning and establish new upper and lower boundaries of comfort and understanding. The guide and mentor sets up a "scaffolding" of support that protects the learner as he or she initially begins to learn a new process or is placed in a new environment. Gradually, the scaffolding is removed as the mentor assesses that the learner is comfortable and able to perform the duties or interactions without support. This dynamic assessment and release of the learner as he or she moves across the continuum of learning and through the zone of proximal development describes the process of mentoring. The theory of social constructivism emphasizes the interaction of the environment and the social structures that support learning. It truly brings the theories of Benner (1984), Kram (1985), and Kanter (1977) into a dynamic whole that provides a strong foundation for continued research and evaluation of outcomes. It, too, however, has not been strongly introduced into the nursing literature at this time (Nickle, 2007).

APPLICATION TO CNS PRACTICE: HOW TO USE MENTORING IN YOUR ENVIRONMENT

Through the mentoring relationships established in residency programs and orientation, the CNS can have direct influence on welcoming, assessment of strengths, identification of areas needing improvement, and ongoing support that ultimately results in retention of the nursing staff. The theories of Lev Vygotsky and his successors are lived on a daily basis in the role of the CNS in the clinical environment. By welcoming, assessing strengths and areas for improvement, and then supporting the neophyte in the clinical environment, the CNS acts as a mentor. It is the CNS who constructs the scaffolding around the new nurse and creates the environment in which the learner feels safe to learn. This protection extends not only to the learner but also to the patients for whom the learner is caring. The expert nurse, in the form of the CNS, is able not only to monitor the learning of the new nurse, but also to provide the safety net for the patient as the CNS assesses the efficacy of the care provided by the neophyte.

Evidence of the strength of this relationship can be indirectly assessed through the role of the CNS in the Magnet movement. CNSs play two pivotal roles in the recent surge of hospitals seeking Magnet status: (a) They are the advanced practice nurses (APNs) who are most visible to the staff and provide the support to new nurses as expert clinicians, and (b) they are most often the individuals who manage and coordinate the Magnet journey (American Nurses Credentialing Center [ANCC], 2013; Muller, Hujcs, Dubendorf, & Harrington, 2010; Walker, Urden, & Moody, 2009).

The key elements of Magnet where CNSs have the greatest impact or influence are in 6 of the 14 forces: Force 1: Quality of Nursing Leadership; Force 3: Management Style; Force 6: Quality of Care; Force 11: Nurses as Teachers; Force 12: Image of Nursing; and Force 14: Professional Development. These six Forces are dispersed across all five of the Magnet Model Components (ANCC, 2013), so the CNS has clear influence across the entire Magnet attainment journey and process. As a leader on the unit or within the facility, the CNS role models the behaviors of leadership and management. As the expert clinician on the unit or in the specialty area, the CNS has a direct influence on the quality of the nursing care,

exemplifies the role of nurses as teachers, and provides a role model for the less experienced nurses. Finally, it is in the professional development force that the CNS has the greatest influence as a mentor.

The three spheres of influence that a CNS functions within are the patient/client sphere, the nursing/nurses sphere, and the systems sphere (National Association of Clinical Nurse Specialists [NACNS], 2010). The one in which the CNS has the greatest role as a mentor is the nursing/nurses sphere of influence. Within the mentor role that the CNS plays, he or she is able to provide the greatest strength to the establishment of clearly defined competencies and evaluation processes to assess whether or not the neophyte has attained these competencies. Regardless of whether or not the initial orientation is called a preceptorship, residency, or internship, the CNS plays a pivotal role. Direct one-on-one interaction in support of both the new and experienced nurses means that the CNS provides a coaching role at the very least and, in many instances, a mentoring relationship with many of the staff over time. This relationship extends not only to the direct relationship with each nurse, but also to the creation of a culture of mentoring by all staff. Grossman (2007) noted that in her vision of a mentoring culture in nursing, "clinical nurse specialists…may allow a mentoring staff to expand the nursing science base in everyday work with patients" (p. 27). The use of evidence-based practice (EBP) principles and sharing of the evidence with staff creates a culture of excellence and quality that can only be attributed to the presence of an APN in the clinical environment (LaSala, Connors, Pedro, & Phipps, 2007).

Additional provisions of mentoring in the CNS influence on the nursing/nurses sphere is the mentoring of masters or doctoral students who are becoming CNSs. A component of the CNS role is the expectation that those who are expert in being the expert clinician will share their lessons learned with the neophyte CNS. Mentoring the next generation of APNs is paramount to the continuation of the role and the direct influence on the quality and safety of the patient care.

In either the mentoring of new staff nurses or the mentoring of new CNSs, the role of the experienced CNS is to assess the learning needs of the nurses/nursing staff and then assist them to move along the continuum of learning within their comfort level and beyond. By stretching the zone of proximal development (Nickle, 2007), the learner moves beyond his or her current capability under the watchful, supportive eye of the CNS.

According to Lakasing and Francis (2005), the characteristics of the most successful mentors include the following: knowledge of how societal systems, processes, or things work; strong values that are parallel to those of the institution and the profession; technical competence; strong character that allows and encourages growth in the mentee; knowledge of how to behave in a social situation; understanding of how to get things done in or through the organization; strong moral standards that encourage the development of same in the mentee; and understanding of other people and their viewpoints. Each of these is an essential competency for the successful CNS. These themes have been reiterated in recent work done in the European Union through the MAITRE project (Miller & Storey, 2007). The MAITRE Project (which is an acronym that stands for Mentoring trAIning maTerials and REsources) is a research collaborative that is looking at what mentor competencies are and how they can be standardized and then measured across multiple disciplines and countries. Maitre is a French word that means "master" and is intended to convey that there is a way to master the art of mentoring as well as to be a master of the protégé.

Within the systems sphere of influence and in relation to mentoring, the CNS works collaboratively with the education and/or nursing professional services department to provide systemwide, consistent programs that will encourage and develop nurses and assist them in feeling supported and mentored by their peers and/or by the CNS. Through a thorough needs assessment and day-to-day interaction with the nursing staff, the CNS is often able to identify the broad learning needs for learners and demonstrate to the systems-level education department what the specific learning needs may be across the facility.

EVALUATION OF MENTORING AND MENTORSHIP

Within the NACNS' *Clinical Nurse Specialist Core Competencies* (2010), the one clear outcome that is addressed in relation to mentoring is within the coaching competency (p. 22). Identification of the necessary knowledge and skill development in nurses is a key outcome of CNS practice (NACNS, 2010). It is unfortunate, however, that very few research studies have been conducted to assess this particular outcome for CNSs, or any other discipline for that matter. Most of the information related to mentoring is anecdotal and not research-based at all.

Buddeberg-Fischer and Herta (2006) conducted a literature review within the medical literature in relation to evaluation of formal mentoring programs for medical students and doctors. They identified that only 16 articles met their criteria for inclusion in the study, and none of them discussed evaluation of the programs. Nursing literature is, as previously stated, confused on the definition of mentoring. This confusion creates a situation where some formal evaluations may have been done in relation to preceptor relationships rather than mentoring relationships, which then focus on the short-term attainment of competencies and skills versus the lasting, guiding relationship of a mentorship (Webb & Shakespeare, 2008).

Outside of nursing and health care literature the situation is similar, whereby authors continue to supply anecdotal information rather than research-based outcomes assessment. Boldra, Landin, Repta, Westphal, and Winistorfer (2008) identify that the benefits of mentoring include improved retention, leadership development, succession planning, and a sense of increased organizational commitment on the part of the mentees. This has not, however, been substantiated through research.

When evaluation has been research based, data that have been collected on the evaluation of mentor programs have been descriptive in nature. Most often, when evaluation of a mentor relationship is discussed, regardless of the perception of it being a true mentorship or preceptorship, the data define the level of satisfaction with the relationship or the program itself (Weiss et al., 2008).

This lack of research data to support the mentor relationship is problematic and needs to be addressed. It is the realm of the CNS to address issues related to the mentoring, coaching, and precepting of new nurses or experienced nurses who have moved into new clinical areas. Perhaps the CNS should lead the way in creation of a sound research process to fully evaluate the outcomes of mentoring, precepting, or coaching and the relative value of each to the organization in which they practice.

ADVANCED NURSING PRACTICE: WHY IS MENTORING AN ADVANCED SKILL?

Regardless of the research base or the anecdotal nature of the perceptions, it is clear that most, both internal or external to the profession, consider mentoring an essential component of current needs to retain and develop personnel. The role of the advanced practice CNS has been defined as an essential element. By being the clinical expert who oversees the quality and safety of the care being provided by the nursing staff and by guiding, coaching, role modeling, and mentoring the staff, the CNS is an element that must be present.

Staff nurses in general do not have the time to mentor other staff nurses. Their role is correctly focused on provision of care to the patient population. They will sometimes assist student nurses or peers who are new to the environment, but typically, if there is something that needs attention beyond the basic assessments, they will refer it to the CNS.

The nurse manager, although he or she carries advanced skills in leadership and management, is not always the clinical expert. The nurse manager refers issues of clinical competence to the CNS to address. Through this assessment and referral the CNS can be both the coach and the guide and potentially address issues of mentorship with promising new nurses. CNSs work in partnership with both the nurse manager and the staff nurse to assist the further development of staff. Working within the nurses/nursing sphere of influence is an essential component of the CNS role and is clearly an advanced skill.

ETHICAL CONSIDERATIONS

The ethics of mentoring are not often discussed in the literature, yet there are many instances of the establishment of a code of ethics associated with mentoring. The code of ethics in most instances outlines the need for mutual respect, confidentiality, and boundaries. It is clear that from the outset there is a power differential in the relationship, with the mentor having more power than the protégé. The power differential can be a cause of concern if it is not used appropriately.

Most often the power differential can cause nothing more than blurring of the lines between being a casual friend versus mentor as the relationship is established and maintained over a long period of time. Unfortunately, the power differential can also lead to a misuse of the relationship for personal gain on the part of the mentor and potentially may even result in the outcome being an inappropriate sexual relationship.

The competence of the mentor is utmost when a mentor/protégé relationship is being considered in either a formal mentoring program or an informal mentored relationship. The mentor has a responsibility to ensure that the protégé has the best opportunity to learn, and that can only be accomplished if the mentor is knowledgeable and can share his or her expertise and network of connections with the protégé. If the mentor knows that he or she is not the correct person who can assist and advance the protégé, he or she needs to acknowledge that and step away.

The CNS is in the unique position of being a clinical expert and guide/coach and mentor to many nurses and nursing staff on the unit. He or she can clearly see the current relationships and the dynamics of those relationships. As a clinical expert and guide, the CNS has the responsibility to ensure that any mentor relationships are healthy and bound by ethical precepts. If they are not, the CNS has a moral and ethical responsibility to bring them to the attention of those who can best address the issues. As a guide and role model on the unit, the CNS is expected to have the highest moral and ethical standards and uphold those expectations in the staff on the unit. As such, he or she represents the best of what professional nursing is and can be.

SUMMARY

It is clear from the literature that mentoring is perceived to have many benefits. Benefits that are expressed are that mentoring allows organizations to grow and flourish by (a) developing, satisfying, and retaining employees; (b) advancing the development of experienced staff by encouraging them to become mentors; (c) improving organizational climate, performance, and image; (d) allowing for the creation of clinical expert networks; and (e) increasing diversity within the discipline.

Although these benefits are not clearly established through research outcomes, the anecdotal benefits have been discussed thoroughly in the literature. The expectation that every professional nurse will guide and mentor another has been firmly implanted in the social fabric of the discipline. The benefits are personal and typically include the sense that the knowledge gained through years of experience will not be lost as one generation transitions and passes responsibility to the next.

The role of the CNS in this process is clear. As an APN working directly in the influence of staff, the CNS has a significant role to play as mentor, guide, and role model. How do we bring this all together? The expectation of being a mentor needs to be incorporated into the education of the CNS as he or she masters the role. The CNS needs to focus on individual development for the staff and themselves. Through the perpetual process of assessing the needs of the staff and then seeking or building the resources needed to further develop the clinical skills, personal attributes, or professional comportment, the CNS plays a key role in the development of nurses and nursing as a profession.

REFERENCES

Allen, T. D., Eby, L. T., & Lentz, E. (2006). Mentorship behaviors and mentorship quality associated with formal mentoring programs: Closing the gap between research and practice. *Journal of Applied Psychology, 91*(3), 567–578.

American Association of Colleges of Nursing (AACN). (2013). *Nurse residency program*. Retrieved September 7, 2013, from http://www.aacn.nche.edu/education-resources/nurse-residency-program

American Nurses Credentialing Center (ANCC). (2013). *ANCC Magnet recognition program—recognizing excellence in nursing services*. Retrieved September 2, 2013, from http://www.nursecredentialing.org/Magnet.aspx

Andrews, M., & Wallis, M. (1999). Mentorship in nursing: A literature review. *Journal of Advanced Nursing, 29*(1), 201–207.

Angelini, D. (1995). Mentoring in the career development of hospital staff nurses: Models and strategies. *Journal of Professional Nursing, 11,* 89–97.

Bally, J. M. G. (2007). The role of nursing leadership in creating a mentoring culture in acute care environments. *Nursing Economics, 25*(3), 143–148.

Bell, C. R., & Goldsmith, M. (2013). *Managers as mentors*. San Francisco, CA: Berrett-Koehler.

Benner, P. (1984). *From novice to expert: Excellence and power in clinical nursing practice*. Menlo Park, CA: Addison-Wesley.

Boldra, J., Landin, C., Repta, K., Westphal, J., & Winistorfer, W. (2008). The value of leadership development through mentoring. *Health Progress, 89*(4), 33–36.

Buddeberg-Fischer, B., & Herta, K. D. (2006). Formal mentoring programmes for medical students and doctors: A review of the Medline literature. *Medical Teacher, 28*(3), 248–257.

Busen, N. H., & Engebretson, J. (1999). Mentoring in advanced practice nursing: The use of metaphor in concept exploration. *The Internet Journal of Advanced Nursing Practice, 2*(2). Retrieved January 12, 2009, from http://www.ispub.com/ostia/index.php?xmlFilePath=journals/ijanp/vol2n2/mentoring.xml

Cahill, M., & Payne, G. (2006). Online mentoring: ANNA connections. *Nephrology Nursing Journal, 33*(6), 695–697.

Collins, A., Brown, J. S., & Holum, A. (1991). Cognitive apprenticeship: Making thinking visible. *American Educator, 15*(3), 6–46.

Dracup, K., & Bryan-Brown, C. (2004). From novice to expert to mentor: Shaping the future. *American Journal of Critical Care, 13*(6), 448–450.

Dyer, L. (2008). The continuing need for mentors in nursing. *Journal for Nurses in Staff Development, 24*(2), 86–90.

Finley, F. R., Ivanitskaya, L. V., & Kennedy, M. H. (2007). Mentoring junior healthcare administrators: A description of mentoring practices in 127 U.S. hospitals. *Journal of Healthcare Management, 52*(4), 260–269.

Fitzgerald, R. (1961) *Translation of Homer: The Odyssey*. New York, NY: Doubleday.

Fulton, J., Bohler, A., Hansen, G. S., Kauffeldt, A., Welander, E., Santos, M. R.,...Ziarko, E. (2007). Mentorship: An international perspective. *Nurse Education Practice, 7*(6), 399–406.

Goran, S. F. (2001). Mentorship as a teaching strategy. *Critical Care Nursing Clinics of North America, 13*(1), 119–129.

Grossman, S. C. (2007). *Mentoring in nursing: A dynamic and collaborative process*. New York, NY: Springer.

Hart, K. (2007). The aging workforce: Implications for health care organizations. *Nursing Economics, 25*(2), 101–102.

Hayes, J. M., & Scott, A. S. (2007). Mentoring partnerships as the wave of the future for new graduates. *Nursing Education Perspectives, 28*(1), 27–29.

Health Resources and Services Administration. (2006). *Preliminary findings: 2004 national sample survey of registered nurses*. Washington, DC: U.S. Department of Health and Human Services.

Hunnerkopf, P. (2007). Clinical learning. *Nursing Standard, 21*(20), 59.

Hyatt, S. A., Brown, L., & Lipp, A. (2008). Supporting mentors as assessors of clinical practice. *Nursing Standard, 22*(25), 35–41.

Kanter, R. M. (1977). *Men and women of the corporation*. New York, NY: Basic Books.

Kram, K. E. (1985). *Mentoring at work: Developmental relationships in organizational life*. Glenview, IL: Scott Foresman.

Lakasing, E., & Francis, H. (2005). The crisis in student mentorship. *Primary Health Care, 15*(4), 40–41.

LaSala, C. A., Connors, P. M., Pedro, J. T., & Phipps, M. (2007). The role of the clinical nurse specialist in promoting evidence-based practice and effecting positive patient outcomes. *Journal of Continuing Education in Nursing, 38*(6), 262–270.

McKinley, M. G. (2004). Mentoring matters: Creating, connecting, empowering. *AACN Clinical Issues Advanced Practice in Acute Critical Care, 15,* 205–214.

McWeeny, M. (2002). The changing mosaic of mentoring. *Creative Nursing Journal, 3,* 3–4.

Miller, A., & Storey, P. (2007). *MAITRE: Mentoring trAIning maTerials and REsources—Appendix 2—Mentor competencies and rationale*. Retrieved January 12, 2009, from http://www.amitie.it/maitre/training/html/comtab_eng.html

Morse, J. M. (2006). Deconstructing the mantra of mentorship: In conversation with Phyllis Noerager Stern. *Health Care for Women International, 27,* 548–558.

Moseley, L., & Davies, M. (2008). What do mentors find difficult? *Journal of Clinical Nursing, 17*(12), 1627–1634.

Muller, A., Hujcs, M., Dubendorf, P., & Harrington, P. (2010). Sustaining excellence: Clinical nurse specialist practice and Magnet designation. *Clinical Nurse Specialist: The Journal for Advanced Nursing Practice, 24*(5), 252–259.

Murray, M. (2001). *Beyond the myths and magic of mentoring: How to facilitate an effective mentoring process* (2nd ed.). San Francisco, CA: Jossey-Bass.

Myall, M., Levett-Jones, T., & Lathlean, J. (2008). Mentorship in contemporary practice: The experiences of nursing students and practice mentors. *Journal of Clinical Nursing, 17,* 1834–1842.

National Association of Clinical Nurse Specialists (NACNS). (2010). *Clinical nurse specialist core competencies: Executive summary 2006–2008*. Retrieved September 14, 2013, from http://www.nacns.org/docs/CNSCoreCompetenciesBroch.pdf

Nedd, N., Nash, M., Galindo-Ciocon, D., & Belgrave, G. (2006). Guided growth intervention: From novice to expert through a mentoring program. *Journal of Nursing Care Quality, 21*(1), 20–23.

Nettleton, P., & Bray, L. (2008). Current mentorship schemes may be doing our students a disservice. *Nurse Education in Practice, 8,* 205–12.

Nickle, P. (2007). Cognitive apprenticeship: Laying the groundwork for mentoring registered nurses in the intensive care unit. *Dynamics: Canadian Association of Critical Care Nurses, 18*(4), 19–27.

Noe, R. A. (1998). *Employee training and development.* Boston, MA: Irwin/McGraw-Hill.

Peddy, S. (2001). *The art of mentoring: Lead, follow and get out of the way.* Houston, TX: Bullion Books.

Pompa, C. (2012). *Literature review on enterprise mentoring.* Retrieved September 4, 2013, from http:// partnerplatform.org/?dk6sxm5w

Poynton, M. R., Madden, C., Bowers, R., & Keefe, M. (2007). Nurse residency program implementation: The Utah experience. *Journal of Healthcare Management, 52*(6), 385–396.

Rhodes, J., Kupersmidt, J., Manza, G., Schineller, K., Stelter, R., Van Patten, D.,… Zappie-Ferradino, K. (2009). *Elements of effective practice for mentoring* (3rd ed.). Retrieved September 7, 2013, from http:// www.mentoring.org/downloads/mentoring_ 1222.pdf

Robert Wood Johnson Foundation. (2004). *Nurse executives fellow program.* Retrieved January 12, 2009, http://futurehealth.ucsf.edu/Program/ rwj

Schweibert, V. (2000). *Mentoring: Creating connected, empowered relationships.* Alexandria, VA: American Counseling Association.

Shea, G. (2001). *Mentoring: How to develop successful mentor behaviors* (3rd ed.). Boston, MA: Thompson Crisp Learning.

Stewart, B., & Krueger, L. (1996). An evolutionary concept analysis of mentoring in nursing. *Journal of Professional Nursing, 12,* 311–321.

Tuohig, G. (2007). *Nurse mentoring: Creating a professional legacy.* Retrieved January 12, 2009, from https://www.nnsdo. org/dmdocuments/ NurseMentoring.pdf

Walker, J. A., Urden, L. D., & Moody, R. (2009). The role of the CNS in achieving and maintaining Magnet status. *Journal of Nursing Administration, 39*(12), 515–523.

Webb, C., & Shakespeare, P. (2008). Judgements about mentoring relationships in nurse education. *Nurse Education Today, 28,* 563–571.

Weiss, L. M., Williams, C. A., Wetzel, D. E., Drake, A. C., Cumberlander, L. B., & Gordon, C. L. (2008). Veterans Health Administration mentoring model for new nurse executives. *Nursing Administration Quarterly, 32*(3), 226–229.

Yoder, L. (1990). Mentoring: A concept analysis. *Nursing Administration Quarterly, 15*(1), 9–19.

Yonge, O., Billay, D., Myrick, F., & Luhanga, F. (2007). Preceptorship and mentorship: Not merely a matter of semantics. *International Journal of Nursing Education Scholarship.* Retrieved January 12, 2009, from http://www.bepress.com/ijnes/vol4/ iss1/art19/

Zucker, B., Goss, C., Williams, D., Bloodworth, L., Lynn, M., Denker, A., & Gibbs, J. D. (2006). Nursing retention in the era of nursing shortage: Norton navigators. *Journal for Nurses in Staff Development, 22*(6), 302–306.

Project Management: A Core Competency for Clinical Nurse Specialists

Stacy Webster-Wharton and Kelly A. Goudreau

Since 2010, U.S. health care expenditures neared $2.6 trillion. This is more than 10 times the $256 billion spent in 1980. While the growth rate in more recent years has slowed, the rate is expected to grow faster than the national income over the foreseeable future (Martin, Lassman, Washington, & Catlin, 2012). Further, until fully implemented, the financial and workload impact of greater access to insurance as a result of the pending implementation of the Patient Protection and Affordable Care Act of 2010 (PPACA) will not be completely known. The current size, complexity, and costs of the health care system in North America necessitates highly effective and efficient nurse management systems (Aorian et al., 1997; Carnevale, 1997; Loo, 2003/2010; Manion, Sieg, & Watson, 1998; Wilmot, 1998). These management systems include the ability to effectively coordinate projects on a large scale. In today's economy, the projects may include both creation and disassembly of services, but in either case there must be a clear path to follow as the services are either provided in a new format or are refocused to an alternate service/facility. Most often, it is the clinical nurse specialist (CNS) who is squarely placed in the position of looking at a project for its feasibility as well as working with the interprofessional team that will bring the project to reality. This chapter provides some tools and resources for the CNS to manage large-scale projects in the day-to-day activities of provision of clinical care and integration of expert nursing knowledge.

PROJECT MANAGEMENT—WHAT IS IT?

Outside of the nursing world, the term project management is often used within an organization in the same manner as program management. In some organizations, the title of program manager is one of seniority or compensation versus project manager. Sometimes there is no meaningful difference within an organization. The key concern with these two terms is if an organization does not have a clear understanding of the difference and the expectations from each manager, it makes it very difficult for the organization to train and develop employees to work at the high performance levels required of a program or project manager level.

Within nursing the responsibilities of program or project manager are assigned as a collateral duty, adjunct to the clinical role. Typically, it will be the CNS who is tasked with the creation, management, and coordination of a major project of a health care nature. The differences in the job focus of the two areas can be simplified to the project manager. According to Peisach and Kroecker (2008), the project manager has the following responsibilities:

- Project activities
- Reduced span of control
- In-depth technical knowledge
- A specific attention to details
- Execution and implementation of project-specific processes

In contrast, the program manager has the following responsibilities:

- Wide span of control and breadth of responsibilities
- Completes portfolio management for the long-term programmatic considerations
- Reviews the tools, systems, and processes from a higher level to see how not meeting one deadline impacts the other projects and milestones as well as the associated risks of the entire program
- Develops processes and manages people while strategically completing business objectives (Peisach & Kroecker, 2008, pp. 37–39)

Recognizing the differences can assist an organization in development of performance management systems that can result in greater productivity and business outcomes as well as health care outcomes in a health care setting.

Arguably, the distinction and span of control of a program manager versus a project manager and the impact to nursing is important. While in one organization, a CNS might be asked to oversee an entire program as a program manager where he or she has individual project managers to implement processes; another organization may require the CNS to oversee not only the program management process development but also the process compliance and implementation. Recognizing the importance of training, understanding the span of authority and control, and having an overall understanding of project management in the nursing environment is imperative in both cases, as it enhances goal orientation, control, and accountability for ensuring the project success, which result in stress reduction and an increase in a successful project completion (Loo, 2003/2010).

The project management approach offers the following organizational strengths:

- Results driven and result oriented to get the job done (Loo, 2003/2010)
- Decisions are made, not in a vacuum, but by set processes and procedures with the results in mind
- Effective leadership to achieve goals successfully. Effective leadership does not mean "autocratic," but rather flexibility to use different styles (Loo, 2003/2010). The leadership style is preferably one with a solid *emotional intelligence* basis where the leader can use a resonating leadership style and a limited amount of the pacesetting and commanding styles if required in challenging cases (Goleman, Boyatzis, & McKee, 2002)
- A single point of contact (POC) for overall communication with upper management, such as the program manager, stakeholders, and staff (Loo, 2003/2010). The project manager does not, and

should not, work alone and complete all the work. The project manager establishes clear points of contact for each implementation phase as outlined in the project management documentation and plans. The project manager is the main gatekeeper of the schedule and brings any unresolved issue to the program manager if an additional "push" is required to keep the team members moving forward

- A team environment where each person on the interprofessional team has ownership of specific aspects to achieve the common goals and quality standards within the project for the overall program management
- Effective planning, quality control, quality improvement (QI), and standard and clear project requirements

Many organizations, including some federal government departments, today are recognizing the power of project management to the success of the enterprise, which has resulted in many education and training organizations offering courses in this field. Some organizations offer in-house project management training (Loo, 2003/2010). Typically, project management training is offered by third-party companies, such as Project Management Institute (PMI); classes range in length from one day to one-week immersive experiences. Universities also understand the power of project management and are providing classes, including online classes that assist in teaching skills to prepare students to take the project management professional (PMP) exam. Available classes vary in length depending upon the ultimate goal, whether that is certification or simply establishing a basic conceptual understanding.

KEY ELEMENTS FOR IMPLEMENTATION OF PROJECT MANAGEMENT

The project management process has some key elements that must be implemented initially and on a continuous basis to be effective. They include (1) project manager leadership, (2) executive leadership and staff impact, (3) training, and (4) continuous effectiveness evaluations.

1. *Project Manager Leadership*
   Project management can be accomplished in a vacuum, where the manager dictates and completes most of the tasks; however, this is a nonsynergistic approach that will reduce potential outcomes, creativity, and staff morale. Effective leadership is essential for project management, and one approach is for the project manager to understand

his or her style and how it impacts the working relationships in the group undertaking the project. Understanding the emotional intelligence of the group, individuals, and herself or himself will help the project manager lead more effectively and achieve a positive project outcome. The project manager's ability to play a primordial emotional role remains an essential aspect. Leaders can expect to see an increase in work accomplished by an emotionally intelligent team versus not (Goleman et al., 2002). The CNS is in an excellent position to be a project manager at either the unit or facility level, as he or she has a clear working knowledge of and relationship with the staff at all levels of the organization. Their understanding of the nuances of dynamics at the unit level can assist with the overall management of the project and assist the other non–health care professionals engaged in completing the project to better understand the needs of the health care environment.

2. *Executive Leadership Commitment and Staff Impact*

Executive leadership support is critical because the overall effectiveness of a project team centers on both an effective project manager and executive leadership. There are a number of articles describing project management results as effective and efficient for a variety of organizations (Johns, 1999; Loo, 2003/2010; Meredith & Mantel, 1999; Stuckenbruck, 1988). Executive leadership's belief in the value of project management and support of project managers is the key to success; otherwise, the staff will see the process as an exercise in futility and will be disenfranchised.

Again, the CNS can play a pivotal role in being the communication linkage between the staff nurse and the executive team and the project team. If issues of a clinical nature arise that must be taken into consideration as the project proceeds, the CNS can be that connection or bridge between those in health care and those who are not.

3. *Training*

Project managers can have all the desire and intention to accomplish a project and to effectively lead people through it to create the best results for the organization, but without the skill acquired through training and coaching, managers will fall short. Loo (1990, 2003/2010) notes that a 1-day course can be effective in organizations, and also that sending one or two nurses to a more detailed, longer course (typically 3- to 5-day courses) can be effective, especially when these nurses are sent to the training with a "train the trainer" scenario in mind. Training one or two nurses within an organization who can come back and train others can be a cost-effective method if the right nurses are

chosen. These "trainer" nurses must have the ability to train, excite, and coach their fellow nurses; otherwise, the outcomes will be less than desirable. The skills needed for training are essential if the project team and the staff nurses are to become engaged in the process. CNSs can again play a key role here, because they understand the strengths and weaknesses of the various staff members and have coached or mentored the staff nurses to some degree. The CNSs' knowledge of the staff is invaluable in this instance.

Courses in project management are also available through academic preparation, either in a face-to-face format or an online environment. These courses give a very detailed education, which may be a preferred method. No matter which training avenue is preferred, leadership must not only train and educate project managers, but should also provide training short courses for team members wherever possible.

4. *Continuous Effectiveness Evaluations*

Project management is centered on improving processes, procedures, and implementation and assessing the outcomes as the project comes to closure. Ongoing evaluation of outcomes is the subject of another chapter in this text. It is imperative that an organization routinely determine if the project management implementation process structure is truly effective in the current setting. This can be accomplished by evaluating assumed or desired outcomes versus actual. Specifically, areas such as life cycle costs in comparison with assumptions or any preproject estimates, effectiveness of projected timelines versus actual completed timelines, how many changes occurred, and many others should be considered.

Another aspect of monitoring continuous effectiveness is to evaluate the working functions and stages of each project team. In 1965, Tuckman first discussed the stages for group development of forming, storming, norming, and performing as a basis for team growth. The model is still used today. Several books and articles discuss this model and the benefits to understanding a team as the team comes together to approach a process or project (Adubi, 2010).

One way for a project manager to evaluate team effectiveness is to determine where the team is in the Tuckman model (Adubi, 2010) and realize that as people transition in and out of teams, stages change as a natural process of any team. The goal of any organization to is to have as many teams working at the performing stage and to understand and appreciate the fact that high-functioning, well-performing teams can go back to the forming stage when membership changes.

PROJECT MANAGEMENT PROCESS

Scope and Planning

A well-defined scope of project and expectations should be clearly discussed before a project is initiated. These discussions must include considerations such as cost and methods of communication that are to be used when issues arise.

Project managers should work closely with stakeholders, subject matter experts (SMEs), the program manager, and project team on establishing the project intention or purpose, key personnel required, and measureable outcomes expected. Input from management or the client should review the strengths, weaknesses, opportunities, and threats (SWOT) analysis in regard to the project team, management, and the proposed project (Loo, 2003/2010).

Work Breakdown Structures (WBS)

A WBS is generally defined in the project management book of knowledge (PMBOK; PMI, 2013) as a decomposition of the work that will be completed by the project team in a hierarchical, deliverable-oriented system. In simpler terms, the WBS is important because it sets up the structure of the scope of the entire project, assigns duties related to the structure, and sets deliverables and requirements. The 100% rule (Haugan, 2002) is the essential principle behind a WBS; this rule basically states that the WBS includes 100% of the scope and all associated deliverables. CNSs must become familiar with this process in order to speak the language of the project engineers and other non–health care professionals who will be engaged in dialogue regarding the project.

The WBS can be presented graphically, textually, or in tabular views and can be described in outline view format, organization chart format, and the tree or centralized tree structure format (Brotherton, Fried, & Norma, 2008). Various examples of WBS formats can be found in various publications and also on various websites. Examples of these types are as follows:

Outline Example: (Does Not Include All Potential Levels and Sublevels)

Level 1. Health Care Management System—Nurse Call System

   1.1 Main Deliverable No. 1—Preliminary

     1.1.1 Activity No. 1—Establish project charter and parameters

     1.1.2 Activity No. 2—Review and feedback on project charter and parameters

     1.1.3 Activity No. 3—Finalized and approved

   1.2 Main Deliverable No. 2—Planning

     1.2.1 Activity No. 1—Draft Team design scope of work requirements

     1.2.2 Activity No. 2—Review scope requirements

     1.2.3 Activity No. 3—Finalized and approved

   1.3 Main Deliverable No. 3—Design

     1.3.1 Activity No. 1—Create Design Project Team

     1.3.2 Activity No. 2—Design project team meetings

        1.3.2.1 Subactivity No. 1—Initial meeting

        1.3.2.2 Subactivity No. 2—Develop meeting schedule and parameters

     1.3.3 Activity No. 3—Preliminary design

There are several more levels and sublevels for this type of project related to implementation, quality control, including equipment testing and end user training, and project process review.

Table Format Example

Level 1	Level 2	Level 3	Level 4
Health care management system	1.1 Main Deliverable No. 1	1.1.1 Activity No. 1 1.1.2 Activity No. 2 1.1.3 Activity No. 3	
	1.2 Main Deliverable No. 2	1.2.1 Activity No. 1 1.2.2 Activity No. 2 1.2.3 Activity No. 3	
	1.3 Main Deliverable No. 3	1.3.1 Activity No. 1 1.3.2 Activity No. 2 1.3.3 Activity No. 3	1.3.2.1 Subactivity No. 1 1.3.2.2 Subactivity No. 2

(Example is not all inclusive.)

Tree Example

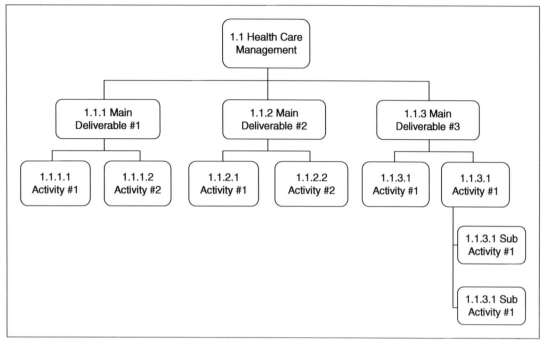

(Example is not all inclusive.)

Time Management and the Schedule

Transition from a WBS to a schedule can be challenging, and one method to ease the transition is to have the lower-level WBS items be more "schedule oriented" (Cioffi, 2004). Various scheduling software tools are available for organizations to use; these are typically Gantt chart–based with critical path components. Critical path items are components that must be completed in order for the project to stay on task. These are essential components to understand and provide to the workforce to complete. They help to keep the project on task and on time. There are times when the schedule can be "resource oriented" or "task oriented." The premise for this type of scheduling is to use resources effectively when there are limited resources available or unique resources are used (Hendrickson, 1998). In the health care industry, resources and time can be scarce or perhaps unique and so either the resource- or task-oriented scheduling perspective may be more appropriate, depending on the situation/circumstances. The CNS needs to understand the differences between these elements and the best use of the time and expertise of the SMEs as a resource that has conflicting needs and requirements competing for their time.

Cost Management Including Nonmonetary Costs

It is imperative for project managers to work with program managers on the cost parameters of a project and to regularly discuss actual costs versus assumed costs. This is an essential element for the CNS to be very aware of. The total cost of a project from a programmatic standpoint to determine cost effectiveness, overall costs, and for cost–benefit analysis is developed by a review of the assumed, projected costs from cradle to grave. For this reason, projected cost estimates are key to success of a project, especially one that is driven by a cost–benefit analysis. SMEs are critical in the planning stages for projecting cost estimates. Also, the CNS position can live or die based on the cost-effectiveness of the role. If projects that are proposed by the CNS are intended to be cost-effective and ultimately save money, but they do not due to poor project management, the credibility of the CNS and his or her role is at stake.

During implementation, the project manager should work closely with the program manager on the actual costs versus projected costs to determine where gaps exist, how to be more cost effective, or when to request additional funding from leadership, if possible. Not all costs are quantifiable, and some may result from a previously unknown risk. This can be true within the health care industry when implementing a project that requires unique resources that may or may not be readily available within geographic areas, or when full project implementation may result in some hard-to-determine outcome such as efficiency improvements. These cost considerations may be difficult to quantify until after full implementation and/or analysis over several years after implementation.

Managing Risks

In an article about the "10 Golden Rules of Project Risk Management" (Jutte, 2010, p. 13), the author describes the rules as follows:

1. Make Risk Management Part of Your Project: do not ignore the fact that there are risks.
2. Identify Risks Early in Your Project: brainstorming potential risks with the team early on in a project is essential.
3. Communicate About Risks: include risk communication in plans.
4. Consider Both Threats and Opportunities: risks are not bad, risks are opportunities.
5. Clarify Ownership Issues: establishing who is responsible for each risk is essential.
6. Prioritize Risks: not all risks are created equal, so risks must be prioritized.
7. Analyze Risks: determine the probability of risks occurring and the level of threat.
8. Plan and Implement Risk Responses: planning responses will minimize negative impact.
9. Register Project Risks: document risks, including who has ownership.
10. Track Risks and Associated Tasks: if you track risk, day-to-day operations will be easier.

Implementation Plan—Quality Plan, Communication Plan, and Procurement Plan

Quality Plan. This plan is developed within the team to look at various quality improvement and control items within the project. The following are some questions to ask in order to outline the plan:

1. How the team can do things better; otherwise, what improvements should be made?
2. How to do the right thing; otherwise, how to maintain control, and
3. How to do things right; otherwise, how to maintain quality

Communication Plan. This plan is dynamic, as the risk management plan changes. The key to a solid communication plan is to plan who will be assigned as the main communication POC, what types of things will be communicated, timelines for communication, any deliverables, and communication methods (e-mails, face-to-face meetings, publications, memos, etc.). Communicating at multiple different venues and using both verbal and oral communication is the key, as everyone learns and hears information differently.

Procurement Plan. Every company or agency has various methods for procurement, and the key for the project manager is to first research to understand his or her company's procedures, rules and regulations, and what actual procurement authority the project manager really has. This may require meetings with the company's procurement and logistics department to understand the procedures, consequences, and expected lead times. Some health care companies will also have a policy for approval for onsite vendor demonstrations for equipment and supplies. If a nurse manager jumps in without the proper company-specific regulations and requirements, the nurse may find himself or herself obligated for unauthorized purchases.

It cannot be stressed enough that the CNS is a key player in project management within health care systems. It is the CNS who often identifies the need for a change in process or performance as determined by patterns and trends in patient outcomes. It is also the CNS who has the skill set needed to ensure that the project goals and objectives can be met in a timely manner, in a cost-efficient way with consideration of both monetary and nonmonetary issues, and with all stakeholder input needed to ensure effective implementation. The CNS can be the strongest link in the chain of quality, communication, and procurement to a successful implementation.

CONCLUSION

The CNS carries with him or her the training, education, and expertise needed to be an excellent project manager. The intention of the project management process is not to be cumbersome and to increase workload, but quite the opposite, as proper planning can reduce workload stresses and provide better outcomes creating win-win outcomes (Loo, 2003/2010). Of course, win-win outcomes are not guaranteed, as win-wins come only with team collaboration and not compromise. The CNS can provide that linkage between the staff nurse, the nurse manager, and the non–health care professionals who need to collaborate on the project. The ultimate outcome is expected to be safer patient care, improved patient outcomes, and increased satisfaction of both patients and staff. The CNS is pivotal to all of these and therefore must understand the role of project manager.

REFERENCES

Adubi, G. (2010). *The five stages of project team development*. The Project Management Hut. Retrieved from www.pmhut.com/the-five-stages-of-project-team-development

Aorian, J. F., Horvath, K. J., Secatore, J. A., Apert, H., Costa, M. J., Powers, E.,...Stengrevics, S. S. (1997). Vision for a treasured resource, Part 1: Nurse manager role implementation. *Journal of Nursing Administration, 27*(3), 36–41.

Brotherton, S. A., Fried, R. T., & Norma, E. S. (2008). *Applying the work breakdown structure to the project management lifecycle*. Denver, CO: Global Congress Proceedings.

Carnevale, F. A. (1997). Perspective: The practice of management in nursing from novice to expert. *Canadian Journal of Nursing Administration, 10*(2), 7–13.

Cioffi, D. R. (2004). Work and resource breakdown structures for formalized bottom-up estimating, cost engineering. *American Association of Cost Engineers, 46*(2), 31–37.

Goleman, D., Boyatzis, R., & McKee, A. (2002). *Primal leadership: Realizing the power of emotional intelligence*. Boston, MA: Harvard Business School Press.

Haugan, G. T. (2002). *Effective work breakdown structures*. Vienna, VA: Management Concepts Publishers.

Hendrickson, C. (1998). Project management for construction (Carnegie Mellon University, Department of Civil and Environmental Engineering). Pittsburgh, PA: Prentice Hall (1st ed.). [Second edition prepared for World Wide Web publication in 2000]

Johns, T. G. (1999). On creating organizational support for the project management method. *Internal Journal of Project Management, 17*(1), 47–53.

Jutte, B. (2010). *10 golden rules of project risk management*. Retrieved from http://www.projectsmart.com/articles/10-golden-rules-of-project-risk-management.php.

Loo, R. (1990). *One-day project management training: Is it possible? 1990 Proceedings of the Project Management Institute Annual Symposium* (pp. 568–574). Newtown, PA: Project Management Institute.

Loo, R. (2003/2010). Project management. In J. Fulton, B. Lyons, & K. Goudreau (Eds.), *Foundations of clinical nurse specialist practice* (pp. 269–273). New York, NY: Springer.

Manion, J., Sieg, M. J., & Watson, P. (1998). Managerial partnerships: The wave of the future. *Journal of Nursing Administration, 28*(4), 47–55.

Martin, A. B., Lassman, D., Washington, B., Catlin, A; National Health Expenditure Accounts Team. (2012). Growth in US health spending remained slow in 2010; health share of gross domestic product was unchanged from 2009. *Health Affairs (Millwood), 31*(1), 208–219.

Meredith, J. R., & Mantel, S. J, Jr. (1999). *Project management: A managerial approach*. New York, NY: Wiley.

Peisach, J., & Kroecker, T. S. (2008, July–August). Project manager and program manager: What's the difference? *Defense AT&L,* 37–39.

Project Management Institute (PMI). (2013). *Project management book of knowledge (PMBOK) guide* (5th ed.). Author. Newtown, PA.

Stuckenbruck, L. C. (Ed.) (1988). *The implementation of project management: The professional's handbook*. Reading, MA: Addison-Wesley.

Wilmot, M. (1998). The new ward manager: An evaluation of the changing role of the charge nurse. *Journal of Advanced Nursing, 28,* 419–427.

Program Evaluation and Clinical Nurse Specialist Practice

Jane A. Walker

Clinical nurse specialists (CNS) frequently establish new programs of care in order to improve patient outcomes (Muller, McCauley, Harrington, Jablonski, & Strass, 2011). These new programs might focus on any or all of the three spheres of influence described by the National Association of Clinical Nurse Specialists (NACNS; 2004): patients, nursing and nursing personnel, and the organization/system. The impetus for initiating new programs may arise directly from CNSs as they intervene to address CNS-identified problems among the three spheres of influence. Other programs may arise through requests from other stakeholders within the organization. Regardless of the source of the request to develop new programs and initiatives, it is useful for CNSs to use a comprehensive process during the program-planning phase that not only addresses the program's structure and processes, but also lays the groundwork for program evaluation. Using a comprehensive evaluation process can help ensure that the program is thoroughly evaluated with respect to its efficacy and outcomes. Documenting evaluation efforts leads logically to the process of disseminating findings of the evaluation. Dissemination of evaluation findings both within and outside the organization is an important professional responsibility that can contribute to our understanding of what works and doesn't work with respect to patient outcomes. Additionally, documenting and disseminating evaluation efforts can be an important CNS contribution for those hospitals that hold Magnet recognition or are in the process of pursuing this recognition (Walker, Urden, & Moody, 2009).

Measuring the results or outcomes of programs and communicating them to organization stakeholders is an important CNS competency. The NACNS *Statement on Education and Practice* (2004) included competencies related to program evaluation. Specifically, the NACNS statement indicated that the CNS "selects evaluation methods and instruments to identify system-level outcomes of programs of care" (NACNS, 2004, p. 37). Other related competencies addressed the need to give feedback about program effects and evaluate policies with respect to program sustainability. Similarly, the CNS core competencies published in 2010 (National CNS Competency Task Force) addressed the CNS role in leading efforts to evaluate clinical programs and process improvement initiatives. Thus, CNSs need to possess skills related to program evaluation, because these skills are important not only to patients and their families but to the health care system as a whole. The purpose of this chapter is to describe select methods of program evaluation and demonstrate how CNSs can use an evaluation model to guide a comprehensive program evaluation.

BACKGROUND

Purpose of Evaluation

Evaluation is a concept that touches upon all aspects of society. Everyone encounters on a daily basis a myriad of evaluative ratings. Examples of the focus of these evaluation efforts include personal, recreational, athletic, academic, or occupational considerations. As health care providers, CNSs are also fully involved with evaluation activities. One example of the focus of these efforts involves using data for evaluating care quality or for benchmarking against other organizations or services. Another focus of evaluation efforts is the degree to which programs are effective and address the needs for which they were created. A number of well-established models and methods exist to guide the process for evaluating programs (Posavac & Carey, 2007; Stufflebeam, 2007). These models are multifaceted and are associated with specific methods to ensure objectivity and rigor. According to Posavac and Carey (2007), program evaluation activities are important because they give necessary feedback to those who can make decisions about the program's structure and processes with respect to improving quality. As Stufflebeam (2003) stated, "Evaluation's **most** important purpose is not to prove, but to improve" (p. 4).

Stufflebeam and Shinkfield (2007) defined evaluation as "the systematic assessment of an object's merit, worth, probity, feasibility, safety, significance, and/or equity" (p. 13). Not only is it important to evaluate programs with respect to merit and worth, programs should also be evaluated with respect to their ethical or moral value. The evaluation process should also address how feasible and safe it is to deliver the program. Finally, programs should be evaluated with respect to their level of significance and potential for generalizability and sustainability over time and distance, as well as the equality of access to society (Stufflebeam & Shinkfield, 2007). This definition and conceptualization of evaluation and related evaluation models originated primarily in the field of education. However, it is apparent that this definition of evaluation and the related values are wholly compatible with the nursing profession.

Differentiating Among Concepts of Evaluation, Research, Assessment, and Audit

The preceding discussion demonstrates the wide-ranging, values-driven nature of program evaluation. It is important, however, to describe evaluation with respect to what it is not. Confusion exists with respect to how basic research, individual assessment, and audit relate to and differ from evaluation (Posavac & Carey, 2007). Part of this confusion may arise from the similarities of methods and instruments that may be used in these activities. For example, both evaluation and research may use comparison groups and rigorous data collection methods. Similarly, instruments used in individual assessment, such as functional ability scales, can also be used in evaluation. Additionally, data collected for quality

improvement (QI) audits might be the same as those collected for formal program evaluation. One way to differentiate among these concepts is to examine the intent for which they are carried out. The primary purpose of basic research is to generate new knowledge, whereas the purpose of evaluation is program improvement. Therefore, although both approaches may share similar methods, the purposes for which they are carried out differ. Individuals might be assessed using a formal assessment tool to monitor the effect of a specific treatment or plan of care. However, data collected for this purpose are quite different from those collected to measure the effectiveness of a program. Finally, ongoing audits of care outcomes provide a measure of unit and/or organizational performance that can be independent of specific program performance.

Formative and Summative Evaluation

When examining the process of program evaluation, it is important to differentiate between formative and summative evaluation. The concepts of formative and summative evaluation were initially described in the late 1960s by Michael Scriven (Stufflebeam & Shinkfield, 2007). The primary aim of formative evaluation is to provide information that can be used to improve a program. Formative evaluation can occur during the program development phase or during its ongoing existence. Data are collected on a prospective basis and thus can be used to assess to what extent program effectiveness is evolving. The role of the evaluator in formative evaluation is to share evaluation data with those who are responsible for program development and delivery for the purpose of improving program quality (Stufflebeam & Shinkfield, 2007).

The primary aim of summative evaluation is to provide information demonstrating the extent to which programs were effective. Summative evaluation activities take place at the end of the program or at designated time periods. Data are collected on a retrospective basis and provide an accounting of program effectiveness. Consumers and sponsors are the primary target of summative evaluation information (Stufflebeam & Shinkfield, 2007). Both types of evaluation, working together, are important in order to fully judge the effectiveness of programs.

General Steps of the Program Evaluation Process

Multiple approaches to engaging in the program evaluation process exist. Some approaches are specific to a particular evaluation model, whereas others are more general and include selection of an evaluation approach or model as a step within the process. One example of a general program evaluation process was developed by the Centers for Disease Control and Prevention (CDC, 2012) for the purpose of evaluating public health programs. The general steps outlined by the CDC (2012) are described in the following section and have potential to be applied to a variety of evaluation efforts.

The first step in the process is to engage stakeholders. At this stage, evaluators clarify expectations and develop a relationship with stakeholders in order to understand their values and concerns. It is important to include as stakeholders those responsible for carrying out the program, direct or indirect recipients of the program's services, and those who will use the results of the evaluation. It is necessary for evaluators to interact on a regular basis with stakeholders throughout the evaluation process (CDC, 2012).

The second step in the process is to describe the program. Evaluators work with stakeholders to ensure that the program to be evaluated is clearly described. This description addresses the need for the program, indicators of program success/effect, program activities, types of resources needed to carry out the program, stage of development, context or environmental influences, and a flow chart or logic model of the program processes (CDC, 2012).

Third, evaluators choose an evaluation design. There are many types of evaluation models or approaches, and the one chosen should match both the type of program to be evaluated and the purpose of the evaluation. For example, evaluation approaches that are appropriate for new programs would be different from those used to evaluate mature programs to assess effects (CDC, 2012).

The next step is to gather information and evidence that is relevant and defensible. Evaluators work with stakeholders to select indicators and to collect information. Considerations of measurement quality, including reliability and validity, are important to the data collection phase (CDC, 2012).

The last two steps of the evaluation process as described by the CDC (2012) justify conclusions and ensure use and sharing of lessons learned. Evaluators justify conclusions by relating them to data collected and making judgments that relate to values and standards. With respect to ensuring use and sharing lessons learned through the process, evaluators help stakeholders with dissemination activities that relate evaluation findings to recommendations (CDC, 2012).

Stufflebeam and Shinkfield (2007) also described a series of evaluation steps that can also be applied to a variety of evaluation models or approaches. These steps represent an operational definition of evaluation and include delineating, obtaining, reporting, applying, and descriptive and judgmental information. The

phase of "delineating" is similar to CDC's "stakeholder engagement" step. The emphasis of and work to be done associated with the "obtaining" phase correlate with the "gathering information" step described earlier. Data collection and management skills are important at this stage to ensure credibility of findings. In the "reporting" step, the focus is on clearly communicating the findings of the evaluation. Stufflebeam and Shinkfield (2007) discussed the importance of excellent writing and verbal communication and presentation skills in order to successfully influence application of evaluation findings. The "application" phase relates closely to "ensuring use and sharing lessons learned." The focus is on the stakeholders actually using the findings of the program evaluation and putting recommendations into place. According to Stufflebeam and Shinkfield (2007), it is helpful for evaluators to offer assistance in this process. Finally, Stufflebeam and Shinkfield (2007) discussed the need for evaluators to include in their reports descriptive information as well as judgments about the information collected. This step is similar to the "justifying conclusions" step described by CDC (2012).

From the preceding discussion, it is apparent that program evaluation is a comprehensive, far-reaching process. It is important for CNSs, as change leaders within an organization, to understand the processes and steps involved in program evaluation activities. Understanding the steps involved may give CNSs additional tools for program management and practice change.

Program Evaluation Categories

Several categories of program evaluation exist and relate to evaluating the need for a program, the process that is being used to meet an identified need, and the extent to which program outcomes are being met (Posavac & Carey, 2007). With respect to evaluating the need for a program, evaluators collect information to determine existing gaps, organization/community needs, program alternatives, and client preferences. This type of evaluation occurs during the program development phase and leads to formulation of the new program's scope and structure. Evaluation of processes determines to what extent the program is being delivered as planned. The program is evaluated during implementation on a continual basis according to predetermined criteria. Data collected can improve program implementation and address questions related to generalizability. Finally, evaluation of program outcomes examines the effectiveness of the program itself. Evaluation occurs at specific endpoints and addresses to what extent projected outcomes were met. Outcomes evaluation information can inform decisions pertaining to overall program effectiveness (Posavac & Carey, 2007).

Evaluation Approaches

Posavac and Carey (2007) identified several general categories of program evaluation approaches. Examples of these approaches include objectives-based evaluation, objectives-free evaluation, naturalistic or qualitative approach, success case method, and the improvement-focused approach.

In the objectives-based evaluation approach, data are collected to determine to what extent program objectives were met. Objectives-based evaluation has historically been the most commonly used approach and is most useful when objectives are clear and easy to assess. The objectives-based approach has been criticized, however, because process is not addressed and evaluation results may be too narrow to draw valid conclusions about the program's effectiveness (Stufflebeam & Shinkfield, 2007). In response to some of the limitations of objectives-based evaluation, Scriven, as described by Stufflebeam and Shinkfield (2007), developed an objectives-free model of evaluation. The focus of an objectives-free model is the consumer and the consumer's needs and perspectives, as opposed to the developers' goals and objectives (Posavac & Carey, 2007; Stufflebeam & Shinkfield, 2007). To guide evaluators through this type of evaluation, Scriven (2007) developed the key evaluation checklist. Evaluators may use the naturalistic or qualitative approach to program evaluation when they desire an understanding that is in-depth and thorough. Methods can include direct observation, in-depth interviews, and review of written documents. Qualitative evaluation information may be collected in addition to quantitative data (Patton, 2003). In the success case method, evaluators obtain a random sample of high performers and low performers and conduct in-depth interviews to identify factors contributing to and interfering with success. Information obtained from the interviews can then be used for program improvement (Brinkerhoff & Dressler, 2003). Stufflebeam and Shinkfield (2007) indicate that the focus of the success case method is somewhat narrow in comparison with more comprehensive evaluation approaches. Finally, improvement-focused approaches guide evaluation efforts aimed to improve programs. These approaches are generally comprehensive and meet the needs of participants and stakeholders (Posavac & Carey, 2007). One example of an improvement-focused approach is the Context, Input, Process, and Product (CIPP) model for evaluation (Stufflebeam, 2003). This approach is described in the following section.

CIPP MODEL FOR EVALUATION

Description of Model

The CIPP model is an improvement/accountability model and has been widely used since its development by Stufflebeam in the late 1960s. The CIPP acronym stands for context, input, process, and product. Stufflebeam (2007) provided a quick description of the focus of each of the four components of the CIPP model by posing four respective questions: "What needs to be done? How should it be done? Is it being done? Did it succeed?" (p. 1). Stufflebeam developed the model as a way to help evaluators make decisions about program quality and effectiveness and to assist with program planning as well as formative and summative evaluation (Stufflebeam, 2007; Stufflebeam & Shinkfield, 2007; Zhang et al., 2011). Following is a discussion of each of the model's components.

Context evaluation refers to the process of examining within a specific situation or environment the presence of needs, gaps/problems, assets, and opportunities for improvement. Decision makers use the results of the context evaluation to establish relevant and realistic priorities and goals. The established goals then provide the basis for judging the effectiveness of the program itself. Methods that can be used to conduct a context evaluation include surveys, interviews, review of documents and standards, benchmarking, and analysis of the system (Stufflebeam & Shinkfield, 2007).

Input evaluation refers to the process of assessing various courses of action with respect to factors such as feasibility, staff availability, budgetary resources, and procedural possibilities/constraints that can influence plans to achieve identified priorities and goals. Those responsible for making decisions use the data from input evaluation to inform the program's structure, processes, and procedures. Methods that can be used to perform input evaluation include conducting an inventory of available resources with respect to staff, budget, and other materials; examining the feasibility of planned interventions with respect to staff acceptance, system constraints, and costs; and performing literature reviews and searches for best evidence (Stufflebeam & Shinkfield, 2007).

Process evaluation refers to the process of assessing to what extent actions are being implemented as planned. Information from process evaluation activities assists planners and those responsible for program delivery to take actions and make adjustments as needed in order to carry out the program plan. As a result of participating in process evaluation activities, a documented record of program implementation is created, which aids interpretation of program outcomes. Methods used to perform process evaluation include monitoring and documenting actual and potential barriers to program implementation; describing and documenting the process; and interacting with those carrying out the program as well as the program's stakeholders (Stufflebeam & Shinkfield, 2007).

Finally, product evaluation refers to the process of assessing the achievement of program outcomes and relating them to program objectives along with context, input, and process. Decision makers use the results of product evaluation to determine if the program met its objectives and goals, whether the program should continue in its current form, continue in a modified form, or be discontinued. Stufflebeam (2007) further divided product evaluation into several subcomponents to increase depth of understanding regarding a program's impact and to provide decision makers with adequate information. Specifically, Stufflebeam (2007) outlined criteria to examine product from the perspective of impact (is the program reaching its target audience?), effectiveness (what is the quality and significance of program outcomes?), sustainability (to what extent is the program institutionalized and continued over time?), and transportability (to what extent can the program be applied in a different setting?). Methods used in the product evaluation phase include obtaining data that correspond with outcome operational definitions; collecting feedback and judgments from stakeholders; and collecting qualitative feedback from relevant sources (Stufflebeam & Shinkfield, 2007).

At the heart of context, input, process, and product evaluation lie the core values upon which respective evaluation efforts are based. Figure 22.1 shows the relationship of the CIPP model components, the focus of each model component, and the recognition of the role values play as the hub or anchor of the program evaluation process (Stufflebeam & Shinkfield, 2007).

Stufflebeam and Shinkfield (2007) provided examples of values that could serve as a core of a program evaluation effort in the field of education. These examples included values such as academic success for all students, meeting the needs of students with special needs, parent involvement, innovation, teacher development, and so forth. Within nursing, the American Nurses Association's (ANA) *Code of Ethics for Nurses* (2010) provides an excellent source of values underlying evaluation efforts in nursing and health care. Examples of values from the ANA Code of Ethics that can anchor program evaluation efforts in nursing include respect for human dignity; primary commitment to patients; protection of patient health, safety, and confidentiality; responsibility and accountability for individual nursing practice, self-respect, and professional growth; responsibility to participate in health care improvement activities; responsibility to collaborate with other health care providers to address health needs; and responsibility to professional integrity (ANA, 2010). According to Stufflebeam and Shinkfield (2007), it is important to clarify core values with stakeholders before beginning the evaluation process.

Another consideration with the CIPP model's four components is that they can be viewed from a formative as well as a summative perspective. When viewed from a formative perspective, data are collected prospectively for the purpose of program improvement. When viewed from a summative perspective, data are collected retrospectively for the purpose of program accountability (Stufflebeam & Shinkfield, 2007). Thus, the model aids decision making for two important purposes. As can be seen from the preceding discussion, the CIPP model is a well-developed, comprehensive approach to evaluation and program development.

Related Literature

The CIPP evaluation model was originally applied to the field of education by Stufflebeam and colleagues. Their goal at the time was to provide an evaluation approach aimed at improving and demonstrating accountability in the country's education system (Stufflebeam & Shinkfield, 2007). Since that time, it has continued to be used extensively, both nationally and internationally, in the field of education (Stufflebeam & Shinkfield, 2007; Zhang et al., 2011).

In addition to its use in the field of education, the CIPP model has also been used to evaluate various aspects of discipline-specific education programs. In the field of medical education, the CIPP model has been used to evaluate a family practice education program

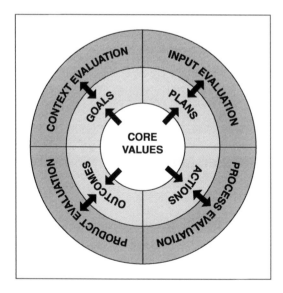

FIGURE 22.1 Key components of the CIPP evaluation model and associated relationships with programs.

CIPP, Context, Input, Process, and Product.

Source: From Stufflebeam and Shinkfield (2007, p. 333).

(Al-Khathami, 2012); faculty development program for the purpose of teaching and evaluating professionalism in medical students (Steinert, Cruess, Cruess, & Snell, 2005); and as a framework to study communication styles in medical education programs (Razack et al., 2007). Similarly, the CIPP model has been used to evaluate education-related projects in nursing education programs. For example, evaluators have used the CIPP model to evaluate the use of anecdotal notes as a way to evaluate nursing student clinical performance (Hall, Daly, & Madigan, 2010) and to evaluate a system for monitoring attendance in undergraduate nursing students (Doyle et al., 2008).

In addition to education applications of the CIPP model, it has been used to evaluate health service-focused programs. For example, the model has been used to evaluate the effectiveness of a suicide prevention program (Ho et al., 2011) and to evaluate the introduction of a quality development program in a nursing department (Petro-Nustas, 1996).

The CIPP model has also been used to evaluate various aspects of CNS practice. Although the articles were published some time ago, they still give useful examples of ways the CIPP model can be used in practice. In the first published article, the authors related the CIPP model to the nursing process and used the model as a framework for measuring CNS productivity (Anderson, McCartney, Schreiber, & Thompson, 1989). With respect to context, the authors discussed the process of CNS collaboration with their directors to establish practice objectives and also described the process of using standards of practice from nursing organizations as guidelines for measuring job performance. Examples of the input phase of evaluation included CNS consideration of the impact of the various issues affecting practice and outcomes. Methods of process evaluation used by the authors included the use of time management instruments: program evaluation and review technique (PERT), and Gantt charts. Finally, with respect to product evaluation, the authors described a product review report (PER) that the organization used to demonstrate achievement of objectives as well as productivity and cost/benefits. The authors concluded that the model was a useful way to document practice and evaluate CNS outcomes (Anderson et al., 1989).

The CIPP model was also used as a way to evaluate indirect care activities performed by CNSs. Kennedy-Malone (1996) defined indirect care as including those activities that are difficult to measure with respect to specific outcomes. Examples of these activities included CNS work as change agents, consultants, and motivators. Kennedy-Malone (1996) adapted the CIPP model as a way for CNSs to evaluate these activities. According to Kennedy-Malone (1996), context evaluation could be performed through methods such as developing surveys and assessing needs. The outcome related to context would include the establishment of priorities. Input evaluation could be accomplished though literature review and collaboration with other disciplines and leaders related to resource management within the organization. The outcome of input activities would be program/project plans that were cost-accountable. With respect to the process component of the CIPP model, methods used by CNSs would focus on documenting CNS activities and actions taken along with copies of correspondence. The process-related outcome would be the implementation and refinement of programs. With respect to product, CNSs would document the attainment of objectives and outcomes, thus demonstrating role effectiveness and accountability (Kennedy-Malone, 1996).

Finally, although not specific to CNSs, Nugent and Lambert (1997) described a variety of evaluation models, including CIPP, and applied them to advanced practice nursing (APN). In an example, the authors used the CIPP model to demonstrate a method for evaluating effectiveness of a school-based nurse practitioner (NP). In this example, *context* referred to NP identification of student health needs; *input* described items to measure with respect to student health and resources; and *process* included measures such as the completion of assessments, the identification of problems, and the development of a plan. Finally, the *product* outcome would be a documented improvement in student health according to key indicators (Nugent & Lambert, 1997).

In summary, the CIPP model is well developed and has been used in a variety of ways over a number of years. Although the model has been used sporadically for CNS practice, it could be useful for future program evaluation efforts. The following section of this chapter focuses on examples of CIPP application to CNS practice and education.

APPLYING THE CIPP MODEL TO CNS PRACTICE AND EDUCATION

Example 1: CNS Practice and New Nurse Orientation

A group of CNSs working in a community-based hospital noticed that problems existed with the hospital's existing nursing orientation program. New nurses had confided with the CNSs that they felt ill-equipped to work on their new units. Many had been working on their units for a month or more before attending orientation. There were few designated preceptors and very little attention was given to long-term follow-up. The managers voiced concerns about the current orientation program, and safety occurrence reports frequently involved nurses who had been at the hospital less than 1 year. Satisfaction among many newly employed nurses was low and preceptors were dissatisfied with the current system. The group of CNSs at the hospital recommended that the current orientation process be modified. The hospital's administrative team agreed and asked the CNSs to lead the efforts to change the current system. The CNSs were asked to lead a newly formed task force to determine goals and expectations, examine the current orientation process, and select an evaluation method. The team decided to use the CIPP model for the remaining planning and evaluation processes.

At the beginning of the planning process, the task force agreed upon the values that would form the core of the evaluation process. They also decided upon the sources of data that they could access and use. Data sources included published evidence, staffing records, human resources reports, education department records, meeting minutes, written statements of support, benchmarking data, best practices, follow-up surveys/interviews with new nurses and preceptors, risk control data, patient and nurse satisfaction results, and skills checklists.

To begin the needs assessment component of the evaluation plan, the task force began the process of evaluating context. The primary objective for this phase was to formally assess the need for an adequate orientation and precepting program for new nursing staff. The group used several methods to carry out the evaluation. These methods included compiling and reviewing best practices and national standards related to new nurse orientation, surveying regional hospitals regarding their orientation practices, surveying high-performing hospitals to find out what their orientation practices consisted of, and interviewing new nurses and their managers to identify concerns and recommendations. The team located high-level evidence, including practice guidelines and a systematic review that they used to form the foundation of their recommendations. The results of the benchmarking interviews were highly useful in pointing out shortcomings of the current system as well as identifying promising features, consistent with the evidence, that the team would incorporate into the new program. Specific features the group decided to implement included a preceptor development program, establishing criteria for preceptor selection, maximizing consistency with preceptor/orientee staffing schedules, holding orientation on a regular basis, ensuring that new nurses attend orientation prior to working on their assigned unit, and extending the orientation time frame. Thus, the task force, serving as decision makers, would use the data collected from the context evaluation phase to develop the goals of the orientation program. These goals would continue to guide the further development of the program. Refer to Table 22.1 for a summary of the objectives and methods corresponding with each phase of the CIPP model.

The primary objective of input evaluation was to plan an orientation program that enhanced patient safety, increased nurse and preceptor satisfaction, and enhanced new nurse confidence and skills. Methods used to achieve this objective included assessing availability of staff to carry out orientation activities; examining best practices related to preceptor development; reviewing staffing schedules to ensure availability of preceptors for development and schedule release; and obtaining a commitment from managers and administration that following orientation program processes would be a priority. The task force and other stakeholders used input evaluation data to create a feasible and realistic program, ensure that the proposed recommendations would meet the identified needs, and use findings to make nursing and hospital staff aware of the needs and issues.

The task force's objective related to process was to identify shortcomings and positive aspects associated with the newly revised orientation program. To carry out evaluation activities related to process, the team reviewed staffing records to determine to what extent recommended orientation practices were being followed; reviewed education records to determine if all preceptors attended preceptor development programs and met predetermined criteria; and conducted surveys and interviews of new nurse and preceptor satisfaction with the process. As program decision makers, the task force and administrative team used the findings to revise processes, adjust nurse responsibilities and expectations related to orientation activities, and determine program progress and costs.

At the outset of the planning process, the task force identified an objective related to product. This objective was to determine to what extent the new orientation program affected patient safety, patient satisfaction, new nurse satisfaction, preceptor satisfaction, and new nurse confidence and competence. In order to measure the product component of the evaluation plan, the task force reviewed reports of medication errors, nosocomial infections, and patient falls; reviewed patient satisfaction surveys; assessed nurse and preceptor satisfaction with orientation at the completion of orientation and 6 months later; reviewed new nurse performance on skills checklists; and discussed manager and preceptor feedback regarding new nurse performance. To assist the decision-making process, product evaluation was subdivided into judgments related to impact, effectiveness, sustainability, and transportability and included a consideration of all evaluation data collected throughout the process. The task force, along with relevant stakeholders, used the data to decide if the orientation program

TABLE 22.1

APPLICATION OF THE CIPP FRAMEWORK TO A NEW NURSE ORIENTATION PROGRAM			
Context	**Input**	**Processes**	**Product**
Objective			
To assess the need for an adequate orientation and precepting program for new nursing staff	To plan an orientation program that enhances patient safety, increases nurse and preceptor satisfaction, and enhances new nurse confidence and skills	To identify shortcomings and positive aspects associated with the newly revised orientation program	To determine to what extent the new orientation program affects patient safety, patient satisfaction, new nurse satisfaction, preceptor satisfaction, and new nurse confidence and competence
Methods			
• Compile and review best practices and national standards related to new nurse orientation • Survey regional hospitals regarding their orientation practices • Survey high-performing hospitals to determine orientation practices • Interview new nurses and their managers	• Assess availability of staff to carry out orientation activities • Examine best practices related to preceptor development • Review staffing schedules to ensure availability of preceptors for development and schedule release • Obtaining a commitment from managers that the orientation procedures will be a priority	• Review of staffing records to determine how recommended practices are being followed • Review of education records to determine if all preceptors attend development programs and meet predetermined criteria • Surveys and interviews of new nurse and preceptor satisfaction with the process	• Review of reported medication errors, nosocomial infections, and patient falls • Review of patient satisfaction surveys • Nurse and preceptor satisfaction with orientation at the completion of orientation and 6 months later • Review of skills checklists • Manager feedback regarding new nurse performance

CIPP, Context, Input, Process, and Product.

was serving the needs of preceptors and new nurses (impact); improved patient safety, patient satisfaction, new nurse satisfaction, preceptor satisfaction, and new nurse confidence and competence (effectiveness); should be continued or not (sustainability); should be expanded to all areas of the hospital and whether the program should be adapted if implemented widely within the hospital (transportability). Finally, a report of the evaluation and recommendations was disseminated to the executive team.

The final outcome of this formative evaluation process was a successful new nurse orientation program. With respect to context, data demonstrated that preprogram orientation methods were inconsistent with best available evidence and best practices. Therefore, need for changing the orientation program was demonstrated and the project team created a new approach. Data from the input evaluation phase provided the project team with the information related to the adequacy of resources and feasibility. As a result of input evaluation judgments, the team was aware that the hospital possessed adequate resources to implement the program housewide if it was deemed successful. However, before committing widespread resources, the team decided to start the program by

pilot-testing it on several units. During the process evaluation phase, the project team was able to determine that all staff were participating in the program and also identified areas for improvement. The CNSs involved in the project collected information related to costs and were able to document that the orientation program was highly cost-effective and resulted in considerable cost savings. Finally, based on their review of impact, effectiveness, sustainability, and transferability, the executive team decided to expand the orientation program to the entire hospital.

Example 2: CNS Education

When initiating a new CNS program or modifying an existing program, the CIPP model can provide a useful framework for planning and evaluating the program. Planners can use the context, input, process, and product components of the model to frame evaluation questions and criteria and to establish program objectives. A useful tool to guide the process of framing evaluation questions and criteria is the CIPP evaluation checklist created by Stufflebeam (2007) and available online at www.scribd.com/

doc/58435354/The-Cipp-Model-for-Evaluation-by-Daniel-l-Stufflebeam. Table 22.2 shows an example of the various components of the CIPP model in relation to planning and evaluating a CNS education program. Beginning with the context evaluation phase of the process, the focus primarily relates to planning.

The objective of this phase of the evaluation was to assess the need for initiating a new adult-gerontology CNS program to meet regional needs for CNS practice. Information collected related primarily to conducting a needs assessment by compiling and reviewing background information related to national and local health goals/needs, trends in evidence-based practice (EBP), knowledge transfer and translation, funding priorities, recognition of CNS contributions to safety and quality, national curriculum standards, and certification and accreditation requirements. Additionally, regional health care leaders and potential employers were surveyed or

interviewed with respect to their needs for CNSs and potential students were surveyed to determine interest. Decision makers used data collected from the context evaluation phase to review and revise goals of the proposed CNS program and ensure that the proposed CNS program would be able to make use of community assets and address regional needs. The results of the context evaluation continued to be used throughout the implementation process as a basis for program evaluation.

With respect to input evaluation, the objective was to plan a CNS curriculum that met national standards, was feasible with respect to available resources, and produced well-prepared graduates. The methods used to evaluate this phase included examining exemplar CNS programs, comparing planned CNS program implementation strategies with current literature and trends, assessing the adequacy of budgetary resources to support the CNS program, assessing curriculum

TABLE 22.2

EXAMPLE OF CIPP MODEL APPLIED TO PLANNING AND EVALUATING AN ADULT-GERONTOLOGY CNS PREPARATION EDUCATION PROGRAM			
Context	**Input**	**Process**	**Product**
Objective			
To assess the need for initiating a new adult-gerontology CNS program to meet regional needs for CNS practice	To plan a CNS curriculum that meets national standards, is feasible with respect to available resources, and produces well-prepared graduates	To identify issues and strengths related to CNS program delivery	To determine that the CNS program is meeting stated outcomes with respect to context, input. and process objectives
Methods			
<ul><li>Compile and review relevant information related to</li><ul><li>National and local health goals/needs</li><li>Trends in evidence-based practice, knowledge transfer and translation</li><li>Funding priorities</li><li>CNS contributions to safety and quality</li><li>National curriculum standards</li><li>Certification and accreditation requirements</li></ul><li>Survey or interview potential employers regarding need for CNSs</li><li>Determine student interest in a CNS program</li></ul>	<ul><li>Examine exemplar CNS programs</li><li>Compare planned CNS program implementation strategies with current literature and trends</li><li>Assess adequacy of budgetary resources to support CNS program</li><li>Assess curriculum and program plans for feasibility and viability</li><li>Determine availability of adequate faculty and education resources, preceptors, and specialty practice opportunities</li></ul>	<ul><li>Review course syllabi and evaluations related to</li><ul><li>Content, objectives</li><li>Teaching strategies</li></ul><li>Survey students and preceptors to determine that</li><ul><li>Course objectives can be met at the practicum site</li><li>Preceptors and students are adequately prepared</li></ul><li>Conduct focus groups with students to identify opportunities for improvement</li></ul>	<ul><li>Examine the extent to which CNS students achieve capstone course objectives</li><li>Measuring how well graduating students rate themselves as achieving program objectives</li><li>Review of preceptor evaluations of student performance</li><li>Surveys and/or interviews of graduating students, alumni, and employers</li><li>Review of certification exam pass rates</li><li>Review of graduate employment patterns</li></ul>

CIPP, context, input, process, and product; CNS, clinical nurse specialist.

and program plans for feasibility and viability, and determining the availability of adequate faculty, education resources, preceptors, and specialty practice opportunities. Decision makers within the program used input evaluation data to devise a strategy for CNS program implementation that meets scientific, economic, social, political, and technologic needs; assure that the CNS program strategy is feasible for meeting needs; support funding requests; and identify potential issues affecting success.

With respect to process evaluation, the primary objective was to identify issues and strengths related to delivery of the CNS program. Examples of methods used to evaluate process included reviewing course syllabi and evaluations related to content, objectives, and teaching strategies; surveying students and preceptors to determine that the practicum site enabled students to meet course objectives and that preceptors and students were adequately prepared for the practicum experience; and identifying opportunities for improvement by conducting focus group interviews with students. Process evaluation data were used by program decision makers to help coordinate and strengthen teaching activities, strengthen the curriculum, and document the cost and integrity of the education process.

Finally, with respect to product, the objective of this phase was to determine that the CNS program met stated outcomes with respect to context, input, and process objectives. The evaluation methods included examining the extent to which CNS students achieved capstone course objectives; measuring how well graduating students rated themselves as achieving program objectives and reviewing preceptor evaluations of student performance; conducting surveys and/or interviews of graduating students, alumni, and employers; reviewing certification exam pass rates; and reviewing employment patterns of CNS graduates. Decision makers used product data to judge to what extent the program produced CNSs who meet societal and employer needs (impact), produced competent CNSs, and ensured student achievement of program goals (effectiveness). Additionally, decision makers used all evaluation data to determine whether the program should continue (sustainability). Depending on the type of program—for example, online versus traditional or single site versus a multiple campus system—decisions regarding transportability may or may not be made.

In the preceding example, the types and sources of data collected were similar, but the purpose for which data were used in the evaluation and decision-making processes differed. In general, evaluation data sources included stakeholder interviews and focus groups. Stakeholders included potential employers and students, patient/community representatives, exemplar

programs, and professional organizations. Other examples of data sources include public health and workforce data, budget information, publications from government, database, and professional organization sources, regulatory/certification bodies, and local and national quality dashboards.

With respect to formative and summative evaluation, the focus thus far has been on the use of evaluation data to continually improve the program. Therefore, the type of evaluation addressed would be considered formative evaluation. If the evaluation were undertaken for accountability or reporting purposes, then the process would be considered summative evaluation. Generally, CNS programs participate in summative evaluations when submitting reports for accreditation or university reporting purposes.

ETHICAL CONSIDERATIONS

As CNSs participate in planning or carrying out program evaluation activities, many ethical implications must be considered. According to Stufflebeam and Shinkfield (2007), The Joint Committee (TJC) on Standards for Educational Evaluation has published a set of standards governing the ethical behavior of evaluators in the field of education. These standards are grouped into the four categories of utility, feasibility, propriety, and accuracy (Stufflebeam & Shinkfield, 2007). The first category, pertaining to utility, addresses the need for evaluations to be useful and to meet the needs of the stakeholders. Evaluators should report strengths as well as opportunities for improvement along with recommendations for applying evaluation results (Stufflebeam & Shinkfield, 2007). The second category refers to feasibility and includes the need for evaluations to be nondisruptive to the program itself. Furthermore, evaluations should be cost-effective and realistic (Stufflebeam & Shinkfield, 2007). The third set of standards, referring to propriety, addresses the need for evaluations to protect the rights of those involved with the evaluation process. Propriety standards also require truthful, balanced reporting of evaluation findings while protecting the welfare of those involved with the process (Stufflebeam & Shinkfield, 2007). The final group of standards, accuracy, addresses the quality, validity, and reliability of the evaluation itself. Evaluators need to use accurate and reliable information and report findings accurately and without bias (Stufflebeam & Shinkfield, 2007).

It is apparent from this overview of evaluation standards that the process of evaluating programs relies heavily upon ethical principles. These ethical principles possess many corollaries with ANA's (2010) *Code of Ethics for Nurses*. Nurses and CNSs involved with program evaluation activities should be familiar with the ANA Code of Ethics as well as TJC evaluation standards.

CNS OUTCOMES RELATED TO PROGRAM EVALUATION

At the beginning of this chapter, CNS competencies related to evaluating programs of care were addressed. The competencies included were published by NACNS

(2004) as well as the National CNS Competency Task Force (2010). In addition to developing and publishing CNS competencies, NACNS (2004) also developed and published outcomes of CNS practice. Many of these outcomes related directly to CNS program evaluation activities. Outcomes of CNS practice organized according to each of the three spheres of influence (patient, nurses/nursing practice, and organization/system) and that relate directly to program evaluation are located in Table 22.3. It is apparent that as CNSs are involved with program evaluation,

TABLE 22.3

NACNS OUTCOMES RELATED TO PROGRAM EVALUATION ACTIVITIES	
Sphere of Influence	**NACNS Outcome**
Patient	4. Innovative educational programs for patients, families, and groups are developed, implemented, and evaluated 10. Collaboration with patients/clients, nursing staff, as well as physicians and other health care professionals, occurs as appropriate 14. Unintended consequences and errors are prevented 15. Desired measurable patient/client outcomes are achieved. Desired outcomes of care may include improved clinical status, quality of life, functional status, alleviation or remediation of symptoms, patient/family satisfaction, and cost-effective care 16. Reports of the new clinical phenomena and/or interventions are disseminated through presentations and publications
Nurses/nursing practice	18. The research and scientific base for innovations is articulated, understandable, and accessible 20. Nurses are empowered to solve patient care problems at the point of service 21. Nurses' career enhancement programs are ongoing, accessible, innovative, and effective 22. Educational programs that advance the practice of nursing are developed, implemented, evaluated, and linked to evidence-based practice and effects on clinical and fiscal outcomes 26. Nurses use resources judiciously to review overall costs of care and enhance the quality of patient care 27. Nurses have an effective voice in decision making about patient care
Organization/system	30. Models of practice are developed, piloted, evaluated, and incorporated across the continuum of care 31. Nursing care and outcomes are articulated at organizational/system decision-making levels 32. Patient care initiatives reflect knowledge of cost management and revenue enhancement strategies 33. Patient care programs are aligned with the organization's strategic imperatives, mission, vision, philosophy, and values 34. Clinical problems are articulated within the context of the organization/system structure, mission, culture, policies, and resources 36. Change strategies are integrated throughout the system 37. Evidence-based, best practice models are developed and implemented 38. Stakeholders (nurses, other health care professionals, and management) share a common vision of practice outcomes 39. Decision makers within the institution are informed about practice problems, factors contributing to the problems, and the significance of those problems with respect to outcomes and costs 40. Patient care processes reflect continuous improvements that benefit the system 41. Staff complies with regulatory requirements and standards 42. Policy-making bodies are influenced to develop regulations/procedures to improve patient care and health services

NACNS, National Association of Clinical Nurse Specialists.

they address outcomes of practice within all three spheres of influence. However, outcomes related to program evaluation derive primarily from the organization/system sphere. Depending upon the nature of the program evaluated, additional outcomes in the patient or nurse/nursing practice sphere might also be addressed. Because program evaluation can be related to such a large number of CNS outcomes, it is apparent that CNS participation in program evaluation efforts is an important facet of CNS practice.

SUMMARY AND CONCLUSIONS

This chapter addressed the topic of program evaluation in a general way and described the CIPP model in more detail. Exemplars of applying the CIPP model to CNS practice and education were presented. The topic of program evaluation is vast and many other models and approaches to program evaluation exist. It is beyond the scope of this chapter to address each model in detail, but many resources exist that can provide additional information to interested CNSs.

In conclusion, program evaluation is an important activity for CNSs to pursue. Models of program evaluation, such as CIPP, can give CNSs tools not only to evaluate innovative programs, but also to assist with the process of planning the innovation. Following a structured format can help to focus the planning and evaluation process. Additionally, CNSs who use a model for evaluation may be better equipped to implement programs that have a lasting positive outcome on patient, nurse, and organizational outcomes at the local level and beyond.

DISCUSSION QUESTIONS

- Why is it important for CNSs to carry out planned efforts to evaluate programs they initiate? What resources exist to help CNSs evaluate programs? What types of barriers interfere with CNS participation in program evaluation activities?
- This chapter discussed the role of values in the evaluation process. As a practicing CNS working with a group that is about to embark upon a program-planning evaluation effort, what primary values would you anticipate being discussed? How would you initiate a discussion on values and who would you engage in this discussion?
- In the exemplar related to new nurse orientation, what ethical implications would be important for the implementation team to consider?
- What are some similarities and differences between QI activities and program evaluation?
- Why is it important to outline an evaluation plan during the program-planning process? Also, during this initial phase, why is it important to identify key stakeholders, and what criteria would you use to identify them?

ANALYSIS AND SYNTHESIS EXERCISES

- This chapter presented the CIPP model as an exemplar. For this exercise, go to the literature and select another evaluation approach such as Michael Scriven's objectives-free, consumer-oriented approach to evaluation. Compare and contrast the model you chose with the CIPP model. Address the type of general approach or orientation upon which the model is based, the types of evaluation methods each uses, the ways stakeholders are involved, and the processes for making evaluative judgments. Discuss strengths and limitations of each.
- At your place of work or study, find out what type of evaluation models or methods are used to guide program evaluation. Interview someone who is responsible for using the models and determine how the model has been used in the past. Determine how the evaluation approach assists with decision making with respect to program adaptation or continuation. Find out how satisfied the organization is with the evaluation approach and what works and what doesn't work.
- Compare and contrast formative and summative evaluation approaches. Locate within your place of work or study examples of formative and summative evaluation. Consider similarities and differences with respect to the purpose, evaluation methods, impact, and evaluative judgments.

REFERENCES

Al-Khathami, A. D. (2012). Evaluation of Saudi family medicine training program: The application of CIPP evaluation format. *Medical Teacher, 34*, S81–S89.

American Nurses Association (ANA). (2010). *Code of Ethics for nurses with interpretive statements.* Retrieved from http://nursingworld.org/MainMenuCategories/EthicsStandards/CodeofEthicsforNurses/Code-of-Ethics.pdf

Anderson, E. L., McCartney, E. S., Schreiber, J. A., & Thompson, E. A. (1989). Productivity measurement for clinical nurse specialists. *Clinical Nurse Specialist, 3*, 80–84.

Brinkerhoff, R. O., & Dressler, D. E. (2003). *Using the success case impact evaluation method to enhance training value and impact.* Retrieved from http://www.kenblanchard.com/img/pub/newsletter_brinkerhoff.pdf

Centers for Disease Control and Prevention (CDC). (2012). *A framework for program evaluation.* Retrieved from http://www.cdc.gov/eval/framework/index.htm

Doyle, L., O'Brien, F., Timmins, F., Tobin, G., O'Rourke, F., & Doherty, L. (2008). An evaluation of an attendance monitoring system for undergraduate nursing students. *Nurse Education in Practice, 8,* 129–139.

Hall, M. A., Daly, B. J., & Madigan, E. A. (2010). Use of anecdotal notes by clinical nursing faculty: A descriptive study. *Journal of Nursing Education, 49,* 156–159.

Ho, W., Chen, W., Ho, C., Lee, M., Chen, C., & Chou, R. H. (2011). Evaluation of the suicide prevention program in Kauhsiung City, Taiwan, using the CIPP evaluation model. *Community Mental Health Journal, 47,* 542–550.

Kennedy-Malone, L. (1996). Evaluation strategies for CNSs: Application of an evaluation model. *Clinical Nurse Specialist, 10,* 195–198.

Muller, A., McCauley, K., Harrington, P., Jablonski, J., & Strauss, R. (2011). Evidence-based practice implementation strategy. The central role of the clinical nurse specialist. *Nursing Administration Quarterly, 35,* 140–151.

National Association of Clinical Nurse Specialists (NACNS). (2004). *Statement on clinical nurse specialist practice and education.* Harrisburg, PA: NACNS.

National CNS Competency Task Force. (2010). *Clinical nurse specialist core competencies.* Retrieved from http://www.nacns.org/html/competencies.php

Nugent, K. E., & Lambert, V. A. (1997). Evaluating the performance of the APN. *Nursing Management, 28*(2), 29–32.

Patton, M. Q. (2003). *Qualitative evaluation checklist.* Retrieved from http://www.wmich.edu/evalctr/archive_checklists/qec.pdf

Petro-Nustas, W. (1996). Evaluation of the process of introducing a quality development program in a nursing department at a teaching hospital: The role of a change agent. *International Journal of Nursing Studies, 33,* 605–618.

Posavac, E. J., & Carey, R.G. (2007). *Program evaluation: Methods and case studies* (7th ed.). Upper Saddle River, NJ: Pearson Education.

Razack, S., Meterissian, S., Morin, L., Snell, L., Steinert, Y., Tabatabai, D., & MacLellan, A. (2007). Coming of age as communicators: Differences in the implementation of common communications skills training in four residency programs. *Medical Education, 41,* 441–449.

Scriven, M. (2007). *Key evaluation checklist.* Retrieved from http://www.wmich.edu/evalctr/archive_checklists/kec_feb07.pdf

Steinert, Y., Cruess, S., Cruess, R., & Snell, L. (2005). Faculty development for teaching and evaluating professionalism: From programme design to curriculum change. *Medical Education, 39,* 127–136.

Stufflebeam, D. L. (2003). *The CIPP model for evaluation.* Retrieved from http://www.scribd.com/doc/58435354/The-Cipp-Model-for-Evaluation-by-Daniel-l-Stufflebeam

Stufflebeam, D. L. (2007). *CIPP evaluation model checklist.* http://www.wmich.edu/evalctr/archive_checklists/cippchecklist_mar07.pdf

Stufflebeam, D. L., & Shinkfield, A. J. (2007). *Evaluation theory, models, & applications.* San Francisco, CA: Jossey-Bass.

Walker, J. A., Urden, L. D., & Moody, R. (2009). The role of the CNS in attaining and maintaining Magnet status. *Journal of Nursing Administration, 39,* 515–523.

Zhang, G., Zeller, N., Griffith, R., Metcalf, D., Williams, J., Shea, C., & Misulis, K. (2011). Using the context, input, process, and product evaluation model (CIPP) as a comprehensive framework to guide the planning, implementation, and assessment of service-learning programs. *Journal of Higher Education Outreach and Engagement, 15*(4), 57–84.

Accountable Care Organizations—New Horizons for Clinical Nurse Specialist Practice

Kimberly S. Hodge, Courtney Federspiel, and Janet S. Fulton

On March 23, 2010, the Patient Protection and Affordable Care Act (ACA), also known as the Healthcare Reform Act or the ACA, was signed into law. This monumental legislation addressed nearly all aspects of the U.S. health care system, from individual insurance coverage mandates to new requirements for health insurers, employers, and providers. Responsibility for implementation of the new law is assigned largely to the Centers for Medicare & Medicaid Services (CMS) of the U.S. Department of Health and Human Services (DHHS). CMS created the Center for Medicare & Medicaid Innovations (CMMI) for the purpose of designing, implementing, and evaluating innovative initiatives consistent with the intent of the ACA (www.cms.gov/About-CMS/Agency-Information/CMSLeadership/Office_CMMI.html). Under CMMI, several new initiatives are being launched. Five top initiatives are accountable care organizations (ACOs), medical homes, retail clinics, dual eligibility, and bundled payments. ACOs are a service and payment model wherein hospitals, medical groups, or other providers agree to manage the total, seamless care of a group of patients for the purpose of achieving improved clinical outcomes and reduced cost. ACOs are at risk for the entirety of their assigned population's health care costs, not simply the costs for services participating providers themselves render. Medical homes are primary care provider groups intended to improve outcomes through care management and coordination. Retail clinics, such as those available in national chain drug stores, are

being reexamined as a way to address minor care needs and divert patients from costly emergency department care. Dual eligibility is a pilot program to improve care and reduce cost for persons covered by both Medicare and Medicaid. The bundled-payments initiative is moving to a fee-for-value system, where the focus is on outcomes and not individual services. Quality is rewarded over volume (Daly, Zigmond, Barr, Robezniels, & Evens, 2013). This chapter discusses ACOs and probes opportunities for clinical nurse specialist (CNS) practice within ACOs.

BACKGROUND

America is experiencing an increase in aged persons as the baby boomer generation—persons born post–World War II between the years 1946 and 1964—is turning 65 years old. Baby boomers segment into two broad cohorts: The Leading-Edge Baby Boomers, born between 1946 and 1955 and representing slightly more than half of the generation, or roughly 38,002,000 people of all races; and Late Boomers, persons born between 1956 and 1964 and representing about 37,818,000 individuals (Live Births by Age of Mother and Race, 1933–1998). The subsequent increase in Medicare enrollment, the health care program for Americans older than 65 years, along with current projected Medicare funding deficits, are a main driver for finding new, more efficient ways to deliver health care. So emphatic was this goal of efficiency that the ACA, under the CMMI, set aside $10 billion dollars in funding over the next decade to pilot new health care delivery and reimbursement models (ACA Section 3021). One of the first programs to come out of CMMI was the Medicare Pioneer ACO, known as the Pioneer ACO program, which began on January 1, 2012.

WHAT IS THE PIONEER ACO PROGRAM?

The Pioneer ACO program was the first Medicare ACO program. The name "Pioneer" is indicative not only of this initiative's position as the first to participate in a Medicare ACO, but also of the participant's status as leader in the field, pioneering new models for coordinated health care delivery and creating best practices to share with future Medicare ACOs such as those participating in the Medicare Shared Savings Program (MSSP).

The Pioneer ACO model has three primary aims: improving the quality of care delivered to patients, improving population health, and lowering/slowing the overall growth in costs of health care. To meet these aims, ACOs focus on collaboration among groups of health care providers. Specifically, an ACO is a group of health care providers spanning the entire continuum of care and including but not limited to physician practices, hospitals, home care agencies, assisted living, and rehabilitation centers, all collaborating to provide coordinated, high-quality care for Medicare patients (www.cms.gov). ACO providers collectively provide Medicare patients with the right care at the right time and in an appropriate care setting. For example, ACOs prevent major health incidents by assuring access to primary care providers, providing home health nurses to work with patients in the home to take medications as prescribed or making available advanced practice nurses to help patients manage stress emotions. If providers in an ACO succeed in improving the health of an assigned population during a performance year (defined as January 1 through December 31 of a calendar year) and meet certain quality and cost benchmarks, they can share in any generated cost savings as a monetary reward.

ACOs: THE MECHANICS

Data

A large differentiator between the ACO model of care delivery and past iterations of health care models is the focus on data. Successful management of patients across care settings depends on an efficient electronic health record (EHR) or data aggregator that facilitates rapid and efficient sharing of health information across ACO providers. EHRs are central to being able to use data to monitor outcomes and link outcomes to savings and ultimately to revenue. McBride (2013) noted that the health care industry has been slow to convert to the network-based models long ago adopted in industry, clinging instead to old communication infrastructures, tools, and methods. ACOs aim to expedite this transition to centralized data and making data available to providers. Providers partnering with Medicare in the Pioneer ACO receive access to 3 years of claims history from CMS on attributed Medicare beneficiaries, unless the beneficiary opts out of data sharing. Additionally, ACO providers receive monthly updates on claims paid on Medicare beneficiaries. Access to beneficiary historical data helps give ACO providers a more comprehensive picture of a patient's health for diagnosis and treatment of conditions, as the provider has an understanding of all visits the patient may have had, not just those made within his or her office or delivery system. This allows tracking and trending of a patient's health history, such as risk factors, diseases treated, how and when services are accessed, and linking these variables to long-term outcomes.

Providers

Provider participation in an ACO is currently voluntary. Providers such as medical doctors, advanced practice nurses, and physician's assistants joining an ACO assume shared responsibility for coordinating and managing care for an assigned population. The roster of participating ACO providers is then used by CMS to attribute, or assign, patients to an ACO.

Provider reimbursement mechanisms in the Pioneer ACO began with the traditional fee-for-service basis, with successful ACOs having the option to migrate to population-based payments in successive years. If, at the end of the year, an ACO succeeds in meeting specified quality measures and slowing the growth in health care costs of its attributed population, providers in the ACO are eligible to receive a portion of the savings achieved through the ACO. Savings are calculated at the end of each performance year by subtracting actual costs for the ACO-attributed population from the cost Medicare expected to pay for these individuals (known as the ACO's "benchmark") based on their claims history.

Beneficiaries

CMS refers to patients covered by Medicare as beneficiaries. ACOs are required to notify all beneficiaries who have been assigned, or attributed, to an

ACO of their attribution and a description of what this means for them. Additionally, beneficiaries must be informed that Medicare will share their medical claims data with the assigned ACO and that they can stop this sharing of data (called "opting out") at any time. As with other beneficiaries in traditional Medicare, beneficiaries attributed to an ACO retain their freedom of choice, which means that they can continue to see providers of choice and decide when and in which setting to seek care. The benefit of the ACO model is that assigned or attributed individuals who do not opt out are provided with additional resources such as complex case management services, coordinated and enhanced communication across their team of care providers, and additional education and support to assist with self-care management of disease and illness states.

Attribution and Shared Savings

To be eligible for attribution to the Pioneer ACO, an individual must have 12 consecutive months of fee-for-service Medicare coverage under Medicare Part A and Medicare Part B. Individuals are ineligible for ACO attribution if Medicare was the secondary payer, they had primary residence outside the United States, or they are enrolled in Medicare Advantage plans. Beneficiaries are assigned to ACOs based on historical primary care–based evaluation and management (E&M) visits[1] with ACO providers. CMS uses its claims database to identify beneficiaries eligible for the ACO, attributes these individuals to an ACO, and gives the ACO an expected cost ("cost benchmark") for the ACO for 1 year (January 1–December 31). In general, a beneficiary is aligned with a Pioneer ACO if he or she received the largest amount of primary care services (under circumstances, selected specialty care services) from physicians and other practitioners who are affiliated with the ACO compared to providers affiliated with any other ACO or any non-ACO-affiliated provider.

Although Medicare's traditional fee-for-service payment system is retained in an ACO model, Medicare creates an additional incentive for ACO providers by offering ACOs a share in any savings achieved while caring for an assigned ACO population. For example, if ACO providers come in below the cost target set by CMS and meet certain quality metrics (www.cms.gov/Medicare/Medicare-Fee-for-Service-Payment/sharedsavingsprogram/Downloads/

ACO-NarrativeMeasures-Specs.pdf), they are eligible to share in those savings. In other words, providers in ACOs are incentivized to keep beneficiaries at an optimal state of health, engaged in preventive care, out of the hospital, and using appropriate settings of service such as an urgent care facility in place of a hospital emergency department. If a Pioneer ACO cannot achieve clinical goals and keep the cost within the benchmark for the attributed population—that is, the cost is greater than CMS had anticipated (ACO goes over its cost benchmark)—the ACO may have to pay Medicare a portion of the amount by which it exceeded the benchmark.

The Approach

ACOs shift the focus of care from episodic, fragmented, high-cost hospital-centric care delivery systems to patient-centered care systems focused on quality outcomes rather than volume. Traditional fee-for-service health care is a well-worn path of escalating volume of care services regardless of quality of care. Providers are incentivized by volume of service, which by definition does not put the patient in the center. Patients are shuttled between care sites and providers with limited to no coordination among clinicians. The more complex the patient problems, the more services are consumed. Thus, a small percentage of patients with chronic health conditions consume a high percentage of the resources (Leaver, 2013). Reducing the cost of a unit of service encourages an increase in the number of units to preserve revenue, which means providers see more patients in the same time and space and initiate more procedures and tests. Silos of care contribute to waste and duplication, multiple billing systems and multiple management infrastructures, and for the patient, a lack of care coordination. The traditional focus is on treating sickness, not keeping people healthy (Baicker & Levy, 2013; Leaver, 2013).

ACOs are expected to provide full range of health care services, eliminate individual billing for services, use data to monitor health outcomes of beneficiaries, and keep people healthy. Central to these changes is complex case management with a focus on transitions of care between providers and among care settings. Providers are incentivized to keep beneficiaries healthy and meet quality targets, so a robust care management strategy should address the needs of patients at multiple levels while engaging them in self-care management, with the goal of ultimately achieving improved population health. Additionally, patient and caregiver education for self-care becomes paramount for managing patients in their home settings (White, 2012).

---

[1] Eligible HCPCS codes include: 99201–99215, 99304–99340, 99341 through 99350, G0402, G0438, G0439. Also included are codes 0521, 0522, 0524, 0525 when submitted by Federally Qualified Health Centers or by Rural Health Clinics. *Source*: www.cms.gov/Medicare/Medicare-Fee-for-Service-Payment/sharedsavingsprogram/Downloads/MSSP_FAQs.pdf

CNS PRACTICE IN ACO ENVIRONMENT

Optimizing safety, achieving quality outcomes, and reducing costs of care are central to CNS practice, making CNSs strategically aligned with the goals of ACOs. CNS practice occurs in three domains: patients/families, nurses/nursing practice, and systems/organizations. ACOs create opportunities for CNSs in all three domains, also called spheres of influence. CNS opportunities within a Medicare ACO system include direct care with the Medicare beneficiary and his or her family, providing and supporting nurses in providing case management, creating programs for disease prevention and management, and enhancing self-care for maximum function and quality of life among persons with chronic illnesses. In clinical care systems, CNSs provide leadership for nurses in the delivery of evidence-based practice (EBP) and use data to monitor outcomes and initiate intervention, program, or system changes. In an ACO system, CNSs will continue to lead teams in care improvement initiatives and remove barriers to delivering best practices. Medicare ACOs are designed to provide care to older adults. The Adult-Gerontology CNS Competencies (www.nacns.org/docs/adult-geroCNScomp.pdf) serve as a guide for the scope of practice for CNSs in a Medicare ACO organization. The following discussion explores the application of CNS practice using the adult-gerontology CNS competencies as a guide to innovative practice within Medicare ACOs.

CNS as Direct Care Provider

The U.S. population of older adults or those 65 years old and older is growing at a rate never before experienced, primarily because of longer life spans and the aging of baby boomers. According to DHHS Administration on Aging (AoA), older adults accounted for 12.9% of the U.S. population in 2009 and by 2030 this number is expected to be 19% (Aging Statistics). It is estimated that two of every three older adults have more than one chronic condition and that treatment for chronic health conditions in the population across all age groups accounts for 66% of the U.S. health care budget (www.hhs.gov/news/press/2010pres/12/20101214a.html). Many older adults experience chronic conditions and many experience more than one. Chronic health problems commonly experienced by older adults include, but are not limited to, osteoarthritis, diabetes, chronic obstructive pulmonary disease, and cardiovascular disease, including hypertension (www.nia.nih.gov/newsroom/features/nih-seeking-strategies-multiple-chronic-conditions-older-people).

A growing older adult population, the presence of more than one chronic condition among older adults, and costs associated with treating chronic conditions combined with age-related changes has resulted in complex health care needs in this population. As direct care providers, CNSs have traditionally worked with patients experiencing complex care needs in inpatient settings to restore health, minimize complications, and reduce length of stay. In ACOs, CNSs will continue to be important providers for patients with complex health problems, with an increased emphasis on minimizing complications, early discharge, and reduced readmission.

CNSs have traditionally led efforts to develop, implement, and evaluate evidence-based protocols designed to prevent hospital-acquired complications such as pressure ulcers, bloodstream and urinary tract infections, and falls. In ACOs, CNSs will continue to be central to these efforts in an expanded leadership capacity. CNSs will lead systemwide initiatives for multidisciplinary teams of providers including system-level monitoring and evaluation. In addition, because CNSs are specialty practice focused, they will adapt evidence-based care routines to meet specialty populations' needs and to monitor outcomes, plan, and evaluate programs of specialty care. To assure success of EBP initiatives, CNSs will teach, coach, and mentor not only bedside nurses, as has been standard practice, but also other providers in an expanded scope of responsibility for the totality of patient outcomes related to these initiatives.

ACOs succeed financially when patients are discharged in a timely manner. Prolonged hospital stays contribute to deconditioning and loss of function and increase the odds for hospital-acquired complications, which are threats to the ACO. As direct care providers, CNS must be leaders in championing early discharge from hospitals to alternative care settings and in transitioning patients throughout the care continuum. Transitional care models, such as Naylor's Transitional Care Model (www.transitionalcare.info) have been tested for effectiveness and have demonstrated ability to meet the needs of patients transitioning from an inpatient setting to home. For complex, specialty patients, CNSs should begin a transitional care plan upon admission. To prepare for postacute needs such as medications, physical and cognitive functioning, symptom burden, and self-care management of preexisting and new problems, CNSs need an assessment toolkit of reliable, clinically valid instruments and techniques for initial assessment and ongoing monitoring of patient progress across time. CNSs will lead the development of specialty assessment toolkits for use by nurses and other providers. One-size-fits-all assessment likely will not provide the level of information needed to address transition planning if we are to keep patients healthy and functioning in home settings.

Once the patient is discharged from the hospital, CNSs extend their direct care practice by following up in the home or other setting. Not all patients will be discharged to home. Some patients may require postacute care in a setting such as a long-term acute care hospital, acute inpatient rehabilitation, skilled nursing facility or subacute rehabilitation, or home health with rehabilitative services. These types of services will be under the ACO; thus, CNSs will be leading a transitional plan of care from the acute inpatient setting to the postacute setting and then to home. Ongoing assessment and monitoring of outcomes in the home setting will alert the CNS to risk factors and impending problems and provide the CNS and the care team with opportunity for early intervention. Patients with complex problems are frequently discharged to the care of a family member. Family caregivers need education, support, and guidance to learn new skills, to develop confidence in using judgment, and to feel secure in having access to a trusted provider. CNSs in ACOs serving as teachers, mentors, coaches, and facilitators for family caregivers will help stabilize patients in their homes, reduce complications, and prevent costly readmissions.

In nonhome settings, CNSs will support achieving the best possible health outcomes by working with facility staff, patients, and their families while avoiding readmission to an acute care facility. Just as CNSs teach, mentor, and coach bedside nurses in inpatient settings, CNSs will likewise be teaching, mentoring, and coaching nurses working with staff to promote continuity as patients transition across settings.

In ACOs, expanded CNSs practice will include leading, mentoring, and evaluating delivery of care and patient outcomes for all providers on a team because all providers share in the risks and benefits of outcomes for a designated population. Communication requirements within the provider team will be heightened, as any individually provided care must be delivered in concert with all care providers. Also, the provider delivering the care may shift from current established practice. The provider with the most appropriate skill set will deliver the care, meaning that CNSs may serve as the team leader for total management of some patient cases where the providers are not nurses or not majority nurses. Or, a CNS may be assigned to deliver care as a member of a team led by a nonnurse provider.

Ambulatory care or primary care settings, not a past common setting for CNS practice, will need CNS specialty practice services. CNSs specialty services such as wound care, stress emotions management, and diabetes education, parenting skills programs, stop smoking initiatives are needed if ACOs are to provide the broadest array of health care services possible. CNSs in these types of specialty services will be focusing on individuals and populations of individuals achieving self-care management skills and abilities for symptom management, functional enhancement, prevention of disease, and improvement of quality of life. Again, a toolkit of appropriately sensitive assessment and evaluation instruments and techniques is needed for monitoring patient progress and outcomes for specialty services in primary care settings. CNSs delivering specialty care services will use diagnostic reasoning competencies to enable correct identification of etiologies of problems for guiding selection of interventions. CNSs, as members of ACO care teams, will consult and collaborate with team members to keep patients well and highly functioning at home.

CNS as Complex Case Manager Consultant

Care management is a primary activity in a Medicare ACO. Registered nurse (RN) complex case managers are team members with the CNS and together they identify patients with complex problems in need of case management and facilitate achievement of safe, high-quality clinical outcomes in a cost-sensitive manner. ACOs are developing predictive models to identify the most at-risk Medicare beneficiaries and assign these patients to an RN complex case manager. Case management is defined by the Case Management Society of America (CMSA) as "a collaborative process of assessment, planning, facilitation, care coordination, evaluation, and advocacy for options and services to meet an individual's and family's comprehensive health needs through communication and available resources to promote quality cost effective outcomes" (www.cmsa.org). In ACOs, complex case managers are focusing on individuals with complex needs, such as the older adult with chronic conditions, to improve health outcomes across the system and providers and not just for a care incident.

In the ACO complex case management structure, the case management staff members are a "unit" of the organization. CNSs will consult with RN complex case managers as they work to assist patients and families with providing care in the home, coordinate care provider visits and families, and problem-solve barriers interfering with desired outcomes (www.nacns.org/docs/CNSCoreCompetenciesBroch.pdf). With specialty expertise, CNSs will be available to the RN complex case managers when they are providing care for beneficiaries with specialty care needs alone or in combination with other health-related problems. Examples of consultation activities by CNSs include reviewing assessment data collected by RN complex case managers, in-depth probing for problem identification, identifying target problem etiologies for interventions, designing interventions, measuring and evaluating outcomes, and modifying the plan of care to meet patient priorities and ACO principles. CNSs will work with the nursing staff and other providers in the complex case management unit in much the same manner as working with staff assigned to a traditional inpatient unit—consulting, coaching, mentoring, teaching, and problem solving.

Other consultation activities include assuring that nursing practice in an ACO complex case management unit is evidence-based best practice. CNSs will lead the development, implementation, and evaluation of evidence-based protocols and best-practice policies. CNSs will assess the staff for ongoing educational needs and, in collaboration with managers, educators, and others, will provide or support the development of educational programs to assure knowledge and skill for quality outcomes.

CNS Leading ACO Quality Monitoring

CNSs will lead quality teams. In order to be eligible for shared savings, a Medicare ACO must decrease the overall cost of care provided to attributed beneficiaries and achieve benchmark performance in 33 quality measures. The measures are divided into four primary areas, which includes the patient and/ or caregiver experience, care coordination and patient safety, preventive care, and at-risk population (www.cms.gov/Medicare/Medicare-Fee-for-Service-Payment/sharedsavingsprogram/Downloads/ACO-NarrativeMeasures-Specs.pdf). See the appendix at the end of this chapter for the four domains and specific measures.

CNSs can and should be leaders in any of the domains. The at-risk domain is where CNSs will affect maximum impact, because it requires engaging patients in self-management of preventive services and stabilization of underlying chronic conditions. An ACO sole strategy of expecting the provider to prescribe treatments and refer to other health care clinicians for specialty services will *not* suffice in achieving CMS benchmarks. Patients have significant responsibility for acquiring and maintaining self-management skills and, in partnership with their primary care provider, to successfully manage chronic health problems. CNSs are knowledgeable about physiological, psychological, and social underpinnings of illness and disease. Successful CNS practice in ACOs requires program initiatives designed to enable patients to achieve self-management and to become active collaborators with their primary care provider to achieve quality benchmark outcomes.

CNS as ACO Systems Leader

CNS systems leader competency is defined as "the ability to manage change and empower others to influence clinical practice and political processes both within and across systems" (www.nacns.org/docs/CNSCoreCompetenciesBroch.pdf). Behaviors of this competency include performing system-level assessments, determining interventions that optimize population safety, promoting the adoption of EBPs, fostering inter- and intraprofessional communication and collaboration, mentoring team leadership competencies, coordinating care delivery across the continuum, and disseminating outcomes of CNS practice that contribute to the ACO's achievement of safety, quality, and cost goals for Medicare beneficiaries.

Health care reform has multiple goals to achieve; however, at the forefront is the need to optimize the safety and quality of the care provided and to lower costs associated with care delivery. Because ACOs will be, by definition, complex systems, CNSs should be able to transfer knowledge and skills developed in traditional inpatient settings and hospital systems to ACOs. An ACO will be composed of macro-level system and many microsystem units. Both macrosystems and microsystems must be understood, evaluated, and managed if the ACO as a whole is to function efficiently and achieve broad overarching clinical and fiscal outcomes. System-level assessment, monitoring, and evaluation will be needed to address immediate problems and ongoing growth. CNSs will need to lead teams, serve on teams, and evaluate teams as they design, test, refine, diffuse, and evaluate programs to sustain the ACO. This work will take place with in the complexity of an ACO, for many identifiable elements and some yet to be discovered.

To date, the circumscribed features of an ACO include coordinated care delivery, complex case management, evidence-based best practices, fiscal responsibility for utilization of services, and at-risk population identification and management. Actualizing an ACO will demand improved communication strategies across settings and providers, creation of evidence-based multidisciplinary order sets, disease management programs, launching of public education campaigns, strategic initiatives for managing population health, and more. CNSs should look for opportunities to engage, support, and lead these initiatives.

ACOs will be establishing a provider office charged with overall care management, making this office the hub of care provision for a patient panel. The Patient-Centered Medical Home is one such strategy being used to reduce fragmentation and improve coordination of care provided to a medical practice's patients and to shift the focus to quality over quantity. Medical Homes provide additional opportunities for CNSs. For example, a CNS can support the care management of a specific group of specialty patients within the practice, such as those with heart failure or diabetes. CNSs can design, implement, and evaluate programs of care for these specialty patients and their family caregivers, making continuous improvements until quality benchmarks are met or exceeded for the specialty population. A natural outcome of such program development will be the creation of best practices that will be shared with other ACOs.

At-risk population identification and management is another area of opportunity for CNSs within ACOs. CNSs can identify an at-risk population using the CMS claims data and collaborate with data analysts to address clinical needs while optimizing predictive models. Once the at-risk population is identified, a CNS creates/determines best practice and creates a delivery model to meet the ACO aims of improving the quality of care delivered, optimizing the health of the identified population, and slowing/lowering the overall growth in costs for the at-risk population.

Other examples of opportunities within the ACO system for CNSs include:

- Creating public health programs focused on prevention or disease management
- Reviewing utilization patterns and designing services to improve care. For example, creating a geriatric assessment unit in an emergency department to assure best practice placement postevaluation
- Participation in population health strategic planning to address pervasive public health problems such as smoking, obesity, and infant mortality

Additional CNS Competencies

Collaboration is central to functioning as a CNS and will be the requirement for successful participation in an ACO. The CNS collaboration competency is defined as "working jointly with others to optimize clinical outcomes" (www.nacns.org/docs/CNSCoreCompetenciesBroch.pdf). Within an ACO environment, every person encountering Medicare beneficiaries has an opportunity to impact their safety, quality, and cost outcomes. Collaboration transcends the continuum and the CNS must practice, mentor, foster, and lead collaboration efforts across the continuum of care.

Coaching will include nurses and will extend to other providers and to other clinicians/nonclinical leaders within an ACO environment. Clinical coaching will occur in the day-to-day activities associated with case management, physician practices, and specialty services. CNSs will also coach patients and families as well as support nurses in improving coaching skills in working directly with the Medicare beneficiary and his or her family and/or caregivers, assisting them in managing symptoms and implementing effective self-care strategies as well as navigating the complex health care system.

Research and clinical inquiry are at the foundation of CNS practice, regardless of setting. Within the ACO, CNSs will participate in the systematic evaluation of programs of care, many of which will be research focused, and will review and interpret evidence for use in clinical care. In an ACO setting, evaluation of the clinical practice environment includes assessment of a beneficiary's postacute setting, home environment, and the primary practice setting. Examples include finding, implementing, and evaluating fall risk and depression screening in complex case management and the primary care practice. The CNS will need to assure that each screening assessment includes interventions, which may be initiated based on findings. The CNS will need to monitor and respond to the outcomes associated with the assessments and subsequent interventions, continuously scanning the evidence for opportunities to improve clinician practice and Medicare beneficiary outcomes.

Oftentimes, existing EBP recommendations are associated strongly with the acute inpatient environment and the CNS is challenged to find evidence generalizable to the new environment. The CNS is presented with great opportunities to create and disseminate new knowledge. Doctoral-prepared CNSs, both PhD and clinical doctorates, are greatly needed within the ACO environment to contribute the tools for addressing knowledge gaps. Additionally, collaborating in multidisciplinary research programs (e.g., nursing, social work, engineering) presents a significant opportunity for the master's prepared CNS to facilitate the achievement of ACO goals and gain increased skill in research.

The ethical decision making, moral agency, and advocacy competency for the adult-gerontology CNS is defined as "identifying, articulating, and taking action on ethical concerns at the patient, family, health care provider, continuity, and public policy levels" (www.nacns.org/docs/CNSCoreCompetenciesBroch.pdf). In an ACO, a CNS's population of interest is the Medicare beneficiary, by definition an older or disabled adult and a member of a group that frequently is experiencing multiple and complex health problems. Care for these individuals carries a high probability of ethical conflict, as these beneficiaries often face situations with no single clear care path or ideal outcome. CNSs will need improved ability to identify, articulate, and resolve ethical conflicts with existing available resources. Examples of ethical conflicts include continuation of futile care, failure to provide evidence-based care, and providers not fully disclosing to beneficiaries and their families expected outcomes of care. Desired outcomes of CNS intervention in ethical decision making, moral advocacy, and advocacy competency include self-evaluating one's own practice, assuming and fostering professional accountability, promoting ethical practice environment, bringing the inter- and intraprofessional team together to address ethical concerns, facilitating full disclosure to Medicare beneficiaries for informed decisions regarding their plan of care, and advocating for safe and fair beneficiary care across the continuum.

Disseminating Outcomes

It is vitally important that the CNS promote both the role and the scope of CNS practice to all participants in the ACO—executive leadership, physicians, beneficiaries, other providers, and staff. And legislators! CNSs must take responsibility for making the link between ACO outcomes and CNS practice, and to widely disseminate this information to all possible audiences. CNSs must prepare and distribute reports reflecting their outcomes on a timely, routine basis. CNSs should take every opportunity to attend CMS learning sessions, professional conferences, and clinical meetings and, while there, engage attendees in discussion about CNS practice and contributions to the ACO. For example, a CNS served in a leadership capacity to facilitate determination of quality measures for documenting outcomes in a newly created continuing care network of postacute providers and home health. At a national learning session for Pioneer ACOs, this CNS shared the process for developing and implementing the measures, and explained the outcomes associated with the interventions in a CMS postacute care setting. As a result, the CNS was invited to participate in a second learning session focused on the collaboration skills used by the CNS for engaging the ACO postacute providers, including competitors, in collectively achieving goals for the Medicare beneficiaries in their settings.

SUMMARY

The ACA and subsequent development of Medicare ACOs is a new horizon for CNS practice. Because Medicare ACOs are designed to provide care to older adults, the NACNS Adult-Gerontology competencies can serve as a guide to practice. The overarching charge to the ACO is to provide patient-focused, comprehensive, coordinated care in place of fee-for-service, episodic, siloed care. Care coordination occurs across settings including acute, subacute, rehabilitation, long-term, and home settings. Opportunities exist for the CNS to fully engage in practice across the three spheres of influence (patient, nursing/nursing practice,

and organization/system) to support achievement of ACO aims. These aims are focused on enhancing the patient experience of care (including quality, access, and reliability) while reducing or at least controlling the cost of care. Within an ACO structure, the CNSs needs to translate the skills used in traditional inpatient settings to the ACO and support the ACO in achieving the transition to a new paradigm of care. CNSs are uniquely educated and positioned to be clinical leaders in ACOs as this delivery model becomes the cornerstone in the achievement of affordable, safe, high-quality care for Medicare beneficiaries. ACOs, in turn, will be providing the national-level leadership necessary to continue thinking and operating in a new paradigm for health care.

▨ DISCUSSION QUESTIONS

- Discuss the purpose of an ACO in health care reform. What are the pros and cons of belonging to an ACO? Will ACOs have a long-term impact on reducing costs and improving the quality of care for Medicare beneficiaries?
- Discuss the role of a CNS in an ACO. Of the three areas of influence, which one (patient/beneficiary, nurse/nursing practice, or system/organization) will have the largest impact on the aims of an ACO? Why?

▨ ANALYSIS AND SYNTHESIS EXERCISES

- Explore the similarities and differences between CNS practice in an acute inpatient setting and CNS practice in an ACO ambulatory complex case management setting.
- Review the historical development and current status of ACOs and consider future opportunities for CNSs as providers (members) of an ACO with attributed lives.

▨ CLINICAL APPLICATION

Review both the National Association of Clinical Nurse Specialist (NACNS) CNS core competencies and the NACNS Adult-Gerontology CNS competencies. In each sphere of influence, identify methods of measuring CNS contribution toward the ACO quality measures in each domain: patient/caregiver experience, care coordination/patient safety, preventive care, and at-risk population management.

APPENDIX

MEDICARE ACCOUNTABLE CARE ORGANIZATIONS QUALITY MEASURES BY DOMAIN AND MEASURES	
Domain	**Measures**
Patient/caregiver experience	• Getting timely care, appointments, and information • How well your providers communicate • Patients' rating of provider • Access to specialists • Health promotion and education • Shared decision making • Health status/functional status
Care coordination/ patient safety	• Risk standardized all condition readmission • Ambulatory-sensitive conditions admissions: chronic obstructive pulmonary disease (COPD) or asthma in older adults • Ambulatory-sensitive conditions admissions: Heart failure (HF) • Percentage of primary care physicians who successfully qualify for an electronic health record (HER) program incentive payment • Medication reconciliation • Falls: Screening for future fall risk
Preventive care	• Influenza immunization • Pneumococcal vaccination for patients 65 years and older • Body mass index (BMI) screening and follow-up • Tobacco use: Screening and cessation intervention • Screening for clinical depression and follow-up plan • Colorectal cancer screening • Breast cancer screening • Screening for high blood pressure and follow-up documented
At-risk population	• Diabetes mellitus: Hemoglobin A1c control (8%) • Diabetes mellitus: Low-density lipoprotein control • Diabetes mellitus: High blood pressure control • Diabetes mellitus: Tobacco nonuse • Diabetes mellitus: Daily aspirin or antiplatelet medication use for patients with diabetes and ischemic vascular disease • Diabetes mellitus: Hemoglobin A1c poor control • Hypertension (HTN): Controlling high blood pressure • Ischemic vascular disease (IVD): Complete lipid panel and LDL control (100 mg/dL) • Ischemic vascular disease (IVD): Use of aspirin or another antithrombotic • Heart failure: Beta-blocker therapy for left ventricular systolic dysfunction (LVSD) • Coronary artery disease (CAD): Lipid control • Coronary artery disease (CAD): Angiotensin-converting enzyme (ACE) inhibitor or angiotensin receptor blocker (ARB) therapy—diabetes or left ventricular systolic dysfunction (LVEF 40%)

Source: Accountable Care Organization (ACO, 2013).

REFERENCES

Accountable Care Organization (ACO). (2013). *Program analysis: Quality performance standards narrative measure specifications.* Retrieved from http://www.cms.gov/Medicare/Medicare-Fee-for-Service-Payment/sharedsavingsprogram/Downloads/ACO-NarrativeMeasures-Specs.pdf

Administration on Aging (AoA). *Aging statistics.* Retrieved from http://www.aoa.gov/Aging_Statistics

Affordable Care Act (ACA Section 3021). Retrieved from http://dhhs.nv.gov/HealthCare/Docs/reimbursement/ACA3021InnovationCenter.pdf.

Baicker, K., & Levy, H. (2013). Coordination versus competition in healthcare reform. *The New England Journal of Medicine, 369,* 789–791.

Case Management Society of America (CMSA). Retrieved from www.cmsa.org

Centers for Medicare & Medicaid Service (CMS). Retrieved from www.cms.gov

Centers for Medicare & Medicaid Innovation (CMMI). Retrieved from http://www.cms.gov/About-CMS/Agency-Information/CMSLeadership/Office_CMMI.html

Daly, R., Zigmond, J., Barr, P., Robezniels, A., & Evans, M. (2013). Redesigning healthcare. *Modern Healthcare, 25*(12), 6–16.

Department of Health and Human Services (DHHS). *HHS issues new strategic framework on multiple chronic conditions.* Retrieved from http://www.hhs.gov/news/press/2010pres/12/20101214a.html

Institute for Healthcare Improvement (IHI). *Triple aim: Better health and better care at lower cost.* Retrieved from http://www.ihi.org/explore/tripleaim/pages/default.aspx

Leaver, W. B. (2013). Volume to value. *Frontiers of Health Services Management, 29*(4), 27.

Live births by age of mother and race, United States, 1933–1998. Retrieved from www.cdc.gov/nchs/data/natality/mage33tr.pdf

McBride, M. (2013, January 10). Four trends to watch in 2013. *Medical Economics*, 36. Retrieved October 10, 2013, from http://medicaleconomics.modernmedicine.com/medical-economics/news/user-definedtags/electronic-health-records/4-trends-watch-2013

National Association of Clinical Nurse Specialists (NACNS). (2008a). *Adult-gerontology clinical nurse specialist competencies.* Retrieved from http://www.nacns.org/docs/adultgeroCNScomp.pdf

National Association of Clinical Nurse Specialists (NACNS). (2008b). *Clinical nurse specialist core competencies.* Retrieved from http://www.nacns.org/docs/CNSCoreCompetenciesBroch.pdf

National Institute on Aging. (2013). *NIH seeking strategies for multiple chronic conditions in older people.* Retrieved from http://www.nia.nih.gov/newsroom/features/nih-seeking-strategies-multiple-chronic-conditions-older-people

Naylor's Transitional Care Model. Retrieved from http://www.transitionalcare.info

White, M. T. (2012). Preparing for the future: What nurses need to know. *Journal of Continuing Education, 43*(2), 55–56.

Economic and Financial Considerations for Clinical Nurse Specialists

Mary L. Fisher, Leeann Blue, Lori D. Stark, and Jan M. Powers

*H*ealth care economics exerts remarkable control on nursing practice in the United States. The American Association of Colleges of Nursing (AACN, 2011) lists health care financing literacy to be an essential core skill for all advanced practice nurses. The U.S. health care system has seen consistent increases in costs, which have resulted in careful and constant government and employer review of the resources expended but have not yet resulted in a major overhaul of the health care system. This environment requires careful consideration of efforts within the system to deliver cost-effective care to individuals and the community. Understanding the value the clinical nurse specialist (CNS) brings to the efficient delivery of quality care is essential to addressing these economic concerns.

The objectives of this chapter are to (a) give an overview of U.S. health care economics and the financial challenges faced by the health care system, (b) define key economic terms associated with the U.S. health care economy, (c) describe how the CNS role can impact or influence the health care economy, and (d) identify methods for tracking and quantifying CNS practice outcomes The chapter closes with conclusions and discussion questions.

ACCESS TO CARE

The U.S. health care system changes over time, but it has reflected a revenue stream from private payer insurance, individuals, and government sources. These sources do not fund all those who require health care services. The uninsured represented 15.2% of our population, or 47.8 million Americans, in 2012. With the passage of the Patient Protection and Affordable Care Act (ACA) in 2010, the federal government has begun to address the issue of uninsured and underinsured Americans. The incremental implementation of the Act over the next few years is projected to reduce the number of uninsured to 7.3% of our population, or 24 million Americans, by 2017 (Centers for Medicare & Medicaid Services [CMS], 2013). CMS has outlined the estimated financial effects of the ACA to reflect an overall net cost of $251 billion through 2019 (CMS, 2010a).

Funding for the uninsured may come from charity sources, self-payment, or cost shifting (charging more to other groups to cover the costs for this group). Medically indigent Americans often seek inappropriate care in emergency room (ER) settings due to lack of access to primary care. By using very costly ER settings inappropriately, overall costs of health care rise, but the individual is shielded from the normal market pressures because there is no intent or capacity to pay for the service.

U.S. HEALTH CARE ECONOMICS

Health care is an important part of the overall economy in the United States and has gained a lot of attention because of increasing costs over the past 40 years. National health care expenditures went from $245.8 billion in 1980 to $2.7 trillion in 2011 (CMS, 2012a). Over the period from 2015 to 2021, health care spending is projected to grow at an average rate of 6.2% annually (CMS, 2012a). Those increased costs will most certainly generate pressure for providing the best value of health care and for new solutions to deliver effective, efficient, and safe health care. Questions about how much health care the country can afford continue to surface, and decisions about what types of services are a fundamental right of all citizens have yet to be addressed. The underlying issue of reform of the health care system is fraught with political roadblocks due to special interests like the insurance industry and health care provider groups.

U.S. health care economics stands apart from our normal understanding of the U.S. free enterprise economic system. Our economy is built on a concept of supply and demand in a market where consumers and traders are free to exchange goods and services for currency. A direct exchange and interchange between purchasers and traders in the purchasing process is fundamental for free enterprise to work. Any system that bypasses that direct exchange stands to limit the free market and undermine our free enterprise system.

One aspect of a purchase decision that is directly undermined by blocks in the direct exchange between purchasers and traders is quality. The extent to which quality is transparent and publicly reported impacts a consumer's ability to make informed decisions. Consumers balance their need for quality with what they plan to pay. In making purchasing decisions based on this balance, consumers serve as a control on the free enterprise system. Their demand for quality at a certain price point drives the market to control costs while still providing a quality product. Without that dynamic, costs can spiral out of control and quality can go unchecked.

Many consumer advocacy groups test products and provide data to consumers to assist their decision making. For example, consulting *Consumer Reports* before making a major purchase or calling the Better Business Bureau to check on a contractor are expected aspects of consumerism.

Separation of the Health Care Consumer From Price

Health care stands apart from these normal consumer–product relationships within our free market. We rarely know the costs of health care before we have consumed the product. This creates an in-elastic demand setting where, in health care, demand is insensitive to changes in price. Consumers, therefore, cannot exert control over quality.

The need for consumers to understand quality outcomes within our health care system is being heard. The CMS now requires all hospitals that receive funding from these sources to share in the public realm their patient satisfaction data and quality core measures for several high-volume diagnoses. This requirement provides consumer transparency related to patient care outcomes, process measures, and patient satisfaction with services delivered in different provider settings and is updated annually by CMS (2010b). This is a very new aspect to our health care environment and is intended to provide the patient/family/community with the information needed to help drive patient care delivery decisions. CMS and private insurers will continue efforts to provide transparency in health care outcomes and satisfaction data as tools to benchmark best practice and to ensure that the consumer has access to data for health care decision making (CMS, 2010).

While health care costs are of increasing concern, the health care consumer is shielded from evaluating quality in relation to cost for health care decisions. Insured consumers are affected because

1. They do not always know the true costs of care delivered.
2. Health care coverage providers may negotiate discounts for health care products or services, which then leads to inconsistent pricing across the health care system.
3. Health care coverage providers may limit access to certain types of care by withholding coverage for certain transactions (e.g., setting limits for psychiatric care).
4. Health care providers may limit access to care by limiting provider participation (e.g., preferred provider organizations [PPOs] reimburse more for in-plan providers than out-of-plan providers; health maintenance organizations [HMOs] only pay for in-plan providers and use gatekeepers to limit specialty referrals).
5. Health care providers may limit access to care by establishing large copays and deductibles.
6. Health care providers may deny coverage, period.

Uninsured consumers are affected as well:

1. Providers engage in "cost shifting" by inflating charges to uninsured people to cover losses from care that is not reimbursed in contractual discounts.
2. If the uninsured cannot pay up-front costs, they may not get nonemergency care or very important preventative care.
3. Clinical providers may limit their exposure to uninsured people by closing their practices to new patients.
4. One of the top reasons cited for bankruptcies in the United States is catastrophic health care costs.

The Health Care Costs as a Percentage of Gross Domestic Product (GDP)

There are many reasons for separation of the consumer from price in our health care system, and those reasons may have helped contribute to a health care price index (HCPI) that has risen faster than other consumer prices for the last 20 years. "As a percentage of Gross Domestic Product (GDP), national health spending reached 17.9 percent in 2012, up from 14.1 percent in 2001" (CMS, 2012b). The next highest percentage of GDP is held by the Netherlands (12%), and the average for industrialized nations is 9.5% (PBS, 2012). Because U.S. health care costs are the highest of any industrialized nation, American products are less competitive on the world market—a real detriment to the United States in the global economy.

Other factors that impact the HCPI include labor costs and inflation, technological advances, pharmaceutical development costs and inflation, malpractice costs, inflation of the cost of medical-related supplies and equipment, building expansion and competition for customers, insurance company profits, and chronic illness in an aging population.

Health Care Consumers' Need for Agency

Consumers usually inform themselves about products before they make a major purchase. For some highly technical purchases, consumers still must rely on experts to advise them. In health care, the majority of our transactions as consumers are technically and medically complex, and our reliance on experts is much more complete. This places a burden of agency on providers. *Agency* refers to authority given to a provider with unique knowledge to make decisions about the care of another and to consume health resources in the process (Propp, Krubert, & Sasson, 2003). Agency carries with it a moral obligation to act in the patient's best interest even when that is not congruent with the provider's best interest. This is a

key precept for the transparency of sharing outcomes by hospitals with the public.

Competition Within Health Care

Another concept inherent in the free enterprise system is competition. While we have a lot of competition in health care, it is often not the normal competition intended to inform consumers and influence their decision making. Much of the competition in health care is aimed at the true decision makers: providers and insurers. Consumers may be targets of advertising, but much of it is of the "ask your doctor about..." type. This type of advertising often does not serve to educate the consumer about a product, but rather to trigger consumers to ask a provider if they need the medication or treatment. This type of marketing is intended to have consumers pressure providers to provide the medication or treatment, even if not required by a consumer's medical needs. Marketing directly to the consumer is becoming more of a focus and will likely continue.

Providers are competing for insurance contracts, often based on cost alone. Until insurers receive pressure from employers (the majority of nongovernmental insurance is employer-sponsored) to negotiate contracts based not only on costs but also on quality outcomes, there is no incentive on the part of insurers to care about quality. There is a trend for employers to begin looking at quality as a factor in insurance negotiations. Offering quality health care can be seen to be in the employer's best interests in order to attract and retain the best employees and to keep the workforce productive. A long-term perspective is needed for employers to take this view, however.

Regulation Mechanisms

There have been many efforts to curb health care spending for over 30 years. As the major payer of health care bills (federal government sources accounted for 37% of health care dollars spent in 2011; CME, 2012b), the federal government has been active in regulating the health care industry. In the 1970s, certificate of need (CON) approval was required before major health care facility building could occur. Prospective payment, a federal program that designed diagnostic-related groups (DRGs) as a mode to reimburse for care, was operational in 1983. This system is still in effect today for Medicare and Medicaid reimbursement. The DRG system is consistently reviewed and changes made to reflect practice utilization and costs. CMS has started a process of consistent auditing of clinical providers' documentation to ensure that they meet the criteria for payments. This effort is called Recovery Audit Contractor audits.

In the 1980s, private industry responded by seeking access controls through development of HMO and PPO models. These so-called capitated models share risk for insurance coverage with providers by paying based on covered lives in a variety of negotiated contract forms instead of paying directly for services provided. This type of contracting provides an incentive to providers to ration care unless quality outcome standards are negotiated at the same time.

The Move to Pay for Performance (P4P) and Values-Based Purchasing

The goal of CMS, beginning in 2008, was to have hospitals and providers share their actual performance data, to provide transparency of the outcomes of care, and to not pay for events caused by errors within the hospital setting that were not anticipated (CMS, 2008). This effort is called the Medicare P4P initiative. The foundation for effective P4P initiatives is collaboration with providers and other stakeholders to ensure that valid quality measures are used. Through these collaborative efforts, CMS is developing and implementing a set of P4P initiatives to support quality improvement in the care of Medicare beneficiaries. Within a hospital setting, these initiatives focus on quality measures by linking the performance of these measures to the payments that the hospitals receive for each Medicare discharge in the new Hospital Values-Based Performance (HVBP) plan; a feature of the phased implementation of the ACA.

The HVBP incentive plan is part of Inpatient Prospective Payment System (IPPS) rules that began to reward hospitals in fiscal year 2013 (CMS, 2013). It is funded by a 1% withholding from participating hospitals' DRG payments and is returned to the most competitive hospitals in relation to the benchmarks of value, patient outcomes, and innovation; rather than simply paying for volume of services rendered (CMS, 2011b). Twelve Clinical Process of Care Measures (CPCMs, representing 70% of the Total Performance Score) and eight Patient Experience of Care Dimensions (PECDs, representing 30% of the Total Performance Score) are monitored and the aggregate Total Performance Scores are compared with peer institutions. Many of the PECDs are nurse-sensitive indicators such as nurse communication, pain management, discharge information, and hospital staff responsiveness. Hospitals are rewarded for both achievement and improvement in each dimension, with the greater set of points being used for the final score. This model now gives competitive incentive to hospitals to outperform not only base standards at the 50th percentile but also their peers' performances to a benchmark in the top decile of performers (as long as a threshold standard is achieved).

To further complicate this formula, consistency points can be earned or lost by a hospital based on its lowest score in comparison to the 50th percentile of base period performance. Spending per Medicare beneficiary measures have been implemented as an added efficiency index. Backsliding in quality or efficiency will be costly! The 1% withholding pool for FY 2013 will increase in the future once the program is normalized, making quality more and more of a focus in payments at the same time that the standards continue to evolve. Hospitals will not be able to budget for this money: it will be warded at the end of the FY cycle.

There are several other pilot P4P initiatives, and most likely this type of incentive-based model will spread to cover most health care delivered within the United States. The Physician Group Practice Demonstration, Nursing Home Values-Based Purchasing, Home Health P4P, and Accountable Care Organization are just a few of the demonstration projects occurring at this time (CMS, 2012c).

Nursing Labor Supply

There is a worldwide nursing shortage and the United States is no exception. By 2020, the Bureau of Labor Statistics projects a shortage of more than 1 million nurses. Because of the continually increasing demand for nurses, health care institutions are in competition for scarce nursing resources. What are the salaries and incentives necessary to attract and retain nurses? How must the work environment improve? The success of Magnet-designated facilities in this area is an example of the extent of competition. One burning question that remains unanswered is "How must nursing practice change if supply continues to be less than demand for nursing services in the future?" CNSs are uniquely positioned as experts in the delivery of care to impact this issue.

CNS Impact on Hospital and Nursing Care

The CNS can provide direct care or help to establish best practice for a patient care population or service that adds value to the care delivery model. The CNS role impacts health care within the patient/client sphere, the nurses/nursing sphere, and the system/organizational sphere (National Association of Clinical Nurse Specialists [NACNS], 2010).

The CNS can impact each of these spheres in several ways:

1. Being the expert direct care provider for complex cases

2. Being the expert for providing evidence-based best practice through:
   a. Educating/mentoring staff nurses on evidence-based practice (EBP) in bridging the gap between what is known and what is done at the bedside
   b. Developing and implementing evidence-based best-practice guidelines
   c. Identifying indicators for and monitoring outcomes of practice within a care setting
3. Conducting clinical inquiries into future care delivery models

Understanding Cost Analysis as an Important Tool

A key skill for the CNS to acquire is a detailed understanding of the financial impact of nursing interventions (equipment, nonpharmaceuticals, and care delivery) on the costs of providing care for patients or a community. One aspect of that financial analysis is how to calculate labor costs associated with nursing care. Early research on cost analysis of nursing care focused on "costing out" nursing services. These studies often were conducted for the purpose of measuring productivity, comparing costs of nursing delivery models, establishing models to directly charge patients for nursing costs, and relating nursing costs to other cost models, most notably DRG categories. Costing efforts have evolved with economic and practice changes to the health care system. For example, most studies in the 1980s were performed in acute care hospitals, whereas more studies now relate to a variety of settings.

"Today, cost analysis of nursing care focuses on justifying the cost-effectiveness of professional practice models, evaluating redesign efforts, and monitoring and controlling nursing costs within an ever-tightening, cost-conscious health care environment" (Fisher, 2006, pp. 112–113). Within the context of rising capitation penetration, cost analysis is essential to accurate capitation bidding and financial viability of the parent organization. As "best practices" benchmarking pushes the envelope of competitive bidding, demonstrating cost-effective nursing practice becomes essential to securing managed care contracts.

Cost-Effectiveness Evaluation

As the U.S. economic picture darkens, with ever-increasing percentages of the GDP being consumed with health care costs, continuing efforts focus on cost containment, quality improvement, and the dynamic between the two. What is the benefit of reducing costs for an episode of care if that care is substandard and results in future health care costs associated with readmission, chronic illness, complications, or death? Analyzing costs, without measuring quality, will not get us where we want to go.

CNS programs and projects designed to improve care must demonstrate cost-effectiveness and be evaluated on the patient/family, personnel, system, and community levels. In cost-effectiveness analysis, we may compare the differences in costs to the differences in outcomes of several possible program choices. This analysis is appropriate where one specific outcome is clear and is expressed as a health status goal, such as percentage loss of excess body weight compared to ideal weight for bariatric surgery. Where multiple outcomes are relevant and must be evaluated in a weighted manner, then a cost-utility analysis is performed. In cost-benefit analysis, health indices are replaced with fiscal measures.

Cost analysis is based on assumptions that must be examined and made explicit when reporting findings. Be leery of studies that describe cost-analyses but fail to report the underlying assumptions of the model.

What are some quality outcome measures that must be considered in a nursing cost-benefit or cost-effectiveness analysis?

1. Length of stay (LOS)—This variable correlates highly with nursing work as measured by such variables as acuity indexes, task/procedure complexity, direct nursing care hours, and patient charges.
2. Quality patient outcomes—patient satisfaction, clinical outcomes appropriate to DRG type and comorbidities, reduction of nurse-sensitive complications and failure-to-rescue, liability costs associated with failed care, CMS P4P measures, and National Quality Forum and National Database of Nursing Quality Indicators measures that are nursing sensitive. The CNS can help teach, review, and set up policies and procedures to structure a foundation for best practice. In addition, the CNS needs to monitor and provide ongoing education to help prevent adverse events from reoccurring.
3. Nurse factors—Adding to cost of care are nurse factors that may be difficult to measure, that is, nurse turnover, ratio of productive to nonproductive hours, training costs, shift fatigue, nurse satisfaction, and education level of the nurse.
4. Patient education outcomes—This area of frequent CNS responsibility can be aided by a model to evaluate the cost-effectiveness of patient education programming, such as that offered by Welch and colleagues (2002). The growth of capitation and cost analysis of nursing services will have to take new directions. As critical pathways (benchmark performance tools) evolve as care guides, the costs of pathway changes on nursing delivery, patient

outcomes, and case costs must be calculated. What are the most efficient *and* effective pathways toward resolution of a given health problem? What practice setting or level of care is appropriate for patients at each step of the pathway? For example, when is it safe to transfer a fresh open heart patient from critical care to a step-down environment? (Earliest transfer to a less costly delivery mode saves money.) These types of calculations may be critical for institutions to secure managed care contracts in a cost-competitive environment. Determining what activities can be safely eliminated from a pathway without negatively impacting care outcomes will have cost and resource savings as we move to "best demonstrated practices."

Finally, we must move toward a cost-effectiveness analysis model that incorporates the outcomes of nursing practice. This aspect has been especially elusive given the generic and group nature of nursing practice. With multiple nursing providers impacting a patient's care, how do we separate the relative contributions of each person or each subspecialty of nursing practice that a patient may experience in the course of his or her care from contributions of other disciplines? Additionally, we need to quantify the costs of increased patient mortality and failure-to-rescue associated with changes in nurse–patient ratios based on landmark studies by Aiken, Clark, and Sloan (2002) and Cho, Ketefian, Barkauskas, and Smith (2003). Kane and associates (2007) performed a meta-analysis on 96 such studies after a systemic review of 2,858 potentially relevant studies. For each full registered nurse (RN) per patient day increase in staffing, the odds of hospital-acquired pneumonia, respiratory failure, and failure-to-rescue were reduced significantly for surgical patients. Additionally, a 9% reduction in mortality for intensive care units (ICUs), a 16% decrease in surgical units, and a 6% decrease in medical units were achieved for each increase in RN full-time equivalent (FTE) per patient day. LOS was shorter by 24% in ICUs and by 31% in surgical patients. Predicted lives saved were 5 per 1,000 hospitalized patients for ICUs and medical patients and 6 per 1,000 for surgical patients. The consistency of observations and RN dosing sensitivity over the large number of studies in this analysis suggests some causality of these measures, but some nurse-sensitive monitors were not reliable predictors (patient falls, pressure ulcers, and urinary tract infections; Kane, Shamliyan, Mueller, Duval, & Wilt, 2007). Their subsequent study (Shamliyan, Kane, Mueller, Duval, & Wilt, 2009) further investigated both societal benefit and institutional advantage of increasing RN ratios through a simulation exercise using the 2007 study data. While the societal net benefits were clearly confirmed, the cost-utility analysis for hospitals did not support sufficient monetary benefit from reduced LOS to validate increasing RN ratios.

More closely linking reimbursement to patient outcomes will help facilities capture more of the benefits from improved staffing "and provide the means to improve quality of care" (Dall, Chen, Seifert, Maddox, & Hogan, 2009, p. 104). This is the premise behind Nurse-Sensitive Values-Based Purchasing (NSVBP). To that end, the 16-member Technical Expert Panel (TEP) that is forming the specifications for the new HVBP includes two PhD-prepared nurses. This is a good start. Understanding the health care current economics and staying on top of these dynamic trends will help the CNS to effectively contribute to patient care cost and quality improvements. Further skills in the budgeting and finance area are essential for contemporary CNS practice.

HEALTH CARE BUDGETING 101

Most CNSs will encounter budgets. In many cases, the CNS will have fiscal responsibility for at least a program budget that falls within an operating budget (see glossary of budgeting terms later in this chapter). Specific budgeting practices are unique to organizations and will not be covered here. The framework for budgeting is described.

All health care organizations practice budgeting discipline. Each year, either on a calendar or fiscal year schedule, the organization decides how to spend its money in relation to its overall goals. It is vital that the budget process be tied to strategic planning for the organization so that scarce resources are aligned with strategic goals. Corporate fiscal officers determine the schedule, format, and processes used in budgeting. Most organizations have budget support resources allocated to assist in the budgeting process.

Each organization will have operating, capital, and cash budgets. The time cycles for these three types of budget will differ.

Operating Budgets

The most complex aspect of budgeting is the operating budget. For most service organizations, the major dollar amount in this category is personnel costs. Also included in the operating budget are supplies and equipment as well as utilities and overhead costs. The operating budget is especially tied to volume and acuity predictions. In addition, inflation factors are often provided by finance based on industry predictions.

Personnel

Health care cannot be provided without an adequate workforce with the right skill mix, experience, and licensure. The organization must be competitive in its salary and benefit structures to ensure a stable workforce. Salary increases must be factored into the personnel budget for the coming year. Salary increases may include cost-of-living adjustments (COLA) and merit increases that are based on performance indicators. Benefit costs have become a challenge for all employers as health care costs have skyrocketed and consumed more and more of the dollars reserved for salaries. Benefits also include life insurance, retirement, travel, paid time off, disability, and family leave. All must be factored for inflation in the personnel budget.

Productive and Nonproductive Costs

A factor that greatly impacts the personnel budget is the nonproductive hours that are paid out. This category includes vacation, holiday, sick time, or a combined flexible paid time off allotment as well as bereavement, military, education, and worker's compensation time multiplied by the hourly salary of each employee.

Regulation of Staffing

Who can do what is regulated by state licensing laws in many cases, so the CNS must be knowledgeable about state laws. Personnel are further broken down into direct care and indirect care providers.

Direct and Indirect Care

Direct care is exactly what the name implies. Those activities that are directly associated with care to the patient, including the documentation of care, are calculated into the direct care hours. Nurses may also have indirect care hours that include orientation, continuing education and in-services, meetings, and other activities that take them away from the bedside. Personnel who support care indirectly, such as unit secretaries and transporters, are considered indirect care providers. How these categories are calculated into budgeted nursing hours per unit of service differs widely across institutions.

Units of Service and Acuity

Institutions often track the amount of care patients receive by looking at the direct care hours per unit of service. A unit of service differs based on the clinical setting. For example, in an inpatient setting, the unit of service used is nursing hours per patient day. In a clinic setting, nursing hours per visit or procedure may be used. In the operating room, the unit of service is nursing hours per case. Often an acuity factor is used in addition to units of service to distinguish that patients require varying amounts of care based on their severity of illness or ability to complete activities of daily living.

Volume Projections

A vital role the CNS can play in budgeting is assisting with volume projections. Because the CNS fundamentally understands the business of care, he or she should know when to expect seasonal variations, what the trends in care are that may impact the business practices of the specialty, and if changes in best practices may impact LOS.

Supply and Equipment

Supplies needed for the operations of the unit are in this category of the operating budget. Again, some supplies are directly linked to care. In those cases, they are considered variable needs because how much is needed depends on patient volume and acuity. Other supplies are fixed in that their use is not dependent on patient volume. Minor equipment that does not meet the definition of a capital expenditure is part of the operating budget. CNSs frequently impact the costs associated with this category by their work related to product comparisons.

Overhead

Each budget center is allocated a share of overhead. This is either done on a prorated cost per square foot of space (if the unit has a physical location) or based on a formula related to volume of service. Overhead often includes administration, utilities, maintenance, housekeeping, and other nonrevenue-generating support services.

Capital Budgets

A plan for proposed expenditures for facilities, equipment, or software over $2,000 (the trigger amount differs by institutional policy) and with a durable life exceeding 2 years is called the capital budget. Capital budgets are often constructed on a different budget cycle from the operating budget. Funds for capital expenditures are considered separate from operating funds and often come from profits. Even in a nonprofit enterprise, revenue in excess of expenditures is created, and that excess profit must be put back into the institution to maintain nonprofit status. Due to budgetary constraints of the institution, it may be difficult to obtain allocation of funds. There are never enough capital dollars to meet the huge demand for updated equipment or facilities. These requests are often adjudicated by a panel of executive officers and board members. It is often a political process. The approved capital request will be assigned a date for availability of funds as part of the cash budget process.

Cash Budgets

Institutions use the practice of encumbering funds to ensure that there will be cash to meet obligations. For example, if employees are accruing sick time, the money to pay for that benefit must be available. Payroll must be met. Other ways institutions control cash flow are to limit their inventory liability (just-in-time supplies), keep their personnel costs in check, schedule their capital purchases, and enhance their debt collection.

Foundation Accounts

Philanthropy assists institutions in serving the public. Donations account for more and more of the program development monies for organizations. An endowment will fund a program off the income from a principal that is not touched. Generally, foundations allot from 4% to 5% of an endowment's total to be used in a given year. Of course, this is dependent on income, and if the market is down, the income may not be there to give a payout on an account in a given year.

Budget Compliance and Monitoring

It is not enough to prepare and approve a budget. It must be tightly monitored and continuously updated to make sure reality meets expectation. Variance reporting is the mechanism most institutions use to monitor the budget on a monthly basis. In this type of report, the manager analyzes why the actual is different from the budgeted amount in each category. This is called exception reporting.

Often, volume and acuity variances account for much of the problem. Sometimes, the variance is due to the fact that the manager failed to budget for an important item, or a new practice has changed the rules. For example, when universal precautions were implemented suddenly in the late 1980s, no one had anticipated their latex glove budgets increasing by $1 million annually.

CNS Impact on Hospital and Nursing Care and Budget Considerations

The CNS can provide or support direct care, establish best practice for a patient care population, and influence practice and/or process change throughout the institution. CNSs are a vital component to the institution for their influence over nursing practice and patient outcomes. The CNS also provides influence across specialty populations, facility, and systemwide programs.

The role of CNS is designed to impact three spheres in health care: patient, nurse/nursing practice, and the system/organization (NACNS, 2010). Through these spheres of practice, improved patient outcomes result with the CNS promoting implementation of evidence-based care in all realms. The CNS may provide direct care to patients while working alongside the staff RN as an expert practitioner to aid in care delivery to complex patients. This also allows the CNS to share evidence-based knowledge with the staff RN in real time to promote best practice at the point of care delivery. The CNS initiates dialogue with those practicing at the bedside to encourage questions as to why certain practices are in place, thus reducing the gap between what is known and what is practiced. If an inquiry results in an absence of evidence-based information in the literature, the CNS is ideal for a mentoring relationship with the staff RN to conduct nursing-based research.

CNSs use their knowledge of EBP to author or make substantial contributions to policies and procedural changes, as well as practice guidelines at the unit, organization, or system level. More recently, CNSs are leading multidisciplinary Six Sigma, Black Belt, and other process improvement models to systematically establish best practices and reduce hospital error-induced mortality and morbidity. Special training and certifications are needed to lead many of these processes.

CNS expertise also lends itself to select the most appropriate products for use in patient care areas, with consideration to safety, effectiveness, and fiscal impact. All of these practice behaviors and efforts may contribute to a reduction in hospital-acquired conditions resulting in potential reduction in LOS. Therefore, it is demonstrated that the CNS is able to have an overall impact on patient outcomes across the organization.

In addition to clinical expertise, it is vital that CNSs understand and contribute to institutional budgetary processes. CNS practice impacts budget through cost avoidance, cost savings, and revenue generation. CNSs are able to review the current evidence in order to provide rationale to support or refute purchasing and contract decisions at all levels in the organization/system. This is inclusive of cost-benefit analysis for product changes, which may include justification for a more expensive product, resulting in less use or improved outcomes and therefore reducing fiscal burden. CNSs are held accountable to their projected impact on annual budgets; therefore, it is imperative that anticipated costs be held within budget expectations.

Multiple CNSs in a system may contribute on a more broad perspective to outcomes. It is therefore of utmost importance for the CNS colleagues within an institution to be able to quantify how they serve as a benefit. Currently, there are no published methods to collect CNS outcomes in a standard manner. Therefore, development of an ongoing mechanism to compile this data is essential for CNS departments in any size organization or system.

Development of a CNS outcomes tracking mechanism is most effectively based on contributions in the advancement of nursing practice, contributions toward meeting strategic goals of the organization, and cost savings or avoidance to the institution. Anecdotally, it has been found effective to record and track outcomes on a consistent basis (i.e., weekly or monthly). This enables the CNS department to effectively compile their contributions to successes and change. Tracking CNS departmental outcomes is a team effort; therefore, all members of the department should be expected to contribute. Establishment of an access-controlled database stored in a manner in which all those participating have privileges is an ideal method of capturing CNS initiatives. This method enables numerous CNSs within a facility or system to record their contributions/initiatives in an ongoing, standardized fashion, with minimal risk of duplication or file corruption. Format and items/initiatives to be tracked should be determined and agreed upon by those participating prior to implementation to prevent misinterpretation or error by those making modifications to the tracking database. The process for data collection and formatting data entry should be considered when developing a CNS tracking tool. Additionally, how a summary of this information will optimally support CNS functions should be addressed. Major areas of contribution to be tracked may include CNS advancement of nursing practice, CNS impact on cost avoidance/cost savings by implementation of standardized evidence-based processes, and revenue generated by the CNS department.

Recording CNS Contributions to the Advancement of Nursing Practice. A major focus of the CNS is to advance nursing practice. The CNS incorporates evidence into practice and mentors nurses on EBP and research utilization in order to improve patient outcomes. These interventions have proven to elevate the level of nursing care provided in hospital settings. Examples of how this is demonstrated may include CNS promotion or facilitation of specialty certification through classes or review sessions, CNS mentorship for advancement of formal nursing education, and CNS facilitation for integrating evidence into practice through activities such as skills fairs, research fairs, or journal clubs. Given the impact that the CNS has on all of the aforementioned activities, items such as these could be beneficial to use as exemplars for the overall impact CNSs have on advancing nursing practice in an organization.

Recording CNS Contributions to Cost Avoidance. It is known that improved patient outcomes are a direct result of best clinical practices. Reduction or elimination of hospital-acquired conditions, reduction in LOS, and reduction in adverse patient outcomes are often influenced by the CNS department in an organization. This may be related to the CNS leading implementation of evidence-based bundles for procedures, or maintenance bundles of care when managing an ongoing condition or device. When rates of a certain condition or adverse outcome are reduced, there is often a "cost avoidance" that can be tied to that outcome. By using available published data describing the cost to an organization for a certain condition, CNS impact may be quantified. For those institutions having a robust financial system, actual costs avoided may be obtained and annualized.

> *Example*: A community hospital reports 20 bloodstream infections (BSI) in 1 year. The CNS department noted this as an increase from previous years and performed a literature search identifying best EBPs in the prevention of BSI. The CNS department then used this information to create a bundle of treatment based on evidence to prevent BSI, and implemented the bundle throughout the institution, incorporating it into the standard of care. The following year, the institution reported only 10 incidents of BSI. In the literature, it had been reported that the cost to a facility for a BSI was $30,000. Therefore, the cost avoidance due to the CNS implementing an EBP change would equate to $300,000.

In addition to avoidance of hospital-acquired conditions, the CNS may have an impact on the improvement of patient population outcomes, such as those with chronic (i.e., CHF) or acute conditions (i.e., hip fracture). Tracking the management of these populations may be based on parameters developed and defined by regulatory bodies (i.e., CMS core measures or The Joint Commission standards). When patients are able to meet or exceed what is defined in the recommendations, improved outcomes, decreased complications, and lower LOS result. The CNS has the authority to influence the management of patient populations, and again, through implementation of evidence-based care practices, this may result in a lowered LOS and optimization of DRG reimbursement.

Example: Over the past year, the CNS in a community hospital noticed that patients admitted with hip fracture have an LOS of 6 days. Upon review of the literature, the CNS notes that early ambulation, adequate pain management, and nutritional supplementation are interventions that may reduce acute care LOS. The CNS works within his or her department to enact nursing protocols for supplemental nutrition, coordinates physical therapy to begin activity the day after surgical repair, and collaborates with the pharmacist to provide an optimal pain management regime. The following year, the CNS notes that the LOS for this population has decreased to 4 days. It is possible for the CNS to quantify this LOS by identifying the average cost per patient day with assistance from the finance department. Therefore, if the cost of care for one hospital day equals $1,000, and this is multiplied by 2 days decrease, it results in a $2,000 cost avoidance per patient. If the hospital treats 200 hip fracture patients per year, the annualized cost avoidance would equal $400,000. This improvement also optimizes DRG reimbursement and improves bed availability within the facility. This avoidance can be attributed to the coordination efforts of the CNS.

Recording CNS Contributions to Cost Savings. Health care organizations are continuing to seek means in which care may be delivered in a safe, effective manner with lower cost. The CNS is in an ideal position to support these efforts through product/equipment evaluation and standardization, and is able to quantify efforts around these initiatives. Product effectiveness may be determined through trials and comparisons of cost and quality.

Example: An intravenous (IV) start kit, which is currently available at one hospital within a five-hospital system, is being recommended for review and possible replacement with another, less expensive product. The CNS department brings their expertise in patient care and treatment to the table for evaluation of all available products. After the CNSs compare kits available, a trial comparing the current $5 kit and a new $3 kit commences. The trial results in the $5 kit being more cost-effective, only having to change the dressing every 7 days, whereas the $3 kit only stayed in place for 2 days. The average LOS for this facility is 5 days. Therefore, on average, each patient would require two of the $3 kits, resulting in a greater expense to the organization. Further, the CNSs were able to increase purchasing power by helping with company negotiations, resulting in the $5 kit being reduced to $4 when the five-hospital system agreed to use the same kit throughout.

Recording CNS Generation of Revenue. Direct billing or reimbursement for consultative services or procedures may often be an overlooked strategy for CNSs to generate revenue for an organization. In many states, the CNS would have authority to bill for services similar to a nurse practitioner (NP). CNSs provide consultative services for complex patients and for direct care nurses, as well as institutional improvement efforts. They are also able to perform direct bedside procedures that require advanced expertise or experience, such as placement of a feeding tube. In the psychiatric arena, many CNSs serve as counselors and have been granted prescriptive authority by their State Board of Nursing. In addition, CNSs working in collaboration with physician partners may provide similar types of service and are able to bill for those services, such as in palliative care. Additional sources of revenue directly tied to CNS practice may be found through the procurement of grants for research activities conducted by the CNS department within their institution.

CONCLUSION

The CNS role can impact our health care economy and has been demonstrated in the research as doing so by reducing hospital costs and LOS, reducing frequency of ER visits, improving care practices through critical review and analysis of care and equipment/supplies required for patient care, increasing patient satisfaction with nursing care, and reducing medical and nursing complications in hospitalized patients. It is critical for CNSs to stay aware of the current health care environment dynamics and their impact on safe, quality, efficient patient care. The ability to quantify ongoing initiatives is essential to demonstrate to senior hospital leadership the value through expertise that the CNS uniquely brings to the organization.

■ DISCUSSION QUESTIONS

• Describe how the current U.S. health care economy is shifting to one of transparency related to health care outcomes and how you, as a CNS, can make a difference in this transparency. Identify the sources you can access to identify national benchmarks for costs of care and cost of complications.
• Why it is so important for the CNS to be aware of the current economic trends within health care?
• List a care process or technology/equipment implementation where you believe the CNS could add value for its adoption within your care setting, and describe the value in terms of dollars and benefits.
• How will you, as a CNS, respond to CMS's P4P initiative: Accountable Care Organizations and NSVBP?
• What do you believe to be the major economic priority for your role as a CNS?
• Describe a manner in which you, as a CNS, might quantify the impact of your work on patient outcomes and costs.

■ GLOSSARY OF BUDGETING TERMS

Capital budget: A plan for proposed expenditures for facilities, equipment, or software over $2,000 and with a durable life exceeding 2 years.

Cash budget: A plan for the cash flow of the organization with special attention to timing the outflow of resources to ensure adequate cash to meet the organization's goals.

Cost-benefit analysis: An economic analysis that compares all of the costs associated with a program, service, or project with the anticipated or real benefits.

Debt: Money owed to any creditor.

Depreciation: The annualized loss of value in a durable piece of equipment or structure that is directly related to its anticipated functional life and need for replacement.

Economy of scale: The optimum scale of operation needed to produce the services at the lowest cost per unit basis.

Fiscal year: The unit of time chosen by an organization for its budgeting and reporting cycle.

Internal rate of return: The annualized, compounded return rate, which can be earned on invested capital or the yield on the investment. This figure assists organizations to make business decisions about which services to offer.

Lost opportunity costs: Costs associated with tying up resources in one area when those resources could produce increased revenues in another area.

This calculation is used to determine priorities for business choices. It is the value of the path not taken.

Operating budget: The annual budget needed for the operations of a unit. It includes equipment, space, utilities, personnel, depreciation, and supplies.

Product line (service line) budget: An operating budget that includes all service areas associated with a product or service; for example, cardiac service line budget would include multiple areas associated with the care of cardiac patients.

Return on investment: The time needed to recoup the initial investment and start-up costs of a new venture.

Variance analysis: A monthly analysis of the variations from budgeted allocations. This analysis often compares actual to budgeted costs and relates them to volume and acuity fluctuations.

REFERENCES

Aiken, L. H, Clark, S. P., & Sloan, D. M. (2002). Hospital staffing, organization and quality of care: Cross national findings. *Nursing Outlook, 50*(5), 187–194.

American Association of Colleges of Nursing (AACN). (2011). *The essentials of master's education in nursing.* Retrieved April 29, 2013, from http://www.aacn.nche.edu/education-resources/MastersEssentials11.pdf

Centers for Medicare and Medicaid Services (CMS). (2008). *Home page.* Retrieved September 1, 2008, from http://www.cms.hhs.gov

Centers for Medicare and Medicaid Services (CMS). (2010a). *Estimated financial effects of the "Patient Protection and Affordable Care Act."* Retrieved April 29, 2013, from http://www.cms.gov/Research-Statistics-Data-and-Systems/Research/ActuarialStudies/downloads/PPACA_2010–04-22.pdf

Centers for Medicare and Medicaid Services (CMS). (2010b). *Fiscal year 2009 quality measure reporting for 2010 payment update.* Retrieved April 29, 2013, from, https://docs.google.com/viewer?url=http%3A%2F%2Fwww.cms.gov%2FMedicare%2FQuality-Initiatives-Patient-Assessment-Instruments%2FHospitalQualityInits%2FDownloads%2FHospitalRHQDAPU200808.pdf

Centers for Medicare and Medicaid Services (CMS). (2011a). *Accountable care organization 2012 program analysis final report.* Retrieved April 20, 2013, from http://www.cms.gov/medicare/medicare-fee-for-service-payment/sharedsavingsprogram/downloads/aco_qualitymeasures.pdf

Centers for Medicare and Medicaid Services (CMS). (2011b). *Open door forum: Hospital value-based purchasing fiscal year 2013 overview.* Retrieved May 1, 2013, from https://docs.google.com/viewer?url=http%3A%2F%2Fwww.cms.gov%2FMedicare%2FQuality-Initiatives-Patient-Assessment-Instruments%2Fhospital-value-based-purchasing%2FDownloads%2FHospVBP_ODF_072711.pdf

Centers for Medicare and Medicaid Services (CMS). (2012a). *National health expenditures 2011–2021.* Retrieved April 29, 2013, from https://docs .google.com/viewer?url=http%3A%2F%2Fwww .cms.gov%2FResearch-Statistics-Data-and-Systems%2FStatistics-Trends-and-Reports%2FNatio nalHealthExpendData%2FDownloads%2FProj2011 PDF.pdf

Centers for Medicare and Medicaid Services (CMS). (2012b). *NHE fact sheet.* Retrieved April 29, 2013, from http://www.cms.gov/Research-Statistics-Data-and-Systems/Statistics-Trends-and-Reports/ NationalHealthExpendData/NHE-Fact-Sheet.html

Centers for Medicare and Medicaid Services (CMS). (2012c). *Demonstration projects listing.* Retrieved April 29, 2013, from http://www.cms.gov/site-search/ search-results.html?q=P4P%20demonstrations%20 projects

Centers for Medicare and Medicaid Services (CMS). (2013). *Hospital value-based purchasing.* Retrieved May 1, 2013, from http://www.cms.gov/Medicare/ Quality-Initiatives-Patient-Assessment-Instruments/ hospital-value-based-purchasing/index.html?redirect=/ hospital-value-based-purchasing

Cho, S. H., Ketefian, S., Barkauskas, V. H., & Smith, D. G. (2003). The effects of nurse staffing on adverse events, morbidity, mortality, and medical costs. *Nursing Research, 52*(2), 71–79.

Dall, T. M., Chen, Y. J., Seifert, R. F., Maddox, P. J., & Hogan, P. F. (2009). The economic value of professional nursing. *Medical Care, 7*(1), 97, 104.

Fisher, M. L. (2006). Cost analysis of nursing care. In J. J. Fitzpatrick (Ed.), *Encyclopedia of nursing research* (2nd ed., pp. 112–114). New York, NY: Springer.

Kane, R. L., Shamliyan, T. A., Mueller, C., Duval, S., & Wilt, T. J. (2007). The association of registered nurse staffing levels and patient outcomes. *Medical Care, 45*(12), 1195–1204.

National Association of Clinical Nurse Specialists (NACNS). (2010). *Clinical nurse specialist core competencies, executive summary.* Retrieved April 30, 2013, from https://docs.google.com/ viewer?url=http%3A%2F%2Fwww.nacns.org%2Fdoc s%2FCNSCoreCompetenciesBroch.pdf

PBS. (2012). *Health costs: How the U.S. compares with other countries.* Retrieved April 29, 2013, from http:// www.pbs.org/newshour/rundown/2012/10/health-costs-how-the-us-compares-with-other-countries. html

Propp, D. A., Krubert, C., & Sasson, A. (2003). Healthcare economics for the emergency room physician. *Emergency Medicine, 21*(1), 55–60.

Shamliyan, T. A., Kane, R. L., Mueller, C., Duval, S., & Wilt, T. J. (2009). Cost savings associated with increased RN staffing in acute care hospitals: Simulation exercise. *Nursing Economics, 27*(5), 302–331.

Welch, J. L., Fisher, M. L., & Dayhoff, N. (2002). A cost-effectiveness worksheet for patient-education programs. *Clinical Nurse Specialist Journal, 16*(4), 187–194.

Technology Management in Complex Health Care Settings

Patricia O'Malley

Over the past 100 years, hospitals have become centers of technology for the diagnosis and treatment of disease. Health care environments increasingly depend on nurses to accept new roles and greater responsibilities with emerging technology to ensure success in patient care and outcomes. Despite nursing's continuous emersion in technology, nursing is generally unaware of the depth of impact of technology on nursing values, practice, and environment of care (Barnard, 2007).

Technological dominance has become a priority in health care. Technology has been described as an instrument and a human activity and defines Western culture (Heidegger, 1977). How technology has extended roles in medicine and nursing continues to be debated. However, history suggests that nursing has afforded no resistance to assuming the responsibility for the knowledge and tasks associated with technology application in health care. Furthermore, technology application is increasingly delegated to nursing, which requires intense education, competency assessment, and time-consuming repetitive tasks (Barnard, 2001). Finally, technology is often accepted and promoted before the limitations and outcomes associated with use are known (Barbash & Glied, 2010).

While technology brings the nurse closer to the patient by virtue of task performance, technology can also provide a path for the dehumanization of the patient. The clinical nurse specialist (CNS) has a unique role in assisting nurses to embrace the human–technology interface in health care *and* preserving the art and science of caring in an age of ever-accelerating technological advancement (Locsin, 2001a; Szczerba & Huesch, 2012).

This chapter explores the relationship of technology and the CNS role in health care. Tools and resources for the CNS to use in any environment where technology application is an integral part of the plan of care are provided. However, before exploring the current state of technology in health care, a brief review of the history of technology in health care is required.

HISTORY OF TECHNOLOGY IN HEALTH CARE

The home was the primary site for medical care in the 1900s. The mean life expectancy was 47 years, and 95% of births occurred at home. Pneumonia, influenza, tuberculosis, and dysentery were the primary causes of death. During this period, medical imaging was introduced. The average time for a head x-ray required 11 minutes of exposure time, and patients generally received large doses of radiation.

Electrocardiogram (ECG) was introduced in 1901, with a string galvanometer that used a magnet weighing nearly 600 pounds (Ridgway, Johnson, & McClain, 2004). Thermometers, anesthesia, blood pressure sphygmomanometers, surgical instruments, and sterilizers were in use in hospitals (Richter, 2004; Welter, 2004).

From 1919 to 1939, increasing work in medical instrumentation was accomplished, and the iron lung and radiation treatment were introduced. The golden years for electronics were 1945 to 1959, and the application of military and university research and development technologies combined with the Hill-Burton Act of 1947 provided the foundation for the transformation of hospitals. Emerging technology for this period included prototypes of heart valves, dialysis, the first pacemaker, oscilloscope, cardiopulmonary bypass, and respirators. Radionuclide technology—the precursor to nuclear medicine as well as ultrasound—was introduced (Ridgway et al., 2004).

The technology "arms race" began in the 1960s. Hospitals raced to purchase emerging technology developed through increased funding by the National Institutes of Health (NIH) to universities for biomedical engineering training. The average battery life for a pacemaker was extended to 12 to 18 months, and the first direct current (DC) defibrillator replaced the 1950s alternating current (AC) defibrillator. Lasers, hyperbaric oxygen therapy, silicone implants, fiber optic endoscopes, fetal heart monitors, and computers were introduced during this period. Multichannel laboratory analyzers were introduced, which provided hospitals a path for profit in laboratory testing. The first heart bypass surgery was performed in 1964, followed by the heart transplant in 1967, and the artificial heart in 1968. The birth of the World Wide Web occurred in 1969, when the U.S. Department of Defense merged four university computer networks and named the network the Advanced Research Projects Area Net (ARPANET), which would expand and eventually become the Internet (Ridgway et al., 2004).

The boom of community hospitals in the 1970s increased the number of hospitals in the United States to 5,875. With the expansion of clinical engineering programs, high-tech digital computer-controlled medical devices emerged. Computed tomography (CT) scan was introduced during this time, as were anesthesia machines and nuclear batteries (Richter, 2004; Ridgway et al., 2004).

The emergence of fixed-price health care reimbursement in the 1980s, coupled with the Medical Waste Tracking Act of 1988 and expensive maintenance contracts for technology maintenance and repairs, slowed technology acquisition as an increasing number of hospitals closed. MRI was introduced in 1984 (Ridgway et al., 2004).

Tight budgets and control of labor expenses resulted in erosion of working conditions in hospitals in the 1990s. During this decade, information technology (IT) began to emerge in the health care environment along with positron emission tomography (PET) and single photon emission computed tomography (SPECT) scanners and gamma knives (Ridgway et al., 2004).

The recent technology explosion of medical informatics may result in the greatest transformation of health care. The electronic medical record and integration with increasingly complex clinical systems and nanotechnology promises to make the environment of care paperless and immediately accessible by every care provider anytime and anywhere (Ridgway et al., 2004). Hidden in the promises of medical informatics are the realities associated with implementation (Shekelle, Morton, & Keeler, 2006). Difficult workflow alterations, culture change, role redesign, programming and design flaws, and new medical errors are just a small sample of the obstacles that the CNS faces in the current health care setting (O'Malley, 2007).

Technology has increased the complexity and cost of health care. The merging of science, technology, and engineering has changed hospitals into technology centers with associated medical specialties rather than a place for the sick (Welter, 2004). Balancing cost with return on investment has become an increasingly difficult issue because technology is refined and modified as soon as it is released (Prasad & Cifu, 2011).

Rising labor costs, declining reimbursement, data-driven patient outcomes, and keeping pace with technology development is the current environment of care. The CNS role in health care is well positioned to discern technological rhetoric from science and determine the risks, benefits, alternatives, and limits of technology for organizations, nursing practice, and patients (Kleinpell, 2013; Vogelsmeier & Scott-Cawiezell, 2009).

NURSING AND TECHNOLOGY

While appearing as no more than a footnote in the history of medical technology, nursing was indispensable for the technological transformation of health care during the 20th century (Barnard & Cushing, 2001). Since the 1930s, nurses have been increasingly linked with technology. Matching equipment to procedures, supervision of use, improvisation, sterilization, troubleshooting, and maintenance continue to contribute to the functional redundancy of many aspects of practice (Sandelowski, 2000). While technology has extended the science around the nursing process, it has also blurred the distinctions between nursing, medicine, and other health professions (Sandelowski, 2000).

As more and more technology enters the environment of health care, the boundaries between patient and machine and technical versus professional nursing have become increasingly blurred. Implicit in the mechanization of health care is that technology can be substituted for a nurse. However, experience suggests that *without* a nurse, the technology–patient interface is fraught with safety issues and significant adverse events (Mytton et al., 2010; Newton et al., 2010; Sandelowski, 2000).

While *purposes* of technology can be clearly articulated in complex health care systems, the *consequences* of technology implementation are rarely adequately factored for the organization (David, Judd, & Zambuto, 2004; Prasad & Cifu, 2011). Whether *instrument* or a *product*, technology organizes human activity, labor, and choices. Technology is defined by structure, purpose, and use. Exhibit 25.1 describes the varied purposes of technology in health care today (David et al., 2004). Exhibit 25.2 describes some of the primary technologies purchased by the health care organizations in the United States (Gaev, 2004). All technology has a predictable life cycle that should be the basis of CNS assessment, planning, and evaluation (Mytton et al., 2010). Figure 25.1 describes the life cycle of technology for any health care organization (David et al., 2004). Exhibit 25.3 describes important elements the CNS may consider when evaluating the interface of medical devices during the life cycle (Gaev, 2004; Newton et al., 2010).

EXHIBIT 25.2

United States—Major Categories of Medical Device Sales

Major Categories	
1.	Incontinence supplies
2.	Blood glucose monitoring
3.	Wound closure products
4.	Implantable defibrillators
5.	Soft contact lenses
6.	X-ray equipment
7.	Orthopedic fixation devices
8.	Pacemakers
9.	Examination gloves
10.	Coronary stents
11.	Ultrasound equipment
12.	Arthroscopic accessory instruments
13.	MRI
14.	Computed tomography
15.	Monitoring systems
16.	Medical information technology
17.	PACS (picture archiving and retrieval systems)

EXHIBIT 25.1

Purposes of Technology in Health Care

1. Diagnostic
2. Therapeutic
3. Rehabilitation
4. Increase efficiency
5. Increase cost-effectiveness
6. Increase reimbursement
7. Decrease risk
8. Decrease error
9. Decrease exposure risk
10. Recruitment of staff

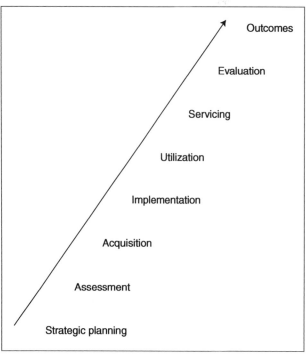

FIGURE 25.1 Life cycle of technology.

EXHIBIT 25.3
Interfaces of Medical Devices

Dyad	Interface Elements
Device–user	Nursing is usually the greatest user of technology; majority of errors with application are user errors; training, competency, and surveillance requirements
Device–patient	Does the device accommodate the physiological variance of human beings? degree of activity/movement restriction
Device–environment	Conditions necessary for storage and use: temperature, humidity, electrical power, shielding from electromagnetic fields, and connections to special gases
Device–accessories	Accessories: cost, strength, average shelf and use life, cleaning requirements compared to disposables

Source: David, Judd, and Zambuto (2004).

TECHNOLOGY PROCUREMENT

Hospitals adopt technology out of clinical necessity, to support operations, or because of market forces, as described in Exhibit 25.4 (David et al., 2004). Successful hospitals link technology acquisition and management with the mission and strategic plan of the organization.

Members from all disciplines should know purposes and objectives of the committee. A proactive approach in seeking emerging technology should underlie the objective of completing a comprehensive impact analysis. Beginning with a formal request for information, the CNS should obtain references from the vendor early. Beware of relying solely on vendor information. Vendor summaries are often biased and designed to attract prospective buyers rather than present a balanced and realistic presentation of the benefits and limits of the device (Keller, 2004). Exhibit 25.5 describes the elements required for a comprehensive analysis necessary for the CNS to make an informed decision about medical devices (Harding & Epstein, 2004; Mytton et al., 2010). Sources of evidence for informed decision making are described in Exhibits 25.6A and 25.6B (Baretich, 2004; Eastman & McCarthy, 2012; Mytton et al., 2010; Rotter, Foerster, & Bridges, 2012).

The CNS must plan for problems associated with technology assessment. Once there is broad acceptance of a medical device based on insufficient evidence, there is little incentive to complete a critical evaluation. However, critical evaluation is necessary for an informed decision and to reduce the emergence of unseen problems in the clinical setting later. Exercise great caution when evaluating clinical trials,

EXHIBIT 25.4
Rationale for Technology Adoption

Rationale	Indices
Clinical necessity	Meet standards of care Increase quality of care Improve quality of life Enhance safety Treat disease Reduce length of stay Support care protocols
Operations support	Increase efficiency Expand or develop services Reduce errors Regulatory compliance Reduce dependence on user skill levels Integrate departments Reduce maintenance loads
Market preference	Increase access to care Improved customer satisfaction Increase return on investment Improve revenue stream Impact market share

which often have small samples, inconsistent procedures across trials, lack of randomization, and focus on *intermediate* rather than *final* outcomes. Then the CNS can bring to the table all the evidence to promote a rational and cost-effective decision for the

EXHIBIT 25.5

Required Elements for Comprehensive Technology Assessment

Factor	Elements
Technology type	Therapeutic, diagnostic, or supportive alternative products
Return on investment—costs	Life cycle of the medical device Purchase versus lease Plan for upgrades Maintenance Replacement Accessories Disposables Reimbursement
Quality	Comparison with like technologies Other user experiences and outcomes Shelf life of associated disposables Parts availability
Safety	Potential adverse events Redundancy Backup systems Competency requirements Biomedical training Monitoring requirements Outcomes of device failure Availability of loaner equipment
Staffing	Surveillance requirements Transport requirements Credentialing
Service line	Acceptance Clinical justification Expected utilization Integration in existing services Communication requirements Market impact and penetration Support of strategic plan and organizational mission
Vendor control	Ability to pace the rate of device introduction Inventory control Shipping, freight, installation costs Duration of price guarantees Vendor support during introduction Staff training support Postdevice introduction support Resources after implementation

(continued)

EXHIBIT 25.5 *(Continued)*

Factor	Elements
Regulatory	Labeling Liability Insurance Consent issues Maintenance requirements Current Food and Drug Administration (FDA) status History of vendor clearance to market the device Local, state, and federal codes
Users	Competency requirements Training requirements Ease of use Human factors Ability to maintain proficiency Associated clinical procedures Available written materials or manuals Staff evaluations
Contract considerations	Warranty details Payment schedules Grounds for cancellation Price protection How future versions of the device will be made available Timetable for implementation

EXHIBIT 25.6A

Selected Sources of Evidence for Technology Assessment

Sources
Manufacturer guidelines
Evaluation/experience of other users
Focused literature reviews
Government patent review
Clinical trials
Expert opinion
News media
Specialty organization guidelines/standards

EXHIBIT 25.6B

Selected Sources of Evidence for Technology Assessment

Name	Web Site	About
The Association for the Advancement of Medical Instrumentation (AAMI)	www.aami.org	Purpose is to increase understanding and beneficial use of medical instrumentation; AAMI provides continuing education, conferences, certification, and publications of technical documents, periodicals, books, and software
U.S. Agency for Healthcare Research and Quality (AHRQ)	www.ahrq.gov	Technology Assessment Clinical Practice Guidelines
National Guidelines Clearinghouse™	www.guideline.gov	An initiative of AHRQ and U.S. Department of Health and Human Services. Resource for evidence-based clinical practice guidelines
National Quality Measures Clearinghouse™ (NQMC)	www.qualitymeasures.ahrq.gov	Public repository for evidence-based quality measures and measure sets
Emergency Care Research Institute (ECRI)	www.ecri.org/Pages/default.aspx	Nonprofit organization that provides independent evidence: standards, rules, and regulations for the use of technology that affects health; medical device hazard and recall information, management tools, guidelines, and customized consulting; information resources for patient safety, technology planning, and assessment, acquisition, and management
U.S. Food and Drug Administration (FDA) Center for Devices and Radiological Health (CDRH)	www.fda.gov/AboutFDA/CentersOffices/OfficeofMedicalProductsandTobacco/CDRH	Provides important information for device evaluation, human factors, safety news, recalls, medical device reporting, recent medical device approvals, and postmarketing surveillance
National Library of Medicine (NLM)	www.nlm.nih.gov	PubMed—a service that includes over 17 million citations from MEDLINE and other journals from the 1950s. Includes full-text articles and related resources; Health Services/Technology Assessment Text (HSTAT)—a free web-based resource of full-text documents that provides information for health care decision making for health care providers, researchers, policy makers, and consumers
National Information Center on Health Services Research and Health Care Technology (NICHSR)	www.nlm.nih.gov/nichsr	To improve the organization and dissemination of results of health services research; includes practice guidelines and technology assessments

acquisition and use of new and existing technology (Banta, 2009; Eisenberg, 1999; Rotter et al., 2012).

Hospitals that are part of a group purchasing organization (GPO) avoid many problems associated with technology acquisition. The ability to negotiate group rate discounts for medical devices helps control cost but limits choice. Products are usually *not* selected for clinical utility, effectiveness, or safety. More often, products are selected based solely on the lowest negotiated price. Even more problems can occur when the contract requires a sustained commitment to purchase a set volume of medical devices to secure a negotiated price (Keller, 2004). Furthermore, individual GPO member hospitals usually do not have direct input in device selection, and products are often chosen without consideration of the unique needs of each GPO member. Technology assessment committees and the CNS can provide invaluable direction to the GPO for appropriate medical device selection. Finally, common problems associated with technology assessment that can be avoided by careful planning are described in Exhibit 25.7 (David et al., 2004).

Clinical trials are an important part of technology procurement, and the CNS often facilitates medical device trials in clinical areas. Before beginning any trial, obtain relevant department and vendor support. After arranging time with manufacturers for use of the medical device, offer in-service training for all staffs impacted by the trial. User and service manuals should be part of the education process and readily available once the device is in use. Schedule any classes in areas with easy access and low distractions. Provide notebooks in trial areas for staff to write questions and concerns when the CNS is not available. To obtain staff evaluation regarding the device (e.g., ease of use), the CNS should consider preparing and administering a short written survey (Canlas, Hall, & Shuck-Holmes, 2004; Eastman & McCarthy, 2012 ; Harding & Epstein, 2004).

Training super users to serve as resources on individual units to extend the expertise of the CNS is a wise intervention for complex medical devices. In-house maintenance from the vendor or manufacturer is critical during the trial. After approval, in-house clinical engineers must also be as well trained as the manufacturer service providers to ensure safety and to complete required preventative maintenance (Canlas et al., 2004; Harding & Epstein, 2004).

In summary, successful technology procurement is based on prepurchase evaluation, expected life cycle, and cost-benefit analysis of maintenance, depreciation, and obsolescence. This knowledge, combined with outcomes from clinical trials and staff feedback, can help the CNS and the organization make the best decision required for technology procurement (Canlas et al., 2004). Every decision must include consideration for the reality of limited resources and increasing demands. The CNS should balance the choice of any technology with the possible loss of choice in the future of more cost-effective devices (Prasad & Cifu, 2011). Once the decision has been made, technology assessment should remain an ongoing effort because future innovations may make the chosen technology obsolete.

TECHNOLOGY IN THE CLINICAL SETTING

Technology has increased the complexity of nursing practice. Increasingly, medical devices require more and more of the nurse's attention and responsibility, which gives rise to an increasingly impersonal environment. Less time to interact with patients results in fewer patients in therapeutic relationships with their caregivers. Additionally, technology is no longer being applied just to the critically ill but also to the chronically ill outside the intensive care unit (ICU). As a result, medical device monitoring becomes more important than monitoring the patient (Bauld, Dyro, & Grimes, 2004; Mytton et al. 2010).

What are the forces driving technology application outside the ICU? First, technology in many situations improves quality of life independent of the diagnosis or prognosis. However, experience suggests that fear of litigation may be the more common reason. Failure to use available technology appears to increase liability even when all the evidence suggests that application is not necessary, and overacting on information gained from a medical device may result in more harm than good. As a result, nurses practice in a clinical setting fraught with legal and ethical dilemmas (Bauld et al., 2004).

EXHIBIT 25.7

Common Problems Uncovered in a Technology Assessment

Problems
1. Technology underused
2. Device inappropriately used
3. Lack of compliance with guidelines or standards associated with use
4. Frequent repairs
5. Disorganized maintenance
6. Failure to monitor and replace outdated technology
7. In-services held at inappropriate times
8. Disorganized implementation plan
9. Slow engineering responses for problems
10. Failure to plan for upgrades

Evidence suggests that the future will be even more complex. New emerging technologies promise to radically change the environment of care. Some emerging technologies include remote monitoring (Nangalia, Prytherch, & Smith, 2010); robotics (Barbash & Glied, 2010; Nangalia et al., 2010); intelligent infusion and centralized medication and intravenous therapy systems (Agius, 2012); smart phone and table integration in clinical care (Broussard & Broussard, 2013); electronic health record and decision support (Carrington & Tiase, 2013); smart beds and smart pills (Suby, 2013); virtual family visitation (Thibeau, Ricouard, & Gilcrease, 2012); biometrics and artificial intelligence (Suby, 2013); radiofrequency identification (RFID; Fahey, Dunn Lopez, Storfjell, & Keenan, 2013; Norten, 2012); virtual world (De Gagne, Oh, Kang, Vorderstrasse, & Johnson, 2013) and avatars (Anderson, Page, & Wendorf, 2013).

With more medical devices in the clinical setting, there are more alarms in a changing geography that increasingly fails to support the visibility of patients (Leeper, 2006). The challenge for the CNS is finding ways to assist nurses to safely respond to multiple alarms in environments saturated with interruptions and competing demands. Exhibit 25.8 describes the factors associated with failure to respond to medical device alarms, which leads to alarms not heard or even ignored and increased risk of negative patient outcomes (National Patient Safety Goal on Alarm Management, 2013; Sendelbach & Jepsen, 2013).

The CNS can help nursing staff gain control over medical device alarms. To begin, list all equipment and alarms in the clinical setting. The list may include the following: emergency call light, nurse call light or signal, ventilator-cardiac-infusion pump alarms, and medical gas alarms. Second, discern all factors that inhibit responding appropriately to alarms. Factors may include staffing, workload, logistics, competency with use of the device, and lack of guidelines to minimize false and meaningless alarms (Sendelbach & Jepsen, 2013). Third, assess the culture within the clinical area. What are the roles, norms, and behaviors associated with clinical alarms? Does the staff work as a team in responding to alarms, or is each nurse responsible only for his or her assigned patient alarms? Based on this assessment, the CNS can develop meaningful guidelines and individual clinical skills to reduce the number of false and irrelevant alarms, which can reduce the likelihood of failing to respond to a true alarm (Sendelbach & Jepsen, 2013). Simulation can help assess the efficacy of guidelines and interventions (Hallenbeck, 2012). Exhibit 25.9 describes a template that could be used to assess competency for medical

---

EXHIBIT 25.8

Factors Associated With Failure to Respond to Medical Device Alarms

Factors
1. Multiple competing alarms
2. Lack of standards for alarm response
3. Failure to customize alarm settings based on patient assessment
4. Lack of backup for primary responders
5. Staffing
6. Workload
7. Frequency of nuisance alarms
8. Frequency of clinically irrelevant alarms
9. Frequency of false alarms
10. Nursing unit culture
11. Disabling or silencing alarms

EXHIBIT 25.9

Medical Device Alarm Competency Assessment

Assessment
1. Customizes alarms based on nursing assessment
2. Checks alarm defaults
3. Knowledgeable of alarm limits
4. Sets the alarm limits when appropriate
5. Alarm audible within the ambient noise of the environment
6. Knowledgeable of the alarm significance
7. Knowledgeable of the implications of nonresponse
8. Demonstrates methods to decrease nuisance alarms
9. Shares responsibilities of responding to clinical alarms
10. Able to explain alarms to patients and families
11. Responds appropriately to clinical alarms

device alarms and can assist the CNS to improve staff response to medical device alarms (Newton et al., 2010; Sendelbach & Jepsen, 2013).

Concomitant with this transformation of patient care is the beginning of the disappearance of the paper medical record. Increased technology at the bedside has created a greater need for more information for an ever-increasing number of specialists providing care who work in ever-widening venues. The electronic medical record promises increased access to information, interconnection of clinicians, improved biosurveillance, and streamlined processes for collecting quality improvement data (Suby, 2013).

Conversion to the electronic health record may be the most complex application health care has ever experienced. Until there is a standard template to structure health care information as well as access, data entry, and data transfer, information systems will remain more a problem rather than a solution for health care organizations. The dream of *integrating* primary, inpatient and outpatient care, lab results, tests, and procedures is still a dream for many organizations. While the electronic record promises to reduce adverse events, evidence suggests that new, subtle, and systematic events will occur related to the linear design of computer programming that as of yet cannot capture the complex multitasking health care environment (O'Malley, 2007; Szczerba & Huesch, 2012). The generally poor customization ability of many IT systems makes adding and linking data fields very difficult. In an organization undergoing conversion to an electronic record, the CNS must be prepared to work intimately with programmers and staffs to enhance training, prevent workarounds, and correct errors in programming and design. The CNS can play an instrumental role in supporting staffs and the organization implementing an electronic record (Carrington & Tiase, 2013).

TECHNOLOGY MAINTENANCE

The average academic medical center has over 10,000 medical devices, and hidden in every technology purchase is the cost of ongoing training and evaluation (Baretich, 2004). Because few basic nursing programs offer technology theory, and most can give only limited clinical experience with medical technology, the burden is further increased on the nurse educator and CNS to educate new and current employees on a limited budget (Hart, 2012).

The goal of all medical device education is that the user must be able to operate or apply the medical device as intended and prevent adverse events associated with use (Bronzino, 2004; Newton et al., 2010).

Education is crucial to prevent improper and inappropriate use of medical devices. Annual staff surveys and critical evaluation of incident and anecdotal reports from risk management and quality assurance can provide the CNS a foundation for planning appropriate education. CNS collaboration with clinical engineers can further identify and eliminate gaps in knowledge or experience that could lead to injury (Bauld et al., 2004; Mytton et al., 2010; Shepherd, 2004).

Educational content may include medical device safety, proper setup, and indications and contraindications for use. Step-by-step demonstrations for small groups with return demonstrations *during* the class and *after* can increase staff confidence in use of the medical device. Use of simulators is another powerful method for training and can uncover latent design errors not uncovered during technology assessment (Hart, 2012). Computer-based training, newsletters, e-mail, video, and audiotapes, combined with superuser resources for clinical staff, can assist the CNS in preparing a competent and confident nursing staff (Bauld et al., 2004; Hallenbeck, 2012).

Despite education, quality control, preuse inspections, and trials of technology in the clinical setting, medical device failures still occur (Institute of Medicine [IOM], Committee on Quality of Health Care in America, 1999; Newton et al., 2010). The vast majority of medical device errors are due to user error rather than medical device failure (Bauld et al., 2004). User errors are a function of the *interaction* of the *user* and the *device in the environment*. Powerful influences include noise, lighting, user fatigue and skills, competing demands, and patient acuity (Mytton et al., 2010). Exhibit 25.10 summarizes factors associated with technology failure in the clinical setting (David et al., 2004; Newton et al., 2010).

Every adverse event investigation requires that the CNS critically evaluate with an unbiased and nonjudgmental attitude (Bauld et al., 2004; Newton et al., 2010). Preservation of evidence and immediate documentation and recollection of the adverse event are necessary. Crucial observations include device settings, placement, accessories used, environmental conditions, condition of the device, and observations from any personnel in attendance. The investigation should be nonpunitive and supportive of the individuals involved, who are often severely traumatized by the event and even more traumatized by the subsequent investigation. The underlying principle of any investigation must be explicit to all involved, and that is: *Every* adverse event offers incredible opportunity for improvement of related policies and procedures associated with the medical device and, ultimately, improvement in nursing care.

EXHIBIT 25.10
Reasons for Medical Device Failures

Reasons
1. Failure to inspect and certify the device before use
2. Failure to have a medical device management program
3. Failure to verify that the vendor will deliver a complete system with necessary accessories and disposables
4. Failure to control risks associated with implementation
5. Lack of technical support
6. Failure to provide education to direct and indirect users
7. Failure to complete preventative maintenance
8. Failure to act on recalls
9. Failure of clinical engineering or biomedical technicians to listen to staff feedback
10. Failure to operate the equipment according to manufacturer's guidelines
11. Failure to complete postimplementation evaluations
12. Introducing medical devices without guidelines for users
13. Failure to ensure competency of users at introduction
14. Failure to ensure competency of users over time
15. Failure to modify guidelines with experience and from staff feedback

THE FUTURE

While technology is often blamed for the rising costs of health care, the market for medical devices continues to expand. Technology has improved health care in terms of access, quality, and efficiency. Technology has also extended the science and practice of nursing. Technology is driving the rising cost of health care (David et al., 2004; Drummond, Tarricone, & Torbica, 2013; Rotter et al., 2012; Squires, 2012).

However, technology also threatens the profession of nursing. Intimate body care and sacred therapeutic relationships are increasingly being replaced with technical intimacy (Sandelowski, 2000; Schoenhofer, 2001). Overemphasis on technological competency has gradually eroded the nurse–patient dyad to the patient–technology–nurse triad. More often than not, the patient–nurse relationship occurs only if there is time left after required actions with technology are completed. Gradually, the nurse–patient relationship, which has the greatest lasting impact on the health care experience, is eroding (Sandelowski, 2000; Schoenhofer, 2001).

The increasing mechanistic view of human beings expressed as sole emphasis on outcomes and benchmarks implies that human beings are predictable and manageable (Mitchell, 2001). The increasing obsession with technology, task, and evidence-based practice (EBP) is changing practice from holism to a biomedical paradigm. Nursing's commitment to honor, care, respect, and help persons under their care is gradually being lost (Mitchell, 2001).

The continuous technological transformation of health care provides promise and risk for nursing. There are four risks the CNS must continuously monitor and be prepared to address now and in the future to preserve the art and science of professional nursing practice.

First and foremost, beware of the promise that the technology permits the nurse to care for *more patients*. Evidence suggests that technology increases the need for *more nurses* related to maintenance, programming, troubleshooting, and differentiation of true and false alarms (Sandelowski, 2000; Schoenhofer, 2001). Furthermore, technology usually restricts patient mobility, thereby increasing the incidence of pressure ulcers, respiratory problems, falls, and stress for patients and families. More rather than less nursing care is usually needed to prevent these unfavorable outcomes (Sandelowski, 2000; Schoenhofer, 2001). Critical evaluation of technology impact on practice and patients can provide necessary evidence that supports appropriate nurse–patient ratios, which in turn supports nurse retention and safe patient care.

Even more dangerous is the assumption that technology can *substitute* for the judgment of a nurse. No technology, no matter how well designed or programmed, interfaced with a human being can discern all the sources of variance in the physiological and health care environments. Because all technology carries some degree of risk *and* error in application, nursing actions should be based on critical evaluation rather than unhesitating acceptance of technology-provided data (Rinard, 2001; Sandelowski, 2000). The CNS can provide critical advocacy for patients and nurses when technology is implemented through education, training, and development of practice guidelines that enhance decision making rather than replace it.

The increasing mechanization of health care is subtle and powerful. Technology has extended practice, but technology has also increased the risk of depersonalization for the patient *and* the nurse. Critical care environments, where nurses are in continuous relationship with multiple technologies and one patient, are particularly at risk. Depending on patient acuity, staffing, experience, and competency, the nurse–patient relationship is often sacrificed along with teaching, providing comfort, and presence to maintain the technology–patient interface safely (Sandelowski, 2000; Schoenhofer, 2001).

The CNS must protect nursing at the bedside. Increasingly, nurses are doing the work of medicine, respiratory therapy, pharmacy, laboratory, and physical therapy, radiology, and nutrition services under the guise of nursing care. Once the novelty of new technology wears off and risks are known, technology once exclusively under the purview of a specific discipline is usually transferred to nursing *after* application to the patient because nursing is with the patient 24 hours a day (Sandelowski, 2000; Schoenhofer, 2001). Recent examples of technology transfer to nursing include extracorporeal membrane oxygenation, cardiac ventricular assist support, vascular sheath removal, renal replacement therapies, weaning from mechanical ventilation, and bedside laboratory analysis. As a result, nursing care increasingly is becoming more surveillance and less comfort, more troubleshooting and less touch, and technology-based outcomes rather than a healing therapeutic relationship.

The promises of technology—convenience, productivity, and access to information 24 hours a day, 7 days a week—have opened a Pandora's box of unimaginable consequences (Miller, 2007; Wallner & Konski, 2008). It is increasingly difficult to separate human beings (patient or staff) from the technology in health care. Constant availability, multitasking, role expansion, and flattening of management hierarchies have nearly eliminated the *time* necessary for critical thinking (Miller, 2007).

Multitasking, which emerged from the computer sciences under the false conclusion that computers multitask, has become the norm for health care organizations. The reality is that while computers appear to be completing several tasks at once, the program only completes *one task at a time*. However, computer recovery *following* task completion is immediate, so the next task is completed without a break and seemingly simultaneously with the previous task.

Nurses multitask, caring for patients and responding to increasing numbers of interruptions, including requests for information, families, and managing technology. However, recovery is not simultaneous, and evidence suggests that up to 23 minutes is required to get back to the primary task at hand after an interruption. The result is a neurologically stressful environment associated with tension, anxiety, and depression (Miller, 2007). In the future, the CNS will increasingly have to find ways to carve out time for nurses to use the nursing process.

Technological proficiency is an expression of nurse caring. Monitoring, interpretation of medical device data, and technological competency are critical elements of nursing care. However, without intentionality, compassion, confidence, commitment, and conscience, the nurse is only a robot, and the patient is only an object within a technology-dense environment (Locsin, 2001b). The CNS must protect and make known nursing's contribution in technology-rich environments so that nurses do not become invisible, undervalued, and perceived only as an adjunct to medical and economic outcomes (Schoenhofer, 2001).

Technology is fleeting and ever changing and is not owned by any one discipline. Some have suggested that in the future technology may free patients from their caregivers (Mitchell, 2001). This would result in an unimaginable transformation in health care. What then would be nursing's mission?

Technology has reshaped the aesthetics, politics, ethics, and roles in health care. Nurses, physicians, respiratory therapists, nurse's aides, patients, and families use stethoscopes, sphygmomanometers, infusion pumps, ventilators, and defibrillators at home, on the road, in the clinic, and the physician office. Cross-training, personnel substitution, and role dilution are gradually rendering nursing invisible (Sandelowski, 2000). The CNS is the best advocate to make visible nursing's contribution to patient outcomes beyond the management of technology. The CNS can help preserve the art and science of nursing practice in technology-rich environments through critical evaluation, advocacy, teaching, role modeling, consultation, and research.

Experience suggests that technology alone cannot heal, care, protect, or comfort. Without a committed, expert nurse able to balance caring and technology management *within* a nurse–patient relationship, patients become machines whose outcomes can be engineered. Patients are more than biology, disease, machinery, or treatment. Nurses are more than technology managers (Barnard, 2007). The CNS is in the best position to preserve nursing practice, protect vulnerable patients, and drive safe technology application that supports the most important relationship in health care: The nurse–patient relationship.

DISCUSSION QUESTIONS

- How does technology impact your nursing practice?
- What percentage of your practice is devoted to technology issues?
- Technological proficiency has been described as evidence of a caring nurse. Do nurses believe this? Do you think patients also believe this?
- In technologically rich environments, what can a nurse do to foster a personal and healing relationship with a patient?

ANALYSIS AND SYNTHESIS EXERCISES

- Increasingly, complex medical informatics (electronic health record, computerized physician order entry, electronic medication record) promise improved information accessibility and fewer errors. With these promises come the realities of monumental changes in health care culture, workflow, workload, and different errors. Locate a hospital in your area that has converted to the electronic health record (EHR). Obtain an interview with a CNS who practiced through the conversion to the EHR. Discuss the following critical elements: staff training, relationships with IT staff, hardware and software decisions, access and integration of information, and changes in workflow. If the process could be done over, what would be different or the same?

- Using the information provided in Exhibit 25.5, complete an assessment of one technology in a clinical setting. Based on your findings, where in the life cycle is the technology? Are upgrades or improved replacement technologies available? What are the implications of upgrading or replacement for nursing, patients, and the organization?

CLINICAL APPLICATIONS

- Locsin (2001b) believes technological competency defines nursing practice. List the core competencies required for nurses where you practice. Which of these competencies requires technology application? For each technology identified, describe the education, training, and competency assessment required for safe patient application. Next, determine whether the technology increased or decreased nursing workload. Does nursing control the technology, or does the technology control nursing? If workload is increased, is this a function of complexity, patient acuity, or improper use? What could be done differently to reduce workload or improve nurse satisfaction?
- Design and administer a survey of nurses regarding all technologies in a defined clinical setting. For each technology, assess the nurse's perceived competency with application, troubleshooting, alarms, and discontinuation. Based on staff feedback, develop interventions, which may include in-services, individual mentoring, developing superusers as staff resources, writing procedures, or designing posters and/or information cards. Include an evaluation for each intervention.

ADDITIONAL HELPFUL RESOURCES

FDA Medical Device Classification System. Retrieved October 19, 2013, from https://www.google.com/#q=fda+medical+device+classification+system

Biomedical Instrumentation and Technology, http://www.aami.org/publications/BIT

Journal of Clinical Engineering, http://journals.lww.com/jcejournal/pages/default.aspx

PROFESSIONAL SOCIETIES

Association for the Advancement of Medical Instrumentation, http://www.aami.org

American Society for Healthcare Engineering, http://www.ashe.org

REFERENCES

Agius, C. R. (2012). Intelligent infusion technologies: Integration of a smart system to enhance patient care. *Journal of Infusion Nursing, 35*(6), 364–368.

Anderson, J. K., Page, A. M., & Wendorf, D. M. (2013). Avatar-assisted case studies. *Nurse Educator, 38*(3), 106–109.

Banta, D. (2009). What is technology assessment? *International Journal of Technology Assessment in Health Care, 25*(Suppl. 1), 7–9.

Barbash, G. I., & Glied, S. A. (2010). New technology and health care costs: The case of robot-assisted surgery. *The New England Journal of Medicine, 363*(8), 701–704.

Baretich, M. (2004). Equipment control and asset management. In J. Dyro (Ed.), *Clinical engineering handbook* (pp. 122–123). Boston, MA: Elsevier Academic Press.

Barnard, A. (2001). On the relationship between technique and dehumanization. In R. C. Locsin (Ed.), *Advancing technology, caring and nursing* (pp. 96–105). Westport, CT: Auburn House.

Barnard, A. (2007). Advancing the meaning of nursing and technology. In A. Barnard & R. C. Locsin (Eds.), *Technology and nursing practice: Practice, concepts and issues* (pp. 1–15). New York, NY: Palgrave Macmillan.

Barnard, A., & Cushing, A. (2001). Technology and historical inquiry. In R. C. Locsin (Ed.), *Advancing technology, caring and nursing* (pp. 12–21). Westport, CT: Auburn House.

Bauld, T., Dyro, J., & Grimes, S. (2004). Clinical engineering and nursing. In J. Dyro (Ed.), *Clinical engineering handbook* (pp. 321–327). Boston, MA: Elsevier Academic Press.

Bronzino, J. (2004). Clinical engineering: Evolution of a discipline. In J. Dyro (Ed.), *Clinical engineering handbook* (pp. 3–7). Boston, MA: Elsevier Academic Press.

Broussard, B. S., & Broussard, A. B. (2013). Using electronic communication safely in health care settings. *Nursing for Women's Health, 17*(1), 59–62.

Canlas, J., Hall, J., & Shuck-Holmes, P. (2004). Medical device design and control in the hospital. In J. Dyro (Ed.), *Clinical engineering handbook* (pp. 346–349). Boston, MA: Elsevier Academic Press.

Carrington, J. M., & Tiase, V. L. (2013). Nursing informatics year in review. *Nursing Administration Quarterly, 37*(2), 136–143.

David, Y., Judd, T., & Zambuto, R. (2004). Introduction to medical technology management practices. In J. Dyro (Ed.), *Clinical engineering handbook* (pp. 101–107). Boston, MA: Elsevier Academic Press.

De Gagne, J. C., Oh, J., Kang, J., Vorderstrasse, A. A., & Johnson, C. M. (2013). Virtual worlds in nursing education: A synthesis of the literature. *Journal of Nursing Education, 52*(7), 391–396.

Drummond, M., Tarricone, R., & Torbica, A. (2013). Assessing the added value of health technologies: Reconciling different perspectives. *Value Health, 16*(1 Suppl), S7–13.

Eastman, D., & McCarthy, C. (2012). Embracing change: Healthcare technology in the 21st century. *Nursing Management, 43*(6), 52–54.

Eisenberg, J. M. (1999). Ten lessons for evidence-based technology assessment. *Journal of the American Medical Association, 282*(19), 1865–1869.

Fahey, L., Dunn Lopez, K., Storfjell, J., & Keenan, G. (2013). Expanding potential of radiofrequency nurse call systems to measure nursing time in patient rooms. *Journal of Nursing Administration, 43*(5), 302–307.

Gaev, J. (2004). Technology in health care. In J. Dyro (Ed.), *Clinical engineering handbook* (pp. 342–345). Boston, MA: Elsevier Academic Press.

Hallenbeck, V. J. (2012). Use of high fidelity simulation for staff education/development. *JNSD, 28*(6), 260–260.

Harding, G., & Epstein, A. (2004). Technology procurement. In J. Dyro (Ed.), *Clinical engineering handbook* (pp. 118–122). Boston, MA: Elsevier Academic Press.

Hart, C. (2012). Technology and nursing education: An online toolkit for educators. *Journal of Continuing Education in Nursing, 43*(9), 393–394.

Heidegger, M. (1977). *The question concerning technology and other essays*. New York, NY: Harper & Row.

Institute of Medicine (IOM), Committee on Quality of Health Care in America. (1999). *To err is human: Building a safer health system*. Washington, DC: National Academies Press.

Institute of Medicine (IOM). *The future of nursing: Leading change, advancing health*. Accessed October 14, from http://www.iom.edu/Reports/2010/The-future-of-nursing-leading-change-advancing-health.aspx

Keller, J. (2004). Comparative evaluations of medical devices. In J. Dyro (Ed.), *Clinical engineering handbook* (pp. 366–368). Boston, MA: Elsevier Academic Press.

Kleinpell, R. M. (2013). Measuring outcomes in advanced practice nursing. In R. M. Kleinpell (Ed.), *Outcome assessment in advanced practice nursing* (3rd ed., pp. 1–42). New York, NY: Springer.

Leeper, B. (2006). Monitoring and hemodynamics. *Critical Care Nursing Clinics of North America, 18*(2), xiii–xiv.

Locsin, R. (2001a). Introduction. In R. C. Locsin (Ed.), *Advancing technology, caring, and nursing* (pp. xxi–xxvi). Westport, CT: Auburn House.

Locsin, R. (2001b). Practicing nursing: Technological competency as an expression of caring. In R. C. Locsin (Ed.), *Advancing technology, caring, and nursing* (pp. 88–95). Westport, CT: Auburn House.

Miller, H. (2007). *The siren song of multi-tasking*. Retrieved October 19, 2013, from http://www.hermanmiller.com/hm/content/research_summaries/pdfs/wp_SirenSong.pdf

Mitchell, G. J. (2001). Pictures of paradox: Technology, nursing and human science. In R. C. Locsin (Ed.), *Advancing technology, caring, and nursing* (pp. 22–40). Westport, CT: Auburn House.

Mytton, O. T., Velazquez, A., Banken, R., Mathew, J. L., Ikonen, T. S., Taylor, K.,...Ruelas, E. (2010). Introducing new technology safely. *Quality & Safety in Health Care, 19*(Suppl 2), i9–i14.

Nangalia, V., Prytherch, D. R., & Smith, G. B. (2010). Health technology assessment review: Remote monitoring of vital signs–current status and future challenges. *Critical Care (London, England), 14*(5), 233.

National Patient Safety Goal on Alarm Management-Applicable to Hospitals and Critical Access Hospitals. (2013, July). Effective January 1, 2014. *Joint Commission Perspectives, 33*(7). Retrieved October 13, 2013, from http://www.jointcommission.org/assets/1/18/JCP0713_Announce_New_NSPG.pdf

Newton, R. C., Mytton, O. T., Aggarwal, R., Runciman, W. B., Free, M., Fahlgren, B., . . . Whittaker, S. (2010). Making existing technology safer in healthcare. *Quality & Safety in Health Care, 19*(Suppl. 2), i15–i24.

Norten, A. (2012). Predicting nurses' acceptance of radiofrequency identification technology. *Computers, Informatics, Nursing: CIN, 30*(10), 531–537; quiz 538.

O'Malley, P. (2007). Computerized provider order entry and prescribing and the evidence for safe practice: Update for the clinical nurse specialist. *Clinical Nurse Specialist CNS, 21*(3), 139–141.

Prasad, V., & Cifu, A. (2011). Medical reversal: Why we must raise the bar before adopting new technologies. *Yale Journal of Biology and Medicine, 84*(4), 471–478.

Richter, N. (2004). Evolution of medical device technology. In J. Dyro (Ed.), *Clinical engineering handbook* (pp. 339–341). Boston, MA: Elsevier Academic Press.

Ridgway, M., Johnson, G., & McClain, J. (2004). History of engineering and technology in health care. In J. Dyro (Ed.), *Clinical engineering handbook* (pp. 7–8). Boston, MA: Elsevier Academic Press.

Rinard, R. G. (2001). Technology, de-skilling and nurses. The impact of the technologically changing environment. In R. C. Locsin (Ed.), *Advancing technology, caring, and nursing* (pp. 68–75). Westport, CT: Auburn House.

Rotter, J. S., Foerster, D., & Bridges, J. F. (2012). The changing role of economic evaluation in valuing medical technologies. *Expert Review of Pharmacoeconomics & Outcomes Research, 12*(6), 711–723.

Sandelowski, M. (2000). *Devices and desires: Gender, technology, and American nursing (studies in social medicine).* Chapel Hill, NC: The University of North Carolina Press.

Schoenhofer, S. B. (2001). Outcomes of caring in high-technology practice environments. In R. C. Locsin (Ed.), *Advancing technology, caring, and nursing* (pp. 79–87). Westport, CT: Auburn House.

Sendelbach, S., & Jepsen, S. (2013). *AACN Practice Alert™ alarm management.* American Association of Critical Care Nurses. Retrieved October 14, 2013, from http://www.aacn.org/wd/practice/docs/practicealerts/alarm-management-practice-alert.pdf

Shekelle, P. G., Morton, S. C., & Keeler, E. B. (2006, April). *Costs and benefits of health information technology* (Evidence Report/Technology Assessment No. 132; prepared by the Southern California Evidence-based Practice Center under Contract No. 290–02-0003; AHRQ Publication No. 06-E006). Rockville, MD: Agency for Healthcare Research and Quality. Retrieved January 9, 2009, from http://www.ahrq.gov/down loads/pub/evidence/pdf/hitsyscosts/hitsys.pdf

Shepherd, M. (2004). Systems approach to medical device safety. In J. Dyro (Ed.), *Clinical engineering handbook* (pp. 246–249). Boston, MA: Elsevier Academic Press.

Squires, D. (2012, May). *Explaining the high health care spending in the United States: An international comparison of supply, utilization, prices, and quality.* Accessed October 19, 2013, from http://www.commonwealthfund.org/~/media/Files/Publications/Issue%20Brief/2012/May/1595_Squires_explaining_high_hlt_care_spending_intl_brief.pdf

Suby, C. (2013). Nursing operations automation and health care technology innovations: 2025 and beyond. *Creative Nursing, 10*(1), 30–36.

Szczerba, R. J., & Huesch, M. D. (2012). Why technology matters as much as science in improving healthcare. *BMC Medical Informatics and Decision Making, 12*(1), 103. Retrieved October 19, 2013, from http://www.biomedcentral.com/1472–6947/12/103

Thibeau, S., Ricouard, D., & Gilcrease, C. (2012). Innovative technology offers virtual visitation for families. *Journal of Continuing Education in Nursing, 43*(10), 439–440.

Vogelsmeier, A., & Scott-Cawiezell, J. (2009). The role of nursing leadership in successful technology implementation. *Journal of Nursing Administration, 39*(7–8), 313–314.

Wallner, P. E., & Konski, A. (2008). A changing paradigm in the study and adoption of emerging health care technologies: Coverage with evidence development. *Journal of the American College of Radiology: JACR, 5*(11), 1125–1129.

Welter, L. O. (2004). The health care environment. In J. Dyro (Ed.), *Clinical engineering handbook* (pp. 11–14). Boston, MA: Elsevier Academic Press.

Entrepreneurship and Intrapreneurship in Advanced Nursing Practice

Maria R. Shirey

The United States has approximately 25 million small businesses and 10.5 million self-employed individuals (National Association of the Self-Employed, 2004). Small businesses employ 45% of the total U.S. private payroll and over the last decade consistently generated 60% to 80% of all net new jobs annually (U.S. Chamber of Commerce, 2006). It is obvious that small business owners and entrepreneurs contribute greatly to the social and economic growth of the nation. Collectively, the small business owners' economic power base positions this group as a significant voice shaping national policy decisions. Unfortunately, nurse entrepreneur representation in this influential contingency is virtually nonexistent. Much of the reason for lack of nurse entrepreneur presence has to do with reluctance to new ways of thinking, either as a result of limited knowledge of nurse entrepreneurship, lack of empowerment, or lack of "what if" thinking that challenges the status quo. Nurses in advanced practice have a keen understanding regarding the care needs and gaps evident in today's health care systems. Understanding the clinical nurse specialist's (CNS's) potential to seize the opportunities and bridge those gaps is a first step in unleashing entrepreneurial talent. This chapter explores nurse entrepreneurship as a viable option for the CNS. Seeing nurse entrepreneurship within the realm of possibility provides opportunity to consider new ways of thinking, a new way that positions CNSs to change the status quo, improve health

care delivery for the populations they serve, and to do so in their unique way. Leading a resurgence of nurse entrepreneurship for the profession offers control over nursing practice and ultimately a chance to achieve greater personal and professional satisfaction as well to contribute toward greater societal good.

DEFINITIONS

Entrepreneurship

Entrepreneurship refers to the practice of starting new organizations or businesses generally in response to identified market opportunities. One definition of *entrepreneurship* (there are many) is that it is "a way of thinking, reasoning, and acting that is opportunity obsessed, holistic in approach, and leadership balanced" (Timmons & Spinelli, 2007, p. 79). Central to the entrepreneurship concept is the creation and recognition of opportunities inclusive of the will and initiative to seize those opportunities (Timmons & Spinelli, 2007). Although entrepreneurship often refers to the actual creation of a new and small business, the term goes beyond this narrow conceptualization. Drucker, in his classic book *Innovation and Entrepreneurship* (Drucker, 1985), describes entrepreneurship as a distinct feature of an individual or of an institution. This expanded notion of entrepreneurship takes into account that in order for businesses to remain vital in the marketplace, people within business entities must always search for change, embrace it, and exploit it as an opportunity.

The term *entrepreneurship,* coined by French economist Jean-Baptiste Say (Drucker, 1985), originates from the French word *entreprendre* meaning "to undertake" something. Motivation for entrepreneurship involves the desire to create something new that can exploit opportunities. To be an entrepreneur requires using a distinct skill set that may be learned. The entrepreneurial mind-set includes the ability to deal with uncertainty and the aptitude for taking complex goals and breaking these into manageable sequential steps that an individual can diligently address and systematically complete. Entrepreneurs are conscientious risk takers who are driven by a vision of something better. They make decisions based on intuition and data analysis, assuming full risk and benefit from all aspects of their ventures. Overall, entrepreneurship creates value for society and individuals. It serves as an engine for job creation and economic growth for the future. Success as an entrepreneur also facilitates philanthropy to benefit mankind.

The study of entrepreneurship in the business world dates back to the 18th century and to the early work of French economist Richard Cantillon (Falcone & Osborne, 2005). An understanding of entrepreneurship is credited to the 1950s work of Austrian economist Joseph Schumpeter and to the more contemporary work of multiple scholars, including Peter Drucker (1985) and Jeffry Timmons (Timmons & Spinelli, 2007). Although the scientific study of entrepreneurship is prevalent in the business world, its study is far less prominent in health care. In nursing, only a small body of empirical literature is available to examine entrepreneurship as a phenomenon in the profession (Shirey, 2007).

Intrapreneurship

Intrapreneurship refers to the practice of a person utilizing entrepreneurial skills and approaches within a company. Pinchot and Pellman (1985) define *intrapreneurship* as behaving like an entrepreneur to "turn ideas into realities inside an organization" (p. 16). Intrapreneurs are generally independent thinkers who are known as "the dreamers who do" (p. 16). Fundamental to intrapreneurship is the notion of corporate renewal that involves using innovation and creativity to convert dreams or ideas into ventures yielding tangible results. Large organizations need intrapreneurs in order to retain their innovation edge and, thus, their competitive advantage. As such, these organizations depend on employees to

spawn businesses within the business. The motivation for intrapreneurship is to challenge the status quo. Intrapreneurs and entrepreneurs both share a similar "can do" mind-set.

The term *intrapreneurship,* coined by Pinchot and Pellman (1985), is based on an article in *The Economist* written by Norman Macrae, the journal's editor. Macrae (1982) was of the belief that dynamic corporations of the future needed to experiment with alternative and better ways of doing things to stay "on their toes" and remain in competition with themselves. Based on the success of their original research and crediting Macrae for his influence, Pinchot and his associates (1985) developed the concept of intrapreneurship and published the classic book *Intrapreneuring in Action.*

Intrapreneurship can be a rewarding career in and of itself, or it can be the initial step toward entrepreneurship. In intrapreneurship, the intrapreneur works inside an organization and answers to an authority figure within that organization. The entrepreneur, on the other hand, is self-employed and generally is the person running the company. According to Pinchot and Pellman (1985), intrapreneurship provides the best of both worlds: a smart way to learn entrepreneurship, but doing so using someone else's money and existing supportive structures. Intrapreneurship can be fulfilling for individuals who work within an organizational culture of innovation. In the absence of an innovative organizational culture, the intrapreneur may be at risk for frustration that becomes counterproductive to personal and organizational outcomes.

Nurse Entrepreneur

A nurse entrepreneur is a nurse who is "proprietor of a business that offers nursing services of a direct care, educational, research, administrative or consultative nature" (International Council of Nurses [ICN], 2004, p. 4). Nurse entrepreneurs may also be individuals who invent or patent new products, services, or devices. Regardless of the entrepreneurial activity, nurse entrepreneurs are usually self-employed individuals who have nurse control over practice and are directly accountable to the clients they serve. Nurse entrepreneurship ventures may include independent nursing practices, nurse-owned businesses, or consulting firms. Ideas for nurse entrepreneur ventures emerge from the ability to forecast and respond to health care needs and gaps in services or products. The scope of nurse entrepreneurial practice largely depends on the economic infrastructures (reimbursement systems) and legal/regulatory requirements of the health care industry.

Nurse Intrapreneur

A nurse intrapreneur is a nurse who is a salaried (or hourly) employee within a health care setting "who develops, promotes, and delivers on innovative health/nursing programs or projects" within the employment setting (ICN, 2004, p. 4). Nurse intrapreneurs have control over their practice to the extent that is allowed within their employment arrangement. Nurse intrapreneurship ventures may include establishing a nurse-led clinical service, developing a new product line for a hospital, or championing a Magnet-designation journey for a health care system. Ideas for nurse intrapreneurship ventures emerge in response to or in anticipation of a health care or organizational need. The scope of nurse intrapreneurial practice depends not only on economic infrastructures and legal/regulatory requirements of the health care industry, but also on the organizational culture of the employing agency. For example, an individual with an entrepreneurial mind-set employed within a rigid and hierarchical organization may be assigned responsibility for creating a new service or product. Although the nurse intrapreneur should be able to decide what projects to undertake, the employment relationship may dictate which projects the nurse intrapreneur will pursue. In an organizational culture where innovation is not valued, the nurse intrapreneur with new and enterprising ideas may be seen as more of a liability than an asset. In many ways, a stifling organizational culture can potentially squash the entrepreneurial spirit and derail the related intrapreneurial activities.

Entrepreneurship Versus Intrapreneurship

In summary, entrepreneurship and intrapreneurship are similar yet different concepts. Entrepreneurs are self-employed individuals running their companies, whereas intrapreneurs are still company employees given some degree of freedom to run a particular aspect of a program or subsidiary. Entrepreneurs assume the risks and benefits of a new venture, while intrapreneurs assume some level of risk within the safety net of a larger company. Entrepreneurs generally build organizational structures and processes from scratch, whereas intrapreneurs benefit from the support of existing structures (technical support, finance department, human resources department, existing marketing and sales support).

Although the terms are different, the principles underlying effective entrepreneurship and intrapreneurship ventures in nursing (and business) are very similar (ICN, 2004). Specifically, the mind-set and skill set to succeed as either an entrepreneur or intrapreneur are the same. For this reason, this chapter primarily focuses on entrepreneurship, understanding that the principles presented are also valid for intrapreneurship.

BACKGROUND

Historical Overview

Florence Nightingale is largely credited with founding the nursing profession in 1854 (Dossey, 2000). Her original vision for nursing was one much ahead of her time and one that integrated a sense of service, duty, and nonconformity with the practices of the day. Although Nightingale may not have identified herself as an entrepreneur (women of her social stature could not work for financial remuneration), she in fact met many of the elements of a nurse entrepreneur (minus the remuneration piece). Nightingale was certainly *the* change agent who brought forth a new way of thinking, reasoning, and acting that was opportunity obsessed, holistic in approach, and leadership balanced.

Nurse entrepreneurship, which goes beyond the philanthropic efforts of Nightingale's day, dates back to the turn of the 20th century (ICN, 2004). In the 1870s, formal education for nurses in North America was available only within training schools in hospitals. These hospital programs admitted women for a 2-year program (later 3 years), qualifying them upon graduation to practice as nurses inside the private homes of the sick or, to a lesser extent, to work as superintendents or head nurses in hospitals (Schorr & Kennedy, 1999). Private duty nurses went from case to case, living in the homes of their clients for the duration of their patient care responsibility. In this framework, private duty nurses practiced as independent contractors providing one-to-one nursing care within the scope of practice at the time. Private duty nursing was the main form of work available to nurses for the first 50 years of the profession. In many ways, private duty nursing was the precursor to nurse entrepreneurship as we know it today.

The establishment of public health nursing and visiting nurse associations in the 1890s gave graduate nurses a new venue for paid work and self-sufficiency, one not available through private duty nursing. As the reputation of hospitals improved in the early 1900s, patients went there more readily during times of illness (Schorr & Kennedy, 1999). This increasing shift in care from the home to the hospital resulted in many private duty nurses agreeing to take on "special cases" in hospitals. The nation's economic situation in the 1920s resulted in scarce opportunities for private duty nursing work. By the 1930s, hospital staff nursing (general duty) replaced private duty nursing as the major form of nursing work in the United States (Schorr & Kennedy, 1999). Although private duty nursing continued (as did the evolution of public health and visiting nursing) beyond the 1930s, this form of independent practice was no longer the professional mainstay.

Until World War II, most nursing professionals had been independent private duty nurses. The social and economic changes following World War II led to a shortage of nurses and institutionalization of nursing practice. These dynamics resulted in role and educational setting changes for nurses (Schorr & Kennedy, 1999) as well as increases in governmental funding to produce more nurses to meet postwar demand. In the 1950s, early discussions about entry into practice surfaced, followed by significant advances in nursing and health care in the 1960s. By 1965, the American Nurses Association (ANA) had adopted the position paper on nursing education identifying the baccalaureate degree as the basic foundation for professional nursing practice (Schorr & Kennedy, 1999). Concurrently, there was a boom in hospital building, emergence of specialty nursing practice (intensive care units begun), and introduction of the advanced practice nurse (APN). Although many nurses were now employed within the hospital setting, a new breed of nurse entrepreneurs was emerging in the form of the APN.

The 1980s saw significant reimbursement changes for health care as well as a major nursing shortage. Nurses working long hours of overtime with acutely ill patients and now better educated, more empowered, and wanting autonomy and control over practice began leaving hospitals, some to become entrepreneurs. These nurse entrepreneurs set up their own successful staffing agencies, home health agencies, educational services firms, nursing centers, and private practices. Concurrently, the explosion of nursing research accelerated by the creation in 1985 of the National Center for Nursing Research (now the National Institute for Nursing Research [NINR]) contributed to greater visibility for nursing and to documenting the profession's many contributions to society and to health policy development.

The 1990s and beyond have seen many of the conditions of the 1980s revisited, yet, more accentuated. A more profound nursing shortage is currently evident in the United States. Health care restructuring efforts have further constrained nursing practice in hospitals (where most nurses still work), resulting in nurses caring for more acutely ill patients and working under conditions that threaten health care quality and patient safety. Combined with the aging U.S. population; greater demands on the existing health care delivery system; explosion in science, technology, and knowledge; plus the empowerment of women (95% of nurses are women), these changes provide fertile opportunities for nurse entrepreneurship ventures. The fact that APNs are better educated, more highly valued, and more universally respected uniquely positions them to leverage their talents to advance their passion for quality patient care. Seizing the opportunity to reap the benefits of current social, political, and economic dynamics is the sign of a true entrepreneur. APNs now more than ever are in a position to reclaim their priorities, advance the profession's caring covenant, and do so as nurse entrepreneurs.

Prevalence

Statistical data to quantify the number of nurse entrepreneurs are difficult to obtain because different definitions are used to identify what constitutes a nurse entrepreneur. In general, 0.5% to 1% of working nurses are nurse entrepreneurs (ICN, 2004). Nurse entrepreneurs appear to be more plentiful in geographic areas in which a public demand for nurse entrepreneurs is evident. Nurse entrepreneur–friendly areas include those in which the legal right to practice is not challenged, direct third-party reimbursement exists, and access to support services and a referral base prevail. In geographic areas in which the role of the entrepreneur has been seen and experienced closely, it is more likely that new entrepreneurs will emerge (Veciana, 2007). An example of such an area for nonnurse entrepreneurs exists in California's Silicon Valley. No comparable geographic area, however, is noted for nurse entrepreneurs who appear to be scattered throughout the United States. It follows, then, that nurses who grow up or practice in environments that nurture entrepreneurship (such as in a family business or in a business incubator organization) may be more inclined toward entrepreneurship. This supports the notion that to grow more nurse entrepreneurs means that they must be cultivated within the profession and through interprofessional collaboration. A return to nurse entrepreneurship as a prevalent form of practice, however, demands a major paradigm shift for most nurses.

THEORETICAL SUPPORT

Theoretical Approaches to Entrepreneurship

Entrepreneurship as a field of study is very broad, and to date, the entrepreneurship domain lacks one unifying conceptual framework (Shane & Venkataraman, 2007). No one theory prevails, rather many theories are evident (see relevant literature review for expanded discussion of the evidence in support of theory). Theoretical approaches to the study of entrepreneurship (Veciana, 2007), however, may be classified into a matrix (Table 26.1) consisting of three levels of analysis (micro, meso, macro) and four major approaches (economic, psychological, sociocultural, managerial). An extensive discussion of all the theoretical approaches is beyond the scope of this chapter. For purposes of this chapter, primary focus is given to the individual unit of analysis (micro level) and the combination of both the psychological (who the entrepreneur is) and managerial approaches (what the entrepreneur does). The rationale for selecting the micro level and psychological/managerial approaches is twofold. First, CNS practice and development of the role focuses first on the individual. Because entrepreneurial behavior can be learned, it is important to understand the characteristics that define an entrepreneur (psychological approach) and what the entrepreneur does (managerial approach). Second, providing a fundamental understanding of what entrepreneurs are like and what they do facilitates movement to the next stage in personal development that involves *how* to become an entrepreneur and implement the entrepreneurial process.

The Timmons Model of the Entrepreneurial Process

Overview of the Model. The Timmons Model of the Entrepreneurial Process (Figure 26.1) is one conceptual framework originating in the business academic world and field-tested and refined over several decades of research (Timmons & Spinelli, 2007). This holistic framework incorporates thinking from the economic, psychological, sociocultural, and managerial theoretical approaches as well as from systems theory. The framework derives from the principle that change is dynamic, normal, and healthy. This principle is consistent with research that indicates the major task in society and especially in the economy is to affect sustainability by doing something different as compared to doing better than is already being done (Drucker, 1985).

The Timmons Model (Figure 26.1) consists of a foundation, a founder, key elements, influential forces, important inputs, and one guiding map. The model emphasizes a managerial approach to entrepreneurship that is consistent with the definition that entrepreneurship is opportunity obsessed (economic theory), holistic in approach (systems theory), and leadership balanced (leadership/management theory).

TABLE 26.1

THEORETICAL APPROACHES TO THE STUDY OF ENTREPRENEURSHIP				
Level of Analysis	**Approaches**			
	Economic	**Psychological**	**Sociocultural**	**Managerial**
MICRO (Individual level)	• Entrepreneurial function as fourth factor of production • Theory of the entrepreneurial profit • Theory of occupational choice under uncertainty	• Traits theory • Psychodynamic theory	• Margination theory • Role theory • Network theory	• Leibenstein's x-efficiency theory • Behavioral theory of the entrepreneur • Modes of new enterprise creation • Modes to become an entrepreneur
MESO (Corporate level)	• Transaction cost theory		• Network theory • Incubator's theory • Evolutionary theory	• Modes of new enterprise success and failure • Corporate entrepreneurship
MACRO (Global or country level)	• Schumpeter's theory of economic development • Theory of the endogenous regional development	• Kirzner's entrepreneur theory	• Weber's theory of economic development • Theory of social change • Population ecology theory • Institutional theory	

Source: From Veciana (2007).

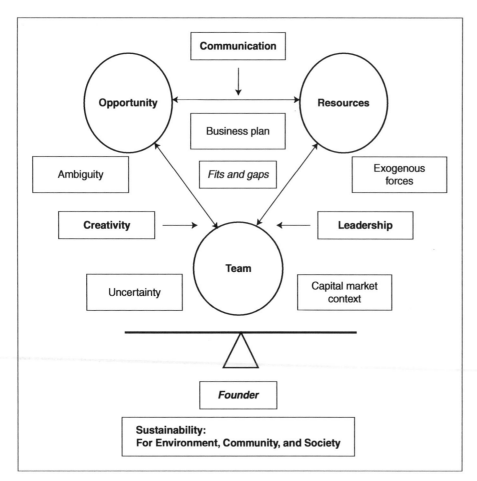

FIGURE 26.1 The Timmons Model of the Entrepreneurial Process.

Source: From Timmons & Spinelli (2007). Reproduced with permission.

The significance of the model is that it provides guidance in executing the entrepreneurial process in venture creation.

Sustainability is the foundation upon which the model is built. Sustainability involves the capacity to endure and to do so in a way that does not harm the environment, the community, or society. A common myth about entrepreneurship is that it only exists for monetary gain. Although wealth creation may be one consequence of entrepreneurship that enhances sustainability, pursuing a passion for achieving greater good is a more powerful motivator.

An entrepreneurial venture originates with the dreams or ideas of the company founder, the lead entrepreneur who starts the business. The founder operates much like a juggler balancing the dynamic interplay of three key elements in the changing environment: the entrepreneurial team, the opportunity, the resources. The entrepreneurial team consists of individuals who will assist the founder in seizing the business opportunity in order to achieve the organizational mission, vision, and goals. The opportunity consists not only of that good idea upon which the business was built but also all other opportunities that will arise within the business environment. The resources refer to the inputs needed to assist the

founder and the entrepreneurial team to maximize the business opportunity. These resources include not only money but also such components as people, raw materials, and technology.

The founder's major job is to take charge of the success equation. That is, this individual is tuned into various influential sources and the changing dynamics created by both ambiguity and uncertainty in the external environment. The founder also tunes into the capital market context to size up competitive challenges, changes in the marketplace, financial risk, and other exogenous forces of a legal or regulatory nature. In effect, the founder manages and redefines the risk–reward equation all with an eye toward sustainability. To do this, the founder uses important inputs of leadership, creativity, and communication skills to execute the conceived business plan (or guiding map) while also balancing the key elements and their related forces within the model.

Interaction of Component Parts. The major driving force of the Timmons Model is value creation (Timmons & Spinelli, 2007). The process is opportunity driven and guided by the lead entrepreneur and the entrepreneurial team. The entrepreneurial process is resource parsimonious and creative and depends on the fit and balance of component parts that are integrated, holistic, and sustainable. Components of the Timmons Model are controllable in that they can be assessed, influenced, and modified at any stage of venture growth. Founders as well as investors in a venture carefully analyze components of the model to determine business risk and improve the venture's chances for success.

The entrepreneurial process begins with first an opportunity. Successful entrepreneurs and investors understand that a good idea is not necessarily a good opportunity (Timmons & Spinelli, 2007). Over time, entrepreneurs learn to identify which ventures to pursue and which to drop. According to Timmons and Spinelli, a good opportunity is one that has four major characteristics. First, the product or service creates or adds value to a customer or end user. Second, the product or service either solves a significant problem or meets a want or need. The customer or end user must also be willing to pay a premium for the product or service. Third, the product or service has robust market size (large enough with reachable customers), significant margins (40% or more), growth potential (20+%growth), and strong and early free cash flow potential (recurring revenue, low assets, and low working capital). Lastly, there is a good fit with the founder, the entrepreneurial team, and the marketplace along with an attractive risk–reward equation.

One of the most common misconceptions among untested entrepreneurs is that all the resources including money must be in place to ensure venture success. In fact, the business literature suggests that thinking money first is a big mistake, primarily because money follows a high potential opportunity conceived and led by a strong management team (Timmons & Spinelli, 2007). Success stories abound of entrepreneurs who start significant businesses out of their garages using minimal resources to grow phenomenal products and services. Frugality in resource utilization at the early stages of a business may indeed provide a competitive advantage.

The entrepreneurial team is a key component of the entrepreneurial process. Success of a good idea rests squarely on the quality of the entrepreneurial team. Finding the right team members and achieving synergy between the business idea, the marketplace, the founder, and the entrepreneurial team are essential. To maximize success of the venture, a leader needs to be authentic (Shirey, 2006), a learner and teacher, resilient, and someone who builds an entrepreneurial culture and organization (this requires cultivating intrapreneurial activities). The entrepreneurial team needs to be competent, confident, motivated to excel, committed, creative, and courageous. Together, all parties need to be passionate about the venture, comfortable with ambiguity and uncertainty, flexible under varying conditions, opportunity obsessed, and receptive to open lines of communication.

Besides the key elements of opportunity, resources, and the entrepreneurial team is the importance of fit and balance between and among forces in the model. It must be noted in the model (Figure 26.1) that opportunity, resources, and the entrepreneurial team are all represented in circles of identical size. The dynamics of the entrepreneurial process are effective when each of the three key elements remain in balance. For example, an opportunity that is too large, has very limited resources, and is directed by a weak entrepreneurial team may not result in a most effective entrepreneurial process. Likewise, the same could result if the opportunity is too small despite adequate resources and a capable entrepreneurial team. The founder ultimately must balance all the elements, being cognizant of not only fit and balance but also of substance and timing. Success in this balancing act requires both analytical ability and intuition (sometimes acting on incomplete information) in order to create and sustain the ideal dynamics consistent with achieving the most effective entrepreneurial process.

Stages of Venture Growth

The entrepreneurial process and the creation of new ventures occurs within the backdrop of five stages in venture growth: research and development, start-up, high growth, maturity, and stability. Venture growth follows a theoretical view of gestation (growth, development, change) manifested by specific stages, distinct boundaries, and crucial transitions. Each stage also has implications for the type of financing commonly seen.

Stage 1, of venture growth, is the research and development (R&D) stage, sometimes called the nascent stage. This stage begins with the discovery of the business opportunity and continues until the business is launched. The R&D stage can be as short as a few months or last years. Research suggests that if the business idea does not become a going concern within 18 months, likelihood that the start-up business will launch falls dramatically (Timmons & Spinelli, 2007). At this stage, the business venture usually includes a single aspiring entrepreneur and a small team exploring the business idea and doing due diligence. Financing at this stage usually comes from the aspiring entrepreneur's personal funds or from some type of seed money (investor, grants, loans).

Stage 2, the start-up stage, covers the launching of the business up to the first 3 years of operation. The failure rate for businesses at this stage exceeds 60% (Timmons & Spinelli, 2007). This explains why this stage is the most risky and thus requires the exhaustive drive, energy, and talents of the business founder and the entrepreneurial team. During the start-up stage, the business interacts with a critical mass of people (customers, vendors, investors, and competitors). It is during this time that customer confidence and competitive resilience are established. Crucial transitions seen in this stage include rapid growth in both sales and employees. The founder and members of the entrepreneurial team support the employee base by doing whatever is needed to grow the business. Financing at this stage is usually from the lead entrepreneur's personal funds (or loans), private investors (friends or family), or venture capitalists.

Stage 3, the high growth stage, usually covers from 4 to 10 years although the length of this stage varies by company. Growth in sales and employees continues. Changes in the management mode are some of the most difficult transitions seen in this stage. As the business grows, the founder finds it increasingly difficult to both grow the company and manage the day-to-day operations. The founder begins to relinquish power and control, delegating more authority to others. Much of the founder's focus is in the short-term strategic planning needed to rapidly meet the overwhelming demands of the marketplace. Financing at this stage may come from the sale of new equity (initial public offering [IPO] or stocks) by the firm to public investors. An IPO allows the company to tap into a wide pool of stock market investors to provide significant capital that gets reinvested into the business. Investors have no further claim over the capital, but they do have a claim to future profits distributed by the company.

Stage 4, the maturity stage, lasts from 10 to 15 years and varies by company. The maturity stage is no longer about survival, but rather about steady and profitable growth. As the business continues to grow and stabilize (Stage 5, beyond 15 years), major crucial transitions include shifts in management (now founder manages managers), potential erosion of founder creativity, and additional working capital needs for renovation, expansion, or reinvention. Without a significant renaissance and corporate energy at Stage 5, the founder's and entrepreneurial team's hard work may be at risk. Company growth at Stage 5 requires corporate renewal or intrapreneurial efforts that should have been in place all along. Financing for company renewal efforts may come in the form of another public offering. In the absence of renewal efforts, the company could position itself for either a sale or be forced into liquidation. In the event of a sale, business owners should ideally have had an a priori harvest strategy in place to capture maximum value from the business.

In summary, the five stages of venture growth bring to bear different time periods, unique conditions, and crucial transitions. Given what is empirically known about the stages of venture growth, the pattern is predictable and informative. Learning from this science, the lead entrepreneur navigating the five stages of growth needs to know these stages are akin to periods of wonder (R&D stage), blunder (start-up stage), thunder (high growth stage), plunder (maturity), and asunder or renaissance of wonder (stability stage; Marram, 2003). During the wonder stage, companies experience great uncertainty about their survival. The blunder stage causes many companies to stumble and fall. The thunder stage allows for significant growth and the evolution of a strong management team. The plunder stage experiences robust cash flow. Lastly, asunder dictates that the company will either renew itself or risk decline.

RELEVANT LITERATURE

The business literature in entrepreneurship is well-grounded in an amalgamation of research and theory that draws from a variety of disciplines. This relevant review of the literature addresses empirical findings at the micro level of analysis (individual) and focuses on the psychological and managerial theoretical approaches (see Table 26.1).

General Entrepreneurship

Micro-Level Psychological Approach. Traits theory, a psychological approach, focuses on who the entrepreneur is and what characteristics define them to identify a profile of the person who decides to create a new enterprise. A synthesis of the literature suggests that the main psychological traits and motivations of the entrepreneur are apparent in a mostly distinct profile (Veciana, 2007). Although there is not an absolute and neat set of behavioral attributes that separates entrepreneurs from nonentrepreneurs, the research shows that the entrepreneur is usually intrinsically motivated and has a higher internal locus of control. Entrepreneurs have a common way of thinking or mind-set that exemplifies a strong need for independence and achievement. They have a propensity for moderated risk taking and the ability to trust their intuition. Entrepreneurs are unsatisfied with the status quo and, because of their high tolerance for ambiguity, can readily navigate in times of turbulence and great complexity.

In exploring motivators for self-employment, particularly in women and specifically addressing the "push and pull" debate, research suggests that women seek self-employment as a result of intrinsic motivation or "pull" factors (Hughes, 2003). Women entrepreneurs are primarily motivated by a desire for challenge, positive work environments, independence, and meaningful work. One third of the 61 participants in the Hughes study were motivated to pursue self-employment as a result of critical economic constraints ("pushed" due to corporate restructuring and downsizing). Although the "pulled" entrepreneurs reported higher levels of satisfaction than did the "pushed" entrepreneurs, overall the levels of satisfaction for both groups were reported to be very high. Interestingly, the "pushed" to self-employment group in this study underwent what the researcher termed an "ideological pull," resulting in the "push" entrepreneurs expressing reluctance to return to paid employment (Hughes, 2003).

The study of the entrepreneur's profile has also led to creation of a taxonomy of entrepreneurs, which further differentiates between high- and low-innovation entrepreneurs (Manimala, 1996). High-innovation entrepreneurs fall into one of seven subtypes: inventor/tinkerer, adventurer, searcher/problem solver, gap filler, social visionary, opportunity grabber, and specialist pioneer. The low-innovation entrepreneurs, on the other hand, fall into one of six subtypes: chance entrant, agent-turned-producer, concession grabber, obsessed producer, ancillary/imitator, and nonpioneer niche holder. The commonality that all entrepreneurs have is that they collectively are innovative. The high versus low distinction within the taxonomy, however, suggests that the high-innovation entrepreneurs are more proactive in executing the entrepreneurial process.

Scientific research in the entrepreneurial area of traits theory was very common in the 1970s, 1980s, and 1990s, but attention to this type of research has declined in recent years. That much is already known about the entrepreneurial psychological profile partially explains the decline in this type of research (Veciana, 2007). What is currently known about the entrepreneur's psychological traits and motivations contributes to the understanding of the skills and abilities that can be taught to foster entrepreneurial behaviors.

Micro-Level Managerial Approach. Behavioral theories of the entrepreneur, a managerial approach, focus on what the entrepreneur *does* rather than what the entrepreneur *is* (psychological approach). Synthesis of the literature suggests that entrepreneurial behaviors demonstrate seven distinct abilities (Veciana, 2007). These entrepreneurial behaviors include the abilities to search and gather information, identify opportunities, deal with risk, establish relationships and networks, and make decisions under uncertainty and ambiguity. Additionally, entrepreneurs have leadership ability as well as the ability to learn from experience and to bounce back quickly from failure.

The entrepreneur's behavior is said to be a reflection of the individual's personal motivations that, in turn, are dependent on environmental characteristics (Stevenson & Jarillo, 2007). This psychosociological point of view was pioneered by David McClelland's (1961) best-selling book, *The Achieving Society*. McClelland's seminal work helped to explain why some societies exhibit high economic and social growth, attributing such growth to the need for achievement. McClelland's research provided the foundation to explain how the environment affects the practice of entrepreneurship.

Beyond the influence of personal motivation on behavior is the understanding that the nature and existence of the managerial team affects the likelihood of positive outcomes in entrepreneurship (Stevenson & Jarillo, 2007). The work by Timmons and Spinelli (2007), as captured in the Timmons Model of the Entrepreneurial Process (Figure 26.1), explains and supports the importance of the managerial behaviors of *both* the lead entrepreneur and the entrepreneurial team. Entrepreneurship within this framework is more than just starting up a new business; it is also a mode of management (beyond traditional management) designed to relentlessly pursue opportunities and achieve desirable results. Accordingly, Timmons and Spinelli identify five broad competencies of entrepreneurial management to include (a) skill in building an entrepreneurial culture (intrapreneurship rises to the top here); (b) leadership, vision, and influence; (c) helping, coaching, and conflict management; (d) teamwork and people management; and (e) other management competencies, including but not limited to marketing, operations/production, finance, law and taxes, project management, negotiations, and information technology.

Nurse Entrepreneurship

Although anecdotal publications on nurse entrepreneurship abound, few research-based articles are available in the literature. A synthesis of the empirical literature on nurse entrepreneurship practice suggests that the first article was published in 1998, and most studies are small ($n = 4$ to 59) and exploratory in nature (Shirey, 2007). The studies available report on nurse entrepreneurship in the United States (Elango, 2007; Roggenkamp & White, 1998), Australia (Wilson, Averis, & Walsh, 2003, 2004), and the United Kingdom (Austin, Luker, & Ronald, 2006). What is empirically known from these studies falls into the categories of the micro-level psychological and managerial approaches. Motivation and traits of the nurse entrepreneur as well as the skill set of the nurse entrepreneur have been studied using qualitative research designs.

Micro-Level Psychological Approach. Motivation for the nurse entrepreneur includes key drivers, business factors, and personal factors (Shirey, 2007). Drivers that motivate nurse entrepreneurs are a love of nursing, self-efficacy as nursing professionals, a desire to make a difference, influence of family (Roggenkamp & White, 1998), and the ability to see opportunities (Elango, 2007). The love for nursing comes from professional experience in traditional practice settings such as hospitals. Most nurses have 3 to 15 years nursing experience before they become self-employed as entrepreneurs (ICN, 2004). The self-efficacy results from professional competence and confidence developed over years of practice. Given their love of nursing and their expertise in the field, nurse entrepreneurs feel they have the unique abilities and strong beliefs that can make a difference in the lives of their clients. Support from family has been shown to be a strong motivator to leave traditional nursing practice settings. A small qualitative study (*n* = 4) by Roggenkamp and White (1998) reported that in 3 of 4 participants, the entrepreneurial shift came as a result of personal reinvention and a desire to have more time with family. Nurse entrepreneurs identified changing demographic trends and opportunities within health care facilities as factors that encouraged their decisions to become entrepreneurs.

The business factors primarily address the perceived enablers and disablers to nurse entrepreneurship. Nurse entrepreneurs report factors that facilitate entrepreneurship are enablers, and these include outside assistance during start-up, mentors, the need to make change (boredom and burnout), and some critical life event (Roggenkamp & White, 1998). A significant disabler or factor that hinders nurse entrepreneurship includes perceived lack of business skills, particularly in the areas of finance, billing and collections, law, regulation, and operational management of a business. Overwhelmingly, nurse entrepreneurs report that their traditional nursing education (at any level) does not prepare them for practice in nontraditional roles such as nurse entrepreneurship. Nurse entrepreneurs report a lack of connectivity between nurse entrepreneurs. Additionally, they report a lack of not only professional and collegial support for private practice but also experiencing negative attitudes of other health care professionals toward nurses in private practice (Wilson et al., 2004).

The personal factors that motivate nurse entrepreneurs include their commitment to a quality mission and their desire to stay close to their clients. These personal factors are identical to the factors that motivated early nurse entrepreneurs to engage in case-by-case care and hold firmly to practice as private duty nurses. This ability to stay close to the client and focus on mission over profit is seen by nurse entrepreneurs as a higher order reward.

The profile of the nurse entrepreneur incorporates characteristics of the traditional business entrepreneur. That is, nurse entrepreneurs are opportunity driven, goal directed, risk taking, creative, assertive, and have strong leadership abilities. Research suggests other important characteristics of the nurse entrepreneur include accountability, commitment, perseverance, good self-esteem, and determination to succeed (Wilson et al., 2003).

The finding by Hughes (2003) in the business world that entrepreneurs follow the "pull" route to entrepreneurship is consistent with the nurse entrepreneurship empirical literature. Most nurses reportedly go into business not because they are unemployable (argument for "pushed" entrepreneurs), but rather because they seek to make a difference in their own way ("pulled" entrepreneurs; Wilson et al., 2003).

Micro-Level Managerial Approach. Nurse entrepreneurs report clinical practice, consultancy, or education as their primary work domain, also identifying research as a less important aspect of the role (Wilson et al., 2004). Consultancy is the most reported nurse entrepreneur activity and is also the most lucrative. Although what nurse entrepreneurs actually do in the role is not mostly managerial, they identify operational and managerial competencies as important for success in the role.

Overall, nurse entrepreneurs report their operational and managerial competencies in venture creation to be weak (Elango, 2007; Wilson et al., 2004). Perceived lack of business skills, particularly in finance, legal issues, and running the day-to-day operations of a business are nurse entrepreneurship disablers. Nurse entrepreneurs may see that knowledge of business is not their forte; nevertheless, they still have the "can do" mind-set to see threats as opportunities and to move forward to correct the perceived deficiencies. Nurse entrepreneurs also realize the difficulty of learning the requisite business skills while simultaneously running the day-to-day operations of a new business (Roggenkamp & White, 1998).

Experienced nurse entrepreneurs suggest the need to improve not only planning and management skills but also networking abilities (Wilson et al., 2004) because these are used daily in the role. To facilitate nurse entrepreneurship, collegial working relationships with peers are essential. The loosely connected and underdeveloped field of nurse entrepreneurship, however, makes executing the role more difficult (Shirey, 2007).

ROLE OF THE NURSE ENTREPRENEUR

Scope of Practice

Nurse entrepreneurs practice in a variety of settings, and the scope of practice is broad. As self-employed nurses, entrepreneurs can legally offer any service that falls within the practice of nursing and does not infringe on the legislated responsibility or the exclusive practice of another health discipline (ICN, 2004). Nurse entrepreneur roles and work settings vary with public demand for services. Increasingly, nurse entrepreneurs use their expertise to develop ventures that not only meet the needs of clients but also are professionally and personally fulfilling.

Roles for nurses as entrepreneurs are diverse and can include being a clinician/practitioner, teacher, consultant, therapist, researcher, case manager, writer, expert witness, business owner, partner, franchise operator, or niche provider. In all roles, nurses combine standard business practices with application of the nursing process to provide a unique product or service that improves the health status of the populations served.

Issues

Ethical Considerations. High ethical standards and integrity are crucial to the long-term success of the entrepreneurial venture. As nurse entrepreneurs, integrity and transparency must guide the multiple roles of business owner, employer, practitioner, and corporate citizen. This obligation requires congruence between the entrepreneur's values and the goals of the business and mandates both a macro and a micro approach. From the macro approach, the nurse entrepreneur establishes the business organization's guiding values and creates an organizational culture that supports ethically sound behavior. The nurse entrepreneur personally models high ethical standards and instills in all employees a sense of shared accountability to uphold those standards. From a micro approach, the nurse entrepreneur as health care provider sets fees for services expecting a profit, but also follows principles of fairness and just value. The nurse entrepreneur realistically presents expected benefits of the business services and follows strict guidelines for open disclosure of any conflicts of interest. Business decisions are patient centered and focus on doing the right thing, while also providing quality services consistent with evidence-based practice and appropriate standards of care. The nurse entrepreneur as employer pays employees fair wages, provides employees with a healthy work environment

for practice, and meets all legal, tax, and regulatory requirements of the business and the industry.

Economic Considerations. Nurse entrepreneurs starting a new venture face an uncertain future with potential fluctuations in income and lack of job security. For this reason, due diligence is an important concept for aspiring nurse entrepreneurs to comprehend. Prior to launching a new venture, the nurse entrepreneur should at a minimum make a determination as to whether the business opportunity meets the criteria for a "good" opportunity. The business concept needs to be explored with the advantages and disadvantages of the potential venture clearly understood. To minimize risk, enhance knowledge and critical thinking about the venture, and to ensure sources of external funding (small business grants or venture capital), the aspiring entrepreneur should develop a business plan. In addition to positioning the entrepreneur for external funding, development of a business plan forces the entrepreneur to consider multiple potential issues and challenges related to the venture.

Nurses considering an entrepreneurial venture must explore any personal turmoil regarding business (money issues) and traditional nursing forces (caring issues). Nurse entrepreneurs "are usually able to reconcile these competing forces by reinforcing their ability to be mission-driven and envision their unique potential for making a difference in the lives of clients" (Shirey, 2007, p. 234). Because traditional hospital-based nursing care does not usually isolate costs, charges, and revenue for nursing services, most nurses have difficulty quantifying the economic value of nursing services. Lack of experience with this cost/charge/revenue equation makes it difficult for nurses to develop an equitable fee for services structure. When calculating fees, the nurse entrepreneur must take into account multiple factors: complexity of the task, professional responsibility implied by the service, level of expertise required inclusive of costs for subcontractors, and time involved to produce the product or service, plus travel, expense for equipment, supplies, and supportive staff needed. When pricing a product or service, the entrepreneur must be cognizant of the fair profit desired and the going market rate for the service. Hard decisions need to be made in terms of which products and services the nurse entrepreneur can afford to provide and still stay in business.

Legal and Regulatory Considerations. Prior to launching a new venture, the nurse entrepreneur should obtain legal advice regarding many aspects of the business. Some legal and regulatory issues to consider include decisions regarding the company name, administrative offices for the business, ownership and protection of technology (trade secrets, patents, copyrights, trademarks), record keeping, security issues, insurance coverage (professional liability, general liability, director's and officer's liability, umbrella coverage, property and casualty, worker's compensation, business interruption, life and disability insurance for key company officers, health, retirement), and permits to operate the business, file claims (provider number), or get paid for services (tax identification number). A full discussion of all the legal and regulatory issues the entrepreneur must consider is beyond the scope of this chapter. For purposes of this section, only the decision regarding the business organizational structure is briefly presented. Selecting the organizational structure for the business (sole proprietorship, partnership, limited liability company [LLC] or corporation) is an important decision that has economic, tax, and liability implications.

A sole proprietorship exists when an individual goes into business for him- or herself (Weaver, 2005–2007). To form a sole proprietorship requires no state or federal filing requirements. The business owner still must comply with all state, local, and/or federal obligations for licensure, business permits, tax payments (property, payroll, sales taxes), and other requirements and regulations. A sole proprietorship is not a separate and distinct legal entity from the owner; in essence, business owners do business in their own name. The main advantage of this type of organizational structure is that it is the easiest way an individual can operate a business. There are no legal formalities to forming or dissolving a sole proprietorship. For tax purposes, income flows on a cash basis directly to the business owner who then reports the income (including business losses and profits) in an individual income tax return and is taxed at the self-employment rate. Setting up a sole proprietorship is inexpensive, proving beneficial for start-ups with limited capital. The major disadvantage of a sole proprietorship is that the business owner is personally liable for all debts and actions of the company. Another disadvantage is that a sole proprietorship will likely have a hard time raising capital for the business.

A general partnership is formed when two or more people operate a business together and share in the profits and losses (Weaver, 2005–2007). Most states require general partnerships to file a certificate of partnership (or its equivalent) with the appropriate state agency. Individuals in general partnerships are taxed as a sole proprietorship. The business owner obligations (in this case multiple partners) are the same as in a sole proprietorship except that with a general partnership, the management responsibilities may be divided. The advantages of a general partnership include having a shared financial commitment, pooling of expertise, and limited start-up costs. The disadvantages include finding a partner who shares a similar vision and goals for the business, partners have personal liability for business debts and liabilities, and there might be difficulties in attracting investors in the business.

An LLC is a separate legal entity that limits the liability of its members (the multiple owners). In an LLC, company profits and losses are passed through the business and taxed on the member's individual tax return. The major advantages of the LLC are that members get the tax advantage of a partnership, while also having the limited liability benefits of the corporation. Members in the LLC can either manage the LLC or hire a management group to run the company. Members also can split the profits and losses any way they wish. Forming an LLC is more complex than a sole proprietorship in that it requires the development of a charter document (Articles of Organization) for filing in the appropriate state. A disadvantage of the LLC is that some states impose income or franchise taxes on LLCs or require payment of state annual fees to operate in that state. The LLC requires the development of a written operating agreement, a document similar to a partnership agreement. Another potential disadvantage of the LLC is that because it is a relatively new type of business entity (Weaver, 2005–2007), there is not much legal precedent available to help owners make predictions on legal disputes.

The corporation is the oldest and most prestigious legal entity, one that is separate from its owners (Weaver, 2005–2007). Like LLCs, corporations limit the personal liability (debts, legal claims, other obligations) of the owners (called shareholders). The major advantage of a corporation is its tax advantages and protection of individual liability. The corporation's debt is not considered that of its owners. The major disadvantage of the corporation is that they are the most expensive to form, and they are subject to complex tax rules. Governance in corporations is more formal, complex, and expensive. Management within a corporation requires officers and directors with their roles specified in the corporation bylaws. Corporations may have shareholders that would require development and adherence to a shareholder agreement. The corporation must be established in accordance with the applicable laws of the jurisdiction in which the entity is formed and will require development of a charter document (Articles of Incorporation).

Personal Considerations. Before individuals decide to be nurse entrepreneurs, they must first ask themselves many personal questions: Is this what I *really* want to do? Do I have it in me to be a nurse entrepreneur? Am I willing to put in the long hours it takes to get this business off the ground and successful? Do I have the necessary support structures in place to help me pursue the nurse entrepreneurship journey?

Given that personal and professional isolation is a possible negative consequence of nurse entrepreneurship, individuals must explore this reality and develop proactive strategies to address this phenomenon. It may be that the nurse entrepreneur can combat the isolation by becoming involved in multiple professional venues that not only keep the nurse entrepreneur socially and professionally connected but also allow for networking that provides exposure and a potential business referral base.

Maintaining a quality professional practice will also require the nurse entrepreneur to stay abreast of standards of practice and health policy matters related to the business and the specific industry. This requires the nurse entrepreneur to actively engage in ongoing professional and career development efforts plus also become involved in specific advocacy issues related to the nurse entrepreneur's business and industry.

APPLICATION TO CNS PRACTICE

At first glance, the role of nurse entrepreneur may appear overwhelming. CNSs, however, have an advantage primarily because their current role as APNs requires many of the elements of entrepreneurship. In looking at the definition of entrepreneurship, CNSs already have a level of proficiency in being opportunity obsessed, holistic in approach, and leadership balanced. CNSs continuously look at ways to improve the health status of the populations they serve. By virtue of their education and experience, CNSs are routinely astute regarding improvements in processes and systems that "raise the bar" for advanced nursing practice. From the holistic perspective, CNS practice addresses the whole of the human experience while also incorporating complexity, systems thinking, and learning from multiple disciplines. Working within all three spheres of influence (patient/client, nurses/nursing practice, and organization/systems), CNSs engage in interprofessional collaboration to achieve desired outcomes (National Association of Clinical Nurse Specialists [NACNS], 2004). CNSs also use their leadership skills on a daily basis to skillfully communicate, educate, and anticipate the future accurately (NACNS).

What CNSs lack and what nurse entrepreneurship research confirms is that aspiring nurse entrepreneurs need a better understanding of the requisite business management skills (finance/managerial accounting, business law, strategic planning, and operations management) to run the day-to-day operations of a business. This skill set certainly can either be taught or found in a capable business partner. Through proper guidance and mentorship, CNSs can gain the requisite business knowledge and savvy to complement their nursing knowledge, further broaden their sphere of influence, and maximize their value as nurse entrepreneurs. Early in the CNS role what aspiring nurse entrepreneurs need is a road map that directs them on *how* to become nurse entrepreneurs. Such a road map, albeit in an abbreviated form, may be found at the end of this chapter.

EVALUATION

Measurement Outcomes

Although CNSs have a long history as health care providers, their unique contributions to patient care and the resultant nurse-sensitive outcomes they generate are not fully understood (Dayhoff & Lyon, 2001). CNS practice affects three spheres of influence, and it is through these spheres that CNS core competencies and actions are thought to affect CNS outcomes (NACNS, 2004).

The nurse entrepreneur outcomes documented include the establishment of nurse-run businesses founded upon the entrepreneur's clinical expertise, business ventures making a difference, desired lifestyle for the entrepreneur, achievement of desired working relationships, emergence of expert status, and leaving a legacy for the profession. Because the nurse entrepreneur studies cited used nurse participants (non-CNSs) with competencies similar to those of the CNS, the study findings could be generalizable to the CNS population of entrepreneurs (Austin et al., 2006; Elango, 2007; Roggenkamp & White, 1998; Wilson et al., 2003, 2004). Further research is needed to study the practices of CNSs who are also entrepreneurs in order to establish the hypothesized relationships.

The more extensive business entrepreneurship (nonnursing) research literature documents additional nonfinancial and financial benefits of entrepreneurship at the various levels of analysis (micro, meso, macro; Luke, Verreynne, & Kearins, 2007). Nonfinancial benefits of entrepreneurship in the business literature include independence, autonomy, competitive advantage, increased market share, employment, and increased standard of living. The financial benefits of entrepreneurship in the business literature include enhanced remuneration from revenue, profits, cash flow, and return on investment. It would also be prudent to study the relationship between CNS core competencies and the entrepreneur outcomes documented in the business literature. It may be hypothesized that the relationships documented for nonnursing entrepreneurs will also hold for the CNS entrepreneur.

CONCLUSIONS

Pursuing nurse entrepreneurship is not an easy professional path, and it is not for everyone. When chosen, the entrepreneurship journey has the potential for having great impact on individuals and communities. That entrepreneurship significantly fuels economic growth is a powerful statement. That it makes a meaningful contribution to society is a profound and sobering reality. CNSs possess a unique skill set, knowledge base, and abilities that position them well for nurse entrepreneurship practice. Taking the step toward CNS entrepreneurship practice offers the opportunity to liberate the CNSs' unique nursing knowledge and to deploy it for potential betterment of both distinct populations and society at large.

HOW TO BECOME A NURSE ENTREPRENEUR: A STEP-BY-STEP APPROACH

Step 1
A. Conduct a self-assessment that compares the knowledge, skills, and abilities (KSA) of the aspiring nurse entrepreneur with that of the established nurse entrepreneur identified in the literature. Use the following parameters for the assessment:
   1. Expertise in area of professional passion for making a difference
   2. Sense of self-efficacy (competence, confidence, connectedness)
   3. Support systems available (mentors, coaches, family) to pursue goals
   4. Business skills and knowledge about finance, law, regulation, general management, and the operation of a business
   5. Ability to see and seize opportunities
   6. Ability to be goal directed, committed, and determined to succeed
   7. Risk-taking abilities, tolerance for uncertainty and ambiguity, and personal resilience
   8. Sense of creativity and innovativeness
   9. Leadership, communication, and networking abilities
   10. Assertiveness, self-discipline, and personal directedness in achieving a desired future
B. Begin self-awareness exercise to identify personal and professional passions that could potentially become a nursing business. Conceptualize the business ideas inclusive of the potential market, resources, and services.

Step 2
A. Develop a self-improvement plan based on findings from the self-assessment.

Note: Nurse entrepreneurs advocate learning the requisite business skills *prior* to and not concurrent with launching a new business. Learning these skills requires tapping into available resources within the community, books, and/or online.

Step 3
A. Identify mentors or a personal coach to help develop or support the aspiring nurse entrepreneur in implementing and critiquing progress with the self-improvement plan.

Step 4
A. Utilize a current employment setting or external community volunteer role as a training site to practice and develop the identified nurse entrepreneur KSA needed. This may involve taking the challenge to be an intrapreneur in the current employment setting and volunteering for projects and assignments that develop the needed skill set.

Step 5
A. Revisit findings from the self-awareness exercise to reconnect with earlier thoughts of the potential nursing business venture.
B. Reassess viability and configuration of this option now that a self-improvement plan, personal coach, and practice with the nurse entrepreneur skill development have taken place.
C. End this step with reconfiguring and shaping the potential business idea inclusive of product or service to be provided and having an idea as to the business name, logo, and color scheme for the business and promotional materials.

Step 6
A. Write the business plan for the proposed venture. If assistance is needed to develop this plan, tap into resources of the U.S. Small Business Administration (SBA), either online or at a local community office.
B. Develop an action plan that addresses each component of the business plan.
C. Identify members of the entrepreneurial team, including a strong management team.

Step 7
A. Seek legal and/or accounting advice regarding what type of organizational structure to pursue (sole proprietorship, partnership, limited liability corporation, corporation) and assistance in ensuring that the appropriate local, state, and federal licenses, permits, and registrations have been accounted for and incorporated into the business plan.
B. Register the strategically conceived (name captures the unique services of the business) Internet domain for the future business website.

Step 8

A. Using information from Steps 6 and 7, determine sources of funding (personal, loan, equity, grant, venture capitalist) for business venture.

B. Proceed to finalize the sources of venture funding.

C. Establish business relationship with a bank and a banker.

D. Open two business checking accounts at the selected bank: a payroll account and a business operations account. Seek assignment of a designated account executive and sign up for minimum account balance protection.

E. Concurrent with opening the checking accounts, an accounting system will need to be developed including a chart of accounts to keep track of business income and expenses. A separate payroll system to keep track of employee hiring documents, time cards, payroll checks for employees, payroll records, payroll taxes, and related reporting systems (weekly, monthly, quarterly, annual) is also needed. A competent individual will either need to be hired or subcontracted to maintain the appropriate record-keeping and accounting systems for both business and payroll functions.

Step 9

A. File for appropriate legal structure for the business, taking into account that the more complex the organizational structure, the longer the lead time to finalize the requirements for the organizational structure.

B. Concurrently submit for the appropriate tax identification (federal, state, local) and provider numbers.

Step 10

A. Establish the business location for the administrative offices. Find the appropriate office space, furniture, equipment, technology (hardware, software programs, data protection and backup protocols, filing systems), and communication (land phones, cell phones, standard phone service, long-distance service, high-speed Internet service, answering service, fax machines, photocopiers, scanners, postage meter) systems for the business start-up. Office, business, and medical supplies will also need to be purchased.

Step 11

A. Commission development of the business logo along with business stationery, business cards, informal note cards, and related promotional materials. Using the business logo, order appropriate building signage and telephone directory advertisements for the business. Concurrently, have available a preliminarily developed website using the preobtained business domain. The nurse entrepreneur should not be too concerned if the initial website is not as elaborate as ultimately desired; there is time later to refine the virtual business presence.

Step 12

A. Design office systems with internal controls to address the various aspects of the business: client services and core operations, business/finance/accounting services and operations, and human resource functions. This will require development of multiple policy and procedure manuals and related forms to address client care (patient flow, standards of practice, quality assurance, documentation of services), business office operations (billing and collection procedures, accounts payable, accounts receivables, financial management and reporting), and personnel policies (employment application procedures, hiring policies, training and education programs, record keeping).

B. Purchase all necessary insurance as specified in the business plan.

Step 13

A. Begin recruiting, interviewing, and screening potential new employees needed for the business start-up.

Step 14

A. Establish a short "soft opening" period for the business as a means to fine-tune operations prior to a "grand" opening.

B. Make necessary improvements following evaluation of soft opening.

C. Have developed and ready to launch the business marketing and advertising campaigns. Launch these campaigns to coincide with the end of the "soft" opening.

D. Aggressively pursue the marketing and advertising campaign to procure new clients and begin establishing a referral base for future clients.

Step 15

A. Hold "grand" opening for the business.

B. Make necessary improvements following evaluation of grand opening.

Step 16

A. Design continuous quality improvement program to regularly monitor key aspects of the operation:

1. Clients: Are patients satisfied? Are those who are sending clients satisfied? What can be done better and how? Are we meeting regulatory standards and/or expected standards of care?

2. Business/accounting: How are we doing with our billing and collections? What are the trends we see? What can we do better and how?

3. Human resources: How are our employees doing? Are they competent and adequately trained? Are they engaged and happy? What could we do better and how?

Step 17

A. Frequently tap into the business support team (attorney, accountant, banker, management team, employees, clients) for advice and suggestions for improvement.
B. Frequently review the business plan and assess progress.
C. Continue to work, work, work, evaluate, improve, and reevaluate.

Step 18

A. Seek advice from potential sources outside of the business support team: advisory board, community representatives.

Step 19

A. Promote the business within the community and beyond through involvement in civic activities and the chamber of commerce.
B. Extend involvement to national venues through speaking and writing engagements.

Step 20

A. Conduct a full-scale evaluation of the business annually and make timely modifications as needed.
B. Plan for the future, following yearly strategic planning sessions and taking into account the stages of venture growth.

▧ DISCUSSION QUESTIONS

- How should entrepreneurship concepts be introduced into the CNS curriculum? To address the learning needs of a CNS considering entrepreneurship as a part of the CNS role, what would you envision the curriculum to look like for the 21st century?
- Conceptualize a business venture, and apply and explain the Timmons Model for the first 5 years of the new venture.
- Think of a successful nurse entrepreneur you know, and identify that individual's KSA. Compare these KSAs with the available nurse entrepreneur empirical evidence in the literature. What additional research questions related to nurse entrepreneur (individual) attributes and actions would you generate? Any other research questions related to the nurse entrepreneur's interactions with groups

(meso level) and organizational systems (macro level)?
- Using the unique CNS lens, identify 10 gaps in patient/client care that could be addressed through CNS intervention. Generate a list of as many possible CNS-related new ventures that could address the identified gaps in patient/client care.
- Identify the entrepreneurial culture at your current organization. What strategies would you utilize to change or enhance the entrepreneurial culture at your current organization? Is it possible? Why or why not?
- Why is the entrepreneurial team/lead entrepreneur relationship so important in the entrepreneurial process? Considering your past experiences leading a team, what strategies as a lead entrepreneur would you contribute to the effective dynamic of the entrepreneurial team? Why?

RESOURCES TO EXPLORE

Books

1. Allen, K. (2002). *Entrepreneurship for dummies*. New York, NY: Wiley.
2. Avillion, A. E. (2005). *Nurse entrepreneurship: The art of running your own business*. Minneapolis, MN: Creative Health Care Management.
3. Bemis, P. A. (2007). *Self-employed RN: Choices, business aspects, and marketing strategies*. Rockledge, FL: National Nurses in Business Association, Inc.

Journals

1. *Wall Street Journal* (online.wsj.com/public/us)
2. *Entrepreneur Magazine* (www.entrepreneur. com)
3. *Harvard Business Review* (hbr.harvardbusiness. org)
4. *Journal of Entrepreneurship* (joe.sagepub.com)
5. *Entrepreneurship Theory and Practice Journal* (www.wiley.com/bw/journal.asp?ref= 1042–2587)

Websites

1. National Nurses in Business Association: www. nnba.net/index.htm
2. National Association of Independent Nurses: www.independentrn.com
3. Nurse Entrepreneurship Network: www.nurse-entrepreneur-network.com

REFERENCES

Austin, L., Luker, K., & Ronald, M. (2006). Clinical nurse specialists as entrepreneurs: Constrained or liberated. *Journal of Clinical Nursing, 15,* 1540–1549.

Dayhoff, N. E., & Lyon, B. L. (2001). Assessing outcomes in clinical nurse specialist practice. In R. M. Kleinpell (Ed.), *Outcome assessment in advanced practice nursing* (pp. 103–129). New York, NY: Springer.

Dossey, B. M. (2000). *Florence Nightingale: Mystic, visionary, healer.* Springhouse, PA: Springhouse Corporation.

Drucker, P. F. (1985). *Innovation and entrepreneurship.* New York, NY: Harper Business.

Elango, B. (2007). Barriers to nurse entrepreneurship: A study of the process model of entrepreneurship. *Journal of the American Academy of Nurse Practitioners, 19,* 198–204.

Falcone, T., & Osborne, S. (2005). *Entrepreneurship: A diverse concept in a diverse world.* Retrieved January 25, 2009, from http://www.sbaer.uca.edu/research/usasbe/2005/pdffiles/papers/21.pdf

Hughes, K. (2003). Pushed or pulled? Women's entry into self-employment and small business ownership. *Gender, Work and Organization, 10,* 433–454.

International Council of Nurses (ICN). (2004). *Guidelines on the nurse entre/intrapreneur providing nursing service.* Geneva, Switzerland: Author.

Luke, B., Verreynne, M. L., & Kearins, K. (2007). Measuring the benefits of entrepreneurship at different levels of analysis. *Journal of Management and Organization, 13*(4), 312–330.

Macrae, N. (1982). *Intrapreneurial now.* Retrieved January 29, 2009, from http://www.intrapreneur.com/MainPages/History/Economist.html

Manimala, M. J. (1996). Beyond innovators and imitators: A taxonomy of entrepreneurs. *Creativity and Innovation Management, 5,* 179–189.

Marram, E. P. (2003). *Managing the growing business: Six stages of growth.* Retrieved January 25, 2009, from http://homepage.cem.itesm.mx/maria.fonseca/master/documents/Growth.pdf

McClelland, D. C. (1961). *The achieving society.* Princeton, NJ: Van Nostrand and Company.

National Association of Clinical Nurse Specialists (NACNS). (2004). *Statement on clinical nurse specialist practice and education* (2nd ed.). Harrisburg, PA: Author.

National Association of the Self-Employed. (2004). *2004 Future entrepreneur: America's young entrepreneurs trend data at-a-glance.* Retrieved October 12, 2007, from http://www.nase.org/fey/youngentrepreneurs_stats.htm

Pinchot, G., & Pellman, R. (1985). *Intrapreneuring in action: A handbook for business innovation.* San Francisco, CA: Berrett-Koehler Publishers.

Roggenkamp, S. D., & White, K. R. (1998). Four nurse entrepreneurs: What motivated them to start their own businesses. *Health Care Manage Review, 23,* 67–75.

Schorr, T. M., & Kennedy, M. S. (1999). *100 years of American nursing: Celebrating a century of caring.* Philadelphia, PA: Lippincott.

Shane, S., & Venkataraman, S. (2007). The promise of entrepreneurship as a field of research. In A. Cuervo, D. Ribeiro, & S. Roig (Eds.), *Entrepreneurship: Concepts, theory and perspective* (pp. 171–184). Berlin, Germany: Springer.

Shirey, M. R. (2006). Building authentic leadership and enhancing entrepreneurial performance. *Clinical Nurse Specialist, 20,* 280–282.

Shirey, M. R. (2007). An evidence-based understanding of entre-preneurship in nursing. *Clinical Nurse Specialist, 21,* 234–240.

Stevenson, H. H., & Jarillo, J. C. (2007). A paradigm of entrepreneurship: Entrepreneurial management. In A. Cuervo, D. Ribeiro, & S. Roig (Eds.), *Entrepreneurship: Concepts, theory and perspective* (pp. 155–170). Berlin, Germany: Springer.

Timmons, J. A., & Spinelli, S. (2007). *New venture creation: Entrepreneurship for the 21st century* (7th ed.). New York, NY: McGraw Hill.

U.S. Chamber of Commerce. (2006). *Work, entrepreneurship, and opportunity in 21st century America.* Retrieved January 25, 2009, from http://www.uschamber.com/NR/rdonlyres/egd6apsvvwg333lvhlomles6lietyvlomlujv4o65b6z7jns4f7nsac6wry5hs6fldzwko5zwt6bwueo4e7gu6pyb2g/21st_final.pdf

Veciana, J. M. (2007). Entrepreneurship as a scientific research programme. In A. Cuervo, D. Ribeiro, & S. Roig (Eds.), *Entrepreneurship: Concepts, theory and perspective* (pp. 23–71). Berlin, Germany: Springer.

Weaver, J. W. (2005–2007). *A start-up businesses guide to choosing the right form of entity (S-Corp, LLC or Sole-Proprietor).* Retrieved January 25, 2009, from http://www.hg.org/article.asp?id=4790

Wilson, A., Averis, A., & Walsh, K. (2003). The influence on and experience of becoming nurse entrepreneurs: A Delphi study. *International Journal of Nursing Practice, 9,* 236–245.

Wilson, A., Averis, A., & Walsh, K. (2004). The scope of private practice nursing in an Australian sample. *Public Health Nursing, 21,* 488–494.

Regulatory and Professional Credentialing of Clinical Nurse Specialists

Brenda L. Lyon

The purpose of this chapter is to provide an overview of credentialing for advanced practice registered nurses (APRNs) and clinical nurse specialists (CNSs), in particular. *Credentialing* refers to the processes by which individuals and agencies are designated by a qualified agent as having met minimum standards and requirements at a specified time (American Nurses Association [ANA], 1979; ICN, 1997). Credentialing processes include both legal or regulatory mechanisms to authorize practice, such as licensure and registration, as well as professional mechanisms, including certification, privileging, and accreditation. The primary purpose of credentialing in health care is to help ensure public safety.

Credentialing is a dynamic and ever-changing area affecting CNSs and CNS practice. Understanding the requirements for various types of credentialing is essential for CNSs to legitimately establish themselves in practice. This chapter presents a discussion of the types of credentialing, including legal mechanisms that authorize an individual to practice, historical context, professional certification, accreditation of schools of nursing, and privileging to practice within an institution. The chapter concludes with a section on current issues and future trends.

LEGAL AUTHORIZATION TO PRACTICE AS A REGISTERED NURSE (RN) AND CNS

The Tenth Amendment to the U.S. Constitution grants states the power to enact laws to protect the public. Thus, states enact laws, also known as statutes. A statute is a formal written enactment of a legislative action that requires or prohibits something. The word *statute* is commonly used to differentiate between laws made by legislative action versus regulations issued by government agencies that have the power of law. A *regulation* is a form of secondary legislation promulgated by a government agency that guides the appropriate implementation of a primary piece of legislation. For example, rules and regulations are issued by state boards of nursing to implement the state's nurse practice act (statute) governing the practice of nursing. The legal authorization to practice can be granted via licensure or registration (Lyon & Minarik, 2001; National Council of State Boards of Nursing [NCSBN], 2005).

Licensure

Licensure is the legal authorization to practice a profession within a designated scope of practice.

Typically, but not always, licensure not only prohibits the use of a designated title, such as RN, or CNS, by an unqualified person, but it also prohibits someone who does not meet the requirements from practicing within the designated scope of practice. The purpose of licensure is to protect the health, safety, and welfare of the public by ensuring a minimal level of professional competence. Licensure requirements include the educational requirements that must be met and the means by which the individual must demonstrate minimal competency to begin practice as a licensed practitioner. Licensure occurs at and is regulated at the state level.

Licensure laws delegate the responsibility for enforcement to state administrative agencies. The agency responsible for regulating the practice of nursing is each state's respective state board of nursing. The statutory law in each state governing the practice of nursing is commonly known as the nurse practice act. Nurse practice acts and related rules and regulations can be accessed via each state board of nursing's website.

History of RN Licensure

Prior to discussing licensure as it pertains to CNSs as APRNs, it is important to discuss the history of RN licensure and the RN scope of practice. Knowing the history helps to put into context the evolution of current interest in and concerns about requiring CNSs to obtain a second license to practice as a CNS.

The first three laws governing the practice of nursing (nurse practice acts) were passed and signed into law in the same year in the following states: North Carolina (March 2, 1903), New Jersey (April 7, 1903), and New York (April, 20, 1903). These statutes established the title RN because these initial laws established the *registration* of nurses. The first recognition of nurses did not specify a scope of practice, but did set out the educational requirements (diploma) to distinguish between the educated nurse and the untrained nurse. The rest of the continental states followed suit over the next 20 years (Driscoll, 1976).

The following sequence of significant events, chronicled by Veronica Driscoll, the executive director of the New York State Nurses Association (NYSNA), provides an informative progression in the evolution of New York's Nurse Practice Act, which led the way for other states. The years of persistent and compelling work by leaders in the NYSNA to advance the definition of registered nursing practice, despite incredible obstacles created by both the medical community and hospitals, was remarkable.

After 8 years of attempts, the 1903 New York Nurse Practice Act was amended in 1920 to require licensure of nurses to protect the title *RN* and to identify trained attendants as a second level of nursing. *Trained attendants* eventually evolved into licensed practical nurses (LPNs) or, in some states, licensed vocational nurses (LVNs). For the next 13 years, NYSNA leaders worked to amend the nurse practice act to define the RN and require licensure for RNs who work for hire. Finally, on April 6, 1938, an amended nurse practice act was signed into law by the New York governor. The definition of a RN was

> A person practices nursing as a registered professional nurse within the meaning of this article who for compensation or personal profit performs any professional service requiring the application of principles of nursing based on biological, physical and social science, such as responsible supervision of a patient requiring skill in observation of symptoms and reactions and the accurate recording of the facts, and carrying out of treatments and medications as prescribed by a licensed physician or by a licensed dentist and the application of such nursing procedures as involves understanding of cause and effect in order to safeguard life and health of a patient and others. (Driscoll, 1976, p. 59)

The 1938 definition of an RN clearly limited the practice of registered nursing to charting and the implementation of delegated medical regimens. All states followed this lead and adopted similar definitions of the RN, limiting the legal scope of practice to delegated activities. From 1969 to 1970, NYSNA leaders recognized the limitations of the definition of an RN in not delineating the independent nature of *nursing* functions in the context of the nursing process. Input was sought from both members of the association and from legal counsel. Legal counsel advised NYSNA that "independence of the nursing function is conditional upon the specification of the diagnostic privilege within the legal definition" (Driscoll, 1976, p. 59). As a result, the Special Committee to Study the Nurse Practice Act proposed the following definition:

> The practice of the profession of nursing as a registered professional nurse is defined as diagnosing and treating human responses to actual or potential health problems through such services as case finding, health teaching, health counseling, and the provision of care supportive and restorative of life and well-being. (Driscoll, 1976, p. 59)

Importantly, the definition shifted from defining an RN to defining the *practice* of an RN. Thus, the definition identifies the autonomous scope of RN practice as "diagnosing and treating human responses to actual or potential health problems." It is interesting to note that this language from 1970 remains essentially the same in the definition of RN practice in the ANA's *Social Policy Statement* (ANA, 2010b): "Nursing is the protection, promotion, and optimization of health and abilities, prevention of illness and injury, alleviation of suffering through the *diagnosis and treatment of human response*, and advocacy in the care of individuals, families, communities, and populations" (p. 100). After considerable interprofessional conflict and challenges to the definition authorizing RNs to carry on an autonomous or self-directed scope of practice in addition to the safe and therapeutic implementation of delegated medical regimens, the legislative bill was signed into law by Governor Rockefeller in March of 1972 (Driscoll, 1976, p. 64).

Just as before, the rest of the states followed the lead of NYSNA and enacted essentially the same scope of practice for RNs over the next 8 years. Thus, the RN scope of practice in each state typically authorizes RNs to practice in an autonomous domain and a delegated domain. *Autonomous* means self-initiated actions, that is, actons not requiring initiation or authorization from another source. The autonomous domain encompasses health assessment, derivation of nursing diagnoses, and the implementation and evaluation of nursing therapeutics/interventions. The delegated domain encompasses the safe and therapeutic implementation of delegated medical regimens. RNs make very important judgments about the medical condition of a patient, but they are not authorized under the RN license to *self-initiate* medical interventions, such as use of pharmacological agents in response to those judgments. However, RNs can and do implement medical therapeutics in response to their judgments regarding the medical condition of patients via delegation from physicians in the form of medical orders, protocols, or standing orders. Although there have been some challenges to the use of protocols or standing orders, the use of these mechanisms remain.

History of APRN Licensure

One of the most significant issues for CNSs and the National Association of Clinical Nurse Specialists (NACNS) from the late 1990s through 2010 has been whether or not to advocate for requiring CNSs to obtain a second license to authorize practice as a CNS. In large measure, the issue was imbedded in confusion arising from two very different definitions of "advanced practice nursing" or "advanced nursing practice" (Lyon, 2004). The first definition emanates from the work of Peplau (1965) and Styles (1996) and is focused on advanced nursing practice within the

domain of nursing's autonomous scope of practice and the "how, when, and where" aspects of implementing medical therapeutics. The advanced nature of nursing practice is reflected in a highly developed and specialized foundation in evaluation and use of theory and research that informs (a) the differential diagnoses of problems that require nursing interventions, and (b) the decisions regarding the "how, when, and where" to ensure that the most therapeutic response is achieved while implementing delegated medical regimens. This view of advanced nursing practice is referred to here as the nursing-focused definition. The second definition of advanced practice nursing, consistent with the ANA's definition contained in the *Social Policy Statement* (ANA, 2003), is focused on expanding the autonomous domain of nursing into the medical domain of practice—that is, defining *advanced* nursing practice as the diagnosis and treatment of disease. This definition is referred to here as the medical-focused definition (Lyon, 2004).

Consistent with the nursing-focused definition of advanced practice, the CNS role from its inception in the 1940s (discussed in Chapter 1) was to improve the quality of *nursing* care provided to patients. The evolution of the nurse practitioner (NP) role began in the mid-1970s. During the late 1970s and through most of the 1980s, the activities of NPs were authorized via "additional acts" clauses added to nurse practice acts. That is, nurse practice acts were amended to include additional activities using such language as "performing acts approved by the board or by the board in collaboration with the board of medical registration" (Lyon, 1983, p. 10). For many years, these clauses were thought to be sufficient in authorizing activities that extended into the medical domain.

In 1986, the NCSBN adopted a position paper on advanced clinical nursing practice recommending that the preferred method of regulating advanced nursing be designation/recognition, also known as registration (NCSBN, 1993). This is the lowest form of authorization/regulation of practice in that it does not require that the state board inquire into the competence of the RN and simply provides the public with information about nurses with special credentials. In 1991, the NCSBN conducted a survey of states to study the regulation of advanced practice nursing (NCSBN, 1993). The study revealed a great deal of variation in the titles for advanced practice nurses and how they were being authorized to practice, that is, varying from "additional acts" clauses to granting a second license with an additional scope of practice. At the same time, there was an increasing desire on the part of NP organizations to enable NPs to diagnose and treat disease independent of physician supervision or collaboration. The 1993 NCSBN position paper recommended a definition of advanced nursing practice to encompass four roles: certified nurse anesthetists (CRNAs), NPs, certified nurse midwives (CNMs), and CNSs. Advanced practice was asserted to be based on the knowledge and skills acquired in a basic nursing education program, licensure as an RN, and a graduate degree with a major in nursing or a graduate degree with a concentration in an advanced nursing practice category such as anesthesia. The position paper also recommended that the title for advanced practice nurses be APRN and presented model legislative language that would require a second level of licensure for NPs and model administrative rules (NCSBN, 1993).

The variation in the forms of authorization and the qualifications to obtain authorization began to create significant state-to-state barriers for advanced practice nurses. During 1995, the NCSBN worked with NP organizations to begin to establish the criteria for professional certification exams to be legally defensible and psychometrically sound, thus enabling certification exams to be used as a proxy for a second license exam for the advanced practice of NPs (NCSBN, 2002, 2008).

In 1998, the legislative/regulatory committee of NACNS conducted a critical analysis of state statutes and regulations governing CNS practice. The analysis found that 26 states had a CNS scope of practice and protected the title *CNS*. That is, the only persons legally authorized to use the title or its abbreviation must have graduated, at a minimum, from a nationally accredited master's degree in nursing program that prepares CNS graduates. Of the 26 states, 10 required certification as a CNS in the CNS's designated specialty area. The remaining states either required certification in the specialty but not as a CNS or provided a waiver of certification option when there was no certification exam available in the specialty or it did not require certification (Lyon & Minarik, 2001).

In 2008 (J. Rust, personal communication, December 1, 2008), another survey of state statutes and regulations governing CNS practice found that 40 states recognize CNSs as advanced practice nurses. An additional 6 states recognize only psychiatric CNSs. Of the 40 states recognizing CNSs, 27 require certification at an advanced practice level, with 6 of those states offering other options for certification if not available to the CNS at an advanced practice level of the specialty. These options include certification in generic practice of the specialty, waiver, presentation of a portfolio, or an appeal process. In addition to the variability in regulatory requirements, there is also variability in titling, including such variations as CNS, APRN-CNS, APN-CNS, APN, APRN, and ANP. In 2012, the NCSBN posted a list of "CNS State Practice Authority by State." (NCSBN, 2012) The list indicated that 22 states have authorized independent practice of CNSs, with 43 states recognizing CNSs as APRNs. However,

it is important to note that "independent practice" is defined by NCSBN as the diagnosis and treatment of conditions requiring independent prescriptive authority without physician supervision or a collaborative agreement. CNSs in all states *have the independent authority to practice nursing at an advanced level*! It is critically important that CNSs become intimately familiar with their respective state's nurse practice act and rules/regulations governing CNS practice as an advanced practice nurse. In states such as Michigan and Kentucky, where CNSs are not legally recognized, CNSs practice nursing in an advanced manner just as we did prior to the move to regulate CNSs. That is, CNSs practice under the authority granted via their RN license. Because the essence of CNS practice is in the advanced practice of *nursing*, there is no authority barrier to CNS practice as long as the CNS does not wish to diagnose disease and/or prescribe pharmaceutical agents. The primary difficulties with a state not legally recognizing CNSs are the inability to obtain third-party reimbursement for eligible CNS services and absence of title protection, meaning that persons not prepared as CNSs are not barred from using the title (Lyon & Minarik, 2001).

Registration

Registration is another form of legal or regulatory recognition of a practitioner whereby a government agency maintains an official roster of qualified individuals. This level of regulation does not require that the state board inquire into the *competency* of the practitioner, but it may require that the person seeking registration meet specified educational requirements and may also designate a scope of practice.

Legal Regulation and Professional Regulation

Legal regulation of the practice of nursing occurs via state boards of nursing and has the power of law. State boards of nursing are charged with the oversight responsibility for the persons it licenses or regulates and may bring sanctions against providers, including, but not limited to, revocation or suspension of a license to practice.

Professional regulation occurs via the ANA's *Social Policy Statement* (ANA, 2010b) and *Scope and Standards of Practice* (ANA, 2010a) along with corresponding certification exams. The ANA scope and standards document spells out both the RN and the APRN scopes of practice, including CNS scope, as well as the standards of practice for both RNs and APRNs. In addition to the ANA standards of practice, many specialty organizations also have standards of practice that are congruent with the ANA standards but are specific to a specialty area of practice.

Professional regulation does not have the power of law; however, scopes of practice and standards of practice are used in courts of law to help determine if a provider was practicing within his or her scope of practice and if the care provider met the standards of practice that would be expected from a reasonably prudent provider in a particular situation.

In addition to a CNS's respective state nurse practice act and the legal delineated scope of practice for the RN and CNS, it is imperative that the CNS be knowledgeable about the standards of practice. The standards for APRN practice provide the overarching framework for competency statements and, therefore, certification exams.

CERTIFICATION

Certification is a process whereby a nongovernmental agency or an association certifies that an individual has met predetermined standards or competencies specified by a profession for a specialty practice (Styles & Affara, 1998). The ANA initiated certification in nursing as an indication of excellence in practice. Certification for nurses to recognize excellence in practice was initiated in the mid-1970s through the ANA and the American Nurses Credentialing Center (ANCC) in the area of medical-surgical (MS) nursing. From the 1970s through the 1980s, many additional nursing organizations initiated certification exams to provide nurses an opportunity to demonstrate excellence in specialty areas of practice. As noted earlier, in the mid-1990s, the NCSBN began to encourage the use of certification exams as proxies for licensure exams that would be required for APRNs to obtain a second license to practice in an APRN role.

When certification exams are used as proxies for licensure exams, a state board of nursing must be assured that the certification exam is both psychometrically sound and legally defensible to be used in regulation. To be psychometrically sound, there must be an adequate number of persons taking the exam to allow psychometric testing for reliability and validity. Many specialties do not have an adequate number of CNSs practicing in the area to be able to demonstrate psychometric soundness of an exam. To be legally defensible, the certification exam must test knowledge at a level corresponding to what is considered safe practice for an APRN who is entering practice after completion of an accredited graduate program. To ensure that exams are both psychometrically sound and legally defensible, certification exams offered by certifying bodies must be accredited by the American Board of Nursing Specialties (ABNS) or by the National Commission for Certifying Agencies (NCCA) for the certification exams to be used by state boards of nursing as a proxy for a licensure exam. The CNS certification exams for use in regulation can be found in Table 27.1. Currently, CNS certification is available through the ANCC in the following areas: adult health, pediatrics, psychiatric–adult, child/adolescent, and gerontology until December 31, 2014. Additionally, the American Association of Critical Care Nurses (AACCN) and the Oncology Nurses Association offer CNS certification exams. However, the only certification exam that currently meets requirements (as of August, 2013) to be used as a proxy for a licensure exam are the AACN's Adult-Gerontology and the Pediatric/Neonatal exams.

Despite the fact that a certification program or exam might be accredited, it is the prerogative of each state board of nursing to determine which exams will be accepted for regulatory purposes. The NCSBN recommends the criteria to state boards of nursing to use when approving the use of a national certification exam to be used for regulatory purposes. Once a CNS has obtained certification, the certification must be renewed at designated time frames, such

TABLE 27.1

ACCREDITED CERTIFICATION PROGRAMS THAT MEET REQUIREMENTS FOR LICENSURE OF CLINICAL NURSE SPECIALISTS (CNSs) AND POPULATION AREAS	
American Nurses Credentialing Center exam; www.nursingcertification.org	Adult Psychiatric Mental Health CNS (until December 31, 2015)
	Adult Health CNS (until December 31, 2015)
	Adult-Gerontology CNS (as of April, 2014)
	Child/Adolescent CNS (until December 31, 2015)
American Association of Critical Care Nurses Certification Board; www.aacn.org	Adult-Gerontology CNS (as of July, 2013)
	Pediatric and Neonatal CNS (as of July, 2013)

as every 3 to 6 years with 5 years being the average (Goudreau & Smolenski, 2008). Most often, the renewal involves presenting proof of continuing education units (CEUs) and additional academic or professional training along with a current curriculum vitae. If an APRN's certification lapses, it is generally necessary to meet any additional/new certification eligibility requirements and to retake the certification exam.

ACCREDITATION OF ACADEMIC PROGRAMS

Accreditation of master's-level programs and soon doctoral-level programs preparing APRNs is required to enable graduates to meet requirements for authorization to practice as an APRN. Accreditation is a voluntary, self-regulating, nongovernmental process that is designed to ensure a designated quality of education. The Commission on Collegiate Nursing Education (CCNE) and the National League for Nursing Accreditation Commission (NLNAC) are the two accrediting bodies that accredit nursing educational programs. Both organizations use criteria for evaluating educational programs. The CCNE uses *The Essentials of Master's Education in Nursing (2011)* approved by the American Association of Colleges of Nursing (AACN, 2011). The NLNAC has endorsed the NACNS Statement for its use in the accreditation of programs preparing CNSs.

CREDENTIALING AND PRIVILEGING IN A HOSPITAL OR OUTPATIENT SETTING

Credentialing and privileging processes initially developed for physicians are now applied to APRNs, including CNSs, when a CNS desires the use of prescriptive authority within a health care organization. *Credentialing* is the process by which professionals provide evidence that they are qualified to perform clinical activities within a designated scope of practice. Although credentialing and privileging may occur within the same time frame, they are related but different operations. The primary intent of credentialing is to determine if the applicant will be authorized to practice within an organization, whereas the purpose of *privileging* is to outline the scope of practice activities that can be provided (Kamajian, Mitchell, & Fruth, 1999).

The responsibility for credentialing rests with the governing body of the institution, such as the board of directors or senior executive committee such as the medical staff executive committee. Decisions are based on review and verification of information gathered in the credentialing process and recommendations of the medical staff regarding appointment and privileging.

CNSs, like other APRNs, are bound by internal and external mechanisms. Internal mechanisms influencing credentialing include an organization's mission, values, practice standards, multidisciplinary operations, and position descriptions. External mechanisms include nurse practice acts (scope of practice for APRN role), state board of nursing rules and regulations governing practice, the ANA (2010), specialty organization standards of practice, and the ANA Code of Ethics (2001). The Joint Commission (TJC) requires its over 15,000 accredited health care organizations to assess and affirm the competency of all providers. Additionally, the Accreditation Association for Ambulatory Health Care (AAAHC) and the National Committee for Quality Assurance (NCQA) for managed care require affirmation of competency. TJC requires that the processes, policies, and procedures of credentialing and privileging be well defined, including specific time frames for response to applications (TJC, 2012).

Every hospital or other health care agency is responsible for ensuring that all practice providers including APRNs are appropriately credentialed and privileged. TJC clearly spells out the requirements for both credentialing and privileging. Typical requirements for credentialing and privileging for CNSs are: (a) licensure as RN and/or as APRN/CNS or CNS, with a license that is in good standing; (b) proof of national certification as a CNS in specialty; (c) proof of education (graduate program transcript); (d) Drug Enforcement Agency (DEA) number; (e) summary of employment history; (f) membership in professional associations; (g) written collaborative agreement with physician if required in board of nursing rules and regulations; (h) photograph; (i) competency assessment; and (j) references. As of 2007, competencies encompass patient care that is compassionate/appropriate, clinical knowledge, practice-based learning/improvement, interpersonal and communication skills, professionalism, and systems-based practice. Privileges to perform well-delineated diagnostic and/or therapeutic services are granted based upon each state's practice act that sets the scope of CNS practice, license, education, demonstrated competence, judgment, and the organization's clinical regulations.

Also as of 2007, TJC initiated a requirement for "ongoing professional practice evaluation." Hospitals must conduct ongoing evaluations of providers. In 2008, a requirement was added for more intense evaluations, referred to as "focused professional practice evaluations." These evaluations occur for the first year that a provider is newly credentialed and privileged and when a provider is requesting a new privilege or a "trigger" is activated, such as low volume of procedures, higher complication rates, or a departure from evidence-based practice (EBP).

It is the responsibility of the CNS to acquire and maintain all records that may be required as proof of meeting any credentialing requirements. A good practice is to keep a file folder in a safe place that contains all original documents. In addition to documents from outside sources, such as academic institutions, continuing education, and certification agencies, it is good practice to keep your curriculum vitae or resume updated yearly.

The ANA (Summers, 2012) recommends peer review within the credentialing and privileging process. As a requirement for the Magnet Recognition Program of the ANCC, "[t]he CNO or his or her designee participates in credentialing and privileging and evaluating advanced practice nurses" (p. 10). Health care facilities use a variety of models for credentialing and privileging. Regardless of the model used, it is imperative that CNSs work to ensure representation on credentialing and privileging bodies.

CURRENT ISSUES AND FUTURE TRENDS

After 4 years of collaborative effort by representatives from multiple nursing organizations on the APRN Consensus Work Group and the NCSBN, the *Consensus Model for APRN Regulation: Licensure, Accreditation, Certification and Education* was published (2008). The work was stimulated by the fact that there is no uniform model of regulation of APRNs across states. States vary in terms of legal scopes of practice, the APRN roles recognized, and criteria for entry into practice, including how competency is demonstrated. The Consensus Model defines APRN practice, including CNS practice; describes a uniform APRN regulatory model; identifies titles to be used (includes CNS); defines specialty; describes emergence of new roles and population foci; and presents strategies for implementation.

There are several important issues inherent in the model that will continue to be grappled with by various APRN groups, including NACNS and state boards of nursing, over the coming years. One central issue is the requirement that all APRNs (including CNSs) obtain a second license to enter into practice as an APRN. Is a second license warranted and justifiable when a CNS's scope of practice does not include the independent diagnosis and treatment of disease? Additionally, the Consensus Model proposes that APRN certification exams accepted as regulatory exams for initial licensure for each APRN role

will only focus on one of six populations: family/individual across the life span, adult–gerontology, neonatal, pediatrics, women's health/gender-related, or psychiatric–mental health. Therefore, CNS specialty areas other than adult and pediatrics or women's health would not be accepted for licensure purposes. Is testing a critical care CNS or an oncology CNS in adult–gerontological competencies sufficient for legal defensibility?

Regarding educational preparation of APRNs, the model has prescriptive curricular components, such as requiring (a) that educational preparation be limited to one of the six population foci; (b) that three separate graduate-level courses be taken in physiology/pathophysiology, advanced health assessment, and advanced pharmacology; and (c) that graduates be prepared with competencies to prescribe pharmacological agents even if such activities will not be part of the APRN's actual scope of practice or position responsibilities. Will these prescriptive educational requirements be accepted by the academic and regulatory communities? How will such prescriptive educational requirements be managed by graduate programs in nursing while maintaining the integrity and adequacy of curriculums in the preparation of CNSs?

Certification exams in specialty areas such as oncology may continue to exist, but will likely only be acceptable for regulatory purposes if built on the preparation for one of the population foci like the acute-critical care exam. The absence of specialty exams raises important social responsibility questions for state boards of nursing in assuring the public that CNSs are competent in their respective specialty areas. It is anticipated that the status of certification exams will be in flux for some time. Many states may opt to continue to recognize specialty areas of practice. For example, in 2013 Rhode Island passed legislation with some language that is consistent with the Consensus Model but also included the opportunity for CNSs to be licensed in their specialty area by portfolio when there is not a certification exam in their specialty area.

It is critical to recognize that the NCSBN and the APRN Consensus Group are not regulatory agencies. The NCSBN is a member association with each state board of nursing holding membership. The APRN Consensus Group is an informal group of representatives from various organizations. Neither the NCSBN nor the APRN Consensus Group can mandate changes in the regulatory arena in any state. In order for the regulatory recommendations contained in the Consensus Model for APRN Regulation to take effect, each state would have to enact those recommendations in statute and in corresponding rules and regulations. This is and will be a massive undertaking. Furthermore, each of the other areas of certification, accreditation, and education would also have to comply.

It is imperative that CNSs are active participants in monitoring and shaping statutes and regulations that govern their practice at the state level. The NACNS has a legislative/regulatory tool kit entitled "Starter Kit for Impacting Change at the Governmental Level: How to Work with Your State Legislators and Regulators" posted on its website (www.nacns.org).

The Consensus Model document contains recommendations for a LACE (licensure, accreditation, certification, and education) structure to facilitate the collaboration of each area to assist in making the recommendations a reality. Representatives from each of the four prongs of LACE comprise the structure to facilitate communication. It is hoped that the LACE mechanism will help in coordinating efforts to implement the Consensus Model recommendations. It remains to be seen if it is possible to actualize the recommendations as they now stand in all 50 states. As previously mentioned, Rhode Island has deviated from the recommendations and it is anticipated that many other states will follow.

In addition to current trends and issues regarding credentialing of CNSs and including demonstration of competence, there is also the issue of continued competence. Credentialing for continued competence has been a long-standing regulatory issue. In 1995, the Per Health Professions Commission called for the implementation of mechanisms to assure the public of health care providers' continued competency. To date, a practitioner is determined to be competent on initial licensure or entry into practice, be that as an RN or as a CNS, NP, nurse midwife, or CRNA. However, 26 states require a designated number of CEUs for relicensure as an RN, and 27 states require certification to be recognized as a CNS, thereby requiring that the licensee meet the CEU requirements of the certifying body to renew certification.

Demonstration of continued competence is a thorny issue. Important aspects of the issue yet to be resolved include: (a) What is a legally defensible way for the practitioner to demonstrate continued competence? Some proposed mechanisms fraught with potential problems in legal defensibility include reexamination, peer review, client/case reviews, supervised practice, computer simulation testing, and employer skills testing; (b) Should basic competence or specialty competence be measured, and how do expected competencies differ based on years of experience? (c) How will competency measurement be used in the workplace? and (d) What role does the employer have in ensuring continued competence?

SUMMARY

Credentialing is a dynamic and ever-changing policy arena affecting CNSs and CNS practice in particular. Legal and regulatory credentialing includes licensure and rules and regulations that have been promulgated by state boards of nursing as state agencies to implement statutes. Professional credentialing includes certification, accreditation, and institutional credentialing for practice privileges. Understanding the history of RN licensure and the legal authorization of nursing's autonomous scope of practice helps to illuminate some of the issues around whether or not CNSs who do not have or need prescriptive authority should be required to obtain a second license to practice. Currently, there is tremendous variation in the manner in which states legally recognize CNSs, in titles, and in requirements to obtain authorization to practice, including whether or not a certification exam is required.

The foundation for professional certification lies in the profession's standards of practice and the standards of practice for each of the CNS specialty areas. Historically, states requiring CNSs to be certified in their respective specialties as a requirement for authorization to practice has presented problems for CNSs in specialty areas where there are not a sufficient number of CNSs to make the creation of a certification exam economically feasible. Recognizing the need for a core CNS exam that would test for competencies generic to the CNS role regardless of specialty, NACNS has worked collaboratively with ANCC in the development of a core CNS certification exam.

Current developments and recommendations embodied in the Consensus Model for APRN Regulation are, in part, directed at trying to create more uniformity in the regulation of APRNs, including CNSs. It is yet to be determined if this effort will be successful.

It is the responsibility of the CNS to be familiar with his or her respective state nurse practice act, all applicable rules and regulations, and national standards for RNs and APRNs, specifically CNSs. It is also the responsibility of each individual CNS to maintain all documents related to credentialing, including proof of meeting requirements for certification and recertification, such as copies of CEU certificates (Joel, 2004).

It is hoped that every CNS will be actively engaged in staying abreast of both state and national level developments regarding CNS credentialing. The area of credentialing offers multiple opportunities for CNSs to become actively engaged in shaping the direction of the discipline and in the regulation of CNS practice in particular.

▓ DISCUSSION QUESTIONS

- Are CNSs legally recognized in your state? If so, what is the statutory language in the nurse practice act recognizing CNSs? Is the CNS scope of practice delineated in statute and/or in rules and regulations, and what is the scope of practice? What are the requirements to be recognized as a CNS in your state, and is the CNS title protected (that is, limited to only those who meet the requirements)?
- What is the difference between legal/regulatory and professional credentialing?
- How can you access other states' nurse practice acts as well as rules and regulations?
- What certification exam will you be taking, and what are the requirements to be eligible for the exam?
- What are current issues in your state regarding credentialing of APRNs and CNSs in particular? Identify what local, state, and national level organizations you can join to remain informed about and influence developments in regulatory and professional credentialing of CNSs.

REFERENCES

American Association of Colleges of Nursing (AACN). (2011). *The essentials of master's education in nursing.* Washington, DC: Author.

American Nurses Association (ANA). (1979). *The study of credentialing nursing: A new approach.* St. Louis, MO: Author.

American Nurses Association (ANA). (2001). *Code of Ethics for nursing with interpretive statements.* Washington, DC: American Nurses Publishing.

American Nurses Association (ANA). (2003). *Nursing: Scope and standards of practice.* Washington, DC: American Nurses Publishing.

American Nurses Association (ANA). (2010a). *Nursing: Scope and standards of practice* (2nd ed.). Silver Spring, MD: American Nurses Publishing.

American Nurses Association (ANA). (2010b). *Social policy statement.* Silver Spring, MD: American Nurses Publishing.

Consensus model for APRN regulation: Licensure, accreditation, certification & education (2008, July 7). Retrieved December 1, 2008, from www.nacns.org. membersonly

Driscoll, V. M. (1976). *Legitimizing the profession of nursing: The distinct mission of the New York State Nurses Association.* New York, NY: New York State Nurses Association Foundation.

Goudreau, K. A., & Smolenski, M. (2008). Credentialing and certification: Issues for clinical nurse specialists. *Clinical Nurse Specialist, 22*(5), 240–244.

International Council of Nurses (ICN), (1997). *ICN on regulation: Towards 21st century models.* Geneva, Author.

Joel, L. A. (2004). Credentialing and clinical privileging. In L. A. Joel (Ed.), *Advanced practice: Essentials for role development* (pp. 136–154). Philadelphia, PA: F. A. Davis.

The Joint Commission (TJC). (2012). *The Joint Commission E-Edition: Medical staff.* Retrieved July 20, 2013, from https://e-edition.jc.ino.can/chapters aspx?c=14

Kamajian, M. F., Mitchell, S. A., & Fruth, R. A. (1999). Credentialing and privileging of advanced practice nurses. *AACN Clinical Issues, 10*(3), 316–336.

Lyon, B. L. (1983). *Nursing practice: An exemplification of the statutory definition—Indiana* [Monograph]. Birmingham, AL: Pathway Press.

Lyon, B. L. (2004). The CNS regulatory quagmire: We need clarity about advanced nursing practice. *Clinical Nurse Specialist, 18*(1), 9–13.

Lyon, B. L., & Minarik, P. (2001). Statutory and regulatory issues for clinical nurse specialist (CNS) practice. *Clinical Nurse Specialist, 15*(3), 108–114.

National Council of State Boards of Nursing (NCSBN). (1993). *NCSBN subcommittee to study the regulation of advanced practice: Position paper on the regulation of advanced practice nursing with model legislative language and administrative rules.* Chicago, IL: Author.

National Council of State Boards of Nursing (NCSBN). (2002). *Criteria for APRN certification programs.* Chicago, IL: Author.

National Council of State Boards of Nursing (NCSBN). (2005). *Nursing regulation and the interpretation of nursing scopes of practice.* Retrieved October 23, 2008, from https://www.ncsbn.org/364.htm

National Council of State Boards of Nursing (NCSBN). (2008). *History of APRN.* Retrieved January 11, 2009, from https://www.ncsbn.org/428.htm

National Council of State Boards of Nursing (NCSBN). (2012). *APRN maps, January 2012.* Retrieved July 14, 2013, from https://www.ncsbn.org/2567.htm

Peplau, H. (1965). Specialization in professional nursing. *Nursing Science, 3*, 268–287.

Styles, M. M. (1996). Conceptualizing of advanced nursing practice. In A. C. Hamric, J. A. Spross, & C. M. Hanson (Eds.), *Advanced nursing practice: An integrative approach.* Philadelphia, PA: Saunders.

Summers, L. (2012, January/February). Clinical privileges. *The American Nurse, 10.*

Student Clinical Experiences: Responsibilities of Student, Preceptor, and Faculty

Florence Myrick and Diane Billay

*I*n the current health care environment, the role of the clinical nurse specialist (CNS) may be described as undergoing a significant renaissance in its evolution (Heitkemper & Bond, 2004). Indeed, there is considerable renewed interest regarding this particular role within the context of the nursing profession and the scope of practice that it entails. The CNS assumes a key position in various facets of health care delivery (Elliott, Gauthier, Mitchell, Oates, & Purdy, 2004; Gurzick & Kesten, 2010). The nurse who is a CNS is required to possess not only a breadth but also a depth of knowledge and skill in a specialized area of clinical practice that can include gerontology, pediatrics, and oncology, to name a few. Key to that knowledge and skill is the preparatory process involved in educating individuals for this advanced role, and integral to that process is the preceptorship experience.

In this chapter, we provide an overview of the preceptorship approach to clinical teaching and learning. In particular, we discuss the roles and responsibilities of the *student*, the *CNS preceptors*, and the *faculty*, or the triad of players integral to the context of the preceptorship experience, and address specifically how preceptorship contributes to the practical preparation of the CNS role.

PRECEPTORSHIP: A CONTEXTUAL PERSPECTIVE

Although preceptorship is often considered to be a recent educational phenomenon within the context of clinical teaching in the nursing profession, historically this is not an accurate reflection of its development and emergence as a viable teaching model (Backenstose, 1983; Myrick & Yonge, 2003). Indeed, one could describe preceptorship as having its roots in Florence Nightingale's day when "it was expected that the first-year practical training of nurses would occur in the hospital setting under the direct guidance of those nurses who had been trained to train" (Myrick & Yonge, 2003, p. 92). Nursing students were taught in hospital schools of nursing in which the apprenticeship approach to the clinical preparation of nursing students was provided. While this particular approach to the clinical preparation of nursing students was considered to be an effective one, a concern began to emerge recognizing that the educational needs of the students were often regarded as secondary to patient care needs. Thus, a move commenced to transfer the education of nurses from the hospital setting to the postsecondary environment so that student learning needs could take priority in the educational process and in the preparation for professional nursing practice. In the 1950s and the 1960s, the transfer of nursing education to postsecondary institutions thus became a reality, with students beginning to be taught in universities, colleges, and technical institutions (Myrick & Yonge, 2003, 2005). And, with this transfer from the hospital setting to the postsecondary institutions, there began to emerge a different set of challenges to the nursing educational process.

Because nursing students were now being prepared away from the clinical practice setting, challenges began to develop in the form of inadequate clinical preparation. Employers began to voice their concerns and educators their frustrations. In her seminal work on this issue, Kramer (1974) coined the phrase "reality shock" to describe the comparative inability of nurses to assume full patient care responsibility immediately upon graduation. A major thrust thus commenced to resolve this particular dilemma. Out of these developments emerged the preceptorship model, a model designed to facilitate and enhance student learning in the clinical practice setting and socialize students successfully into the professional role of the registered nurse (Myrick & Yonge, 2005). The preceptorship experience evolved into one that would make a key contribution to the clinical preparation of registered nurses, not only in undergraduate nursing education but also in advanced practice roles such as the CNS and the nurse practitioner (NP).

PRECEPTORSHIP: THE TRIAD

Educationally, preceptorship is an approach to teaching and learning that affords individual students the opportunity to work directly with expert practitioners or nurses in the clinical or community practice setting. It provides a one-to-one relationship with an expert in the field who can act as a resource, role model, facilitator, and guide throughout his or her entire clinical or practicum experience. "Such pairing intends to foster professional socialization, enhance learning, promote critical thinking, cultivate practical wisdom, and facilitate competence" (Myrick & Yonge, 2005, p. 3). The National Association of Clinical Nurse Specialists (NACNS, 2004) concurs that, through peer review and the establishment of a network of CNS colleagues who can serve as resources for continuing development and professional collaboration, preceptorship socializes the CNS student to professional practice. Key to the success of the preceptorship approach to clinical preparation is the triad of individuals who are directly involved in the experience. This triad includes the student, the preceptor, and the faculty.

The Student

The student in the preceptorship relationship is often referred to in the literature as the *preceptee* (McCarthy & Murphy, 2010; Udlis, 2008). For the sake of clarity of discussion, however, the authors use the term *student* throughout this chapter. The role of the CNS student is central to preceptorship. In this approach to their educational preparation, graduate students are socialized directly into the advanced role of the CNS. In their role, students are required to assume particular responsibilities germane to the context of the preceptorship relationship.

CNS students who enter into a preceptorship experience at the graduate level present with a different demographic than do their counterparts in the undergraduate program (Lewandowski & Adamle, 2009). For example, graduate students "tend to arrive at the [preceptorship] experience with a certain level of expertise and a measure of respect in their own right" (p. 378). In their prior roles, these students have proven themselves to be valuable members of the health care team, and thus they function more effectively in situations that afford them the respect and recognition for the experience with which they arrive to their student role. In a study carried out to examine the process used to enhance the critical thinking ability of graduate students in the preceptorship experience, such respect and value by the preceptor in particular figured prominently in the success of the experience. Conversely, the lack of such respect and valuing on the part of the preceptor was found to be responsible for an unsuccessful experience. This observation was reflected in the comments of a student in the study who stated, "I do think the relationship is seminal to the whole process...without that, forget it. There's no learning. I think it's the relationship first and foremost" (Myrick & Yonge, 2004, p. 374).

Over time, it has often been assumed that a teacher, in this case a preceptor, teaches or tells while the CNS student listens or takes the role of a passive recipient of the knowledge and expertise that is being relayed. Such an assumption is, however, an erroneous one. In order for a learning experience to be an authentic one, both the teacher/preceptor and the student must assume active roles in the teaching and learning process (Dewey, 1933, 1938; Hagler et al., 2012).

> Learning is about being actively involved in what could be described as a discovery process. [Learning] is about being introduced to new ideas and different ways of doing things or about acquiring a new way of looking at an old idea. (Myrick & Yonge, 2005, p. 105)

Being an active participant requires considerable commitment on the part of both the student and the preceptor (Knowles et al., 1998).

Students in the CNS preceptorship experience are being prepared at the advanced practice level and are thus required to be well prepared prior to arriving at the nursing unit to provide advanced patient care. It is important that they be clear about the learning goals to be achieved throughout the practicum and at the completion of the preceptorship experience. Each CNS student needs to discuss these goals with the preceptor immediately upon commencement of the experience so that there is no ambiguity on the part of both the student and preceptor regarding one another's expectations. While this may appear to be a commonsense statement, it is surprising how often confusion can arise as a consequence of discrepancies between student expectations and those of the preceptor. In administering their advanced nursing care under the tutelage of the preceptor, CNS students are required to use various sources of knowledge. They need to be clear about the specific objectives of their care, prioritize appropriately, and carry out patient care in a safe and competent manner reflective of an advanced practitioner (Lewandowski & Adamle, 2009; McClelland, McCoy, & Burson, 2013). They also need to demonstrate effective communication and engage in reflective practice. Students need to demonstrate a strong sense of commitment to their role in the preceptorship experience. They are expected to adhere to ethical and nursing standards of practice; be respectful in their interactions with colleagues, patients, and families; be knowledgeable about their scope of advanced practice regarding their student role; and demonstrate prudent judgment in their clinical decision making.

The CNS as Preceptor

In the study previously alluded to (Myrick & Yonge, 2004), it was found that the preceptor–student relationship is pivotal to a successful preceptorship experience. In the same study, it was also found that preceptors who are flexible, trustworthy, who create an environment that fosters student questioning, and who themselves are open to different ways of approaching a particular situation were found to be facilitative in their role. In light of such findings, it is thus incumbent upon the preceptor to draw on such behaviors to promote a successful and effective experience.

In preceptorship, the preceptor assumes a multifaceted role that entails role modeling, facilitating, guiding, and prioritizing (Myrick, 2002; Myrick & Yonge, 2005), while at the same time demonstrating the following characteristics: clinical expertise; leadership; collaboration and consultation skills; professional attributes such as honesty and personal integrity, confidence, willingness to take risks and be

wrong, self-review, and the ability to value and support diversity; and providing professional citizenship for the specialty (NACNS, 2004). The impact of preceptor behavior on student learning cannot be overestimated. Even at the graduate level, the preceptor is regarded as the role model to whom students look for guidance to inform their thinking and practice. For example, in the study alluded to on graduate student preceptorship, one of the students was heard to state the following:

> When I have the opportunity to watch her work, I'm constantly thinking about what is she doing, how did she think about this, what are the beliefs informing this. How would I do it differently, do I agree, do I disagree, all of those kinds of things. (Myrick & Yonge, 2004, p. 376)

Another student in the same study intimated, "She's [preceptor] a master clinician and my learning and my development come from watching her" (p. 376).

In facilitating student learning in preceptorship, the preceptor essentially paves the way for the various experiences throughout the clinical practicum (Myrick & Yonge, 2001). What this means is that together with the student, the preceptor draws on both of their previous experiences to provide meaningful learning in teaching and in validating psychomotor competencies, promoting enhancement of clinical judgment and decision making, and in providing immediate feedback that is constructive and affirming (Myrick & Yonge, 2005). Facilitating the student experience entails preceptor collaboration with the student by discussing and delineating specific goals that must be accomplished. It is not about direction, it is about collaboration, which is achieved when the CNS preceptor role models the three CNS practice spheres of influence, specifically the patient/client sphere, in which the goal of care is to decrease or prevent symptoms/suffering and improve functioning; nurses and nursing practice sphere, in which the role of the CNS is to advance nursing practice and improve patient outcomes by updating and improving norms of care and by using standards of care that direct clinical actions; and the organization system sphere, in which the CNS articulates the value of nursing care at the organizational, decision-making level and advocates for professional nursing (NACNS, 2004).

In guiding the preceptorship experience, the CNS preceptor essentially shows students the way to achieve success in their role through modeling the five domains explicit to this advanced practice role: practitioner, consultant, educator, researcher, and leader (Canadian Nurses Association [CNA], 2009). As the expert practitioner from whom the student seeks guidance, the preceptor acts as a safety net. In a preceptorship study, one student was heard to say, "I guess you'd call her [preceptor] a safety net because if you need help or you need a question answered you have someone right there" (Myrick, 2002, p. 160). Through guidance, the preceptor helps to tailor or shape student assignments to respond to their individual learning goals and expectations. The preceptor is integral to the student's success.

The ability to organize one's patient workload is critical to the success of nursing care. At the graduate level it is no different. Priority setting is a critical feature of competent advanced nursing practice. While the students in the CNS preceptorship may have had previous nursing experience, they are now new to their current role and, thus, need to be provided with the support to be able to learn to prioritize in their new role. Again, it is important that such support be provided with respect and in an affirming manner so that the student can be not only competent but also confident in his or her new role (CNA, 2009; Hagler et al., 2012; Yonge, Krahn, Trojan, Reid, & Haase, 2002).

The preceptor acts as evaluator of student performance. The role of evaluator is often cited by many preceptors as being the most challenging aspect of the role. For example, it is not often comfortable to provide feedback that may be less than flattering; thus, it is important how such feedback is provided. All feedback should be affirming rather than dismissive. Students must come to understand the areas of their performance that require improvement but at the same come away from such feedback with their dignity intact. It is in this role that the preceptor can draw on the experience and expertise of the faculty to assist them in the evaluation process, particularly with regard to giving and receiving feedback (Clynes & Raftery, 2008; Larocque & Luhanga, 2013; Luhanga, 2006).

The Faculty

Frequently, when one thinks of preceptorship, one thinks of the student and the preceptor. The role of the faculty, however, is pivotal to preceptorship. While the faculty is not and should not be in the forefront of the preceptorship experience, the faculty person acts as an important resource to the student and preceptor alike regarding the teaching and learning process. The faculty brings knowledge of the educational process. It is the faculty who must act as liaison between the clinical and the academic settings. It is important that the faculty meet with the preceptor and the student at the commencement of the preceptorship experience and throughout its trajectory. Availability and accessibility are important characteristics of the faculty

role. Although, as previously stated, the faculty is not actively involved in the clinical aspect of the preceptorship experience, faculty members are still responsible for ensuring that the experience is progressing in an appropriate manner, that the learning expectations of the student are being met, and that the educational goals and objectives of the learning institution are being achieved. It is within the purview of the faculty to clarify questions related to the educational perspective, to maintain open lines of communication among all three members of the preceptorship triad, and, if required, discuss any potential teaching strategies that might assist in contributing to the success of the preceptorship experience. The faculty also seeks ongoing feedback from the preceptor regarding student performance, provides feedback to the preceptor regarding his or her performance throughout the experience, responds immediately to any student or preceptor concerns, and provides input to students with regard to how they can best fulfill their role in preceptorship. Lastly, the faculty assumes the ultimate responsibility for the final evaluation and grading of the student's clinical performance. Such evaluation and grading is derived directly from the ongoing and final evaluation of the preceptor.

The Staff

As with the faculty, the role of the staff is often not regarded as being part of preceptorship. The role of staff, however, as with the preceptorship triad, is significant to the success of the preceptorship experience. For example, if staff is not receptive to or accepting of the student to the unit, the preceptorship can prove to be difficult for all involved. On the other hand, when the staff accept the student as part of the team and provide him or her with the appropriate support, the learning experience becomes invaluable. The staff can act as resource to both the preceptor and the CNS student. In their role, staff can facilitate the preceptor in his or her selection of patient assignments and learning experiences for the student. They can provide assistance when required, and they can contribute to the overall success of the preceptorship experience (Myrick & Yonge, 2005).

PRECEPTORSHIP: THE PROCESS

The process that transpires in graduate education can be considered and anticipated to be different from that which occurs in undergraduate education (Myrick & Yonge, 2004). The graduate learner is one who (a) generally presents with professional as well as personal experience; (b) is committed to the pursuit of a career, thus the pursuit of graduate education; (c) is seeking advanced theoretical knowledge and skill; and (d) is pursuing an advanced level of clinical practice. In light of these differences, one must assume that the process that evolves in the preceptorship experience in graduate education is also different from that which occurs in undergraduate preceptorship.

In a study conducted to explore how the critical thinking ability of graduate nursing students is enhanced in preceptorship, the researchers found that a complex interpersonal dynamic occurs between the graduate student and the preceptor that is key to the enhancement of critical thinking and ultimately to the success or failure of preceptorship (Myrick & Yonge, 2004). The researchers termed the process *the relational process*. The findings from this study are used by the authors to provide a theoretical framework for discussing the teaching and learning experience of the CNS student while in the preceptorship relationship.

As with any relationship, preceptorship can be a challenging one fraught with a variety of tensions, not the least of which can be interpersonal. Consider, for example, the fact that the preceptorship relationship essentially brings two complete strangers together to work closely on a day-to-day basis in what can be described at best as one of the most anxiety-provoking and stressful situations that exists vis-à-vis life and death circumstances (Hautala, Saylor, & O'Leary-Kelley, 2007; Myrick & Barrett, 1994; Yonge, Myrick, & Haase, 2002). Thus, it stands to reason that the one-to-one relationship that transpires between the student and preceptor would figure prominently. In the study alluded to (Myrick & Yonge, 2004), several students indicated that the one-to-one relationship between student and preceptor is critical. How that particular relationship evolves determines not only how well the student develops but also how it contributes to his or her sense of professional competence. Both the student and the preceptor alike bring with them their own individual stories, both personal and professional.

In that same study, students expressed a sense of vulnerability in their role. For example, one student observed, "I think just being vulnerable and taking a risk, and then the fear of getting squashed" (Myrick & Yonge, 2004, p. 374). From such a comment, we can ascertain how important it is for preceptors to create a learning environment in which students are affirmed in their role and become empowered as opposed to invalidated. The approach of one preceptor in that same study reflected that supportive role, "I am very much aware of the students'...previous experience. I usually start by exploring some of their experience so that they feel like I am acknowledging and accepting that" (p. 376).

If students are to progress in their preceptorship experience, they must feel that they are being treated with respect and that they feel a sense of safety and trust in their preceptor. In preceptoring students, preceptors who are successful in their role project a respectful attitude toward their students, a respect that is reflected in their authenticity or their genuine appreciation for the experience and knowledge that the students themselves bring to the experience (Brookfield, 2006). Students need to feel that it is safe for them to be able to express their ideas, to ask questions, and to challenge the different ways of doing things; for such a process to occur, the students need to feel that they can trust their preceptors (Myrick & Yonge, 2004). It is through the approach and demeanor of the preceptor that the student gauges exactly how safe it is to be able to enter into the process in a legitimate way. If such an approach is lacking, it is possible that the student will essentially shut down or present in a manner that is not indicative of his or her actual potential. For example, a graduate student was heard to say the following, "[Y]ou have to feel safe and then you can feel challenged, and then you can be challenged, because it's not about the person, it's about the ideas" (p. 377).

To facilitate the process of teaching and learning within the context of preceptorship, the preceptor can avail himself or herself of several strategies (Myrick & Yonge, 2005). Some of these include such approaches as the use of one-to-one preclinical discussions with the student. Such discussions allow both the preceptor and the student to review the nursing care that will be required for the shift, delineate expectations for the day, address any questions or concerns of both parties, and clarify any areas of confusion regarding nursing care. Postclinical discussions are also important. Such discussions provide an opportunity to evaluate the achievements of the day, extrapolate the positive aspects of the student's performance, examine areas that need improvement, and again, deal directly with any questions or concerns that may arise (McCarthy & Murphy, 2010).

PRECEPTORSHIP: THE OUTCOMES

The goal of preceptorship is to prepare the CNS student for competent advanced nursing practice. To that end, in this section specific outcomes of the CNS preceptorship experience are discussed, in particular (a) socialization into the CNS role, (b) clinical proficiency, and (c) leadership, collaboration, and consultation.

Socialization Into the CNS Role

As preceptor, the CNS is integral to socializing the student into the role of an advanced practice nurse. The preceptor achieves this socialization process by (a) demonstrating the art of advanced nursing practice, (b) fostering student critical thinking, (c) role modeling effective communication, (d) exhibiting effective time management while working concomitantly with his or her caseload and the student, (e) acting as an example for appropriate conflict resolution skills, and (f) nurturing and encouraging the CNS student to achieve success.

Demonstrating the Art of Nursing

Key to the CNS preceptorship is the preceptor's ability to demonstrate and articulate the art of nursing within the context of advanced nursing practice. Such practice reflects the values, attitudes, and beliefs of the discipline and profession of nursing as evidenced throughout the provision of nursing care. Such practice also accommodates the personal and emotional aspects of care and the unspoken, intuitive, and immeasurable facets intrinsic to humane nursing care (Billay, Myrick, Luhanga, & Yonge, 2007; Myrick, Yonge, Billay, & Luhanga, 2011). The art of nursing encompasses not only the everydayness of advanced practice, such as the completion of a detailed history and physical examination of a patient or the determination of a series of treatments for a patient, but also the unspoken aspects of care, such as the intricate nature of performing a bed bath, wiping a fevered brow with a face cloth, or comforting a delirious elder just by the placing on of hands. In other words, the CNS preceptor daily mirrors the intricacies germane to the art of nursing indicative of CNS best practice.

Fostering Student Critical Thinking

A second important student-centered outcome associated with professional role socialization entails the fostering of student critical thinking (Myrick & Yonge, 2002; Sorensen & Yankech, 2008). Learning is an active process that involves student engagement in all aspects of the clinical learning environment. This active engagement involves preceptor questioning for the purpose of ascertaining the student's ability to be able to analyze/deconstruct, synthesize, and evaluate various patient situations. Indeed, it is incumbent upon the preceptor to ask the student "why" questions in order to develop insights into the thought processes used by a student in different clinical situations. Interwoven throughout this questioning process is an expectation that the student will retain a healthy skepticism about knowledge acquisition

(Freire, 1983; Shor & Freire, 1987). Stated differently, while it is important to ask probing questions, it is also important to remain skeptical about the answers. For example, just because a preceptor/physician/professor states something as fact, it is prudent for the student to be able to be confident enough to also question, a confidence that contributes to safe, competent, and humane nursing care.

Role-Modeling Effective Communication

Communication may be described as "a reciprocal sharing of ideas, opinions, information, and emotions. However, unless knowledge or information is presented and received, communication cannot and will not occur" (Myrick & Yonge, 2005, p. 123). Thus, to be an effective communicator must have the ability to articulate clearly and directly, for it is through effective communication, the preceptor that the preceptor and the student can develop an understanding and appreciation of one another. Indeed, effective communication is important to a successful preceptor–student relationship.

The preceptor must be able to demonstrate and role model effective communication skills if he or she is to encourage the same in the student. *How* the preceptor communicates is an important component of the role, particularly in influencing the student's preceptorship experience. Primarily, there are three types of communication: verbal, nonverbal, and paraverbal. In the preceptor–student relationship, it is important that the preceptor be always aware of the manner in which he or she verbally communicates with the students who, despite the fact that they are experienced nurses, can still feel vulnerable in the student role. Because of this vulnerability, students can be predisposed to greater sensitivity with regard to verbal communication. Interestingly, however, nonverbal communication comprises 55% to 65% of all communication (Cantor, 1992). Body language, gestures, and facial expressions are critical to effective communication. Paraverbal refers to "the way you make words sound—angry, happy, determined, sad, etc." (Cantor, 1992, p. 18). These three forms of communication are integral to the professional socialization of the student in the practice setting.

Efficient Time Management Skills

While working with a patient and student, the preceptor faces many professional challenges, one of which involves efficient time management: in particular, balancing the role between preceptor and caregiver. Each of these roles is discretely time consuming and complex. It is the ability of the preceptor in the situation that leads to a successful balancing of these complex roles through efficient time management. The ideal would be a reduction of the preceptor caseload so that the preceptor can effectively nurture the student in an appropriate manner and thus socialize the student effectively. The reality of the hospital/learning environment, however, is such that the preceptor workload tends not to be lessened but rather is often increased as a result of working with a student. Staff support thus becomes even more important to the success of the preceptorship experience in this instance. How well the preceptor balances his or her own workload is also reflected in how well the student develops and enhances his or her own ability to manage time effectively. Because the preceptor is an experienced practitioner, he or she can facilitate the student in contending with the ongoing patient assignments. As already discussed, effective communication is central to the relationship and, indeed, is critical in facilitating and guiding students in developing their time management abilities.

Promoting Conflict Resolution

"The word conflict refers to discord or friction, and is something that often cannot be avoided" (Myrick & Yonge, 2005, p. 114). Owing to the nature of preceptorship—two strangers working closely together in a one-to-one relationship in what could be described as dire circumstances—it is not surprising that conflict can occur. Such conflict can derive from but is not limited to differences in working, personality, and learning styles. When confronted with a conflictual situation, it is important for the preceptor and the student to (a) address the problem directly, (b) discuss their individual understanding and interpretation of the situation, (c) ensure that the preceptor and the student both have an opportunity to be heard, (d) seek clarity based on preceptor and student feedback, (e) jointly develop a plan specifically outlining each other's expectations, (f) delineate timelines for change to occur, and (g) resolve the conflict constructively (Myrick & Yonge, 2005). Do not ignore the conflict.

Supporting the CNS Student

The unwavering support of the preceptor in the practice environment is integral to student socialization. As previously alluded to, the relationship between the student and the preceptor is critical to the success of preceptorship. To that end, the preceptor assumes a supportive role and, in that role, acts as facilitator and guide. As a facilitator, the preceptor draws on his or her experience and expertise to assist students in achieving their objectives. The preceptor needs to adopt a collaborative approach when instructing,

ensure that the students are well prepared for patient assignments, adopt a positive attitude toward the student, and encourage open communication. In guiding the student, the preceptor (a) provides appropriate patient assignments; (b) advises on the best way to improve competencies; (c) helps in developing problem-solving and clinical decision-making skills; and (d) paves the way for new experiences (Myrick & Yonge, 2005).

Clinical Proficiency

The attributes that distinguish a CNS from a registered nurse are many and varied. One such attribute is clinical proficiency within the context of advanced nursing practice (NACNS, 2004), which is a key focus in preceptorship. According to NACNS, the CNS possesses clinical expertise in the specialty, conducts himself or herself in a professional manner, adheres to the Code of Ethics delineated for nursing practice, and demonstrates professional citizenship. The CNA (2003) also identifies similar attributes, including expertise, leadership, consultancy, educator, and researcher.

According to the CNA (2003), the CNS demonstrates proficiency through his or her ability to readily assess clients and intervene in complex health care situations within the selected clinical specialty. While engaged in preceptorship, the CNS student observes and learns from the preceptor by participating in and conducting assessments and by using an evidence-based approach to the provision of care (NACNS, 2004). In the preceptorship experience, the CNS student is facilitated and guided in making differential diagnoses and in providing treatment in the most effective and clinically proficient manner. Preceptorship provides the CNS student with the opportunity to learn best practice regarding the promotion of quality client care and the advancement of nursing practice (CNA, 2003). The preceptorship experience promotes disciplined inquiry through the use of critical thinking, advanced decision making, and the synthesis of knowledge in the practice setting. Opportunities are also provided that allow for exposure to the research process and innovative patient care practices.

Leadership, Collaboration, and Consultation

According to NACNS (2004), the CNS provides clinical leadership by acting as a resource, facilitator, coordinator, role model, and advocate, as well as being a skilled communicator and educator. Fundamental to preceptorship is a focus on these CNS capabilities, as well as the provision of opportunities for students to enhance their ability to work collaboratively with others. The preceptor role models, facilitates, and guides students in developing their leadership skills and in working collaboratively with nursing colleagues and members of other disciplines for the betterment of the client (Myrick & Yonge, 2004). The preceptor also fosters collaboration through active teamwork with others and, in that context, promotes students' ability to develop consultation skills to give and receive professional assistance (NACNS, 2004). The preceptor promotes the use of advanced knowledge, skills, and judgment to enhance client care and deal with complex and challenging clinical and social situations (CNA, 2003). Consultation is directed toward a multifaceted range of needs, including patient-related issues, staff education, program development, development of best-practice guidelines and

professional practice models, system change strategies, and professional development (NACNS, 2004).

The preceptorship experience is apropos for CNS students in developing professional integrity, promoting self-confidence, and increasing an awareness of their own strengths and areas that require further development with regard to clinical competence. It also affords students opportunities to cultivate the ability to embrace and support diversity (NACNS, 2004). Fundamental to the nursing care provided throughout preceptorship are the following principles: respect for individual uniqueness, an appreciation for patient autonomy, a belief in the patient's right to a dignified life and death, and the delivery of safe and equitable patient care (NACNS, 2004).

CASE STUDY

The scope of CNS practice is reflected in three spheres of influence and includes (a) the patient/client, (b) the nurses and nursing practice, and (c) the organization/system (NACNS, 2004). According to NACNS, the goal of CNS practice is to achieve effective and efficient patient/client-centered care while at the same time also influencing the practice of other nurses and health care organizations to support nursing practice.

The three spheres of CNS influence provide an organizing framework with in which to describe core

CNS competencies. To explicate these fundamental core competencies and to provide practical knowledge, or "how to" guidance, related to each sphere, three interwoven case studies are presented within the context of the preceptorship experience, and they appear in *italics* throughout this next section. These exemplars highlight the specific outcomes for each sphere. Each case study involves *Steven*, a 30-year-old CNS student engaged in his final practicum experience prior to graduating with a master's of nursing (MN); *Yvette*, a preceptor with 15 years experience as a master's-prepared CNS who has preceptored 10 CNS students during her CNS career; and *Mr. C.*, the patient.

Patient/Client Sphere of Influence

In this sphere of influence, the goal is to decrease or prevent symptoms and improve a patient's functioning. The preceptor role models for the student appropriate advanced-level knowledge and skills necessary to assess, diagnose, and treat the ill patient and, as appropriate, the family and/or community. Depending on the student's learning style, learning can occur through a variety of modes. It can happen via direct, hands-on experience, which can be achieved by performing a targeted history and physical examination and then relaying the findings to the preceptor. Students also can learn through observation, which is achieved when the student directly observes, for example, the preceptor gathering swabs necessary to rule out a sexually transmitted infection. At the completion of the physical examination,

the student and preceptor then discuss the case as a postconference. The student could learn by listening and discussing. Thus, an appropriate approach of the preceptor in this instance would be to discuss with the student a specific case to determine whether or not the student is adept at diagnosing and treating a complex patient. Perhaps the student is a kinesthetic learner, which implies that he or she learns best through movement. Whether the movement is related to tracing objects or making notes and then rewriting them, the preceptor should acknowledge this learning style and accommodate the student accordingly.

Scenario 1

Steven is acquiring considerable knowledge and practical experience throughout this preceptorship placement. He finds Yvette, his preceptor, to be knowledgeable, enthusiastic, an excellent patient educator, and an exceptional facilitator of his learning. Today, he and Yvette are facing a particularly busy day. Yvette has informed Steven that Mr. C., a single 50-year-old male, is a newly admitted patient to the surgical unit and is to be treated with intravenous antibiotic therapy for multiple abscesses to both of his forearms and his left calf, and he requires a multifaceted approach to his nursing care needs. For the past three years, since his wife died, Mr. C. has injected morphine, and the nursing staff on the surgical unit feel that their collective knowledge regarding the effective care of a patient such as Mr. C. is limited. They have, therefore, requested that Yvette and Steven provide them relevant evidence-based information about injection drug users.

Patient/Client Outcomes of CNS Practice

According to NACNS (2004, p. 28), 16 outcomes of CNS practice are listed under the patient/client sphere of influence. These include the following:

1. Phenomena of concern requiring nursing interventions are identified
2. Diagnoses are accurately aligned with assessment data and etiologies
3. Plans of care are appropriate for meeting patient needs
4. Nursing interventions target specified etiologies
5. Programs of care are designed for specific populations (e.g., vulnerable groups such as injection drug users, geriatrics, oncology)
6. Prevention, alleviation, and/or reduction of symptoms, functional problems, or risk behaviors are achieved
7. Nursing interventions, in combination with interventions by members of other disciplines, result in synergistic patient outcomes
8. Unintended consequences and errors are prevented
9. Predicted and measurable nurse-sensitive patient outcomes are attained through evidence-based practice (EBP)
10. Interventions have measurable outcomes that are incorporated into guidelines for practice
11. Collaboration with patients, nursing staff, as well other health care professionals, occurs as appropriate
12. Desired measurable patient outcomes are achieved
13. Innovative educational programs for patients, families, and groups are developed, implemented, and evaluated
14. Transitions of patients are fully integrated across the continuum of care to decrease fragmentation
15. Reports of new clinical phenomena and/or interventions are disseminated through presentations and publications
16. Interventions that are effective in achieving nurse-sensitive outcomes are incorporated into guidelines and policies

Mr. C.'s well-being and recovery are contingent upon nurses understanding the intricacies involved in caring for a patient who uses drugs as a means of coping. Steven knows that caring for Mr. C. will be a challenge because he has never cared for an injection drug user before, so his learning curve will be great. As Steven develops a nurse–patient relationship with Mr. C., he understands he will have to identify (a) care need requisites specific to Mr. C.; (b) care plans and interventions appropriate to Mr. C.'s needs; (c) relevant consultation with other health care professionals/specialists to reduce/address Mr. C.'s needs; (d) achievement of measurable, patient-centered outcomes; (e) specific appropriate educational initiatives needed to ensure humane, ethical, and nurturing manner; (f) care needs of each family member; and (g) available policies and/or position statements that address patients in Mr. C.'s situation.

Application of CNS Outcomes to Scenario 1

The outcomes addressed in this scenario include diagnosis, planning, and identification of outcomes; interventions; and evaluation.

Steven and Yvette enter Mr. C.'s room and immediately Steven begins his assessment of Mr. C. Because Steven knows the competencies of CNS practice as outlined by NACNS, he understands that his assessment will include the following (NACNS, 2004, pp. 29–30): (a) conducting comprehensive, holistic wellness and illness assessments using known evidence-based techniques, tools, and methods; (b) obtaining data about context, such as disease, culture, and age-related factors, along with data related to etiologies necessary to formulate differential diagnoses; (c) identifying the need for new or modified assessment methods or instruments within a specialty area; and (d) before designing new programs, identifying, collecting, and analyzing appropriate data on the target population (in this case, injection drug users) that serve as the basis for demonstrating CNS impact on program outcomes.

Mr. C. is sitting in bed with several pillows propping his back, his face is clean-shaven, and his hair is neatly combed. Steven looks at Mr. C.'s bright blue eyes and observes that Mr. C. is staring intently at both him and Yvette. Mr. C. is frowning. Both Yvette and Steven have smiles on their faces, and their postures are relaxed. Yvette introduces herself as the

CNS for the surgical units and introduces Steven as the CNS student working with her. Mr. C. allows both Yvette and Steven to shake his hand. Steven notes that Mr. C.'s skin feels smooth and warm to touch. Yvette begins speaking with Mr. C. and explains both their roles in his care and that they are there to obtain a health history and to conduct a physical exam. During the brief time Yvette speaks with Mr. C., Steven notes that both of Mr. C.'s hands are clenched on the bed sheets and he wonders if Mr. C. is in pain from the abscesses located on his limbs. Steven remembers that a history can be unreliable when obtained from someone who chronically uses morphine. With that in mind, Steven sits down on a chair next to Mr. C.'s bed and begins his assessment.

The questions Steven asks Mr. C. about the abscesses include the following: when the abscesses first formed; location; presenting symptoms; quality; radiation; setting; timing, including onset, duration, and frequency; severity, noting if the abscesses are getting better, worse, or staying the same; aggravating factors; relieving factors; associated symptoms; and meaning for the patient. Additional components of the health history that Steven assesses include past health, including childhood illnesses, accidents or injuries, hospitalizations or operations, allergies, and current medications; family history; a review of systems; a functional assessment, including asking questions related to self-esteem/self-concept, activity/ exercise, sleep/rest, nutrition/elimination, interpersonal relationships/resources, coping and stress management, personal habits, environment/hazards; and Mr. C.'s perception of his health status. The answers elicited by asking questions related to interpersonal relationships/resources, coping and stress management, personal habits, and perception of health provide for Steven and Yvette a good snapshot into the past and current life of Mr. C. Specifically, this information provides Steven with insights into Mr. C.'s level of education, coping skills, social roles, support systems, past and current stresses in Mr. C.'s life, the last time Mr. C. injected morphine, how much he injected and where, how frequently Mr. C. typically injects in a day, how the morphine makes Mr. C. feel, and whether Mr. C. has tried any other drugs, such as marijuana, amphetamines, cocaine, and so forth.

As a CNS student, Steven is knowledgeable about the six CNS competencies as outlined by NACNS (2004, p. 30). Specifically, Steven knows he must complete the following processes: (a) synthesize and assess data, and develop differential diagnoses of illness problems; (b) draw conclusions about individual or aggregate patient problems with etiologies amenable to nursing interventions; (c) describe problems in context, including variations in normal and abnormal symptoms, functional problems, or risk behaviors inherent in disease, illness, or developmental processes; (d) plan for systematic investigation of patient problems needing clinical inquiry; (e) predict outcomes of interventions relative to prevention, remediation, modification, and/or resolution of problems; and (f) anticipate ethical conflicts that may arise in the health care environment and plan for resolution.

Results of the health history include the following pertinent information about Mr. C. History of present illness: There are a total of five abscesses located on his four limbs. Specifically, there is one abscess located on each of the following: his right forearm, left forearm, and right calf; and there are two abscesses located on his left calf. This is the first incidence of abscess formation for Mr. C., and he is worried about the condition of his skin and the pain he is experiencing as a result of the wounds. Mr. C. acknowledges that just recently he used one of his own dirty needles and then a few days later his abscesses began to form and have since become worse over these past several weeks. Mr. C. denies any history of childhood illnesses, accidents or injuries, allergies, or current use of prescribed medications. As well, Mr. C.'s family history is unremarkable. A review of systems reveals an unremarkable history except for the following: head—experiencing frequent severe headaches; skin— he has problems concealing his track marks from his coworkers and parents; neurological—Mr. C. states he is sad but denies any thoughts of killing himself.

The results of Mr. C.'s functional assessment were unremarkable except for the following: sleep/rest— Mr. C. indicated to Steven that he has been suffering from insomnia for the past 6 months; nutrition/ elimination—Mr. C. acknowledges a poor nutritional intake; interpersonal relationships/resources—Mr. C. reports a strained relationship with his two parents and informs Steven that his wife of 30 years died 3 years ago, and since then his life has been "hell on earth." Since his wife's death, Steven states that he has just wanted to be "left alone"; coping and stress management—Mr. C. reluctantly acknowledges his inability to feel happy and appears to be in constant emotional pain. Mr. C. has not sought counseling; personal habits—Mr. C. admits to his morphine use, which involves injections three to four times a day, injecting each time between 30 mg and 60 mg to whatever vein is available, yet surprisingly, his using has not yet significantly affected his work life. Mr. C. always uses sterile needles and supplies except for the one time. He tells Steven that on the anniversary of his wife's death he goes on a "bender" and will inject multiple times, usually until his parents come to his house to "smarten him up"; perception of health—Mr. C. states he is ready to accept help to deal with his morphine use and wants to attend a residential rehabilitation program.

Upon a comprehensive examination of all systems, no abnormalities are detected except with the following areas: mental status, specifically his mood and affect, and skin. Regarding Mr. C.'s mental status, his appearance, behavior, cognition, and thought processes are examined. Specifically, he is alert, oriented, cooperative, and shows signs of acute distress because he is clenching at his bed sheets with both hands and is frowning. He appears clean, and when asked "how do you feel today?" Mr. C.'s facial expression changes to a frown, tears gather in his eyes, and he states, "I am sad and also in pain from these sores on my body." Mr. C. denies any thoughts of suicide. His speech is appropriate, and his recent and remote memory is intact.

The examination of his skin reveals the following: color is light brown, warm to touch; turgor is good. Lesions are noted to the following: Right and left arms reveal one lesion to each region; to the left calf there are two lesions evident. A detailed description of each lesion will not be provided.

Steven is pleased that his assessment and physical examination of Mr. C. only took 1 hour. Upon completion of the session, Mr. C. was looking tired. Now that the assessment and physical examination are complete, Steven must determine the differential diagnosis and the interventions required for Mr. C.'s care. In terms of differential diagnosis, the following are discussed with Yvette: anxiety, ineffective individual coping, impaired adjustment, as well as damaged skin integrity, pain, and increased risk for infection. Based on the results of Steven's assessment and physical examination of Mr. C., Yvette agrees with Steven's differential diagnoses.

In accordance with approaching a patient intervention, Steven reviews NACNS's five competencies of CNS practice, which include (a) selection of evidence-based nursing interventions for patients/clients with a focus on the etiologies of illness or behaviors; (b) development of interventions that enhance the attainment of predicted outcomes while minimizing unintended consequences; (c) implementation of interventions that integrate the unique needs of individuals, families, groups, and communities; (d) collaboration with multidisciplinary professionals to integrate nursing interventions into a comprehensive plan of care for the enhancement of patient outcomes; and (e) incorporation of evidence-based research into nursing interventions within the specialty population (2004, pp. 30–31).

Based upon these competencies, Steven, together with Mr. C.'s input, determines that appropriate interventions regarding Mr. C.'s treatment will include the following:

1. *Wound care including a course of intravenous antibiotic therapy followed by oral antibiotics* as well as appropriate dressing choices for abscesses.
2. *Pain control appropriate to his level of pain. Mr. C. will require higher than usual doses of analgesic.*
3. *A consult to psychiatry to ascertain the appropriate medications necessary to treat Mr. C.'s anxiety; referral to a residential drug treatment program to help Mr. C. address and appropriately cope with the death of his wife.*
4. *A dietician to help Mr. C. remain nutritionally fit.*
5. *Patient education regarding safe injection of drugs—choosing a vein, how to keep veins healthy, how to stay healthy while injecting, and so forth.*
6. *Staff education involving knowledge about the injection drug user, information pertinent to sexually transmitted infections, specifically HIV and hepatitis C, and pain control for the person involved with illicit drug usage.*
7. *Social support or resources provided to the family, in particular, the names of agencies that can be accessed by the family to help them cope with Mr. C.'s illnesses, which may include respite, support groups such as Narcotics Anonymous, and so forth.*

The final competency of CNS practice is evaluation (NACNS, 2004, p. 31). Just as it is vital to assess, plan, and implement care for a patient, it is also vitally important to evaluate the outcomes of the care provided. NACNS details six competencies of CNS related to evaluation of care. These include (a) selection, development, and/or application of appropriate methods to evaluate outcomes or nursing interventions; (b) evaluation of the effects of nursing interventions for individuals and populations of patients/clients with regard to clinical effectiveness, patient responses, efficiency, cost-effectiveness, patient satisfaction, and ethical consideration; (c) collaboration with patients and other health care professionals, as appropriate, to monitor progress toward outcomes as needed; (d) evaluation of the impact of nursing interventions on fiscal and human resources; (e) documentation of outcomes in a reportable manner; and (f) dissemination of the results of innovative care, as appropriate.

Steven understands that once Mr. C. is discharged from the surgical floor for admittance to the residential drug treatment program, he will not be able to follow up with Mr. C.'s medical or emotional progress. Mr. C., however, has not yet been released from the surgical unit, so Steven will continue to monitor Mr. C.'s health status based upon the evaluation competencies as stated previously.

Nurses and Nursing Practice Sphere of Influence Outcomes of CNS Practice

Nursing is a practice profession. To that end, the CNS advances nursing practice by improving patient outcomes and by updating and improving norms and standards of patient care. Vital areas in which the CNS exerts influence include development of policies, procedures, and protocols that ensure nursing practice is evidence based; role modeling best practice to colleagues and nursing personnel; consultation; and education, all of which directly influence patient care outcomes (NACNS, 2004).

Scenario 2

Steven is amazed at how quickly the practicum is progressing, to the point at which he cannot believe he has only 2 weeks left with which to learn from Yvette. Mr. C.'s healing is progressing well. During the course of the past 2 weeks Mr. C. has made great progress with his wound care and, beginning 2 days ago, he even now carries out his own dressing changes. The wounds have almost healed, so he is now taking oral antibiotics. Other aspects of his care have progressed as well: two members from the acute pain service—the physician and the NP—have visited Mr. C. and have written orders indicating what narcotic he should receive, the appropriate dosage, frequency, and so forth. Observing the physician and NP working together was a great learning experience for Steven because he was able to witness how members of this service positively interact with Mr. C., the nursing staff, Yvette, and the physicians on the surgical unit. In addition, this experience provided a great opportunity for Steven and the pain service NP to begin staff education regarding appropriate pain control measures for injection drug users such as Mr. C.; Steven consults the dietician twice a week, and together they have devised a realistic plan to continue improving Mr. C.'s nutritional status, even while attending the residential drug rehabilitation center; every Monday, Wednesday, and Friday morning Mr. C. speaks with the psychiatrist about all aspects of illicit drug use, positive coping strategies, and his grief about his wife's death, to name a few; the unit-assigned social worker has been consulted to refer Mr. C.'s mother and father to a Narcotics Anonymous support group. The social worker has proved invaluable to his parents and their road to recovery.

Outcomes of CNS Practice

According to NACNS (2004, p. 31), there are 13 outcomes of CNS practice related to this particular sphere:

1. Knowledge and skill development needs of nurses are delineated
2. EBPs are used by nurses
3. The research and scientific base for innovation is articulated, understandable, and accessible
4. Nurses are able to articulate their unique contributions to patient care and nurse-sensitive outcomes
5. Nurses are empowered to solve patient care problems at the point of service
6. Desired patient outcomes are achieved through the synergistic effects of collaborative practice
7. Nurses' career enhancement programs are ongoing, accessible, innovative, and effective
8. Nurses experience job satisfaction
9. Nurses engage in learning experiences to advance or maintain competence
10. Nurses use resources judiciously to reduce overall costs of care and enhance the quality of patient care
11. Competent nursing personnel are retained due to increased job satisfaction and career enhancement
12. Educational programs that advance the practice of nursing are developed, implemented, evaluated, and linked to EBP
13. Nurses have an effective voice in decision making about patient care

Application of CNS Outcomes to Scenario 2

During Steven's interactions with Mr. C., the NP, and the physician, he determines that his knowledge is lacking in the area of injection drug use and sexually transmitted infections. After discussing with Yvette his intention to access seminal peer-reviewed journals addressing addictions and epidemiology, Steven visited the university library. There was nothing Steven enjoyed more than to perform hand searches of the library stacks because he usually found exciting articles relevant to the topic he was searching. In this case, Steven found four seminal articles addressing the psychology of addictions, and he found three excellent articles addressing current research findings on sexually transmitted infections. The discovery of the articles greatly informed his current knowledge in these areas and helped him to better understand Mr. C.'s reality.

To fulfill one practicum objective, Steven proposed to Yvette that he would provide for the unit's health care team a 40-minute in-service on best practices related to the following topics: the culture of drug use and current knowledge on sexually transmitted infections, specifically HIV and hepatitis C. Yvette was in total agreement, as was the unit manager (UM). As a result, Steven prepared, with input from Yvette, one newly hired staff nurse, and Mr. C.'s psychiatrist, a PowerPoint presentation addressing these topics.

The in-service went well. In attendance were 25 staff, including the unit pharmacist, the pastor, 3 newly hired nurses with various levels of clinical experience, the unit dietician, 2 physiotherapists, 4 interns, 2 medical residents, and 11 staff nurses, including nurses from the emergency department (ED) and the medical units. After the in-service, the 3 newly hired staff nurses approached Steven and congratulated him on a job well done. They told Steven that if this in-service reflects the caliber of future in-services, they were going to enjoy working on the surgical unit. Yvette was proud of the scholarly presentation Steven presented to the attendees because she knew that the information shared and discussed with the group would ultimately benefit patients who experience care-related situations similar to Mr. C.

This outcome includes assessment; diagnosis, outcome identification, and planning; intervention; and evaluation of the effects. Under "Assessment: Identifying and Defining Problems and Opportunities," NACNS (2004, pp. 32–33) delineates six competencies:

1. Uses/designs methods and instruments to assess patterns of outcomes related to nursing practice within and across units of care
2. Uses/designs appropriate methods and instruments to assess knowledge, skills, and practice competencies of nurses and nursing personnel to advance the practice of nursing
3. Identifies, in collaboration with nursing personnel and other health care providers, needed changes in equipment or other products based on evidence, clinical outcomes, and cost-effectiveness
4. Gathers and analyzes data to substantiate desirable and undesirable patient outcomes linked to nursing practice
5. Identifies interpersonal, technological, environmental, or system facilitators and barriers to implementing nursing practices that influence nurse-sensitive outcomes
6. Collaborates with nurses to assess the processes within/across units that contribute to barriers in changing nursing practices

The UM on Yvette's surgical floor was very encouraging of Steven. Indeed, the UM understood that many nurses on the surgical unit lacked knowledge related to caring for injection drug users and people who engage in a high-risk lifestyle, so she wanted these nurses updated on current best practices related to these areas of care. To that end, the UM knew Steven would present an excellent, evidence-based discussion regarding these topics because he had direct access to resources such as the library and clinical experts in the area of drug use, and he could access practice leaders at the state board office to ascertain the legal/ethical knowledge required to care for patients experiencing similar realities to Mr. C. Steven would also visit one local inpatient rehabilitation facility and speak with an addictions counselor about typical plans of care withdrawal, the psycho-social aspects of addictions, and so forth. Because the UM wanted this topic addressed with the nursing and allied health staff, she asked two of the newly hired nurses to accompany Steven when he visited the addictions counselor.

It was advantageous that the UM had the full support of the hospital administration and the staff nurses, because if she did not have that support the in-service would likely not occur, due to barriers such as staff bias related to injection drug use and a mistaken belief that injection users should not be given narcotics because doing so would contribute to drug use, to name a few. Yvette knew that there were some nurses who were judgmental toward this vulnerable population, but she hoped that with time and education these nurses would see things her way, which, in essence, was to be patient-centered.

Under "Diagnosis, Outcome Identification, and Planning" (NACNS, 2004, p. 33), seven competencies are identified:

1. Drawing of conclusions about the evidence base and outcomes of nursing practice that require change, enhancement, or maintenance
2. Identification of desired outcomes of continuing or changing nursing practices
3. Anticipation of both intended and unintended consequences of change
4. Incorporation of clinical and fiscal considerations in the planning process for product and device evaluation
5. Plans for achieving intended and avoiding unintended outcomes
6. Plans for using facilitators and overcoming barriers for changing nursing practice and incorporating new products and devices
7. Consideration of resource management needs when weighing the benefits of changing practices

The day after the in-service, Steven met with Yvette and the UM to discuss the completed evaluation forms he had recently received. Several key themes were identified that would be addressed *by the unit nurse educator at a later date. The five themes pertained to (a) a pervasive lack of knowledge on the part of the nurses related to "what is an addict," specifically, how one defines an addict and what might an addict medically resemble; (b) treatments a person who uses drugs should receive while in hospital, what does withdrawal look like; (c) the amount of analgesic that a person who uses drugs can receive for pain control; (d) services that are available in the community for people who use drugs; and (e) what the names of commonly abused substances are and the concomitant signs/symptoms of (over)use.*

Under "Intervention: Developing and Testing Solutions," NACNS (2004, pp. 33–34) identifies eight competencies:

1. Anchors nursing practice to evidence-based information to achieve nurse-sensitive outcomes
2. Mentors nurses to critique and apply research evidence to nursing practices
3. Works collaboratively with nursing personnel to implement innovative interventions that improve outcomes
4. Implements interventions that are effective and appropriate to the complexity of patient care problems and the resources of the system
5. Develops and implements educational programs that target the needs of staff to improve nursing practice and patient outcomes
6. Assists staff in the development of innovative, cost-effective patient programs of care
7. Mentors nurses to acquire new skills and develop their careers
8. Creates an environment that stimulates self-learning and reflective practice

Yvette was proud of Steven. The in-service was well received by all who attended because he set up the room so that the tables/chairs were arranged in a circle, engaged the participants by encouraging everyone to ask questions, encouraged participants to discuss individual experiences of caring for patients who inject drugs and who live a high-risk lifestyle, and provided opportunities for participants who were less likely to speak up to engage in the in-service by asking them to write responses on the white board. At the completion of the in-service, Steven challenged all attendees to reflect on the goal of the in-service and the content discussed. Steven requested that each participant determine at least one strategy he or she would use to humanely and effectively care for a person who uses drugs, but he realized that realistically some attendees would not follow his suggestions. Some would, however, and those individuals would be the catalysts for change.

Under "Evaluation of the Effects," NACNS (2004, p. 34) identifies four competencies:

1. Evaluates the ability of nurses and nursing personnel to implement changes in nursing practice, with individual patients and populations
2. Evaluates the effect of change on clinical outcomes, nurse satisfaction, and collaboration with other health care disciplines
3. Documents outcomes in a reportable manner
4. Disseminates results of changes to stakeholders

This is Steven's last week of his preceptorship experience. He and Yvette just completed a meeting with the faculty/tutor, and everything went well. There were no surprise revelations from Yvette or the faculty member, as should never be the case. This week Steven will work with the nurse educator and Yvette to determine if the in-service actually resulted in a positive outcome: specifically, was the desired effect achieved, that is, a better understanding of injection drug use by the health care team members?

Yvette has a long and collegial history with the nurses and other health care staff on the unit, so she knows which natural leaders to approach to ascertain if the in-service was beneficial. If it was, she wanted to know why and how so, but if it was not, she would want to know why and why not, and how the in-service could be improved. For all intents and purposes, the in-service was highly regarded, but there were two key areas to improve. First, the nurses would have liked a handout detailing the kinds of drugs typically abused, their side effects, withdrawal symptoms, and a discussion regarding the differences between the culture of acute care facilities and the culture of the street or people involved with high-risk lifestyles because they note that while Mr. C. does live a risky lifestyle, he is not a typical "user." Normally, the patients who the nurses treat are more immersed in the "street" lifestyle (drug-seeking behavior) to the point at which the acute care culture clashes with the culture of the street.

Organization/System Sphere of Influence

This sphere "is critically important in the complex health care systems of today" (NACNS, 2004, p. 19). The role of the CNS is to communicate the value of nursing care at the organizational level where decisions are being made that affect patient care. In addition, he or she promotes and advocates for the profession of nursing (NACNS, 2004).

According to NACNS (2004), "the CNS influences the trajectory of care from admission through to discharge in order to assist the patient in achieving the desired outcomes after discharge and to minimize recidivism and readmission" (p. 20). Indeed, once a patient is admitted to a health care facility it is the focus of the CNS to ensure that all patient care needs are competently managed and to plan for all immediate and potential care needs for when the patient is discharged back to the community. However, in order to provide the necessary services and care that patients require, administration must provide the CNS with mechanisms by which the CNS can collect and analyze data to document the impact of nursing practice on outcomes (NACNS, 2004). Another focus of the CNS is to develop and then establish health care policies so that effective and efficient patient-centered care occurs.

Scenario 3

On the day of his admission, Mr. C.'s discharge planning began. As previously illustrated, Yvette and Steven, along with Mr. C. and other members of the health care team, were busy planning for Mr. C.'s eventual discharge from the surgical unit to a residential rehabilitation facility. However, along the way many care concerns had to be addressed, such as the rehabilitation facility to which Mr. C. would be discharged and the earliest intake date.

Resulting from Mr. C.'s time spent on the unit, several policies were developed by Yvette and Steven. Each of the new policies addressed the care needs of the injection drug user/street-involved person and specifically addressed pain control, stigmatization, and preconceived ideas of health care workers regarding this vulnerable population, wound care, withdrawal from narcotics, grief/grieving, social networking, and psychiatric consult.

Outcomes of CNS Practice

According to NACNS (2004, p. 34–35), there are 13 outcomes of CNS practice:

1. Articulation of clinical problems within the context of the organization, mission, culture, policies, and resources
2. Continuous patient care processes that benefit the system
3. Integration of change throughout the system
4. Policies that enhance the practice of nurses individually as members of multidisciplinary teams
5. Innovative models of practice that are developed, piloted, evaluated, and incorporated across the continuum of care
6. Development and implementation of evidence-based, best-practice models
7. Articulation of nursing care and outcomes at organizational decision-making levels

8. A common vision of practice outlines shared by stakeholders, such as nurses, other health care professionals, and management
9. Decision makers within the institution who are informed about practice problems, factors contributing to the problems, and the significance of those problems with respect to outcomes
10. Patient care initiatives that reflect knowledge of cost management strategies
11. Patient care programs that are aligned with the organization's strategic imperatives, mission, vision, philosophy, and values
12. Staff adherence to regulatory requirements and standards
13. Policy-making bodies that are influenced to develop regulations/procedures to improve patient care and health services

Application of Outcomes to Scenario 3

As mentioned previously, Steven in consultation with Yvette identified the following clinical issues associated with Mr. C., their 50-year-old patient who has been an injection user for less than 5 years: multiple abscesses located on all of his limbs that required antibiotic treatment; a consult with a psychiatrist who will assist him in dealing with his immediate addiction and the grief experienced because of his wife's death; the unit nutritionist, who will assist Mr. C. in maintaining his nutritional status; and the pain service team, who together with Mr. C. will help to ensure that appropriate pain control measures are used in his care. In addition, Steven developed, implemented, and evaluated an in-service targeted toward all health care disciplines, but in particular targeting frontline nurses who would care for injection drug users.

As a result of Steven's in-service, the hospital administration developed several policies and procedures reflecting evidence-based, best-practice models when caring for injection drug users in inpatient units as well as in the ED. Indeed, given the inner-city location of this hospital, and with the implementation of the policies and procedures, the administration has seen a decline in patient admissions to the hospital as well as a decreased patient stay by this vulnerable population. The reasons for these outcomes are ED health care staff appropriately administering narcotic analgesics, instead of underadministering same; frontline nurses choosing appropriate, cost-effective wound care products to treat abscesses; frontline health care workers markedly improving their understanding of the complexities involved in caring for this population, the immediate need to consult psychiatry to treat dual diagnoses (treat mental health issues as well as drug use–related issues), and to consult the dietician upon admission to a hospital unit;

and the understanding that this population group must be treated humanely and with respect.

This outcome includes assessment; diagnosis, outcome identification, and planning; intervention; and evaluation of the effects. Under "Assessment: Identifying and Defining Problems and Opportunities," NACNS (2004, pp. 35–36) delivers six competencies:

1. Uses system-level assessment methods and instruments to identify organization structures and functions that impact nursing practice and nurse-sensitive patient care outcomes
2. Assesses the professional climate and multidisciplinary collaboration within and across units for their impact on nursing practice and outcomes
3. Assesses targeted system-level variables, such as culture, finances, regulatory requirements, and external demands, that influence nursing practice and outcomes
4. Identifies relationships within and external to the organization that are facilitators or barriers to nursing practice and any proposed change
5. Identifies effects of organizational culture on departments, teams, and/or groups within an organization
6. Monitors legislative and regulatory health policy that may impact nursing practice and/or CNS practice for the specialty area/populations

During the planning phase for the in-service, Steven benchmarked with several national and international organizations whose mandates for the treatment of drug use are imbedded in the philosophy of harm reduction. Specifically, Steven wanted to produce an in-service that focused on the humane treatment of people who use illicit drugs. To that end, Steven contacted two Canadian harm reduction programs and one European-based program, as well as two U.S.-based programs, and asked each program manager to e-mail/mail him copies of their program's philosophy of care, mission statement, program expectations/outcomes, and any educational reference materials, such as pamphlets, videos, and so forth, that were free of charge, to assist him in planning for the in-service. Because the in-service would be videotaped, Steven knew that all staff who could not attend could view the video at a later date. As well, the administration along with the nurse educator guaranteed that every newly orienting staff member would view the video during organization orientation.

Under "Diagnosis, Outcome Identification, and Planning," NACNS (2004, p. 36) identifies five competencies:

1. Diagnoses facilitators and barriers to achieving desired outcomes of integrated programs of care across the continuum and at points of service

2. Diagnoses variations in organizational culture (e.g., values, beliefs, or attitudes) that can positively or negatively affect outcomes
3. Draws conclusions about the effects of variance across the organization that influence outcomes of nursing practice
4. Plans for achieving intended systemwide outcomes, while avoiding or minimizing unintended consequences
5. Draws conclusions about the impact of legislative and regulatory policies as they apply to nursing practice and outcomes for specialty populations

Yvette is proud of Steven and the video/in-service he produced as part of his preceptorship experience. Not only did he identify the organization-wide need for best practice–related policies and procedures for injection drug users, but he also, then, benchmarked with noted national and international harm reduction programs to learn best practices related to drug use. As a long-term employee of an inner-city hospital, Yvette is very familiar with the players within the system who consistently erect barriers when a patient-centered initiative is implemented that might be perceived by those individuals as risky and "outside the box." Yvette was not worried that Steven's educational initiative would fail because she was a recognized practice leader in the hospital and would "spread the word" that the video must be reviewed by all nurses, and hopefully all other disciplines, because the content was patient-centered, educated the frontline staff on an important topic, and, from an ethical and moral standpoint, was the right thing to do.

Under "Intervention: Developing and Testing Solutions," NACNS (2004, p. 36–37) identifies 11 competencies:

1. Develops innovative solutions that can be generalized across differing units, populations, or specialties
2. Leads nursing and multidisciplinary groups in implementing innovative patient care programs that address issues across the full continuum of care for different population groups and/or different specialties
3. Contributes to the development of multidisciplinary standards of practice and evidence-based guidelines for care, such as pathways, care maps, benchmarks
4. Solidifies relationships and multidisciplinary linkages that foster the adoption of innovations
5. Develops or influences system-level policies that will affect innovation and programs of care
6. Targets and reduces system-level barriers to proposed changes in nursing practices and programs of care

7. Facilitates factors to effect program-level change
8. Designs strategies to sustain and spread chance and innovation
9. Implements methods and processes to sustain evidence-based changes in nursing programs of care, and clinical innovation
10. Provides leadership for legislative and regulatory initiatives to advance the health of the public with a focus on the specialty practice area/populations
11. Mobilizes professional and public resources to support legislative and regulatory issues that advance the health of the public

The wonderful aspect of this video, in Yvette's opinion, is that it can be used across differing units, ethnic populations, and specialties. Indeed, the video is an excellent teaching tool, not only for the inpatient units but also for outpatient services and community settings as well. Just the other day, a CNS from a hospital in another part of the city called wanting access to the video: This CNS wanted it so she could teach frontline nurses involved in community outreach about drug use by patients. As well, an emergency NP at the hospital, after viewing the video, began to develop pathways and care maps specifically addressing this vulnerable population. Yvette has also contacted the faculty member contact and insisted that together with Steven they submit abstracts to present at conferences related to harm reduction, clinical evidence-based best practice, education-focused best practice, and leadership-focused best practice.

Under "Evaluation of the Effects," NACNS (2004, p. 37–38) identifies seven competencies:

1. Selects evaluation methods and instruments to identify system-level outcomes of programs of care
2. Evaluates system-level clinical and fiscal outcomes of products, devices, and patient care processes using performance methods
3. Uses organizational structures and processes to provide feedback about the effectiveness of nursing practices and multidisciplinary relationships in meeting identified outcomes of programs of care
4. Evaluates organizational policies for their ability to support and sustain outcomes of programs of care
5. Evaluates and documents the impact of CNS practice on the organization
6. Documents all outcomes in a reportable manner
7. Disseminates outcomes of systemwide changes, impact of nursing practice, and CNS work to stakeholders

Yvette, Steven, and the faculty member have just finished discussing the content of Steven's final evaluation. Needless to say, Steven passed his final

preceptorship experience with honors. At this meeting, Steven disclosed to Yvette that prior to being a BScN-prepared registered nurse he was a teacher at an inner-city high school, which, in hindsight, did not surprise Yvette. Yvette believes that not only is Steven an excellent CNS clinician, but he is a superb educator, as well: two qualities that will enhance the care he provides to and for his future patients/families.

It was evident by the quality of the in-service Steven provided to the health care staff that he had read and synthesized the contents of the NACNS (2004) document. Steven clearly demonstrated the need for: the hospital administration to "buy in" to the education initiative; benchmarking with seminal organizations, to clearly advocate for the principles of harm reduction; Yvette to positively influence all frontline staff and advanced practice nurses to attend the session and view the video; effective evaluation methods to be used to identify strengths and areas for improvement of the in-service and video; and the evaluation of current policies and procedures related to the care of vulnerable populations, such as injection drug users.

SUMMARY AND CONCLUSION

This chapter has provided an overview of the preceptorship experience within the context of CNS student education. Preceptorship is an important approach to teaching and learning in the clinical/community practice settings. It provides a connection between the theoretical and practical aspects of advanced practice nursing, and in so doing, it continues to further strengthen the profession and discipline of nursing.

REFERENCES

Backenstose, A. G. (1983). The use of clinical preceptors. In S. Stuart-Siddall & J. M. Haberlin (Eds.), *Preceptorship in nursing education* (pp. 9–20). Rockville, MD: Aspen Systems.

Billay, D., Myrick, F., Luhanga, F., & Yonge, O. (2007). A pragmatic view of intuitive knowledge in nursing practice. *Nursing Forum, 42*(3), 147–155.

Brookfield, S.D. (2006). *The skillful teacher* (2nd ed.). San Francisco: Jossey-Bass.

Canadian Nurses Association. (2003). *Achieving excellence in professional practice: A guide to preceptorship and mentoring.* Ottawa: Author.

Canadian Nurses Association (CNA). (2009). *Position statement: Clinical nurse specialist.* Ottawa, Ontario, Canada: Author.

Cantor, J. A. (1992). *Delivering instruction to adult learners.* Toronto, Ontario, Canada: Wall & Emerson.

Clynes, M. P., & Raftery, S. E. C. (2008). Feedback: An essential element of student learning in clinical practice. *Nursing Education in Practice, 8,* 405–411.

Dewey, J. (1933). *How we think.* Boston: Health.

Dewey, J. (1938). *Experience and education.* New York: Macmillan.

Elliott, H., Gauthier, P., Mitchell, M., Oates, S., & Purdy, N. (2004). The clinical nurse specialist. *Registered Nurses Association of Ontario (RNAO) Practice Page, 4*(3). Retrieved January 9, 2009, from http://www.rnao.org/Storage/13/726_Practice_Page_CNS.pdf

Freire, P. (1983). *Pedagogy in process.* New York: Continuum.

Gurzick, M., & Kesten, K. S. (2010). The impact of clinical nurse specialist on clinical pathways in the application of evidence-based practice. *Journal of Professional Nursing, 26*(7), 698–703.

Hagler, D., Mays, M. X., Stillwell, S. B., Kastenbaum, B., Borrks, R., Fineout-Overholt, E., . . . Jirsak, J. (2012). Preparing clinical preceptors to support nursing students in evidence-based practice. *Journal of Continuing Education for Nurses, 43*(11), 502–508.

Hautala, K. T., Saylor, C. R., & O'Leary-Kelley, C. (2007). Nurses' perceptions of stress and support in the preceptor role. *Journal for Nurses in Staff Development, 23*(2), 64–70.

Heitkemper, M. M., & Bond, E. F. (2004). Clinical nurse specialists. State of the profession and challenges ahead. *Clinical Nurse Specialist, 18*(3), 135–140.

Knowles, M., Holton III, E. F., & Swanson, R. A. (1998). *The adult learner.* New York, NY: Elsevier.

Kramer, M. (1974). *Reality shock. Why nurses leave nursing.* St. Louis, MO: Mosby.

Larocque, S., & Luhanga, F. (2013). Exploring the issue of failure to fail in a nursing program. *International Journal of Nursing Education Scholarship, 10,* 1–8.

Lewandowski, E., & Adamle, K. (2009). Substantive areas of clinical nurse specialist practice: A comprehensive review of the literature. *Clinical Nurse Specialist, 23*(2), 73–90.

Luhanga, F. (2006). *The challenges for preceptors in dealing with nursing students engaging in unsafe practices (Unpublished doctoral dissertation).* University of Alberta, Edmonton, Alberta.

McCarthy, B., & Murphy, S. (2010). Preceptors' experiences of clinically educating and assessing undergraduate nursing students: An Irish context. *Journal of Nursing Management, 18*(2), 234–244.

McClelland, M., McCoy, M. A., & Burson, R. (2013). Clinical nurse specialists: Then, now and the future

of the profession. *Clinical Nurse Specialist, 27*(2), 96–102.

Myrick, F. (2002). Preceptorship and critical thinking in nursing education. *Journal of Nursing Education, 41,* 154–164.

Myrick, F., & Barrett, C. (1994). Selecting clinical preceptors for basic baccalaureate nursing students: A critical issue in clinical teaching. *Journal of Advanced Nursing, 19,* 194–198.

Myrick, F. & Yonge, O. (2001). Creating a climate for critical thinking in the preceptorship experience. *Nurse Education Today, 21*(6), 461–467.

Myrick, F. & Yonge, O. (2002). Preceptor behaviours integral to the promotion of student critical thinking. *Journal for Nurses in Staff Development, 18*(3), 127–133.

Myrick, F., & Yonge, O. (2003). Preceptorship: A quintessential component of nursing education. In M. H. Oermann & K. T. Heinrich (Eds.), *Annual review of nursing education* (vol. 1, pp. 91–107). New York, NY: Springer.

Myrick, F., & Yonge, O. (2004). Enhancing critical thinking in the preceptorship experience in nursing education. *Journal of Advanced Nursing, 45*(4), 371–380.

Myrick, F., & Yonge, O. (2005). *Nursing preceptorship. Connecting practice and education.* Philadelphia, PA: Lippincott Williams & Wilkins.

Myrick, F., Yonge, O., Billay, D., & Luhanga, F. L. (2011). Preceptorship: Shaping the art of nursing through practical wisdom. *Journal of Nursing Education,* (3), 134–139.

National Association of Clinical Nurse Specialists (NACNS). (2004). *Statement on clinical nurse specialist practice and education* (2nd ed.). Harrisburg, PA: Author.

Shor, I., & Freire, P. (1987). *A pedagogy for liberation: Dialogues on transforming education.* New York: Bergin & Garvey.

Sorensen, H. A., J., & Yankech, L. R. (2008). Precepting in the fast lane: Improving critical thinking in new graduate nurses. *Journal of Continuing Education in Nursing, 39*(5), 208–216.

Udlis, K. A. (2008). Preceptorship in undergraduate nursing education: An integrative review. *Journal of Nursing Education, 47*(1), 20–29.

Yonge, O., Krahn, H., Trojan, L., Reid, D., & Haase, M. (2002). Supporting preceptorship. *Journal for Nurses in Staff Development, 18*(2), 73–79.

Yonge, O., Myrick, F., & Haase, M. (2002). Student nurse stress in the preceptorship experience. *Nurse Educator, 27*(2), 84–88.

29

Hospital-Based Clinical Nurse Specialist Practice

Ginger S. Pierson

As a career certified critical care nurse of 32 years, with 21 of those years as a critical care clinical nurse specialist (CNS), I had no idea of what opportunities might lie ahead to utilize my CNS clinical expertise and yet also challenge me to grow further professionally. During the past 2 years, I have had a special opportunity: to serve as the CNS for a busy 58-bed emergency department (ED) in a nonprofit community hospital. Changing to a related, yet very different specialty clinical area, the ED, has allowed me to bring a fresh perspective as a CNS to a new continuum of clinical needs and process improvement opportunities. The challenging ED environment has a constant need for teamwork, efficiency, and flexibility and is a perfect environment for a CNS to facilitate clinical outcomes. I have become so impressed with and more fully appreciate the unique contributions made by emergency nurses to provide care to such a vast array of patients with specialized needs and am privileged to serve as their CNS. The case exemplar presented will highlight the impact of CNS practice in clinical improvement processes of care. These affect all three spheres of influence of CNS practice, which include the patient, nurse/nursing practice, and the organization/system (National Association of Clinical Nurse Specialists [NACNS], 2004).

As a CNS in a 510-bed, not for profit community-based hospital, I have dual reporting and clinical practice responsibilities. I report to both the nursing education department and to the ED. Consistent involvement with the nursing education department allows for collaboration with education coordinators and other CNSs. We work together to innovate and then standardize educational programs, nursing orientation, conferences, and specialty certification review courses and provide refinement of evidence-based practices related to policies and standardized procedures. Continual assessment of compliance with state and national regulatory requirements, including the identification of gaps and improvements needed to achieve and maintain compliance, are other key roles of collaboration with all staff throughout the organization. Nursing education clinical leaders are also challenged to then ensure consistent communication of key practice changes and updates regarding clinical care across the organization and mentor and support nursing colleagues to provide world-class care. Approximately 30% of my time is involved directly with nursing education and about 70% of my time is dedicated to my clinical area of practice in the ED.

The ED is a 58-bed, Level-2 (nontrauma) county base station directly serving approximately 200 to 220 patients per day. Approximately 22% of these patients are admitted to the hospital for further care. This ED has been designated as a ST-elevation myocardial infarction (STEMI) and neuro (stroke) receiving center by the county in order to serve our community with these specialized services.

CNSs are important members of several shared governance councils and eagerly support Magnet nursing excellence throughout our hospital system. CNSs and nurse practitioner colleagues form the advanced practice council. Clinical outcomes for each of our specific CNS or nurse practitioner (NP) practices are shared and supported in this advanced practice registered nurses' (APRN) council and are reported on a monthly rotational basis with nursing leadership and as requested in organization-wide performance excellence councils. APRNs from our council consult with all core measure teams and value index teams, and are represented on each of the nursing shared governance councils. Recently, APRNs have been invited to be regular guests to the medical staff quarterly meetings to facilitate awareness and visibility of CNS and NP roles in the hospital system, and to promote collaboration and consultation opportunities.

Another important role for our APRNs is involvement and service to the nursing research council. As a CNS, I formally represented our APRNs on the research council for many years. Opportunities for APRN support coordinated through the nursing research council include collaboration with staff nurses and leadership colleagues on organization-wide clinical practice changes utilizing evidence-based research/best evidence, nursing grand rounds, and nursing research forums. Additional consultation and support are shared through service as mentors for individual staff nurses, developing and implementing evidence-based practice and research projects through the translating research into practice (T.R.I.P.) program. APRNs are selected as mentors by the staff nurse T.R.I.P. Fellow, the PhD researcher, and the nursing director based on the APRN's current or recent clinical practice specialty to help complete the team. This collaborative team is intended to support the staff nurse in achieving success in his or her research or evidence-based practice project.

EMERGENCY NURSING PRACTICE: TEAMWORK TO ADDRESS CONTINUOUS IMPROVEMENTS IN PATIENT CARE

The ED of a large community, nonprofit hospital is an amazingly complex environment for nurses and other health care workers to provide care to patients from the time of birth through death. It takes a special team of health care professionals to deal with emergencies of all levels, with patients of all ages and outcomes, and for patients in whom death comes too early and occurs from a variety of unexpected circumstances. Patients and their families come to the ED for urgent and emergent care. This visit is a crisis in their lives, and they are often unsure of what the outcome will be and what to expect. They are in need of care, support, and guidance. Nurses are often the key persons that patients trust and identify with the most, to meet these needs. What a privilege it is to serve and advocate for patients and their families in the ED as a nurse and as a CNS. Immediate attention to the patient and his or her family to determine needs is of utmost importance for prioritization of the level of care needed to lead to a correct and timely diagnosis with subsequent appropriate treatment options. As a CNS in the ED, I have come to appreciate the critical qualities ED nurses and other team members possess—unlike any others: teamwork, flexibility, innovation, and a commitment to continuously improving care at every opportunity. I will focus attention on a case exemplar in which I had the privilege as the ED CNS to lead the collaborative work with an interprofessional team, including several ED and in-patient nurses, pharmacists, and educators, to improve patient care as a result of a complication of IV therapy. These improved processes will help to prevent and reduce risks of critical IV infusion therapies for current and future patients throughout the organization.

CASE EXEMPLAR

A patient was admitted to the ED with hyperkalemia (potassium level 6.4 mm/L) as a complication of worsening renal impairment while on a complex medication regime for multiple medical conditions. There was difficulty in obtaining large vessel IV access rapidly, despite several different ED nurse attempts at peripheral IV cannulation. A successful IV was placed above the wrist in a moderately large vein. Emergency medications of dextrose 50%, insulin, and a calcium chloride infusion were administered to treat the patient per physician collaboration and implementation of the hyperkalemia order set protocol. The calcium chloride was administered slowly per continuous IV infusion over approximately 2 hours. At the end of the infusion, the patient complained of pain at the IV site; when reevaluated by the nurse, the site appeared to be edematous and discolored, with suspected extravasation of some of the calcium chloride medication into the forearm and hand tissues. Dextrose 50% IVP had also been administered, without difficulty, through this IV site prior to the calcium chloride infusion. Team collaboration occurred immediately with ED and hospitalist physicians, a pharmacist, and nurses to assess the situation, prescribe, and treat the site with the evidence-based extravasation-specific vasodilators and implementation of other comfort and treatment measures—including ongoing reassessments. The original hyperkalemia and renal impairment diagnoses improved with emergency care treatment as planned and delivered, but the unintentional extravasation of a potentially irritant medication (calcium chloride and dextrose 50%) created pain, tissue damage, and a need for prolonged hospitalization to treat the complication. The patient did well eventually with medical care and surgical debridement treatments and was discharged home approximately 2 weeks later. The patient's hospitalization was required for treatment of the existing primary hyperkalemia, worsened renal impairment at time of admission, and other comorbid medical conditions, as well as care for the resultant IV medication complication. This case, and potential risks for others, highlighted a need to reassess and look for additional opportunities to innovate current processes to prevent, collaborate, and coordinate care to optimize treatment outcomes. This hyperkalemia treatment protocol and other IV irritant and vesicant medications to treat emergent and critical care situations are frequently used throughout the organization. Any of these identified known irritant or potential vesicant medications could potentially extravasate and cause tissue damage complications, whether or not recommended vasodilators or specific antidotes (where applicable) are administered immediately upon recognition. We are committed to do all we can collaboratively to prevent or at least minimize risks for our patients—with a focus on proactive, continual improvement of our care processes.

As the CNS, I had the opportunity to lead an interprofessional team with staff nurses (ED and in-patient representatives), educators, charge nurses, pharmacists, and physicians for these multiple improvement strategies to collectively prepare a comprehensive plan for ongoing assessment and care for this patient and the IV extravasation site. Additionally, I thoroughly reviewed all documentation of care delivered in the ED and interviewed all nurses involved in care of the patient (ED nurses and intermediate care inpatient nurses). Opportunities were identified to improve and positively impact care for future patients receiving IV medication with high-risk potential to cause tissue damage should extravasation occur. Bedside nurses are the experts at identifying patient needs and challenges that may occur, which can positively or negatively impact care. CNSs are the clinical experts in the facilitation of identification and implementation of clinical process improvements through the use of multidisciplinary teams to make changes and improved outcomes happen. Commitment to innovate and continuously improve care openly is evident in this ED clinical setting. A discussion of specific improvements implemented throughout the organization as process improvements related to this case exemplar will include:

- Modification in the handoff report between the ED nurses and inpatient nurses
- Policy changes, including a thorough review of select high-risk IV medications
- Suggested specialty consultations should a suspected extravasation occur
- Photographic requirements to monitor site/wound stability or progression
- Electronic medication administration record (eMAR) enhancements
- Education for nurses on this case study—resultant policy enhancements and expectations
- Advanced clinical nursing skills—ultrasound-guided peripheral IV therapy

HANDOFF REPORT

Modification in the handoff report between the ED nurses and inpatient nurses caring for patients who are being held in the ED awaiting admission (bedside handoff report) can present challenges. Many fast-paced processes are occurring around the ED environment and distractions may entice nurses from different units to modify the handoff report process. This change can lead to missed opportunities to visualize and discuss key aspects pertaining to ongoing care needs. Among the expectations for organization-wide bedside report, patient involvement (as possible) in report is encouraged, and the nurses' collaborative assessment of any wound/skin impairment is key. This bedside report involves the patient and electronic medical record, which provides an opportunity to discuss current treatments performed to date, any pending test results, or orders/interventions needing follow-up. Hourly rounding (minimum) on all patients is also an expectation for patient satisfaction and safety, and is implemented organization-wide, including in the ED, with much success.

POLICY CHANGES

Policy changes were implemented after a thorough review by pharmacy and nursing of commonly used high-risk IV medications (irritants and vesicants) that have potential for tissue damage upon extravasation. Pharmacist experts reviewed the current policy list of IV medications identified in this high-risk category at the time of the case exemplar, as well as the specific vasodilators/treatments recommended by best available evidence in the literature for those medications. No changes were recommended for the medications that this case exemplar patient received. A few additional medications were added, which include dextrose 25% and 10% concentrations (used in pediatrics), radiopaque IV contrast, and TPN and PPN (total and peripheral parenteral nutrition) infusions. These additions centralized medications with potential extravasation risks to one (nonchemo) policy for assessment and treatment guidance. Chemotherapy and biotherapy IV infusions, with their very specific antidotes and treatment guidelines, are addressed in a separate policy and are cross-referenced. Nurse experts—bedside nurses, CNS and educators, and certified wound nurses (CWON)—collaborated and reviewed the IV extravasation policy and enhanced nursing recommendations for extravasation site monitoring, assessment guidelines, photographic documentation recommendations, and specialty consultation services to be considered for an individualized collaborative plan of care. Open, regular communication involving the interprofessional team (pharmacy and nursing) when policy changes occur was reinforced and adopted as an additional safety outcome recommendation.

eMAR ENHANCEMENTS

Critical patient situations often exist where these potential high-risk IV medications for extravasation may be administered. Patients frequently have several simultaneous IV infusions and documentation may be lacking on the eMAR as to which specific IV site a medication was administered through. Though our case exemplar patient was not affected by this problem, as having one good IV site was our challenge, the interprofessional improvement team felt this could be important for future patients. It is important to properly identify and treat the correct IV site where the irritant or vesicant IV medication extravasated to safeguard or minimize tissue damage. Signs and symptoms of extravasation may be delayed for up to 48 hours or longer; this often means that care providers must rely

on documentation to identify what IV site the medication was given through. If the nurse who administered the medication is not available for contact or does not specifically remember (potentially several days later) which specific IV site the medication of concern was given through, a site could go untreated or receive delayed treatment. Our recommendation, a work in progress, is to enhance the eMAR to force documentation of the specific IV site at the time of medication administration/documentation, and additionally, that IV site assessment and patency be confirmed prior to administration. Warning messages alerting the nurse to each specific high-risk medication for extravasation (per policy list) has previously been incorporated on the eMAR medication instructions, but nurses now want a screen "pop-up message" to better warn them of potential risks and requirements. Pharmacy, IT experts, and clinical documentation advisors continue to work together to optimize these desired eMAR enhancements.

EDUCATION FOR NURSES

Education regarding policy highlights and process enhancements continues to occur for all implemented improvements. Nurses, pharmacists, pharmacy interns, and radiology technicians (who administer IV radiopaque contrast) have been included in this focused education and serve as contributors as we continue to innovate and improve processes. Revised policies and accompanying treatment tables and a computer-based training module on IV extravasations for nurses have been assigned to all registered nurses currently employed in the organization and upon hire. This ensures focused attention to important processes, policy review, and expectations of care for patients receiving these potentially high-risk medications. Resources for immediate consultation (physician, CNS, pharmacist, CWON-wound nurse specialist) are included in policies and in all educational materials. Education provided and enhanced attention to processes have been well received by all and have further unified collaborative efforts to improve care.

ENHANCED IV ACCESS OPPORTUNITIES

ED nurses, true IV experts, have identified the occasional to frequent need of rapid peripheral IV access in difficult-to-access patients in our ED setting. Placement of a large-bore peripheral IV with verifiable blood flow is key in minimizing extravasation risk and resultant tissue damage should it occur. A proposed solution by our ED nurses was to have a core group obtain the advanced clinical nursing skill of implementing ultrasound-guided peripheral IV therapy. This skill would allow nurses trained to utilize ultrasound technology to rapidly identify and guide peripheral IV cannulation in difficult IV start situations. This solution was supported by me (the CNS), the ED nursing director, and the nurse manager of interventional radiology (who coordinates the ultrasound-guided IV therapies and certifications for the organization). Plans are currently in progress to provide skill acquisition to a select group of experienced ED nurses on day, mid, and night shifts to allow a rapid IV access solution for immediate IV needs of ED patients. Educational classes, precepted skill acquisition, and competency completion are provided in collaboration with our interventional radiology/PICC (peripherally inserted central catheter) team IV experts for standardization of practice.

SUMMARY

Working together to continually improve patient care, enhance patient satisfaction, and achieve best outcomes is part of our nursing commitment to our patients as their advocates. We as CNSs and as nurses need to proactively look for opportunities to improve the safe, effective, and efficient care delivered to our patients. When complications or near misses occur, we must utilize expert resources, such as the CNS, to collaborate and to lead appropriate care teams to design, implement, and evaluate evidence-based interventions and strategies to improve care at all levels. CNS contributions in this case exemplar and many others provide opportunities for high-value outcome achievement affecting the patient, nurses/nursing care, and the organization/system. CNSs must look for those seemingly small opportunities to make a big impact to improve care. There are many opportunities just waiting to be discovered where CNS-led processes could improve care and outcomes. This is the work CNSs do best.

REFERENCE

National Association of Clinical Nurse Specialists (NACNS). (2004). *Statement on clinical nurse specialist practice and education*, 2 ed. Harrisburg, PA: Author.

Clinical Nurse Specialist in Collaborative Private Practice

Jeffrey S. Jones

The purpose of this chapter is to briefly describe one type of clinical nurse specialist (CNS) private practice model. It is not meant to be an all-inclusive guide on how to set up your own business. Rather, it is a highlight of key points that are essential to the ongoing success of a private practice. The intent is to motivate and inspire CNSs who desire a private practice by illustrating that such entrepreneurship is achievable.

DESCRIPTION OF POPULATIONS AND PRACTICE

Pinnacle Mental Health Associates, Inc., is a psychiatric CNS business offering primary mental health services for adults based in Mansfield, Ohio. Currently, the business primarily offers mental health services (assessment, diagnosis, therapy, medication management, consultation, and supervision) through contracts with other organizations.

EMPLOYMENT STATUS

The practice is CNS-owned and operates as a professional S corporation (S corp.). A professional S corp. structure was decided upon after study of various business options (LLC, C corp., etc.) and consultation with a local business attorney. An S corp. allowed the owners to share the profits and offered some tax advantages to the owners in that they were able to report gains and losses on personal income tax. An S corp. structure also protected the owner's personal assets in the event of liability. The original two CNS partners divided the duties of president, vice president, secretary, and treasurer. As owners they were also shareholders in the company. The business had a third employee who functioned in a clerical capacity as an office manager and provides administrative support.

WORK ENVIRONMENT

From 2006 through 2011 the business suite was located in a professional office building in the heart of the city's business community. The professional environment was designed by the two owners. In collaboration with the building owner, the suite was redesigned to capture a very open, casual, warm, and homey feel. The intent was to distinctly not have a medical office appearance. Tan, earthy colors were chosen for the walls and carpet. A living room feel was accomplished by placing a modular couch and swivel chair in one corner and a table and chairs at the other. Fresh coffee and iced tea were always available for consumers as they waited to be seen. Numerous plants and other foliage augmented the homey feel. The waiting area was open, with the receptionist in an island in the center where she freely interacted with patrons. The clinician's offices were at opposite ends of the suite and were professionally decorated in continuation of the relaxed homey feel. Plush couches, chairs, and a small but functional desk completed the scheme. Each office had a laptop because all the records were electronic. As the result of purposeful milieu management, the small workforce and comfortable surroundings created a relaxed and intimate environment. In 2011 it was decided to transition the practice into a consultation business primarily. The lease of the office space was not renewed and the one partner left the practice to pursue other opportunities. More on this business decision will be discussed later.

PROFESSIONAL RESPONSIBILITIES

Typical daily duties include overseeing the day-to-day operations of the business. This includes but is not limited to managing cash flow, making decisions regarding the business, marketing, negotiating contracts with entities such as the Department of Rehabilitation and Corrections and local mental health centers, and so forth. The actual clinical work performed may consist of assessment and diagnosis of mental health disorders; engagement in individual, family, or group therapy; prescription and management of medications; and liaison contact with other community linkage support services or referral entities.

PROFESSIONAL SUPPORT STRUCTURE

The structure of the business originally consisted of two CNS partners, an office manager/clerical support person, and a collaborating physician. The collaborating physician is not physically located onsite, but instead collaborates from a distance. The requirements of the collaborative agreement are met via monthly meetings with the physician for the purpose of case review. A third therapist, a licensed independent social worker (LISW), was added as a contract professional prior to closure of the office in 2010.

FUTURE OPPORTUNITIES AND CHALLENGES FOR CNSs

Because advanced practice registered nurses (APRNs) are increasingly recognized as a source of primary care, CNSs have the opportunity and a duty to retain their place among their APRN peers. This is actually very crucial, for even though CNSs are historically recognized as experts in a given area, there is notable resistance from the medical community and nursing entities/APRN colleagues in viewing the CNS as an APRN. This resistance is primarily due to the prevailing, traditional medical model of primary health care delivery and the embrace of this model by the nurse practitioner (NP) discipline.

TAKING THE PLUNGE

As a CNS, you may have arrived at a point in your career where you have worked within an organization and have survived downsizing, rightsizing, and many corporate changes. You may now be ready to make the decision to create your own universe by practicing outside of the established medical model/community. Welcome to the ranks of CNS entrepreneurs who have established their own private practice and given birth to a business.

Those who choose to take this route have several decisions to make. The first choice is whether or not to join an existing practice in a traditional office structure. If you choose this, be forewarned that this type of practice is very likely based on a medical model design. The second option is to open your own business. This option offers control to choose a nursing framework as a practice model. My partner and I chose the latter. Deciding on the second option grew out of past frustrating experiences trying to function as a CNS within a medical-dominated practice model. CNSs think and practice differently than MDs and NPs because of the difference in CNS education. We both had reached a point in our career where we needed to be in an environment that reflected and supported the CNS's three spheres of influence: client, system, and nursing.

The next choice is deciding whether you want to establish a solo practice or work within a partnership. There are positives and negatives to either choice. Establishing a solo practice offers more control and autonomy, which some entrepreneurs need or find attractive. Going it alone, however, means that you shoulder the whole responsibility. This can be burdensome and very lonely. I chose to have a partner because I valued the collegiality and peer support of another CNS. I also preferred starting off with a business model of shared responsibility.

The economic events of 2009 and the upheaval in health care changed this. After three successful profit-producing years of owning and running a business mainly comprised of a private practice in an office setting, it became clear that adjustments had to be made for the survival of the business as unemployment rose and our client numbers dropped. A shift in our income meant that it was now coming primarily from outside contracts, yet we still were paying large overhead for an office suite, clerical staff, and so forth. A reenvisioning of the practice/business took place and throughout 2010 it was decided to morph Pinnacle Mental Health Associates, Inc., into a primarily contract entity that would retain a small private practice option (at the discretion the owners) but mainly be a competitive force in the consulting market. We decided to allow our lease to expire in 2011 and to continue any desired private practice through brief subletting of office space elsewhere, based on caseload flow and geographic need around the state, in other therapists' offices. We also eliminated the role of the clerical staff. While this strategy significantly reduced our expenses and saved the business, the CNS business partner chose at that time to leave the practice and pursue other opportunities. Thus, on May 1, 2001, all shares of stock in the business were transferred to me, and Pinnacle Mental Health Associates, Inc., changed to operating as a business out of my home with me being sole provider of services for the practice. I do still maintain a small private practice as Pinnacle by subletting space out of the collaborative physician office several times a month. Now, however, the primary source of income for the business is through multiple contracts with entities such as the Ohio Department of Rehabilitation and Corrections, various community mental health centers, and speaking engagements.

Whether you choose a solo business model or a partnership model, you may also need to consider a collaborative arrangement with a physician if this is required in your state. The specifics of this will vary from state to state in terms of the language that is used to describe the relationship. The most common terms are collaboration or supervision. In Ohio the relationship language is *collaboration*. Choosing a collaborating physician is equally important as choosing a business partner. This decision should be guided by a sense of like-mindedness. Both the physician and the business partner need to have a clear understanding and appreciation for the scope of practice of CNSs and how it differs from NP-focused practice. It may be helpful at some point to gather information and evaluate personality traits through the use of such tools as the Myers-Briggs Personality Inventory. Additionally, and more specific to you and your business partner, it is important to invest time in evaluation of each other's entrepreneurial traits. A clear understanding of each other's perspective allows each person to know himself or herself, to know how he or she reacts under various circumstances, and to become familiar with his or her own particular strengths and comfort levels. Once these very basic but key steps are taken, you are ready to develop a business plan.

PUTTING IT ON PAPER

The development of a sound, well-structured business plan can open many doors for you as you proceed. When you seek advice and assistance from the local business community or lenders that will help with your financial needs, all will want to review your business plan. There are numerous books as well as free online resources concerning the construction of a business plan. Some have been written specifically for nurses. Whatever source you use, the most common elements of a good business plan are:

1. Executive summary (including your mission statement)
2. Table of contents
3. Description of the practice
4. Products and services
5. Operations
6. Marketing plan
7. Assessment of competition
8. Risks
9. Finances (start-up costs, projected spreadsheets, etc.)
10. Milestones
11. Summary

Our original business was a private mental health practice, which has now evolved in to a consulting/ contract business. As most owners do, we had many choices to make in order to set up the business. Meeting with an attorney who understands business law and the services you plan to deliver is essential in clarifying the advantages and distinctions among these options. After completing this step, our business decided to structure itself as a professional S corp. As previously described, an S corp. allows the owners to share the profits and also offers some tax advantages because each is able to report gains and losses on personal income tax. The other main advantage of an S corp. structure is that it separates and protects the owner's personal assets in the event of liability. This remains true even though the business has now transitioned into mainly a consulting entity.

WHAT ARE NURSING SERVICES WORTH?

Now that you have a business plan and an attorney, the next step is to begin to explore your financial needs. This should start with a meeting with an accountant who has had experience with servicing health care organizations. The accountant will help you refine elements of the business plan that may be unrealistic. This feedback will lead to the development of a more accurate financial spreadsheet. When this step is completed, you are ready to approach a lender.

This phase of the business experience for the CNS can be the most awkward. Nurses are not inherently educated or acculturated to think of nursing services as independent and marketable commodities. More likely, nurses have adapted the identity of who they are and the service they provide from an organization or an MD provider. It is absolutely imperative that these false (and weak) notions about nurses and dependent nursing services be dealt with and refined before the beginning phase. Lenders want to know what experience you have, what has brought you to this point in your career, and what enables you to offer services independent of another entity. They need to see that you have confidence in your abilities, and they need to get a crystal-clear idea of how you plan to succeed. This is precisely the time to drag out the power suit, brush up your presentation skills, and do everything you can to sell yourself.

You may have to speak with several lenders before you find one willing to take the risk of investing in a start-up business. Securing the actual start-up funds should involve two products from the lender. The first should be a term loan to use for start-up essentials. The second should be a line of credit to cover operational costs until your cash flow is steady. Remember that over 50% of new businesses fail in the first year. The main reason this happens is that the business is undercapitalized at start-up.

Finding the right location for your business and beginning to market your services will take more time than you may think. Choosing just the right spot that fits your budget and also is convenient to the population you intend to serve is tricky. Marketing is also complicated. You can spend a lot of money on commercial advertising that may be wasted. Many marketing people will want to help you spend your money on advertising. It is wise to adapt a diverse approach. Here are some helpful tips.

- Know that the most powerful marketing tool is word of mouth, so start networking early.
- Schedule yourself for speaking engagements that target the population you serve.
- Get the local newspaper interested; an in-depth interview about a nurse-run business is usually a newsworthy item.
- Develop a website for the business. This can be relatively inexpensive and a lot of consumers can get their information about you from the Internet.
- Get interviewed on the local radio and TV station.
- Save the costly things such as print ads, flyers, and direct mailings to deploy closer to your opening. A successful marketing strategy is ongoing and

never ends. It takes a long time for a community to remember that a new business is in town.

Set aside some of your budget each month to do some advertising. You may or may not get support from the medical and APRN community. Some communities are more receptive to others regarding CNSs in private practice. The name recognition of APRN is so closely linked with the NP/MD practice model that it may be difficult for other health care providers, including your own colleagues, to understand a practice model that is truly focused on advanced practice nursing.

Another consideration is the decision regarding how you will be reimbursed for your services. Will you apply for and become impaneled on all the major insurance plans? Will you accept Medicare and Medicaid? If so, this process needs to start no later than 60 days prior to opening. Will you accept credit cards? What current procedural terminology (CPT) codes will you use to bill for services, and how much will you charge? After carefully looking at various options, we decided to be a solely fee-for-service/out-of-network practice at the inception. This remains true today. I am not a Medicare or Medicaid provider in the private practice setting, but I do hold Medicare/Medicaid provider numbers and these are used when I'm providing service at a contract agency such as a community mental health center. In a private practice setting, the client simply pays out of pocket. Consumers are charged the same rate for service as the marketable rate in comparable mental health care offices. They are then provided with an invoice with appropriate diagnostic codes and CPT codes for submission to their insurance company. The client is then reimbursed from their out-of-network benefits allowance. This practice model works for the market niche I target when I see clients privately. Your practice may have to operate differently depending on the population you intend to serve.

COVERING YOUR ASSETS

A crucial but often overlooked aspect of owning a private practice is ensuring that you and the business are adequately covered regarding liability. It will be necessary to find an insurance carrier who will provide coverage not only to you and your partner as CNSs, but also to the building or office suite for claims not related to malpractice. An essential aspect of this is finding a carrier that recognizes the CNS category in the APRN role. Some of the more prominent nursing malpractice carriers only recognize NPs, nurse midwives, and nurse anesthetists, placing CNSs under the NP category. If pressed, some of these carriers will write what is called a rider, acknowledging that you are a CNS and not an NP. While this may suffice in a court of law, from a legal perspective you would be better advised to procure a company that clearly recognizes the scope of practice of a CNS as unique and distinct from that of other types of APRN.

Finally, the day-to-day operations of the business will ebb and flow as the weeks go by. You will make daily decisions and the next week change your mind after learning from your mistakes. There are only a few absolutes in managing your own practice. As your business matures, it will become part of the community. Your business will develop a rhythm, and your attentiveness to that rhythm will provide cues as to when to make changes to meet changing economic, business, and community needs. This may include augmenting services or implementing different marketing strategies or (as in our case) reenvisioning the business in order to survive.

TRUE AUTONOMY

The opportunity to function independently as a business in a private practice setting can be an incredibly powerful and liberating experience for CNSs. Free from the hospital structure that sometimes is unsupportive of the role of the CNS, you may find yourself wondering what took you so long to make the decision to become an entrepreneur. To be sure, this chosen path is not without its risks. Managing a business is a time-consuming, 24/7 job, and unless you have a large sum of money invested and available, you will potentially have to use your home and car for collateral. Relationships can be strained both personally and professionally. You may find days when you wonder if you have done the right thing. Then you will get together with your colleagues and listen to the frustrations that are currently born out of struggling to practice as a CNS in today's health care climate. You will reflect on the path you have chosen that has now afforded you complete control over how and when you choose to practice. You will be reminded that you are offering true advanced practice nursing services to clients, systems, and other nurses and you will be reminded of why you became a nurse in the first place and a CNS in the second place. A smile will cross your face and you will come to the quiet realization that you "have arrived."

SUGGESTED READING

Abernathy, S. F., & Adams, L. T. (2011). *Nursing entrepreneurship for the 21st century: Starting a nurse-operated business.* Columbus, OH: Zip Publishing/The Educational.

Dayhoff, N. E., & Moore, P. S. (2004). Entrepreneurial dimensions of CNS practice. CNS entrepreneurship: Marketing 101. *Clinical Nurse Specialist, 18*(3), 123–125.

Dayhoff, N. E., & Moore, P. S. (2005). CNS entrepreneurs: Innovators in patient care. *Sourcebook for Advanced Practice Nurses, 30*(1), 6–8.

Fine, S. (1997). *Developing a private practice in psychiatric mental health nursing.* New York, NY: Springer.

Fitzpatrick, J. J., Glasgow, A., & Young, J. N. (2003). *Managing your practice: A guide for advanced practice nurses.* New York, NY: Springer.

Woodreuff, D. (2003). The metamorphosis of a CNS entrepreneurial business. *Clinical Nurse Specialist, 17*(6), 290–291.

Clinical Nurse Specialist Entrepreneurship: A Journey From Idea to Invention, Leading to a Consulting/Education Business

Kathleen M. Vollman

*I*n your nursing career, have you come across a product or service that you thought could be improved upon or changed? Perhaps you have even thought of something totally new that would help meet a health care need. What barriers exist that prevented you from exploring it further? As clinical nurse specialists (CNSs), we are presented with many unique opportunities to pursue entrepreneurial adventures—and we possess the necessary skill set to make it happen. What questions need to be asked and answered in order to motivate you to pursue your idea? A nurse entrepreneur is considered to be an owner of a business that offers nursing services of a direct care, educational, research, administrative, or consultative nature (International Council of Nurses, 2004). They are innovators who drive visions that lead to change, safer health systems, and creative models of care (Raine, 2003). The major attributes of a nurse entrepreneur include a decision maker, visionary, problem solver, risk taker, self-starter, and great communicator. They have to be confident, committed, determined, creative, well organized, flexible, but most of all passionate and persistent (Dayhoff & Moore, 2002; Palmer, 1996; Price, 2004; Wilson, Whitaker, & Waterford, 2012). I would like to share my journey of creating and marketing a positioning frame to help turn and support a critically ill patient with acute

respiratory distress syndrome (ARDS) into the prone position to help improve their oxygenation, and from that the launch of a consulting career. The journey is a fascinating, challenging, sometimes exhausting, and rewarding life event that shows what can happen when you take a product from the idea stage to market and then serve as an expert consultant.

CRITICALLY ILL PATIENTS WITH ARDS: MAKING PRONE MOBILIZATION SAFE

Discovering the impact of positioning on oxygenation in critically ill patients occurred early in my career. Because of a review of the literature and my clinical experience, I discovered that a strategy of a 30-minute interval positioning from side to side for a patient with ARDS improved the patient's gas exchange (Ray et al., 1974). Therefore, when introduced to the concept of the prone position, several of the nursing staff were excited to try it. In the early 1980s, we were reaching for any treatment strategies that could assist a population with a 70% mortality rate. The challenge of positioning a critically ill patient with extensive tubes and lines without risking major complications posed a large obstacle to use of the prone position. I saw this challenge as an opportunity to make a patient care process better. My passion for the idea joined with the foundational information served as a strong basis for me to believe I could pursue this idea and actually make it work (Vollman, 2004). Ideas for successful inventions usually arise from solution development surrounding problems that exist in our everyday work and personal life. The concepts or ideas created need to come from our current knowledge, skills, or abilities. If an invention is launched in order to learn new skills the chance of success diminishes significantly (Zagury, 1993).

What is usually missing from most CNSs' toolkits, as it was in my case, are the general knowledge and skills of business planning and financial management. However, there are many resources that can help CNSs, such as small business associations, local community colleges, professional associations, and Internet sites (Biel, 1994; Levy, 1995; Vollman, 2001, 2004). I took advantage of each of these to move from passion about an idea to product development. With considerable advice from family, friends, and colleagues, I developed a plan to further examine the concept of prone positioning. I designed and developed a support frame and procedure for prone positioning as part of my master's thesis, and then tested it with critically ill patients as described in this chapter.

PRACTICE INNOVATION

Producing the Prototype

A prototype is a workable model that can be tested and further developed. If you don't have the time, money, skills, or commitment to build or get your idea turned into a prototype, the odds of licensing or bringing that idea to market are small (Levy, 1995). There are a number of ways to get prototypes built, including university engineering schools, prototype development businesses, and talented extended family members. A local inventors group may be an additional resource to help you find prototype makers within your community (Levy, 1995). I was fortunate enough to have a relative who was a mechanical engineer and believed he could build the frame I had in mind. The engineering schools may also be an economical way to develop your idea. Each semester engineering classes have projects they must design and develop. Why not have one of those project ideas be yours? In addition, many universities outside of the engineering department have formal programs designed to assist inventors with their ideas or patents. Whatever strategy you choose, remember you

will move farther in the process with a tangible product that can be tested versus just an idea on paper (Biel, 1994).

The prone positioner's first prototype was built out of wood. Blueprints were developed from that model and changes were made to accommodate the technology of critical care during the turning procedure. The second prototype was manufactured together with a plastics company that works with prototypes. This prototype was used in a product evaluation study conducted at California State University in Long Beach with nursing students in a simulated critical care environment as the first phase of my master's thesis. The third prototype was made after changes in the design occurred based on the results of the product evaluation study, and was used in the second phase of my thesis with critically ill patients.

Intellectual Property Protection

Once the idea is formulated, it must be analyzed to determine the level of protection that is required. There are three levels of protection for intellectual property (ideas). A copyright protects the tangible expression of an idea. A trademark provides the owner with the right to exclude others from using confusingly similar product identification in commerce. A patent provides the owner with the right to exclude others from making, using, or selling the invention throughout the United States. A patent is the granting of intellectual property rights (Biel, 1994; Vollman, 2004). Think seriously before giving away an idea. Remember, an idea is intellectual property, or your brain trust, and any consideration of sharing that idea should be classified as a consultation that requires a fee.

I started protection of my intellectual property regarding the prone positioner idea very early in the process, with documentation of the initial idea development and crude drawings. I had read somewhere about keeping an inventor's log that included a detailed description of the idea and drawings, and having the document witnessed by two people. Later, my patent attorney shared with me that this document was actually my first form of protection. Since June 8, 1995, the U.S. Patent and Trademark Office (USPTO) has offered inventors the option of filing a provisional application for patent, which was designed to provide a lower-cost first-patent filing in the United States. Applicants are entitled to claim the benefit of a provisional application in a corresponding nonprovisional application filed no later than 12 months after the provisional application filing date. The USPTO reminds inventors that any public use or sale in the United States or publication of the invention anywhere in the world more than one year prior to the filing of a patent application on that invention will prohibit the granting of a U.S. patent on it (USPTO, n.d.). The clearer your description and drawings, the stronger your protection will be. In addition, my attorney and I had the prototype manufacturer, the student nurse participants, and my research assistants all sign five-year confidential disclosure agreements before participating in the testing of the prototype in the product evaluation part of the study. A confidential disclosure agreement provided us with a way to protect the idea while working on the patent submission.

There are different types of patents, including design, plant, and utility patents (Levy, 1995). The prone positioner got a utility patent. A utility patent is granted for a new, useful, and nonobvious process, machine, manufactured article, composition, or an improvement on any of these. In the patent process, there are four steps to move through: a patent search, preparation of a file application, processing the application, and issuing the patent (Levy, 1995).

When I began the search for a patent attorney, I knew the process was expensive. My resources and family financial support were already being stretched by graduate school and prototype development. I was fortunate to be introduced to an attorney who was willing to take a student and work creatively to meet my legal needs in a cost-conscious manner (Vollman, 1999). The patent search found several patents that could be considered similar, making it necessary to document how the prone positioner was different. That step was successfully completed, and the utility patent was filed for in 1987. At that point, the positioner had patent-pending protection and could then be used in the second phase of my master's thesis to examine the effect on oxygenation in critically ill patients using the prone positioner (Vollman & Bander, 1996).

The Cross Roads: A Crucial Decision-Making Point

As you are designing a plan to bring your idea to market, you will reach a crossroads. Do I produce the product myself, license it to a company, or seek out a company that helps inventors move their product to the market? Be cautious of taking your idea to an invention marketing company. Reputable invention marketing companies usually will not require any up-front fees and do not advertise on TV or radio, or in newspapers, direct mailers, or magazine ads (Levy, 1995). If you choose the do-it-yourself road, you will need to raise money and dedicate yourself to one single enterprise. If you decide on the licensing option, there are a number of strategies that can help make the pitch to a company stronger. Some of those strategies include a working prototype, patent

protection, data on market size, selling impact, and potential cost to produce. The more homework done prior to the licensing pitch, the stronger your negotiating platform (Biel, 1994).

The preparation homework was done for the prone positioner. Abstracts, publications, and regional and national lectures to share the information about the science of positioning and the prone positioner were prepared. The mechanical engineer and I formed a company called HosTech Inc., which housed the patent. Because of potential product liability issues, we chose the road of a subchapter S corporation so that we would be individually protected. The road to licensing was hilly and full of curves, taking almost 7 years from completion of the study to signing a contract. I chose the licensing road because I knew I still wanted to be a practicing CNS and not a manufacturer. I began discussions with Hill-Rom, an international company that manufactures and distributes beds, support surfaces, and furniture in early 1996. HosTech, Inc., licensed the invention to Hill-Rom, and the Vollman Prone Positioner went on the market in January of 1997. I have maintained involvement through a consulting agreement in the marketing and education of the device and the science of prone positioning. The device is no longer being manufactured; however, organizations around the world who have the device are still using it to help facilitate the turning and prone positioning of critically ill patients. The knowledge gained from this experience was invaluable in my role as CNS for the medical critical care service in a large urban hospital setting. I was heavily involved in evidence-based new product acquisition and standardization for materials that helped make it more efficient for the bedside nurse to deliver nursing care. Part of the strategy to help get the product to market was submission of scientific abstracts for presentations at local, regional, national, and international conferences, as well as numerous publications covering a wide variety of topics. As my comfort in those CNS competencies increased, I was able to help the staff submit papers and develop and present data on the care practice improvements we created, while helping them to develop professionally. The competencies developed during this process helped prepare me for a consultation business, but more importantly, they allowed me to excel as a unit-based CNS in changing processes and practices to improve patient outcomes (Dayhoff & Moore, 2002; Sao Lan, 2005).

Outcomes: Defining Success

I frequently get asked the questions, "How successful is the positioner?" and "Do you make a lot of money from it?" Every person defines success in a different way, and I would like to share with you how I define success with an e-mail I received from a patient who experienced use of the Vollman Prone Positioner.

> My name is JM and I had been admitted to the hospital with a severe case of *Streptococcus pneumoniae* this past January, which resulted in some serious complications, including ARDS. Among the interventions that saved my life was the use of the prone positioner you invented, which had been procured but never had the chance to be used. It was the hospital's first use of the technique. I responded very well to it and survived the ordeal. I just wanted to drop you a note to thank you for your innovation. I am expected to make a full recovery and am well on the way to doing that now. I thought it might do you good to hear from a beneficiary of your device. Thanks again, and I wish you every success as you continue to make a difference in people's lives.

In addition to the personal rewards, the professional rewards were beyond anything I ever dreamed. As part of the inventing and licensing process, I created a consulting agreement for further refinement of the prone positioner and utilization of my expertise regarding the science of positioning critically ill patients. Through this process I have learned many skills, including contract negotiation, outcome measurement, cost–benefit analysis, and long-term project management. The experience served as a strong foundation for my CNS role in a large urban hospital setting. It also helped launch the next chapter of my career as a CNS consultant and educator (Vollman, 1999; Vollman & Bander, 1996). The product is no longer being manufactured and sold as of May 2011. While the end is sad, the device did what was originally intended: to demystify the fact that we can prone-position critically ill patients safely and make a difference.

The Next Chapter: A CNS Consultation and Education Business

All my previous work and experience helped to prepare me for the next phase that I like to call the "virtual CNS role." The virtual CNS extends the impact of the role beyond the walls of an institution to offer the CNS's expertise, skills and resources to staff nurses and organizations who want to make a difference but are unsure of how to get started. This role provides the CNS with another strategy to empower the bedside practitioner while advancing the profession of nursing outside the walls of a single institution.

During my time as a CNS at a large urban medical center, I was able to gather a wealth of knowledge

and experience around leadership, frontline and organizational change in large systems, lean technology, teamwork, process management, and a passion for creating safe work cultures that empower nurses to own their practice. I also recognized a significant deficit in the practice of basic nursing care. At the time, most health care systems dictated that nurses focus on the technological/medical aspects of patient care rather than basic nursing care activities. Evidence of the lack of focus on the fundamentals was clear in the 1999 IOM report that stated 95,000 patients die each year from medical errors that included medications, infections, falls, and pressure ulcers all falling within the domain of nursing (Kohn, Corrigan, & Donaldson, 1999). Therefore, a significant part of the journey focused on reintroducing the value and evidence around fundamental nursing care and finding the right resources and developing systems to make it easy for the nurse to perform the care (Vollman, 2013). An essential part of the process was engaging frontline staff and the organization in the change as well as measuring clinical and financial outcomes. During the 13 years spent working within acute care, I reached out beyond the walls to share the learning we had experienced. I wrote abstracts to present at local, regional, and eventually national conferences. I published articles on my areas of expertise. Through this work, I began to develop a worldwide reputation for speaking and consulting on various pulmonary/ critical care and professional nursing topics. This help set the foundation for the development of an independent consultation and education business. In 2003, I officially launched the company Advancing Nursing, LLC, which focuses on creating empowered work environments for nurses through the acquisition of greater skills and knowledge to advance the profession of nursing.

Drawing on skills and experience from the Vollman Prone Positioner development, as well as intrapreneurial work performed at the hospital (which included design of a business and marketing plan to launch a systemwide wound care program), I set up the new business (Vollman, 1999; Vollman & Bander, 1996). There are many things to consider when you are deciding on a business, the first being what type of business you want to start. While I had already made the decision regarding the type of business, educational and consultative, it was critical to outline the scope to ensure a realistic expectation of what I could achieve (Leong, 2005). This parallels the issue of the CNS role within a hospital system. If the expectations are unrealistic, the ability of the person to achieve the expected outcomes is limited. Through my nurse journey, I had developed four areas of expertise that serve to guide the scope of the education and consultation product/service. They include a clinical critical care section in care of pulmonary and septic patients, an area focused on "back to the basics using evidence-based nursing care to prevent patient harm," a third section on care of the nurse and work environment, and the last focus on CNS role development and entrepreneurship (Table 31.1). In each of these a common thread exists. The goal and the vision for the business is to provide frontline nurses with the necessary knowledge, skills, and resources to enable them to advocate for their patient and family and be fulfilled in their professional work. The next step is to set up a business structure, which can be a sole proprietorship, general partnership, or a corporation (including S corporation, limited liability company or a limited liability partnership; Dayhoff & Moore, 2003). The structure that best suited Advancing Nursing was a limited liability corporation. A limited liability company is a hybrid type of legal structure that provides the limited liability features of a corporation and the tax efficiencies and operational flexibility of a partnership. The "owners" of an LLC are referred to as "members." Depending on the state, the members can consist of a single individual (one owner), two or more individuals, corporations, or other LLCs. There are six general principles to forming an LLC. They include naming the business, filing articles of incorporation, creating an operating agreement, obtaining licenses and permits if required, hiring employees (optional), and announcing your business. Three rules must be followed when naming your LLC: the name must be different from any existing LLC in your state, it must indicate that the business is an LLC (such as "LLC" or limited company), and it must not include words restricted by your state (Small Business Association, 2013). Once I received the submission document from the state that the business name was official, I set up a separate business checking account at the bank. Minimal capital was required for business startup and overhead was very low. I set up an office in my home and prepared and submitted all the invoices, expenses, travel, lecture, and consultation project prep work.

Developments of a graphic representation of the business and communication strategies were the next steps. Having developed the mission statement made designing the graphic image easier. The image is an inert triangle going from dark to lighter representing growth as the nurse gains knowledge and skill to increase his or her personal power to take care of patients and advance the profession of nursing (Figure 31.1). Most often the web address reflects the type of business, but with an already established professional name it was easy to choose a name: www.vollman.com

One of the lessons learned in starting a business is the importance of networking and being comfortable in admitting your limitations. Through networking, I found a very skilled individual who was starting a web design business (while still having a day job) to design the website to reflect the mission, outline the business, make it easy to navigate, and provide the ability to contact me. Marketing was done by word of mouth, scientific publications, networking, and ensuring that someone could always connect with me to ask questions, request a talk, or visit or to comment. Other types of marketing can include paid advertising to targeted groups, flyers, free web education, discounts, and creating niche markets like education for certification exam prep. As a CNS, we are taught to measure outcomes and that is true in business as well. I measured both process components as well as actual outcomes in a variety of ways, including business growth (new clients), revenue versus expenses, invitations to speak, hits on the website, number of downloads, e-mail follow-through, conference evaluations and posters, individual clinicians, and organizational feedback. I am truly blessed to be able to do what I love and earn a good living.

TABLE 31.1

SCOPE OF SERVICES			
Critical Care Clinical Focus	**Evidence-Based Nursing Care**	**Nurse and Work Culture**	**CNS Role and Intra-entrepreneurship**
Example: Acute respiratory distress syndrome Severe sepsis/ septic shock (implementation management) Prone positioning	Example: Reducing health care–associated infections (HAIs) through oral care, bathing, dressing management Reducing complications of immobility Preventing skin injury	Example: Creating healthy work cultures to impact patient outcomes Nurturing the nurse Shared decision making Safety cultures	CNS role redesign Process of product invention Nurse intra- and entrepreneurship CNS graduate program development

Source: ©Advancing Nursing, LLC (2013).

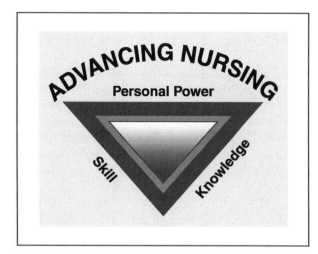

FIGURE 31.1 Advancing Nursing LLC graphic image.
Source: ©Advancing Nursing, LLC (2003).

One of the largest hurdles I had was determining fee structures for various activities. Determining your worth and asking to be compensated for it is difficult for most nurses, me included. My colleagues across the country were instrumental in this area because the information is not published anywhere. Through discussion with clinicians who were doing similar work nationally and internationally, I was able to come up with a fee I was comfortable with and that was accepted well by customers. When asked the question "How much do you charge?" instead of naming a fee that may be too low or high, consider asking the following: "Sounds like a great program and I would love to be involved" "What type of budget have you set aside for this role?" "Whom shall I discuss my fees with? I am really excited to participate and it sounds like a big project, what have you paid in the past for these services?" If you received the business through a referral, you can say "Was anything said about my rates?" The general rule to follow is to try to get the customer to provide a price first. As the business grows, remember to increase your rates based on demand, success of your product/service, and what the market can bear.

There were some decisions I made early on. I chose not to be the continuing education provider. I prepare all the materials necessary but allow the inviting organization to perform the submission. When I add interactive education via the website, I will move to become a provider. I made a conscious decision to work with selected industry. Companies that I formed relationships with had product and services that supported the nurse's ability to perform the research-based care in an effective and efficient manner. Processes developed to help ensure customer satisfaction and referrals included updating talks as soon as new science was available and responding to e-mail requests within a two-week period for clinical questions and within two days for a request for services. Keeping the curriculum vitae up-to-date, as well as maintaining a current professional photo, made it easy to respond to requests even while on the road. I purchase an ongoing Internet-based service for a small monthly fee for remote access to my computer while traveling, providing full availability of all files to respond to e-mail requests. If handouts are not provided by the sponsoring organization, I am able to post the PDF-protected PowerPoint document on the website under the download section. To help maintain life balance, about five years into the business, I added a two-days-a-week assistant to help manage invoices, accounting, article retrieval, and some additional activities.

I feel I am one of the most fortunate people in the world because I am living my dream and sharing my passion of questioning the status quo with other nurses and health care practitioners to make an impact in patient's lives. The key is to be yourself and continue to be creative and adventuresome. It is true what they say: If you love what you do you will never work another day in your life. Take the chance of being an entrepreneur; you will never regret the journey.

REFERENCES

Biel, M. H. (1994). Nurse inventors: Turning ideas into products. *Dimensions of Critical Care Nursing, 13*(4), 202–206.

Dayhoff, N. E., & Moore, P. S. (2002). Entrepreneurial clinical nurse specialists: Innovators of patient care. *Clinical Nurse Specialist CNS, 16*(5), 274–276.

Dayhoff, N. E., & Moore, P. S. (2003). Entrepreneurship: Start-up questions. *Clinical Nurse Specialist CNS, 17*(2), 86–88.

International Council of Nurses. (2004). *Guidelines on the nurse entrepreneur–partner providing nursing service.* Geneva, Switzerland.

Kohn, K. T., Corrigan, J. M., & Donaldson, M. S. (1999). *To err is human: Building a safer health system.* Washington, DC: National Academy Press.

Leong, S. L. (2005). Clinical nurse specialist entrepreneurship. *Internet Journal of Advanced Practice Nursing, 7*(1).

Levy, R. C. (1995). *The inventor's desktop companion.* Detroit, MI: Visible Ink Press.

Palmer, J. W. (1996). Thoughts on becoming a nurse entrepreneur. *Journal of Emergency Nursing, 22*(6), 534–535.

Price, R. W. (2004). *Roadmap to entrepreneurial success: Powerful strategies for building a high profit business.* New York, NY: American Management Association.

Raine, P. (2003). Promoting breast-feeding in a deprived area: The influence of a peer support initiative. *Health & Social Care in the Community, 11*(6), 463–469.

Ray, J. F., Yost, L., Moallem, S., Sanoudos, G. M., Villamena, P., Paredes, R. M., & Clauss, R. H. (1974). Immobility, hypoxemia, and pulmonary arteriovenous shunting. *Archives of Surgery, 109*(4), 537–541.

Sao Lan, J. I. (2005). Clinical nurse specialist entrepreneurship. *Internet Journal of Advanced Nursing Practice, 7*(1).

Small Business Association. (2013). Retrieved June 27, 2013, from http://www.sba.gov/content/limited-liability-company-llc

U.S. Patent and Trademark Office (USPTO). (n.d.). *Provisional application for patent*. Retrieved October 1, 2007, from http://www.uspto.gov/web/offices/pac/provapp.htm

Vollman, K. M. (1999). My search to help patients breathe. *Reflections, 25*(2), 16–18.

Vollman, K. M. (2001). Be an entrepreneur: Create opportunities for a new life adventure. *AACN News, 18*(4), 5.

Vollman, K. M. (2004). Nurse entrepreneurship: Taking an invention from birth to the marketplace. *Clinical Nurse Specialist CNS, 18*(2), 68–71.

Vollman, K. M., & Bander, J. J. (1996). Improved oxygenation utilizing a prone positioner in patients with acute respiratory distress syndrome. *Intensive Care Medicine, 22*(10), 1105–1111.

Vollman, K. M. (2013). Interventional patient hygiene: Discussion of the issues and a proposed model for implementation of the nursing care basics. *Intensive and Critical Care Nursing, 29*, 250–255.

Wilson, A, Whitaker, N., & Waterford, D. (2012) Rising to the challenge of healthcare reform with entrepreneurial and intrapreneurial nursing initiatives. *Online Journal of the Issues in Nursing, 17*(2).

Zagury, C. S. (1993). *Nurse entrepreneur: Building the bridge of opportunity*. Long Branch, NJ: Vista Publishing.

The Clinical Nurse Specialist in Industry/Business

Jane L. Bromund, Mary A. Short, and Kathleen C. Solotkin

The clinical nurse specialist (CNS) in the pharmaceutical or medical device industry has far-reaching spheres of influence that encompass the client, nurse, and organization (Goudreau et al., 2007; National Association of Clinical Nurse Specialists [NACNS], 2004). Industry utilizes the CNS's skill set in a multitude of roles and settings that are often virtual. The CNS must have deep therapeutic knowledge of the patient population being served as well as how the pharmaceutical or medical device affects the patient. The patient population, under stringent privacy protection, is served from afar. Opportunities abound and most often focus on the patient with disease amenable to intervention in such areas as neuroscience, oncology, cardiovascular, critical care, women's health, endocrine disease including diabetes, and infectious disease.

Functioning in a global market, the emphasis is to understand the effects of the therapy across a vast and diverse population. The CNS is called upon to implement strategies in a wide variety of countries, cultures, and health care systems under different regulatory authorities around the world. Because the patient and provider are not located at the primary work site, the CNS must adapt to virtual methods of assessment and communication. Telecommunication is common and the industry CNS utilizes e-mail, web conferences, and teleconferences as primary modes of interaction. Face-to-face interactions often require travel with significant time zone changes and adaptation to different cultural environments, languages, and traditions. At all points of development, safety and quality are at the forefront in the work of the industry CNS. The goal

remains to achieve the best possible outcome for the patient by ensuring the right drug for the right patient at the right time, reinforcing the adage that what is good for the patient is good for the business.

The pharmaceutical and medical device industries have two primary functional divisions relevant to the roles a CNS might pursue: sales/marketing and medical. In addition, various other functional areas support the medical and marketing divisions, including regulatory, data management, and governmental affairs. Work in any of these divisions can be within the scope of the industry CNS practice.

In the sales/marketing environment, one area of focus for the CNS is ensuring medical and scientific accuracy in promotion of approved drugs or devices. The CNS affects the patient through consulting with marketing personnel on the development of materials such as educational brochures, websites, and advertisements directed to the patient or health care professional. The CNS is uniquely qualified to help the sales and marketing staff understand the disease state and the impact the therapy has on efficacy, safety, and quality of life. Sales/marketing associates for an industry CNS may be analogous to the nursing staff for a CNS in a hospital-based practice setting. An industry CNS may be called upon to advance the knowledge level of these associates from basic to advanced in a limited time frame, despite geographical constraints and often without the benefit of health care education or experience. As a marketing team prepares to launch a drug/device in a new indication, the CNS may collaborate with them to develop a "patient journey," which highlights key decision points of care from diagnosis through treatment (U.S. Department of Health and Human Services, 2009). The CNS illuminates important strategic considerations regarding patient and practitioner issues to enhance marketing's ability to positively impact health care.

In the medical division, the CNS has a key responsibility to protect patients' rights and safety in the development of clinically relevant research to address unmet medical needs. Deep therapeutic expertise, a core competency of the CNS role, is necessary to support product development and a clinically relevant research strategy (American Nurses Association [ANA], 2004; NACNS, 2004). The CNS's understanding of the patient population aids in the design of "patient-focused" clinical trials that address clinical trial subject/patient satisfaction and engagement in clinical research (Kole, 2012).

The need for medications/devices to be cost-effective while improving patient outcomes is increasingly important to governments, payers, and patients. Many companies have specific health outcomes and access/reimbursement divisions. The CNS may participate in development and application of the patient-reported outcome (PRO) assessment instrument analysis of data, and presentation of findings (U.S. Department of Health and Human Services, 2009).

Data dissemination is another key responsibility of the CNS in the medical division. The CNS uses the ability to assimilate and communicate large volumes of complex information accurately to produce external scientific publications and regulatory documents. Examples of scientific data dissemination include abstracts, posters, manuscripts, and other medical response documents. Examples of regulatory documents include protocols, informed consent documents, clinical study reports, annual reports, and clinical trial registry summaries.

Developing relationships with key medical experts is another critical role of the CNS in industry. The CNS must establish and maintain contact with investigators and other leaders in the medical community. To do this, it is important for the CNS to maintain scientific expertise in order to provide deep and advanced disease state and product information. The CNS uses the feedback and insights gathered from medical experts to better inform research and overall strategic direction.

Within the organizational sphere, both the medical and marketing divisions use the leadership skills of the CNS to contribute to process improvement initiatives with the goal of decreasing the time and cost of bringing drugs and devices to the market. Leadership, knowledge, and communication skills are needed to influence large multidisciplinary development teams and ultimately to communicate with the health care practitioners. The ability of the CNS to skillfully interpret the health care environment for the organization is highly valued. In industry, the CNS's spheres of influence are very similar to those in a hospital-based practice (Zuzelo, 2003). Figure 32.1 illustrates

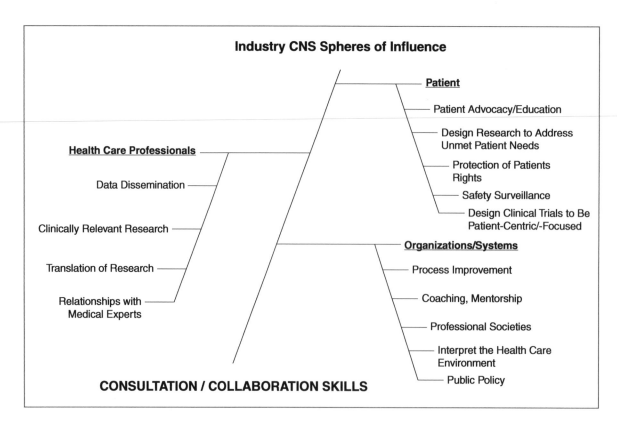

FIGURE 32.1 Industry CNS spheres of influence.
CNS, clinical nurse specialist.

the adaptation of the CNS's spheres of influence to the industry environment and provides examples of key modes of influence.

EXPLORING CNS OPPORTUNITIES IN INDUSTRY

Industry is looking for individuals with advanced health care–related degrees to provide technical or therapeutic expertise, support research, assist in data dissemination, develop important relationships with health care professionals, and provide leadership across functional areas. Potential candidates include individuals with an advanced degree in a scientific discipline such as pharmacy, nursing, or other fields. In addition, several years of hands-on experience in a scientific field, clinical setting, research setting, or pharmaceutical/device industry is often required. It

is important to recognize that individuals with these qualifications are your competitors for industry positions and eventually your colleagues within industry. Highlighting your skill set as a CNS in your curriculum vitae, during the interview process, and eventually when collaborating with your industry colleagues is essential to success.

The CNS is uniquely prepared to function in a variety of roles in industry. The actual title of the roles may vary between companies, but most have a career ladder similar to the clinical ladder in nursing. In general, these roles all require sound clinical judgment, demonstrated problem-solving experience, and an appreciation of drug/device development and clinical research. Strong interpersonal skills, including negotiation, communication, and presentation skills, and an ability to operate in a multicultural environment are highly valued. Some examples of industry roles that may be of particular interest to advanced practice nurses are included in Table 32.1.

TABLE 32.1

EXAMPLES OF ROLES AND RESPONSIBILITIES	
Role	**Responsibilities**
Medical information associate	Reviews pertinent literature and communicates information with team Develops response documents to answer questions from health care professionals Trains business partners such as call center agents and sales representatives
Medical liaison	Serves as a field-based liaison between the company and key opinion leaders Reviews pertinent literature and communicates latest research
Clinical research scientist	Participates in the design and support of clinical trials in the target disease state Provides strategic input into data dissemination and medical/marketing needs Interacts with consultants and investigators Facilitates/develops publications Conducts medical review and approval of marketing and regulatory documents
Scientific communications/ medical writing	Coordinates/develops abstracts, posters, and manuscripts Authors regulatory documents such as protocols and clinical study reports
Regulatory affairs consultant	Acts as a liaison between the company and key regulators such as the Food and Drug Administration Participates in development of the product label and other documents Reviews marketing materials for compliance with regulations
Drug/product safety consultant	Monitors reports of adverse events and product complaints Participates in surveillance and risk management programs
Health outcomes liaison/ research scientist	Functions as a liaison between the company and key payer organizations and health technology assessment agencies Participates in development of formulary dossiers Conducts research on drug utilization and economic modeling/evaluation
Medical education consultant	Develops and coordinates education for industry business partners and health care professionals Evaluates applications for grant support of continuing medical education.
Central risk-based monitor	Assesses the risk level of a clinical trial based on clinical program, trial design, attributes of investigational product, and investigative sites. Identifies critical data points and risk indicators with thresholds of action to direct the monitoring plan of a study to ensure patient safety and data integrity

Therapeutic expertise is a core component of the CNS role and that expertise is valued by industry. Pharmaceutical, medical device, and start-up biotechnology companies may have a narrow therapeutic focus. The key to success in gaining employment, as well as professional satisfaction in an industry role, is aligning CNS therapeutic expertise to industry need. Table 32.2 provides suggestions for the industry application and interview process.

CHALLENGES TO THE CNS ROLE WITHIN INDUSTRY

Industry is a highly regulated environment. While the hospital-based CNS is regularly involved in preparation for inspections by The Joint Commission (formerly the Joint Commission on Accreditation of Healthcare Organizations) and other agencies, audit preparedness is an even more constant focus in industry. The CNS in industry must develop the regulatory mindset critical to protection of patient safety and patient rights as well as the concepts of fair and scientific balance in reporting research results and developing promotional materials. Presentations and publications are critiqued by medical, legal, and regulatory authorities at a level of detail that is not often found in a clinical environment.

The CNS in industry rarely has direct patient contact. The patient remains the most important customer within industry; however, because the patient is further removed, one must be mindful to maintain a patient focus. You may find that many of your industry colleagues do not have a clinical background and may not fully appreciate patient needs. Keeping the team focused on the patient is an area where the CNS can make a significant impact; however, the need to do so can also be a source of frustration.

Historically, clinical trials were conducted primarily in North America and Europe; recently, though, clinical trials expanded to include developing countries. Typically, a CNS has a deep understanding of the standard of care and needs of the patient population of the region in which he or she practiced. Successful medical industries must operate efficiently in the global market. The CNS working in industry must develop and maintain a global mindset.

Maintaining clinical expertise is an area of challenge for the advanced practice nurse in industry. Generally, outside employment must be reviewed for potential conflict of interest. Similarly, even scholarly work (manuscripts, presentations, etc.) completed

TABLE 32.2

INTERVIEWING FOR AN INDUSTRY ROLE	
Activity	**Reason**
It is important to do thorough research before applying for a position in industry	This will help you determine if a particular position interests you and if you have the qualifications necessary Do not arrive for the interview unprepared
Gain an in-depth understanding of the company's areas of interest, approved products, investigational products, and its product pipeline prior to interviewing for a position	The company's website is a good place to start to gather this information The investor section on the company website often contains a brief description of the product pipeline Data on investigational products can often be obtained from clinical trial registries in the public domain, such as clinicaltrials.gov, or from company registries
Update your curriculum vita (CV)	Include all aspects of research and data dissemination in which you have participated Ensure that your leadership strengths are clearly outlined in your resume Describe your previous roles in terms of project management/oversight, organizational, analytical, negotiation, and decision-making skills Highlight situations where you created and maintained relationships with clinical or scientific thought leaders Include any involvement in professional organizations or patient advocacy groups
Provide a portfolio of your written work	Include abstracts, posters, manuscripts, and patient education materials
During the interview	Be prepared to critique a research article or to demonstrate your presentation skills. As you discuss your experience, be as specific as possible about *your* key contributions to and results of the projects highlighted

outside of employment must be reviewed to ensure protection of the company's intellectual property. Like many areas of innovation, bringing a pharmaceutical or a medical device to market takes many years and significant expenditure. Most pharmaceuticals in development do not become approved therapeutic agents. A CNS supporting early phase development may never experience a product "success" because most compounds do not move forward into Phase 3. If a compound moves into Phase 3, clinical trials may take years to complete and additional time is required for regulatory review prior to making an impact for the patient. In contrast, successes in the clinical role may come at a more rapid pace and be more tangible.

The likelihood that a CNS can remain in a specific therapeutic area is less in an industry setting compared to a clinical setting. When compounds do not meet expectations, entire therapeutic areas may be realigned or disbanded. Flexibility is required, and the learning agility of the CNS serves one well as a new area of therapeutic expertise must be developed to retain employment.

SUPPORT STRUCTURE IN INDUSTRY

Like the clinical environment, the industry environment will have a medical director, physicians, and colleagues of diverse allied health backgrounds. In many respects, navigating those interactions will feel familiar. However, the nonmedical, business colleague interactions may be more challenging. It is helpful to establish an informal network of individuals within the company who have a nursing background. Mentoring and coaching are expected behaviors of the CNS in industry, so networking is part of employment expectations. Continuing your involvement in nursing professional organizations is also important to maintain your therapeutic expertise and professional relationships.

CONCLUSION

As in the clinical setting, the role of the CNS has broad application in industry. The need for a professional who can integrate the systems of care and ensure patient safety exists in industry as well as in the clinical setting. The CNS is uniquely prepared to be successful in that role, and many opportunities exist in the industry environment for the CNS to optimize patient outcomes.

REFERENCES

American Nurses Association. (2004). *Nursing: Scope and standards of practice*. Washington, DC: Author.

Goudreau, K., Baldwin, K., Clark, A., Fulton, J., Lyon, B., Murray, T.,...Sendelbach, S. (2007). *A vision of the future for clinical nurse specialists*. Retrieved January 26, 2009, from http://www.nacns .org/LinkClick.aspx?fileticket=7AX5Ga5RbTg%3 d&tabid=117

Kole, T. (2012). Patient centric clinical trials: Fad, trend or future? *PharmaVOICE*, 78.

National Association of Clinical Nurse Specialists (NACNS). (2004). *Statement on clinical nurse specialist practice and education* (2nd ed.). Harrisburg, PA: Author.

U.S. Department of Health and Human Services (DHHS). (2009). *Guidance for industry: Patient reported outcome measures use in medical product development to support labeling claims*. Retrieved June 26, 2013, from http://www.fda.gov/downloads/Drugs/Guidances/ UCM193282.pdf

Zuzelo, P. R. (2003). CNS practice: Spheres of influence. *Association of Perioperative Registered Nurses Journal, 77*, 361–372.

33

Providing Pediatric Palliative Care in a Regional Children's Medical Center

Patricia O'Malley

PRACTICE OVERVIEW

Cindy Brown has provided expert clinical nurse specialist (CNS) practice at the Children's Medical Center in Dayton, Ohio, for nearly 30 years. Ms. Brown received a bachelor of science degree in nursing from Wright State University (Dayton, Ohio) and a master of science degree in nursing from the University of Cincinnati (Cincinnati, Ohio). Recognized as a local and regional expert for pediatric palliative care, her influence stretches from the bedside to the boardroom. This CNS drives best practices at end of life where time is short and the patient/family are extremely vulnerable. Within this acute care environment the needs of the child, family, and staff for comfort, meaning, and safety are overwhelming. Ms. Brown demonstrates how CNS practice meets these critical needs through evaluation, consultation, mentoring, education, and advocacy.

CNS PRACTICE: THE FIRST TWO DECADES

Ms. Brown cared for children and families through the myriad changes in the CNS role. As a novice CNS, primary responsibilities were education and development of nursing staff. Over time, the boundaries dissolved between the classroom and bedside, between nurses and physicians, between caregivers and management, and between staff and families. Years of dedicated practice and careful cultivation of professional relationships across the spectrum of care have allowed her to move freely across all levels of the organization to meet common goals of providing the best care to acutely ill children.

Pediatric practice, like adult care, has changed dramatically. Medical and surgical units provide care for children who were once cared for only in the pediatric intensive care unit (PICU). Children in the PICU require complex technology-based care. With changes in reimbursement and expanding outpatient services, children once hospitalized are increasingly cared for at home.

Societal changes have dramatically impacted pediatric nursing practice. Increasing numbers of blended and nontraditional families with deep economic or social needs drive the character of pediatric admissions. Children with insurance are more likely to be managed as outpatients. Children without insurance or poor social environments are more likely to be admitted. Ms. Brown has observed a rise in depression and emotional problems in children, insured or not. Providing care for the body, mind, and spirit at a variety of developmental levels has become more intense and difficult.

Like adult settings, safety has become the core focus at all levels of care. Coupled with safety is a concentration on increasing regulation by accrediting agencies. Her focus is integration of safety interventions in the fabric of care within the reality of the human condition or error.

CURRENT CNS PRACTICE

Ms. Brown's office is in the middle of the fray. Initially offered an office outside the inpatient units, she decided to maintain her position close to staff and patients to be accessible to patients, families, and staff. Daily patient rounding provides infinite opportunities for mentoring staff, patient advocacy, and bringing best practices to the bedside. Staff advocacy is very important because she believes CNS roles support and facilitate the expert practice of clinical nurses. Staff seek her consultation, information, reassurance, and assistance in solving problems. Particularly satisfying is the mentoring of graduate students to the pediatric CNS role.

Holding on to gains made during continuous change and balancing availability to staff and patients with writing, teaching, research, and education best describes Ms. Brown's current practice. Meetings and paperwork consume precious time yet are necessary parts of the CNS role. Multitasking is required in order to balance organization and personal goals with day-to-day demands.

PEDIATRIC PALLIATIVE CARE

Palliative care began at Children's Medical Center within an endowed bereavement team. Over time, focus has changed from attention to outpatient palliative care with the goal of dying at home to increasing services for children who require inpatient care due to severity of symptoms and/or lack of human or material resources at home. The pediatric palliative care CNS provides pain and symptom consults within the interprofessional team to preserve the relationships of child and family with the primary nurse and to keep the child on his or her unit. Monthly education and development of end-of-life order sets for children with any life-threatening or life-ending process supports clinical nurses and physicians on any unit to provide the evidence-based end-of-life care. Certainly, this is strong evidence of how the CNS role supports and extends the practice of the clinical nurse and facilitates desired patient outcomes.

Specialized education by the CNS is extended across the spectrum, from medical students to residents. Partnership with local medical centers and statewide groups such as the Ohio Pediatric Palliative End of Life Network helps drive best practices, federal and state funding, and grant writing. As a member of the board of directors for the Society of Pediatric Nursing, Sigma Theta Tau, and the American Society of Pediatric Nursing, Ms. Brown is changing the landscape of end-of-life care for children—one bedside at a time.

Ms. Brown further supports nursing practice by individual and group debriefings for staff and families during difficult cases or critical incident reviews. Staff can call a hotline 24 hours a day for any incident or difficulty. The CNS role is pivotal in helping staff respond to grief in themselves or others and to manage the stress of end-of-life care. As necessary, Ms. Brown consults Employee Care for issues beyond end-of-life nursing care.

THE FUTURE

Ms. Brown's goals for the future are full of promise and obstacles. However, this CNS is undaunted. Pediatric palliative care must become more comprehensive and care more formalized to obtain reimbursement and funding to meet community needs. More CNSs are needed to meet staff and family needs. More children are experiencing chronic pain and outcomes of care that are amenable to intervention as nurse-sensitive outcomes—pressure ulcers, ventilator-associated pneumonia (VAP), and infection require vigilance and creative problem solving with nursing staff.

Five years ago, Ms. Brown carefully reviewed the curriculum for the doctor of nursing practice (DNP) program. She was not convinced that the DNP was required for the CNS role and feared that a DNP requirement could reduce the number of future CNSs so desperately needed for practice, as the nurse practitioner (NP) programs have done over the past 20 years. While Ms. Brown believes the NP role is very important to patients, families, and clinical nurses, the CNS role, which ranges freely across the endless networks in health care to drive expert nursing practice and positive patient outcomes, is also very important.

Since her evaluation of DNP programs in 2009, she changed her decision and is pursuing the DNP. Ms. Brown also obtained prescriptive authority to further extend her practice. In the midst of electronic health record implementation, developing a chronic pain care service, facilitating multidisciplinary simulation training, mentoring CNS students, and working on development of a *Pediatric Early Warning Score* to predict transfers to PICU, she maintains relationships with local schools of nursing. Her practice is rich and full of promise for the future.

Ms. Brown is an example of expert CNS practice. Her practice is based on the maxim that excellent nursing care is embedded in relationships and nurses find satisfaction and purpose through these sacred relationships. Her dedication to the dying child and his or her family during the terminal phase of illness creates meaning, strength, and a sense of security for all involved in the child's journey. She empowers rather than takes over for clinical nurses at end of life to protect the nurse–child relationship where safety and security rest. Her understanding of suffering, her ability to address unvoiced needs, and her competence and experience provide a rich foundation for end-of-life services and pain treatment at the Children's Medical Center now and in the future. This CNS personifies caring, compassion, and presence in a dark journey made light through the best nursing care.

Implementing a Comprehensive Bariatric Care Protocol

Kathleen D. Wright

PRACTICE OVERVIEW

While my primary responsibilities as a wound ostomy continence (WOC) clinical nurse specialist (CNS) include providing direct services to patients, I also serve as clinical leader for a team of three board-certified WOC nurses with administrative accountability for our service line. Direct patient care is provided by the WOC team across a continuum of care from preventative to restorative in a community hospital with 150 acute care beds and an active outpatient setting. Additional services are provided on a contractual basis for two long-term care settings, two home health agencies, and a hospice. Indirect patient care activities include management of the service area's human and fiscal resources, and participating in organizational team meetings and committees such as product standardization and evaluation, health education, service excellence, and leadership coordination committees.

Direct patient care remains a central focus of this specialty practice, but all three CNS spheres of influence are crucial to successful outcomes. The WOC nurses facilitate implementation and evaluation of preventive skin care and wound management programs. The WOC nurses also provide individual bedside education as well as formal staff development programs to ensure appropriate implementation of patient-specific treatment recommendations. As research advances the science of the specialty and generates innovative interventions and products,

systemwide policies and procedures are reviewed and revised to ensure state-of-the-art specialty care.

The setting's WOC nurses are all members of the Wound Ostomy Continence Nurses Society. The society provides the membership with an annual conference, professional best-practice documents, and online membership forums to facilitate clinical problem solving and "group think" on timely topics. There is a regional and local affiliate of the national specialty organization, which provides opportunities for networking on a regular basis. Membership in the National Association of Clinical Nurse Specialists (NACNS), the American Nurses Association, and Sigma Theta Tau provides a well-rounded perspective of the nursing profession with valued insights from other specialties and practice settings. The aging population and the increasing number of complications associated with diabetes and obesity provide both a challenge and opportunity to effectively address the demands for CNSs with an expertise in wound and skin care.

PROBLEM IDENTIFICATION

Obesity is epidemic in our country, with two-thirds of adult Americans overweight or obese. It is estimated that over 72 million adults in the United States suffer from obesity (National Center for Health Statistics) and 9 million are morbidly obese

(American Obesity Association). Obesity is reported as the second leading cause of preventable death, killing approximately 400,000 Americans annually, and it is associated with more than 30 medical problems, including various dermatological conditions. This chapter discusses the WOC CNS's involvement in developing a bariatric care program in the community hospital setting.

The community hospital initiated the first bariatric surgery program in the state following extensive planning by a multidisciplinary team, which included the bariatric surgeons, CNSs, registered dietitians, certified social workers, and exercise specialists. Hospital-wide staff education and competency development focused on morbid obesity as a chronic illness with associated comorbidities, surgical risks and complications, postoperative care, cultural sensitivity, and access to size-appropriate equipment.

As the volume of bariatric patients increased, the WOC CNS identified a need to further standardize care for this population. Staff frequently requested consultations for specific information regarding equipment, such as weight limits on equipment and nursing interventions for the morbidly obese patient. One emergent weekend call came to the WOC CNS concerning a 750-pound patient scheduled to arrive in the emergency department whose ambulance stretcher was already bending beneath his weight. Another morbidly obese patient under the care of WOC CNS services for management of erythematous lower extremities due to chronic lymphedema became tearful as he told of being "wedged into a bedside chair" and of delays in toileting because staff could not access a bariatric commode. Safety issues were also identified. The extrawide bariatric bed that had to be constructed in a patient's room would not fit through the doorway or onto the elevator; thus, a transport stretcher or wheelchair had to be constantly available to prevent delays in testing, treatment, or potential emergency evacuation.

GOALS FOR PRACTICE INNOVATION

The CNS's goal was to develop and implement a comprehensive bariatric care protocol. The bariatric care protocol was holistic and addressed the multiple common clinical needs of this patient problem. In addition, the protocol promoted safety concerns for patients and staff by outlining the use of specially modified equipment. The protocol also promoted patient dignity, as issues of stigma, shame, and embarrassment are common for this patient group.

INNOVATION SPECIFICS

The WOC CNS collaborated with the bariatric program director to develop a comprehensive bariatric care protocol (Table 34.1).

The bariatric protocol outlines important assessment parameters to be considered upon the patient's entry into the facility's care. On admission, patients are assessed for weight and height. Body mass index (BMI) charts are available with the protocol for staff reference; patients with a BMI greater than normal are expected to be assessed for abdominal/hip girth related to ability for safe lateral repositioning or chair sitting. Caregiver risk for injury is closely linked to the patient's level of activity, with greater risk associated with lower patient activity, so this parameter is critical for planning both patient care and staffing assignments.

As with all patients admitted to the hospital, a comprehensive head-to-toe skin assessment is completed on the bariatric patient. Staff are expected to be particularly alert for common obesity-related skin complications, including candidiasis in the perineum area or skin folds, incontinence-related dermatitis secondary to inability to perform personal hygiene, pressure ulcers (including sites other than bony prominences), venous insufficiency/ulceration, and/or lymphedema in the lower extremities. After assessment, staff make note of urgent equipment needs, such as continuous positive airway pressure (CPAP) machine for preventing respiratory comorbidities, a bariatric walker to facilitate mobility, or a bariatric bedside commode for toileting.

After completing a comprehensive patient assessment, specific treatment plans and management guidelines are developed to address individualized patient needs. For patients heavier than 204.6 kg (450 lbs) and/or those with significantly widened hip girth interventions might include obtaining size-sensitive equipment, including a bariatric bed. The protocol provides a guideline that the standard hospital frame is 39 inches in width and accommodates up to 204.6 kg (450 lbs). A bariatric bed, stored in the postanesthesia care unit, can be accessed at all times for nonsurgical bariatric patients' admissions as needed. The protocol delineates the location of a wheelchair-accessible bariatric scale that can accommodate up to 454.4 kg (1,000 lbs), which is available in the day surgery unit.

To help ensure safe clinical care and patient dignity, staff in all patient care areas have access to bariatric blood pressure cuffs, bariatric patient gowns, and bariatric sequential compression boots. For patients requiring total or partial assistance with mobility, appropriate size-sensitive lift,

TABLE 34.1

BARIATRIC CARE PROTOCOL POLICY	
Title: Bariatric Care	Policy No.
	Database No. 1965
Category: Protocol	Page: 1 of 3
Owner: Kathy Wright	Effective: 10/20XX
Manual: Care of the Patient, DO-WOCN	Reviewed/Revised:
Committee Review: CCLC	
Signature: Penny Short, 08/11/12	Required review: Every 3 years

Purpose:

To meet the physical needs of the bariatric patient promoting clinical safety and dignity. Note: The word *bariatric* pertains to weight and is used in the field of health care to describe the treatment and management of weight. Weight is measured in kilograms. When referenced with a person's height it can be described in terms of body mass index (BMI) and categorized accordingly: normal (BMI 20–25), overweight (BMI 26–29), obese (BMI 30–39), morbidly obese (BMI >40)

Personnel:

All NMH patient care providers

Desired patient outcome:

To ensure patient and caregiver safety, patient dignity, and emergency preparedness

Areas of responsibility	Care directives
Assessment	On admission, patient should be assessed for
	1. Weight/height
	2. Estimated abdominal/hip girth related to ability for safe lateral repositioning or chair sitting
	3. Level of dependency
	A. Total assist
	1. Cannot support own weight and/or is uncooperative
	2. Little to no upper body strength
	B. Partial assist
	1. Able to bear weight but needs assistance more than supervision/instruction
	2. Upper body strength
	C. Independent
	1. Requires only supervision/instruction
	2. Performs tasks safely with or without assistive devices
	4. Skin complications
	A. Candidiasis within perineum or skin folds
	B. Incontinence-related dermatitis secondary to inability to perform personal hygiene
	C. Pressure ulcers
	D. Venous stasis/lymphedema
	E. Presence of or needs for specialized equipment, for example, glucometer, CPAP, walker, bedside commode

(continued)

TABLE 34.1

BARIATRIC CARE PROTOCOL POLICY (CONTINUED)	
Treatment/management	1. For patients weighing more than 204.6 kg (450 lbs) and/or significantly widened hip girth, consider the use of appropriate size-sensitive equipment:
	A. Bariatric bed (see Procedure No. 922: Specialty Bed Rentals). Standard hospital frame is 39″ in width and accommodates up to 204.6 kg (450 lbs)
	B. Bariatric bedside commode
	C. Bariatric scale (wheelchair accessible and accommodates up to 454.4 kg [1,000 lbs], available from Day Surgery)
	D. Bariatric blood pressure cuff
	E. Bariatric patient gowns
	F. Bariatric sequential compression boots, for example, Flowtrons, if ordered
	G. Gradient sequential compression boots. Consult WOCN for appropriate placement
	2. For patients requiring total or partial assistance with mobility, appropriate size-sensitive lift, transfer, ambulation, and transportation equipment should be used:
	A. Stretcher chair—Camtec Converta Litter available in ICU
	B. Bariatric transport stretcher—Standard hospital stretcher up to 227.2 kg (500 lbs)
	C. Bariatric wheelchair
	D. Bariatric walker
	E. Hover Matt—accommodates up to 363.3 kg (800 lbs). Available on all acute care areas
	F. Vertical lift device—Sit-to-stand device available on PCU and MSU
	G. Bariatric Hoyer/overhead lift device, available from PACU upon completion of Specialty Equipment Requisition form (see Patient Care Specialty Equipment policy and procedure)
Consultation/referral	1. Wound ostomy continence nurse
	2. PT/OT
	3. Social worker/case management
	4. Registered dietician
	5. Bariatric program coordinator
Documentation	1. Clinical notes
	2. Patient education form
	3. Specialty equipment requisition form
Patient education	1. Educate family/caregiver on safe and effective use of equipment

CPAP, continuous positive airway pressure; ICU, intensive care unit; PACU, postanesthesia care unit.

transfer, ambulation, and transportation equipment is available. The protocol notes that the standard hospital stretcher accommodates up to 227.2 kg (500 lbs); both bariatric transport stretchers and bariatric wheelchairs are available. Patient lateral transfer devices can accommodate up to 363.3 kg (800 lbs) and are available on all acute care areas. The bariatric protocol also notes that an overhead lift device is available from the postanesthesia care unit.

EVALUATION AND OUTCOMES

The bariatric protocol is available in the hospital policy and procedure manuals, accessible in each patient care area. Regardless of whether a facility has a surgical bariatric program, ongoing attention to staff education and the organization's physical environment is central in identifying potential areas of risk and opportunities for improvements in meeting the needs of this special patient population. Providing care for morbidly obese patients will continue to present unique challenges to staff and patients, not only for surgical bariatric patients but also for all patients across the continuum of care. Access to equipment sensitive to a person's weight and habitus for purposes of mobility, lift/transfer, and testing is an important consideration for patient care staff. Development of an organization-wide protocol specifically designed to meet the needs of the bariatric patient was found to facilitate safe and dignified care for both patient and caregiver.

Many CNS competencies were operationalized in the design and development of this practice innovation. *Theoretical foundations* enabled the CNS to incorporate the obese patients' perspectives of care delivery into a protocol that would facilitate safe and effective self-care with dignity. Recognition of significant *phenomena of concern*, including potential skin breakdown, mobility limitations, and ineffective coping related to self-image prompted the use of validated measurement tools, for example, the Braden Skin Risk Assessment Tool and other evaluation methods to guide cost-effective patient care. Effective *teaching and coaching strategies* were utilized to facilitate synthesis of the bariatric protocol into staff practice patterns. Clinical inquiry and knowledge of technology, products, and devices combined with interprofessional consultation and systems thinking to move toward positive outcomes for the hospitalized bariatric patient.

SUGGESTED READING

American Obesity Association. *AOA Fact Sheets*. Retrieved June 26, 2013, from http://obesity1.tempdomainname.com/subs/fastfacts/aoafactsheets.shtml.

Camden, S. (n.d.). Obesity: An emerging concern for patients and nurses. *OJIN: The Online Journal of Issues in Nursing, 14*(1). Manuscript 1. Retrieved July 1, 2013 from http://www.nursingworld.org/MainMenuCategories/ANAMarketplace/ANAPeriodicals/OJIN/TableofContents/Vol142009/No1Jan09/Obesity-An-Emerging-Concern.html

Camden, S. (2012). Skin care needs of the obese patient. In *Acute and chronic wounds* (pp. 477–484). St. Louis, MO: Elsevier.

Gray, M., Black, J., Baharestani, M., Bliss, D., Colwell, J., & Goldberg, M. (2011). Moisture-associated skin damage overview and pathophysiology. *Journal of Wound Ostomy Continence Nursing, 38*(3), 233–241.

Harris, H. (2008). Nursing care of the morbidly obese patient. *Nursing Made Incredibly Easy,* 34–44.

National Association of Clinical Nurse Specialists (NACNS). (2004). *Statement on clinical nurse specialist practice and education* (2nd ed.). Harrisburg, PA: Author.

National Center for Health Statistics. *Prevalence of overweight and obesity among adults: United States*. Retrieved June 26, 2013, from http://www.cdc.gov/vitalsigns/AdultObesity

Popovich, K., Tohm, P., & Hurd, T. (2010). Skin and wound care excellence: Integrating best practice evidence. *Healthcare Quarterly, 13*(Spec. No.), 42–46.

Price, P. (2013). Psychological impact of skin breakdown. In M. Flanagan (Ed.), *Wound healing and skin integrity* (pp. 102–113). Oxford, UK: John Wiley & Sons.

Sen, C. K., Gordillo, G. M., Roy, S., Kirsner, R., Lambert, L., & Hunt, T. K. (2009). Human skin wounds: A major and snowballing threat to public health and the economy. *Wound Repair & Regeneration, 17*(6), 763–771.

Reducing Central Line–Associated Bloodstream Infections Through a CNS-Led Systemwide Approach

Mary Pat Johnston

STATEMENT OF THE PROBLEM

Central line–associated bloodstream infections (CLABSIs) are a significant concern due to the high utilization of central lines in both inpatient and outpatient settings for patients requiring long-term venous access. Serious consequences, such as increased costs, longer length of stay, and risk of morbidity are also associated with a central line infection (Richardson & Tjoelker, 2012). According to the National Healthcare Safety Network (NHSN, 2006) and the Centers for Disease Control and Prevention (CDC, 2013), a central line is a catheter whose tip terminates in a great vessel, including the superior or inferior vena cava, internal jugular veins, subclavian veins, pulmonary artery, femoral artery, or aorta. Based on this definition and often missed in clinical practice, a peripherally inserted central catheter (PICC) is a central line. A CLABSI is defined as a laboratory-confirmed bloodstream infection, meaning at least one positive bacterial or fungal blood culture, in a patient with a central line, within the 48-hour period prior to the development of the infection; clinical manifestations of infection, such as fever, chills, and/or hypotension; and no apparent source for the bloodstream infection except the central line catheter (CDC, 2011, 2013).

CLABSI prevention became a priority when external factors, such as the U.S. Deficit Reduction Act (2005), required identification of hospital-acquired central line bloodstream infections and the Centers for Medicare & Medicaid Services (2008) limited reimbursement for patients experiencing a CLABSI during their hospitalization, as these infections could have been prevented through the implementation of evidence-based practices (EBPs; Kuper & Septimus, 2009; Richardson & Tjoelker, 2012). CLABSI prevention initiatives, John Hopkins University and Michigan Key Stone Project, a statewide initiative, demonstrated significant decreases in CLABSI rates in critical care and intensive care units (ICU) through the introduction of the central line bundle (Berenholtz et al., 2004; Pronovost et al., 2008; Schiffer et al., 2013). The central line bundle consists of:

1. Hand hygiene prior to line insertion
2. Maximal barrier precautions during line insertion, including cap, mask, sterile gown, gloves, and head-to-toe sterile drape on the patient
3. Chlorhexidine skin antisepsis prior to line insertion
4. Optimal catheter site selection, avoiding femoral vein for central venous access in adult patients
5. Daily review of line necessity, with prompt removal of unnecessary lines

However, the Institute for Healthcare Improvement (IHI) recognized that CLABSI prevention requires more than a central line bundle focused on insertion of the central line (IHI, 2012). Other health care–related factors, such as site care and dressing material, are important components of prevention of central line infections, and the outcomes are influenced by the clinicians, patients, and caregivers who are the end users of the central line providing care for the catheter every day. IHI recommends that clinicians consider utilization of other guidelines and EBPs for comprehensive CLABSI prevention. Prior to 2012, the focus was on the initiation of the central line bundle and in some instances this was the sole intervention for prevention of CLABSI (Richardson & Tjoelker, 2012). A more comprehensive CLABSI prevention plan is warranted.

At my institution, nursing-sensitive patient outcomes (NSPOs), such as falls, pressure ulcers, catheter-associated urinary tract infections (CAUTIs), and CLABSIs were led by a manager or director and were predominately hospital- or unit-based until 2012. Much of the focus was on the intensive care unit (ICU), where databases existed and reports were easily generated supporting the implementation of the central line bundle in ICU, but we were limited in our ability to implement best practices in other clinical areas. Useful tools for implementing this bundle were the standardization of the central line insertion cart and a central line insertion checklist. However, there were limitations when central lines were inserted at the bedside outside the ICU, and these changes did not facilitate daily evaluation of central line indication beyond the ICU. If hospitals knew their CLABSI rates in the ICU, it was considered a predictor of the rates in the rest of the hospital. Population- or case-specific focus led to implementation of reactive strategies, which resulted in disconnected processes for a community-based health system. While initiatives were launched in the ICUs at two hospitals, there was project team work on CLABSI prevention in the larger hospital. These separate initiatives were ongoing 12 to 18 months prior to the launch of the CNS-led team to standardize, coordinate, and share key learnings across the system. An experienced clinical nurse specialist (CNS) was identified as team leader by the director of clinical practice, based on his or her clinical expertise. The CNS assumed the role to leverage data-driven EBP and guidelines across the system to improve patient outcomes. While four teams were simultaneously established, the focus of this practice innovation is on the CNS lead of the CLABSI team.

GOALS AND OBJECTIVES FOR THE INNOVATION

The goal was to design and implement effective structures and processes to improve organizational outcomes related to CLABSI among inpatients and hospital-based outpatient clinics in two hospitals, Home Care/Home Infusion Services and Hospice. At the onset of the project, the physician-based clinics, extended care facilities, and a rehabilitation hospital in the system were excluded from the initiative, due to an already expansive scope. The CNS developed the following CLABSI team objectives to:

1. Evaluate the current state of unit-based and system outcomes related to CLABSIs
2. Evaluate processes and work flows that lead to these outcomes
3. Determine EBPs to optimize outcomes as compared to organizationally determined benchmarks
4. Conduct a gap analysis between current and evidence-based and best practices
5. Propose recommendations to close gaps to evidence-based and best practices
6. Prioritize recommendations to improve practice
7. Determine structure, process, and outcome metrics of success
8. Review recommendations from case reviews to determine if applicable to other clinical areas
9. Revise central line–related policies as necessary
10. Create education materials and collaborate with appropriate groups to coordinate staff and patient education
11. Implement EBPs and guidelines to prevent central line–associated bloodstream infections
12. Evaluate practice changes against metrics and organizational outcomes

For the first 18 months, the metrics were set based on the inpatient population, expanding from the ICU to other inpatient units in both hospitals. While the ultimate goal for any institution is a CLABSI rate of zero, the metric was evaluated and set by the Systemwide Quality Council, associated with other clinical initiatives and with input from CNS lead, infection control registered nurse (RN), director of clinical practice, and performance excellence leader. The CLABSI rate is calculated by dividing the number of CLABSIs by the number of central line days and multiplying the result by 1,000 (Dudeck et al., 2011). To support a system approach, data from the two hospitals were combined and reported as a hospital-system CLABSI rate, with the goal set at 0; threshold at 0.4; and stretch was 0 central line bloodstream infections per 1,000 catheter days (established with consideration of the previous quarters of 2011). In addition, the central line utilization rates were tracked from October 2010 (beginning of fourth quarter) to December 2012 (end of fourth quarter).

DESCRIPTION OF THE INNOVATION

The CNS developed a team charter to describe purpose, scope, team membership, key deliverables, and timeline, sponsored by the chief nurse executive. She collaborated on the metrics; identified evidence-based assessment and interventions; developed and maintained visibility on the system intranet through a SharePoint page; and planned for celebrating successes. The team composition included five frontline staff nurses from ICU, interventional radiology, medical-surgical unit, oncology clinic, and home care; three infection control RNs, representing each hospital and the clinics; one unit educator; one CNS; and ad hoc members (a frontline nurse from a neonatal intensive care unit and an information technology analyst) for a total of 12 members. The CNS and four of the team members were involved in practice, quality, clinical inquiry, and education councils of Nursing Shared Governance Model, establishing key linkages. The CNS was the owner of the central line–related policies and advance practice nurse (APN) facilitator of the Patient Care Policy and Procedure Committee. This team reported to the Nursing Quality Council and Systemwide Patient Safety and Quality Councils. The CNS utilized performance improvement tools to conduct meetings and facilitate progress, focusing the team on the metrics. Examples of these tools included establishing ground rules and expectations for the team, brainstorming techniques for identifying gaps and potential solutions, setting priorities, decision making, and developing an implementation plan with timeline and responsible person assigned. The CLABSI Team Charter was discussed and approved by the team and then sent to the appropriate system teams and executive sponsor for approval. Key deliverables of the team included revision of policies to embed evidence-based interventions, redesign of documentation tools, and standardization of education for nurses and patients. Within the first year, focusing on an infrastructure, central line–related policies and procedures were revised to emphasize nine EBPs:

1. Using Central Line Insertion Protocol (CLIP) for central line placement (CDC, 2011; Infusion Nurses Society [INS], 2011; Scottish Intensive Care Society Audit Group, 2012)
2. Educating patient about rationale for central line, risks and benefits, and the role of the patient in preventing central line bloodstream infections (National Patient Safety Goal, 2012)
3. Assessing the need for the central line daily, based on criteria (CDC, 2011; IHI, 2012; Scottish Intensive Care Society Audit Group, 2012)
4. Applying antimicrobial dressings, meaning 2% chlorhexidine transparent dressings for central venous catheters and PICC; transparent dressing for implanted port (Camp-Sorell, 2011; CDC, 2011; INS, 2011)
5. Changing dressing every 7 days and when necessary, if loose, wet, bloody, or soiled (Camp-Sorell, 2011; CDC, 2011; INS, 2011)
6. Standardizing intravenous (IV) tubing changes, such as IV tubing changes for continuous, standard solutions every 96 hours (CDC, 2011; INS, 2011)
7. Changing intermittent barrier caps once per week and as necessary when removed, if blood residue observed in cap, or cap appears to be damaged or leaking (CDC, 2011; INS, 2011)
8. Applying antiseptic barrier caps to exposed, unused ports on catheter and IV tubing (Menyhay & Maki, 2008)
9. Instructing hospitalized patient with a central line on daily showering or bathing with 2% chlorhedixine liquid soap (CDC, 2011; IHI, 2012)

To build a systemwide infrastructure, supported by EBP, the first key deliverable was to revise the central line–related policies into 3 system policies, archiving 12 entity or department-specific policies. A communication tool was developed to describe changes in the policies and was distributed to staff through unit educators via unit meetings and e-mail. A staff education plan was developed and implemented, including central line class for RNs and licensed practical nurses (LPNs) during orientation; annual computer-based learning (CBL) program on central lines for all RNs and LPNs who care for central lines; back-to-basics poster on central line care and maintenance, distributed to the clinical areas; and three competency planning tools to validate demonstration of flushing central lines and dressing changes through direct observation or simulation. In addition, the policy on "Central Lines: Declotting with Alteplase to Restore Patency" was revised to integrate EBPs into this related policy. Key points on when to use alteplase to declot a central line were added to the annual CBL for staff training. An "Introduction to Central Lines" patient teaching sheet was revised to include pertinent messages with description and rationale for central line, risks and benefits, and the role of the patient and family/caregiver in preventing central line infections. It was made electronically available and distributed to clinical areas for the physician or nurse to review with the patient prior to placement of the central line.

Another significant key deliverable was revised clinical documentation in the electronic health record, condensing 17 flow sheets with different central line content into 3 flow sheets (i.e., central venous catheter, PICC, and implanted port), aligned by EBP and guidelines for best practices, utilizing similar language or terms to describe assessments and interventions. The content to assess the daily indication for a central line, using language from the Scottish Intensive Care Society Audit Group (2012) criteria, was aligned on these flow sheets. In addition, a component was added to the standardized Interdisciplinary Patient Care Rounds template in the electronic health record to review criteria for necessity of a central line during these rounds. If not or no longer indicated, the physician is notified to obtain order for removal. Of note, this intervention is one contributing factor to a decline in utilization of central lines in our system. With clinical documentation redesigned, clinical informatics resources allocated, and new documentation flow sheets built and implemented in August 2013, more specific metrics and electronically generated reports can be developed to monitor key components of CLABSI prevention, thus moving toward a more comprehensive and inclusive approach for the other clinical areas in our system and increasing sustainability of these changes over time. While individual patient reports related to care and maintenance of central lines were available in fall 2012, the revised, evidence-based clinical documentation provides nurses with a tool that matches the key changes, and subsequent reports will provide a broader perspective to measure success and sustainability of these changes over time.

Another key deliverable was to conduct a case review for each central line bloodstream infection that met the definition of CLABSI as previously described, in the clinical area with the staff providing direct care to the patient, manager/director and unit educator for the area, infection control nurse, and a frontline nurse and CNS lead from the CLABSI team. Recommendations from the case reviews were discussed and evaluated for potential system changes by the CLABSI team. Case reviews were held wherever the CLABSI occurred; both inpatient and outpatient areas were included in case review. An example of a process change from these recommendations was the implementation of a standardized central line dressing kit to maintain sterility of dressing changes across all clinical areas of the system.

EVALUATION AND OUTCOMES

The outcomes are presented in the tables below. Table 35.1 describes the CLABSI rate from October 2011 to March 2013.

The red, yellow, green stoplight concept was used to display data on the intranet for a quick glance at the progress. From October 2011 to March 2012, patients identified with central line bloodstream infections were reported from medical–surgical and specialty units. The case review process and subsequently recommendations provided insights into infrastructure to build in policy and staff education and further identified processes that warranted change. From April 2012 to March 2013, there were four consecutive periods without a CLABSI. From October 2010 to December 2012, the utilization of central lines steadily decreased, as demonstrated by the utilization ratio of total number of patient days to the total number of central line days. These numbers were counted every day for each quarter and then the ratio was calculated. The central line utilization ratio decreased from 0.23 to 0.16 in the larger hospital and from 0.14 to 0.1 in the smaller hospital; the combined hospital central line utilization ratio was reported as 0.15 at the end of 2012. A systemwide, coordinated approach led by a CNS, based in evidence, data, and communication, thus drove improvement in patient outcomes. This CNS-led, systemwide approach has been utilized for other NSPOs, such as falls, CAUTIs, and pressure ulcers, and a Pain Team was subsequently initiated in June 2013. The leadership of the CLABSI team transitioned from an experienced CNS to a novice CNS in April 2013 through a planned

TABLE 35.1

CLABSI RATE FOR HOSPITAL DIVISION	
Time Period	CLABSI Rate Hospital Division
October–December 2012	0.68
January–March 2012	2.6
April–June 2012	0
July–September 2012	0
October–December 2012	0
January–March 2013	0

CLABSI, central line-associated bloodstream infection.

three-month transition, providing a mentored experience in leadership of systemwide teams.

DISCUSSION OF CNS CORE COMPETENCIES AND OUTCOMES

This chapter describes core CNS competencies in action, building on the foundation of clinical expertise in central lines, evolving into leadership for a systemwide initiative, and demonstrating use of power and influence through EBP and utilization of data among all of the CNS spheres of influence (National Association of Clinical Nurse Specialists [NACNS], 2004). The CNS has the knowledge, skills, and competencies to lead systemwide initiatives in NSPO. Although clinical expertise in the NSPO is beneficial, mentoring leadership behaviors in practice is even more valuable. While CNSs coach and mentor frontline staff nurses, opportunities can be created to mentor novice CNSs in developing and refining their leadership skills and competencies to foster the growth of the next generation of CNSs.

REFERENCES

Berenholtz, S., Pronovost, P. J., Lipsett, P., Hobson, D., Earsing, K., Farley, J.,... Perl, T. M. (2004). Eliminating catheter-related bloodstream infections in the intensive care unit. *Critical Care Medicine, 32*(10), 2014–2020.

Camp-Sorell, D. (2011). *Access device guidelines: Recommendations for nursing education and practice* (3rd ed.). Pittsburgh, PA: Oncology Nursing Society.

Centers for Disease Control and Prevention (CDC). (2011). *Guidelines for prevention of intravascular device related infections: Recommendations and reports.* Retrieved September 2, 2013, from http:// www.cdc.gov/hicpac/BSI/BSI-guidelines-2011.html

Centers for Disease Control and Prevention (CDC). (2013). CLABSIs. Retrieved September 2, 2013, from http://www.cdc.gov/nhsn/pdfs/pscmanual/4psc_clabscurrent.pdf

Dudeck, M. A., Horan, T. C., Peterson, K. D., Allen-Brudson, K., Morell, G., Anttila, A.,... Edwards, A. R. (2011). *National healthcare safety network (NHSN) data summary report 2011, device-associated module.* Retrieved September 3, 2013, from http://www.cdc .gov/nhsn/PDFs/dataStat/NHSN-Report-2011-Data-Summary.pdf

Infusion Nurses Society (INS). (2011). Infusion nursing standards of practice. *Journal of Infusion Nursing, 34* (Suppl. 1S).

Institute for Healthcare Improvement (IHI). (2012). *How-to guide: Prevent central line-associated bloodstream infection (CLABSI).* Retrieved September 2, 2013, from www.ihi.org

Kuper, K. M., & Septimus, E. J. (2009). Health-care associated infections: The legislative perspective and the pharmacist's role. *American Journal of Health System Pharmacy ,* 66(5), 488–494.

Menyhay, S. Z., & Maki, D. G. (2008). Preventing central venous catheter-associated bloodstream infections: Development of antiseptic barrier cap for needleless connectors. *American Journal of Infection Control, 36*(10), S174.e1–S174.e15.

National Association of Clinical Nurse Specialists (NACNS). (2004). *Statement on clinical nurse specialist practice and education* (2nd ed.). Harrisburg, PA: Author.

National Healthcare Safety Network. (2006). *National Healthcare Safety Network (NHSN) surveillance definitions: Central line associated bloodstream infection (CLABSI) and related sites.* Retrieved September 2, 2013, from http://www.msic-online.org/ pdf/NHSN_Definitions_CLABSI.pdf

National Patient Safety Goal. (2012). *The Joint Commission.* Retrieved September 2, 2013, from http:// www.jointcommission.org/assets/1/6/NPSG_Chapter_Jan2012_HAP.pdf

Pronovost, P. J., Berenholtz, S., Goeschel, C., Thom, I., Watson, S. R., Holzmueller, C.G.,... Sexton, J. B. (2008). Improving safety in intensive care units in Michigan. *Journal of Critical Care, 23,* 207–221.

Richardson, J., & Tjoelker, R. (2012). Beyond the central line-associated bloodstream infection bundle: The value of the clinical nurse specialist in continuing evidence-based practice changes. *Clinical Nurse Specialist, 26*(4), 205–211.

Schiffer, C. A., Mangu, P. B., Wade, J. C., Camp-Sorell, D., Cope, D. G., El-Rayes, B. F.,... Levine, M. (2013). Central venous catheter care for the patient with cancer: American Society of Clinical Oncology clinical practice guideline. *Journal of Clinical Oncology, 31*(10), 1357–1370.

Scottish Intensive Care Society Audit Group. (2012). *Central line insertion bundle.* Retrieved September 2, 2013, from http://www.sicsag.scot.nhs.uk/HAI/ SICSAG-central-line-insertion-bundle-120418.pdf

Improving Clinical Care for a Specialty Surgical Oncology Population

Colleen O'Leary and Taletha M. Askew

*I*t is well accepted that the clinical nurse specialist (CNS) is a clinical expert, an educator, a researcher, and a consultant who influences the three spheres of practice: patient care, nursing, and systems (National Association of Clinical Nurse Specialists [NACNS], 2013). Based on the NACNS's core CNS practice competencies, our institution developed areas of practice for the CNS, which included clinical expert, researcher, educator, consultant, and leader. Although this exemplar illustrates several of these areas, its focus is mainly systems leadership. According to the NACNS's core competency, this encompasses the ability to manage change and empower others to influence clinical practice both within and across systems (NACNS, 2010).

Review of unit-specific quality data on a surgical oncology unit by the CNS identified failure to recognize acute changes in postsurgical patients' condition, such as increased oxygen requirement and mental status changes, as early warning signs of an acutely decompensating patient. Limited use of the emergency response team (ERT) led to a subsequent increase in code events, with poor communication between the medical team and the nursing staff cited as a contributing factor. The medical team stated that significant patient status changes were not always urgently communicated, especially on the evening and night shifts. The CNS also noted communication concerns during clinical rounds and when reviewing

past code and ERT events. The CNS held a meeting with the nurse manager, unit staff development coordinator, and nurse educator to discuss critical clinical events and feedback from clinical partners, and to review clinical data. It was concluded that a plan was needed to assess, develop, and evaluate a unit-specific plan to improve nurses' performance in addressing critical changes in patient status.

The CNS developed a program to assess nurses' learning needs, design interventions, and evaluate outcomes in order to improve nurses' initiation of appropriate interventions and decrease the episodes of failure to rescue. Initial areas needing improvement included (a) responding to early changes in patient condition, (b) communicating up the physician chain of command, (c) using emergency equipment correctly, (d) obtaining and following treatment orders, and (e) calling for additional resources, particularly the early response team. High-fidelity simulation was chosen as a teaching strategy. High-fidelity simulation in clinical education helps improve self-confidence and clinical judgment, promotes team cohesiveness while enhancing problem-solving abilities, and offers opportunities for unlimited practice of critical events in a safe, controlled environment without risk to patients (Classen, 2010; Decker, Sportsman, Puetz, & Billings, 2008; Ellis et al., 2008; Friese & Aiken, 2008). A simulation scenario was created based on a thoracic surgery oncology patient recently cared for on the unit. Simulation exercises were offered over a 4- to 6-week period. All nursing staff members were required to participate. During the exercise, nurses were paired in teams of two to three nurses, with the staff development coordinator and nurse educator serving in the supportive personnel role and the CNS overseeing the exercise. Nurses were given pre- and postsimulation surveys to determine their perception about simulation experiences.

The scenario began with nurses receiving report on the patient. One nurse was designated in the charge nurse role. As the scenario unfolded, the nurse manager and CNS observed and evaluated the team using a structured evaluation tool. After the exercise, they led the debriefing session. In the debriefing session, nurses were asked to reflect on the level to which the exercise helped in recognizing and responding to critical changes in patient conditions. They were also asked to identify additional learning needs. Additional learning needs included improving performance in a full code and greater familiarity with the contents and operation of the code care equipment and drugs with application to the thoracic surgery patient population. The CNS identified several learning needs based on observational evaluation of simulation exercise.

After completion of the simulation exercises, the CNS, staff development coordinator, and nurse educator formulated a comprehensive education plan tailored to the specific nursing unit. The plan was rolled out in phases. It integrated didactic content with skill building and case study activities focused on the unit's patient population. The didactic content consisted of 12 hours on topics such as failure to rescue, respiratory failure, postthoracic surgery nursing care, and management of cancer pain. Skill building took place in the skills lab and focused on working with equipment and administering therapies related to oncology patients undergoing thoracic surgery. Case studies addressed sepsis and respiratory failure and were based on typical unit patients. Respiratory therapists and the CNS provided brief lectures about various oxygen treatment modalities and nursing management.

The education plan was implemented over 8 months. The CNS was an integral part of each phase, including developing the comprehensive education plan, teaching specific specialty content, coordinating the various activities, and evaluating the outcomes. In addition, the CNS frequently reinforced learning at the bedside in real time.

Within 2 months of beginning the education, the ERT and code data reflected major improvement. ERT initiation increased and code events dropped to zero. This trend held for several months posteducation. Between January 2010 and September 2011, code events remained decreased by 300% and ERT events remained increased by an average of 60%. These data suggested that staff not only recognized the acutely decompensating patients but also were able to intervene quickly and use the ERT effectively. One year after the education plan was completed, a thoracic surgeon commented on how well the nurses on the unit functioned, particularly in a code event. He relayed these comments to the nursing staff, CNS, and the chief nursing officer. The nurses validated they were more confident and knowledgeable about caring for the specialty patient population on the unit and therefore demonstrated improved performance in critical and code situations.

This exemplar demonstrates CNS practice in consultation and coaching competencies. The CNS now is routinely consulted by the surgical oncology nursing staff and the thoracic surgery medical team regarding complex patient needs. She continues to teach classes on care of the thoracic surgery oncology patient, mentor nurses and other providers, and support skill acquisition. Moreover, this exemplar illustrates CNS leadership at the system level. Through her efforts, this CNS was able to manage practice change and empower others to influence clinical practice improvement. She facilitated the provision of clinically competent care using education, role modeling, team building, and quality monitoring. She provided leadership in promoting interprofessional collaboration for improved clinical outcomes, and she disseminated reports of these outcomes both internally and externally.

REFERENCES

Classen, J. L. (2010). Is failure to rescue really failure to communicate? Champion the move from reactive process to proactive model. *Nursing Management, 41,* 38–41.

Decker, S., Sportsman, S., Puetz, L., & Billings, L. (2008). The evolution of simulations and its contributions to competency. *Journal of Continuing Education in Nursing, 39,* 74–80.

Ellis, D., Crofts, J. F., Hunt, L. P., Read, M., Fox, R., & James, M. (2008). Hospital, simulations center, and teamwork training for eclampsia management: A randomized controlled trial. *Obstetrics and Gynecology, 111,* 723–731. doi:10.1097/AOG.0b013e3282637a82

Friese, C. R., & Aiken, L. H. (2008). Failure to rescue in the surgical oncology population: Implications for nursing and quality improvement. *Oncology Nursing Forum, 35,* 779–785. doi:10.1188/08.ONF.779–785

National Association of Clinical Nurse Specialists (NACNS). (2010). *CNS core competencies.* Retrieved October 8, 2013, from http://nacns.org/docs/CNSCoreCompetenciesBroch.pdf

National Association of Clinical Nurse Specialists (NACNS). (2013). *What is a CNS?* Retrieved October 8, 2013, from http://nacns.org//html/cns-faqs.php

Facilitating a Programmatic Approach to Children With Special Health Care Needs

Jo Ellen Rust

PRACTICE OVERVIEW

*I*am a pediatric clinical nurse specialist (CNS) with a clinical focus in pediatric neuroscience. I facilitate a program, *Children with Complex Care Needs*, at a Midwestern quaternary/tertiary children's hospital/ referral center in a large metropolitan city. Children with special/complex health care needs often have multibody system involvement leading to complex care scenarios. These children require health services more or less continuously across their life span, from both generalist and specialist providers, and are frequently hospitalized. As a group, they represent one of the most frequent recipients/consumers of pediatric health care services. We envisioned the concept of a multidisciplinary program to meet the particular needs of this population. Our program was developed to implement a system of care for the child with complex health care needs that is seamless, supportive, and safe—a program that brings the child's identified care providers and resources, including child/family, into "a circle of care." Program goals include the following:

1. Normalize the life of the child in a family and community
2. Minimize the disruptive impact of the child's condition
3. Foster the child's maximum growth and development

4. Foster family-centered care
5. Foster the *medical home* concept
6. Enhance cross-discipline and cross-service communication and collaboration
7. Improve both patient/family and provider satisfaction
8. Maximize patient safety

A criterion for referral is that a child be followed by two or more medical services/providers and hospitalized three or more times per year. Referrals are sometimes made on the basis of family need and can come from any provider, including nurses, social workers, physicians, speech therapists, or others. For each patient, the CNS assists the patient and family with a variety of needs, including but not limited to:

1. Direct patient care, synchronization between admitting and consulting services and with nursing staff, and confirmation that patients are admitted to a consistent unit as much as possible
2. Access to physicians from the multiple services seeing the patient
3. Coordination and management of medical information pertaining to the patient
4. Education of family members regarding the diagnosis, treatment, and management of the patient's health condition

5. Identification of and access to hospital and community-based resources according to the families' needs (social, educational, financial, and medical)
6. Resolution of patient and family complaints
7. Facilitation of communication between multiple services, staff, and the family
8. Management of multiple sources of input for the development of care plans

Problem Identification

The Epilepsy Foundation (n.d.) reports 300,000 people have a first convulsion each year: 120,000 occur in persons younger than 18 years, with between 75,000 and 100,000 involving children younger than 5 years who have experienced a febrile (fever-caused) seizure. About 200,000 new cases of epilepsy are diagnosed each year, with 45,000 cases in children younger than 15 years. Prevalence of active epilepsy (history of the disorder plus a seizure or use of antiepileptic medicine within the past 5 years) is estimated to be approximately 3 million in the United States, with 326,000 school children through age 15 having epilepsy. By 20 years of age, 1% of the population can be expected to have developed epilepsy. The basic, underlying risk of developing epilepsy is about 1%. Individuals in certain populations are at higher risk. For example, it is estimated that epilepsy can be expected to develop in:

- 25.8% of children with mental retardation
- 13% of children with cerebral palsy
- 50% of children with both disabilities
- 8.7% of children of mothers with epilepsy
- 2.4% of children of fathers with epilepsy
- 33% of people who have had a single, unprovoked seizure

Among patients in the *Children with Complex Care Needs* program, the second most frequently affected body system is the nervous system. The third most commonly occurring patient problem across all body systems is a seizure disorder. During the early months of program development, while meeting with patients and families, I identified that education regarding seizures and the management of seizures in children was rudimentary and inconsistent across providers. Resources available through our outpatient pediatric neurology program were not well known by the inpatient staff and therefore not utilized for patient and family education.

GOALS FOR PRACTICE INNOVATION

In addressing educational needs of patients and families related to epilepsy and seizure management, goals were created based on past comments on patient satisfaction questionnaires. The current goals are written from the patient/family perspective:

1. I will have all my questions answered to my understanding.
2. I will receive all necessary training to care for my child.
3. I will know who to contact for concerns.
4. I will know what my child will need at home, have the supplies I need, and know how to provide care.
5. I will know all others who will be helping me if needed at home.
6. I will understand effects of medications.
7. I will understand how to troubleshoot my child's care.

INNOVATION SPECIFICS

I contacted the pediatric neurology nurse clinician about jointly developing a class on the management of seizures in children for our patients and families. The clinical pharmacist, family resource center librarian, and our patient education coordinators were contacted to assist. With input from the pediatric neurologists, a 1-hour class designed to meet the parental/family expectations noted previously was developed.

The class content was designed to meet patients' and families' concerns through the following objectives:

- Understand the basic anatomy of the nervous system
- Describe what a seizure is
- List common causes of seizures
- Describe how we diagnose a seizure disorder
- Describe different types of seizures
- List risk factors that might trigger seizures
- Understand how seizures are treated with medicine
- Identify other treatment options for seizures
- Know how to care for your child during a seizure
- Work with your doctor to manage your child's seizures
- Know how to discover reliable resources
- Have access to contact information for providers

Our hospital is fortunate to have a family resource center, which includes the family education center. The center's goal is to foster and facilitate the independence of our patients and families. Our patient education coordinators facilitate a schedule of classes designed to meet this goal. They assisted in the implementation of the new class within the existing calendar; the course is offered twice a week, every Tuesday afternoon from 3 p.m. to 4 p.m. and Thursday morning from 10 a.m. to 11 a.m. (except holidays). Our content was tested for learner readability. The educational content was calculated at a Flesch-Kincaid grade level of 7.5. The content is presented primarily by the neurology outpatient nursing staff, although we rotate responsibility as our schedules require modification. The Spanish-language patient educator has attended the course and can now provide the content to our Hispanic/Latino population as needed, or we arrange for an interpreter and extra class time if a family with limited English proficiency wishes to attend one of our regular sessions. The class is provided informally in a small, quiet, well-appointed room around a table and chairs. This format provides a relaxed atmosphere for learning away from the bedside. It can be presented at the bedside upon request via a laptop, based on presenter availability. In addition to a copy of the PowerPoint slides used in the classroom, patients/families in attendance receive a "Parents' Guide to Seizures and Seizure Medicines", a seizure diary, a glossary of terms, a list of available books on epilepsy, and a list of reputable websites on epilepsy/seizure disorders. Additional materials available include drug information sheets as desired, information on video EEG, and managing seizures at school.

A teaching record was designed to document the education within the classroom. This record is placed in the inpatient medical record where education can be reinforced by the inpatient staff prior to discharge. If the attendees are outpatient, the record is sent to the health information management department for placement in the patient's medical record. The patient education record will now be transitioned to be located within our electronic medical record patient education design as appropriate.

EVALUATION AND OUTCOMES

The class is offered to the families and patients with a new diagnosis of seizure disorder as well as our long-standing families who were previously diagnosed. The class has been well received by both groups. Families are encouraged to send grandparents or other family members as well as others who interact with their child, such as babysitters or teachers. The class often stimulates discussion or questions between families and their health care team as reported to us by medical providers.

All participants are asked to anonymously evaluate the class upon completion. Early feedback indicated that the content was not presented in an interesting manner. To address this concern, we added video streaming of various seizure types to the educational presentation. Subsequent feedback demonstrated that

this addition corrected the problem, and evaluations are now stellar.

Class attendance can vary. The class is marketed by the family resource center through its flat-screen communication boards, parent bulletin boards on patient care units, and the daily hospital e-newsletter. Additional marketing strategies include a pocket-size invitation to the class with class schedule, contact information, and location. This card is distributed to the inpatient families via the pediatric neurology faculty, residents, and the CNS. An additional card advertising available family resource center classes and time schedule is made available for use with all children with complex care needs and their families. Upon identifying its availability through the online marketing efforts or through one of our system employees, adult patients and families have also availed themselves of the class.

DISCUSSION OF THE CNS CORE COMPETENCIES

CNSs have as their principal focus nursing's unique scientific and practical contributions in the management of symptoms and functional problems to meet distinctively different societal needs at the individual, group, community, and health care institution levels. Within the patient/client sphere of influence, CNSs develop, implement, and evaluate innovative educational programs for patients, families, and groups. Access to health information and knowledge acquisition through patient/family education enhances the attainment of predicted outcomes while minimizing unintended consequences for patients and families. Within the nursing sphere of influence, the teaching record provides a collaborative guide for the synergistic effect of the classroom method with the educational reinforcement by the bedside nurse at the point of care. This work continues to solidify relationships between patients, families, and their providers by helping families better understand their child's condition and treatment plan, encouraging participative decision making, and increasing open, honest dialogue between all. Within the organizational sphere, variation in patient family knowledge acquisition was identified. Facilitators in the organizational structure, such as the family education center and existing patient education materials, were utilized. Content development and implementation required multidisciplinary linkages across medicine, nursing, pharmacy, patient education, and families. This class also provides a generalizable patient education program applicable across differing units, diagnoses, populations, or medical specialties along the full continuum of care (National Association of Clinical Nurse Specialists [NACNS], 2004).

REFERENCES

Epilepsy Foundation. (n.d.). *About epilepsy: Epilepsy and seizure statistics*. Retrieved September 30, 2013, from http://www.epilepsyfoundation.org/aboutepilepsy/whatisepilepsy/statistics.cfm

National Association of Clinical Nurse Specialists (NACNS). (2004). *Statement on clinical nurse specialist practice and education* (2nd ed.). Harrisburg, PA: Author.

The Clinical Nurse Specialist in Primary Care

Jeannette Richardson

The Institute of Medicine (IOM) defines primary care (PC) as "the provision of integrated, accessible health care services by clinicians who are accountable for addressing a large majority of personal health care needs, developing a sustained partnership with patients, and practicing in the context of family and community" (IOM, 1996, p. 1). PC is delivered through both the private sector and government agencies such as the Veterans Health Administration and the Health Resources and Services Administration (HRSA). Both private and public sector models deliver care that is person- rather than disease-focused, provides a point of first contact for the patient, and is comprehensive and coordinated (IOM, 2012).

Until recently, it was unusual to hear of a clinical nurse specialist (CNS) employed in the PC setting. It is still relatively uncommon. This may partially be explained by the fact that PC has historically been undervalued and underfunded in the United States (CMS, n.d.). Past emphasis for distribution of health care resources has been on acute care and large-volume or high-cost procedures rather than on health promotion, disease management, and prevention strategies. In comparison to hospitals, outpatient care settings have been seriously lacking in the staffing and infrastructure necessary to support implementation and sustainability of evidence-based practice (EBP) processes. Many office settings have not employed any nurses at all and have relied on partnerships between physicians and medical assistants as the predominant patient care dyad. Recent health care reform efforts are putting the spotlight on the need to shift the emphasis on U.S. health care funding to more public health-conscious preventive strategies and to more fully incorporate nurses and their unique contributions into the PC setting.

However, there is also controversy within the CNS community whether the role of generalist PC provider is appropriate for an advanced practice registered nurse (APRN) who cares for a *specialty* population. The National Association for Clinical Nurse Specialists (NACNS) is the professional organization representing CNSs. The organization's 2004 statement on CNS practice and education reports that

> [t]he essence of CNS practice is clinical nursing expertise in diagnosis and treatment to prevent, remediate, or alleviate illness and promote health with a defined specialty population—be that specialty broad or narrow, well established, or emerging. (p. 5)

Does this description allow for the role of the CNS within PC? The purpose of this chapter is to explore controversial issues and to describe possible current and future roles for the CNS in the PC setting.

BACKGROUND/LITERATURE REVIEW

Bodenheimer and Grumbach (2007) note that within the field of medicine, the task of PC practice falls to several different types of providers: family physicians, general internists, general pediatricians, PC nurse practitioners (NPs), and physician assistants. They refer to this group collectively as PC clinicians. However, APRNs, including NPs, CNSs, certified nurse midwives (CNMs), and certified registered nurse anesthesists (CRNAs), have not been universally accepted as providers by all members of the health care team.

Within PC, turf battles are being fought over the necessary qualifications to be an independent health care provider. NPs have traditionally been the predominant APRN role integrated into PC, and they are now taking on more responsibilities. The American Association of Nurse Practitioners (AANP) reports that 89% of NPs are educationally prepared with a PC focus (AANP, 2013); they practice autonomously and in collaboration with other members of the health care team to manage patients' health needs. The IOM (2010) and the National Governors Association (2012) support examining and encouraging NP practice based on research, which suggests that NPs can perform many PC services as well as physicians do and achieve equal or higher satisfaction rates among their patients. Studies that are most often cited in support of independent NP practice are Mundinger et al. (2000) and Newhouse et al. (2011).

Alternatively, various physician organizations have come forward with statements warning that independent NPs should not be substituted for PC physicians. The American Academy of Family Physicians (AAFP) published a report noting that family physicians receive 11 years of college and graduate-level education (including residencies), whereas NPs receive 5.5 to 7 years of schooling. They propose that NPs are less-qualified health professionals by virtue of this gap in educational preparation (AAFP, 2012). The AAFP reports that they are supported in their conclusions by the American Academy of Pediatrics, the American Medical Association, and the American Osteopathic Association. The AANP counters this argument by stating that NP education is competency based, not time based (AANP, n.d.).

Much of this debate is occurring now due to implementation of the Affordable Care Act (ACA) and a projection for up to 32 million more insured patients who will be seeking health care. According to the Association of American Medical Colleges, there will be a projected shortage of 45,000 PC physicians by the year 2020 (AAMC, n.d.). Health care policy experts note that options for improving the ability to care for the increased number of patients could be enhanced through increased Medicare funding of resident physicians, increasing physician productivity through the use of team-based care models (AAMC, n.d.), expanding the role of the NP, and optimizing electronic communication (Green, Savin, & Lu,

2013; Poghosyan, Lucero, Rauch, & Berkowitz, 2012). Others argue that even with aggressive training scenarios for physicians, NPs, and physician assistants as independent providers, demand will still exceed the supply of clinicians (Sargen, Hooker, & Cooper, 2011).

Why is this professional debate of importance to CNSs? The NP has been and continues to function as a generalist provider within the PC setting; CNSs have not typically assumed this role. But as efforts to standardize education and certification standards for all types of APRNs are ongoing, it makes sense that administrative decisions affecting one subset of the APRN will affect others. If NPs are allowed to function as independent providers in PC, it is more likely that these privileges will be extended to CNS work in their own specialty areas.

CNS Roles in PC

NACNS recently published a statement on specialty competency, which describes specialty practice as the principal element and hallmark of CNS practice. NACNS recommends achievement of both population and specialty education as competencies for the CNS (NACNS, 2013).

NACNS also published a briefing paper in June, 2010, which describes the contribution of CNSs to PC practice. CNS services might "include but are not limited to: prenatal services, transitional care from hospital or rehabilitation facility to home, psychoeducational self-care counseling and coaching to manage chronic disease, gerontological services, palliative care in the promotion of comfort/quality of life, foot care, wound care, and stress-related illness counseling, mental health counseling and psychotherapy" (p. 1). Also, "[i]t is important that CNSs are recognized as contributing to the care of patients as providers to whom PC practitioners can easily refer patients or as members of established PC teams" (p. 3). This implies that the role of the CNS within PC is to receive referrals for specialty care and/or to work in specific care subsets of PC patient populations rather than as generalist providers (NACNS, 2010).

The three spheres of CNS practice shown in Exhibit 38.1 can be used to help distinguish how the CNS can play a role in the PC of patients (NACNS, 2004).

- *Client Direct Care*—As noted earlier, the CNS does not typically function as the generalist care provider in PC, but rather works within some specialty area. This practice is supported by Bodenheimer and Grumbach (2007) who note that, in fact, many specialists do not appreciate doing PC; they most likely lack PC competencies, and they are

EXHIBIT 38.1
Three Spheres of CNS Influence

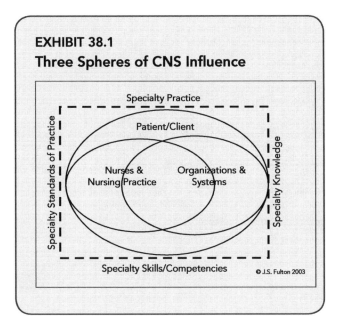

Specialty Practice

Specialty Standards of Practice

Patient/Client

Nurses & Nursing Practice

Organizations & Systems

Specialty Knowledge

Specialty Skills/Competencies

© J.S. Fulton 2003

less effective in providing preventive care services. In this sphere, the CNS may serve as a direct care specialty provider in cardiology, diabetes, wound care, and so forth and accept referrals for this care from the PC team. They may, in fact, be embedded inside PC themselves and so might technically be considered "PC providers" even though they continue to provide specialty care.

- *Nurses and Nursing Practice*—The CNS can influence nurses and nursing personnel within PC by assessing practice and providing supportive education, examining and developing competencies necessary for patient care, and coaching for improved performance. An example is the emerging practice of transitional care for patients. The CNS can review the evidence base, consider the role of the RN in the transitional care of patients, develop competencies tailored to the process within the relevant health care organization, and model and educate staff on best practices for the practice and documentation.

- *Organizations and Systems*—In the previously underfunded PC setting, there are many opportunities for the CNS to effect change within systems to improve efficiency and effectiveness. As health care organizations are restructuring PC settings, they are considering different options for improving care while limiting costs. Group visits are one methodology used as an alternative to individual patient visits. They consist of various members of the health care team working with a group of patients to increase efficiency. Some of the group visits are based on patients with similar disease processes; others provide a scheduled drop-in visit open to a large group of patients based on interest (Bodenheimer & Grumbach, 2007). The CNS can lead organizational changes necessary to provide

the infrastructure for these different options for patient care and may even participate as a specialty provider within the group visit.

CONCEPTUAL FRAMEWORK

Currently, the most frequently noted example of a conceptual framework within the PC practice setting is that of the patient-centered medical home (PCMH). The PCMH is not an actual house or a home; rather, it is a philosophy for the delivery of team-based PC based upon a partnership between the patient and his or her health care team. The focus of care has shifted away from the episodic treatment of disease and is now on the holistic care of the patient. The goal of the PCMH model is to reach the patient in the right place, at the right time, and in the manner that best suits the patient's needs (Patient-Centered Primary Care Collaborative [PCPCC], 2013).

This model of care promotes the use of an interprofessional team to improve preventive health services, chronic disease management, access to services, and clinical effectiveness (Klein, 2011). Within the PCMH, expanded care delivery options for patient visits (telephone visits, nurse-managed medication protocols, postdischarge transitional care, etc.) are emphasized in order to achieve adequate access and improved patient outcome measures. Stronger, more proactive team-based PC is expected to decrease hospitalizations and visits to the ED through better care coordination and chronic illness management.

In recent years, the PCMH model for providing care has become increasingly popular and has been endorsed by multiple professional organizations, including the U.S. Department of Veterans Affairs (Shinseki, 2009), the AAFP (2012), and The Joint Commission (TJC, 2013). The National Committee for Quality Assurance (NCQA, 2013) and the Utilization Review Accreditation Commission (URAC) are among a growing group of organizations that have developed certification and recognition programs for designation of a specific organization as a PCMH according to a group of standards (National Center for Medical Home Implementation, n.d.). Use of the PCMH framework is foundational to current health care reform efforts as a required component of an Accountable Care Organization (Longworth, 2011).

The PCMH Model

The PCMH model of care is operationalized differently from one organization to the next, but several key features span almost all definitions (see Exhibit 38.2; PCPCC, 2013).

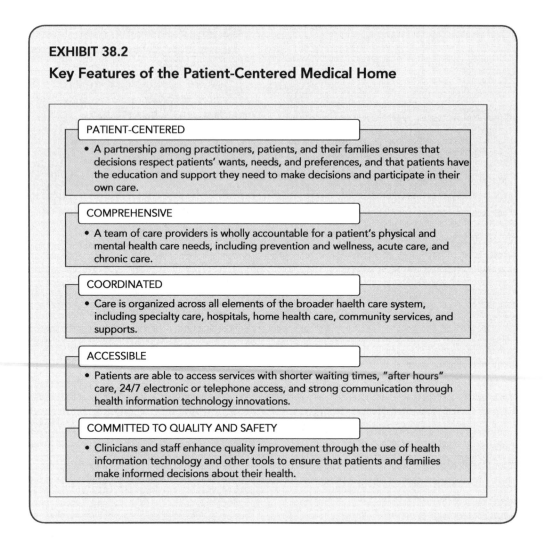

EXHIBIT 38.2

Key Features of the Patient-Centered Medical Home

PATIENT-CENTERED

- A partnership among practitioners, patients, and their families ensures that decisions respect patients' wants, needs, and preferences, and that patients have the education and support they need to make decisions and participate in their own care.

COMPREHENSIVE

- A team of care providers is wholly accountable for a patient's physical and mental health care needs, including prevention and wellness, acute care, and chronic care.

COORDINATED

- Care is organized across all elements of the broader haelth care system, including specialty care, hospitals, home health care, community services, and supports.

ACCESSIBLE

- Patients are able to access services with shorter waiting times, "after hours" care, 24/7 electronic or telephone access, and strong communication through health information technology innovations.

COMMITTED TO QUALITY AND SAFETY

- Clinicians and staff enhance quality improvement through the use of health information technology and other tools to ensure that patients and families make informed decisions about their health.

Early results on the effectiveness of the PCMH model show mixed effects. When considering study results individually, the PCPCC (Nielsen, Langner, Zema, Hacker, & Grundy, 2012) noted impressive outcomes of decreased health care utilization with decreased cost of services associated with the PCMH model. These outcomes derive from numerous PCMH initiatives launched by state and agency organizations.

In a separate systematic review sponsored by the Agency for Healthcare Research and Quality (Peikes et al., 2012), the authors were looking for improved outcomes associated with the Triple Aim Initiative (Institute for Healthcare Improvement [IHI], 2013a), including:

1. Improving the patient experience of care (including quality and satisfaction)
2. Improving the health of populations
3. Reducing the per capita cost of health care

Results from this systematic review indicate that most interventions tested the addition of a care manager within the PC practice and targeted patients who were older and sicker than average. There were some favorable effects on all three triple aim outcomes, a few unfavorable effects on costs, and mostly inconclusive results due to insufficient sample sizes or uncertain statistical analyses. The report concludes that since improving PC is the linchpin of achieving triple aim outcomes, stronger evaluations are needed to provide guidance for modification and adaptation of the PCMH model. A newer review is slated to be published soon.

As noted earlier, there is much controversy over who is considered to be the team leader in the PCMH model. Interestingly, a recent study examined perspectives of NPs and physicians regarding PC practice. Physicians worked longer hours and saw more patients but earned higher incomes than NPs. NPs were more likely than physicians to believe that they should lead medical homes, be allowed hospital admitting privileges, and be paid equally for the same clinical services. When asked whether they believed that physicians provided a higher quality examination and consultation than NPs, 66% of physicians agreed and 75% of NPs disagreed (Donelan, DesRoches, Dittus, & Buerhaus, 2013).

APPLICATION TO CNS PRACTICE

Critical and controversial topics, mostly related to education and practice, surround the role of the CNS in PC. In a previous section, the NACNS perspective on education and competencies was presented. The national organization recommends achievement of both *population* and *specialty* education and competencies for the CNS (NACNS, 2013). This presents both challenges and opportunities. In an adult PC setting example, the CNS might specialize in cardiology. This would require education as an adult-gerontological CNS with a specialty in cardiology (APRN Consensus Work Group & the National Council of State Boards of Nursing APRN Advisory Committee, 2008). In this scenario, the CNS could be functioning as a specialty direct care provider on cardiac conditions, but what would happen if the CNS was asked to lead a project on transitional care for *all* PC patients within the organization? Is this CNS considered adequately educated and with the appropriate competencies to perform in this role? If not, who would be the appropriate choice? These questions related to education and competencies for the CNS in PC will require ongoing discussion and decision making from the national perspective.

Functioning within the more generalist world of PC, there are specific areas of responsibility that the CNS can address. Care coordination and transitional care are becoming common and standardized roles for nurses in PC; CNSs can provide organization and structure for implementation and sustainment of these activities.

Care Coordination

The American Nurses Association (ANA, 2012) notes that RNs and APRNs have been performing care coordination since the turn of the last century and, for many patients, the RN is the appropriate care coordinator. It is foundational to health care reform efforts to improve the quality of care and maximize efficiency in the utilization of resources through coordination of care; the CNS can take this work to the advanced practice level. In fact, APRNs have been used in care coordination models, which require advanced practice skills in physical assessment for identification of exacerbation of comorbidities, medication management, and development of interventional strategies as well as organizational change projects (Naylor, 2012).

The National Quality Forum (NQF) defines care coordination as

a function that helps ensure that the patient's needs and preferences for health services and

information sharing across people, functions, and sites are met over time. Coordination maximizes the value of services delivered to patients by facilitating beneficial, efficient, safe, and high-quality patient experiences and improved health care outcomes. (NQF, 2006)

The NQF goes further to explain that care coordination is composed of five domains:

- Health care "Home"—the source of usual care selected by the patient and serving as the medical home. This medical home should be the central point for coordinating care around the patient's needs and preferences
- Proactive Plan of Care and Follow-Up—a current care plan that actively tracks the patient's progress toward health care goals
- Communication—available to all members of the care team, including the patient and his or her family
- Information Systems—well-integrated electronic records
- Transitions or "Handoffs"—care processes for improved patient safety between settings of care

The ANA (2012) reports that nursing involvement in care coordination activity has impacted health care indicators by

- Reducing ED visits
- Decreasing the cost of medications
- Reducing inpatient charges
- Increasing survival rates with fewer readmissions
- Increasing the ability for patients to manage their self-care
- Increasing safety during transitions
- Improving patient satisfaction overall

The optimal coordination of patient care across care settings accomplished proactively throughout the patient's lifetime is an intuitive health care population need, which has not received adequate attention in past decades. This aspect of both nursing and APRN care is now helping to articulate the value of nursing in PC.

Transitional Care

In the past, health care professionals were employed in specific practice settings and provided care for their patients while they resided within that setting. Best practices included preparing the patient for discharge from that practice setting by providing education on medications and ongoing medical concerns—but once the patient was sent out the door, there was little if any participation in patient care. Gradually, it became apparent to administrators and clinicians that patients were experiencing adverse events when they transitioned from one care area to another. Patients discharged from the hospital to home were noted to have significant medication discrepancies (Coleman, Smith, Raha, & Min, 2005) and, in one study, almost one in five patients experienced an adverse event within two weeks of hospital discharge (Forster, Murff, Peterson, Gandhi, & Bates, 2003). Adverse health outcomes have also been noted to occur after discharge from the emergency department (ED), resulting in repeat visits to the ED, readmission, and even death in a small percentage of patients (Hastings et al., 2007).

To address the problems that can arise when patients travel between care settings, an emerging study of transitional care has developed; transitional care can be thought of as a specific type of care coordination. The National Transitions of Care Coalition (NTOCC) remarks that "Transitions of Care refer to the movement of patients between health care locations, providers, or different levels of care within the same location as their conditions and care needs change" (2008). Specifically, they can occur:

1. Within settings; for example, PC to specialty care, or intensive care unit (ICU) to ward
2. Between settings; for example, hospital to subacute care, or ambulatory clinic to senior center
3. Across health states; for example, curative care to palliative care or hospice, or personal residence to assisted living
4. Between providers; for example, generalist to a specialist practitioner, or acute care provider to a palliative care specialist

The actions undertaken for the purpose of transitional care should be designed for optimal care coordination and continuity. A comprehensive care plan should guide that care and it should be supported by practitioners who have access to information within the care plan indicating the patient's treatment goals, preferences, and health or clinical status (Coleman & Boult, 2003).

EVALUATION

The evaluation of the role of the CNS within PC reflects the outcome measures associated with the interventions discussed earlier in this chapter. To some extent, outcomes will be tailored to a specific project, its implementation, and the outcomes for the specialty populations, nurses, or systems that the CNS is working with. However, it is important to use standardized outcome measures when possible in order to make any comparisons across work settings and regarding the population as a whole.

Triple Aim Initiative

The IHI emphasizes that, to optimize health system performance, all three of the following dimensions should be pursued simultaneously. Corresponding outcome measures include:

- *For Population Health* → Health function status, risk status, disease burden, and mortality
- *For Patient Experience* → Standard questions from patient surveys and a set of measures based on key dimensions
- *For Per Capita Cost* → Total cost per member per month, and hospital and ED utilization rates

Specific information related to these outcomes is available on the IHI website (IHI, 2013b).

Care Coordination

The NQF (2010) published a consensus report of recommended performance measures for measuring and reporting care coordination. These performance measures are quite specific and, in some cases, specialty oriented. To some extent, these measures reflect the limitations and challenges associated with our current processes for data collection based upon those aspects of care that are reimbursable and, subsequently, counted. They do advocate for use of the three-item Care Transitions measure (CTM-3), which would require a change in practice for most facilities (Coleman, n.d.; see Exhibit 38.3).

Transitions in Care

The NTOCC (2008) reports that appropriate structures, processes, and outcomes are all required for optimal health care system functioning. Outcome measures should include:

1. Patient's and/or family's experience and satisfaction with care received
2. Provider's experience and satisfaction with the quality of interaction and collaboration among providers involved in care transitions
3. Health care utilization and costs (e.g., readmissions, etc.)
4. Health outcomes consistent with patient's wishes (e.g., functional status, clinical status, medical errors, and continuity of care)

EXHIBIT 38.3

National Quality Forum Recommended Performance Measures for Care Coordination

Performance Measure	Measure Description
Cardiac rehabilitation patient referral from an inpatient setting	Percentage of patients admitted to a hospital with primary diagnosis of acute myocardial infarction or chronic stable angina or who during hospitalization have undergone coronary bypass surgery (CABG), a percutaneous coronary intervention (PCI), cardiac valve surgery (CVS), or cardiac transplantation who are referred to an early outpatient cardiac rehabilitation/secondary prevention program
Cardiac rehabilitation referral from an outpatient setting	Percentage of patients evaluated in an outpatient setting who in the previous 12 months have experienced an acute myocardial infarction or chronic stable angina or who have undergone CABG, PCI, CVS, or cardiac transplantation who have not already participated in an early outpatient cardiac rehabilitation/secondary prevention program for the qualifying event, and who are referred to an outpatient cardiac rehabilitation/secondary prevention program
Patients with a transient ischemic event ED visit who had a follow-up office visit	Patient(s) with a recent ED encounter for a transient cerebral ischemic event who had any physician visit within 14 days of the acute event
Biopsy follow-up	Biopsy performed, entered into tracking log, reviewed, and communicated to patient or patient's guardian/caregiver and to patient's primary care physician and/or other physician/professional responsible for follow-up care
Reconciled medication list received by discharged patients (inpatient discharges)	Percentage of patients discharged from an inpatient facility to home or any other site of care, or their caregiver(s), who received a reconciled medication list at the time of discharge
Transition record with specified elements received by discharged patients (inpatient discharges)	Percentage of patients discharged from an inpatient facility to home or any other site of care, or their caregiver(s), who received a transition record (and with whom a review of all included information was documented) at the time of discharge
Timely transmission of transition record (inpatient discharges)	Percentage of patients discharged from an inpatient facility to home or any other site of care for whom a transition record was transmitted to the facility or primary physician or other healthcare professional designated for follow-up within 24 hours of discharge
Transition record with specified elements received by discharged patients (ED discharges)	Percentage of patients discharged from an ED to ambulatory care or home health care, or their caregiver(s), who received a transition record at the time of ED discharge
Melanoma continuity of care –recall system	Percentage of patients with a current diagnosis of melanoma or a history of melanoma who were entered into a recall system with the date for the next complete physical skin exam specified, at least once within the 12-month reporting period
Three-item Care Transitions Measure (CTM-3) (Coleman, n.d.)	Unidimensional self-reported survey that measures the quality of preparation for care transitions (scoring strongly disagree → strongly agree) *The first statement is about when you were in the hospital...* 1. The hospital staff took my preferences and those of my family or caregiver into account in deciding what my health care needs would be when I left the hospital. *The next statement is about when you were preparing to leave the hospital...* 2. When I left the hospital, I had a good understanding of the things I was responsible for in managing my health. *The next statement is about your medications...* 3. When I left the hospital, I clearly understood the purpose for taking each of my medications

ADVANCED PRACTICE NURSING

Although the role of the CNS in PC is relatively new and untested, there have been some examples of how advanced practice nursing skills are utilized in ways that can be integrated into PC. As described earlier, the CNS does not typically function as the generalist direct patient care provider within PC, but there are many organizational needs related to the nursing and systems spheres that could benefit from the intervention of the CNS. Muller, McCauley, Harrington, Jablonski, and Strauss (2011) relate their experiences emphasizing the role of facilitator of EBP and quality improvement. The CNSs provided clinical support and multiple opportunities for the professional development of nurses. They also influenced practice through identification of best practices and implementation of change efforts and tracking of outcomes. The PC setting, which has been lacking in supportive resources in the past, desperately needs advanced practice nursing skills to help all members of the health care team standardize and streamline organizational and patient care efforts based on the evidence.

Tringali, Murphy, and Osevala (2008) describe care coordination activities in which they worked from each of their three specialty practice areas—cardiology, gerontology, and oncology. Working within all three spheres of CNS practice, the authors coordinated care for high-volume, complex patients with the goal of impacting the quality of nursing care and facilitating systems change to improve patient outcomes. The CNSs worked across practice settings and incorporated aspects of transitional care.

Finally, one of the most prominent nursing research efforts in transitional care has been led by Naylor, who has spearheaded development of what has evolved into the Transitional Care Model (TCM). The TCM incorporates comprehensive discharge planning and home follow-up care for chronically ill, high-risk, older adults. The transitional care nurse who visits the patient and his or her family both in the hospital and in the home is an APRN with expert training, knowledge, and skills in the care of chronically ill older adults. The TCM model has been effective in reducing readmission rates, improving health outcomes, enhancing patient satisfaction, and reducing total health care costs. The TCM has been proposed as a means for bridging acute care and the PC medical home; challenges to wider implementation are related to the need for a more proactive health care organizational culture and the financial backing that would be required to initiate the model (Naylor, 2012).

ETHICAL CONSIDERATIONS

The ACA was constructed based on many ethical justifications. Health care insurance will be expanded to many more individual Americans, insurance companies will be more accountable for the value of their policies, and the individual patient will be much more in control of his or her health care dollars and choices (Lachman, 2012).

However, one of today's greatest challenges within the PC setting is meeting the needs of all the patients with health care concerns; that is, access to basic care. With the advent of the ACA, there will be an estimated 32 million more Americans looking for health care (AAMC, n.d.). As noted earlier, there are not enough PC physicians to take care of the current patient census, much less those millions enrolling in the near future. Adding all possible NPs and PAs to the provider rolls may (or may not) meet the need. Despite the noble intentions of the ACA in assisting uninsured patients to receive health care, it is not clear how and for whom care will be prioritized. Team-based care allows PC to have a longer reach by having nursing and other support staff take on some of the responsibilities previously shouldered by the provider alone, but will this be enough? Can the CNS in PC help build nursing care processes and systems that can assist care teams to increase access? Will specialty CNSs off-load some of the care burden noted in PC? Will quality and safety be sacrificed for the sake of efficiency?

A related topic of ethical concern involves the allocation of limited resources. Some medications are extremely expensive but can also be lifesaving or life preserving. In a limited economic situation, how will decisions be made regarding the distribution of these medications? At the same time, some less expensive generic medications have been in short supply because there may not be enough economic incentive for manufacturers to produce the drug. Durable medical equipment and supplies will experience similar cost limitations and shortages. These concerns require high-level discussions and solutions, but it may be the individual organizations and PC teams who must initially problem-solve for their own solutions. Will the CNS serve as an EBP expert and/or patient advocate in these situations? Is there a role for the CNS in development of policies or protocols regarding distribution of limited resources?

CONCLUSION

From the content covered within this chapter, it is clear that the emphasis being placed on preventive care and chronic disease management by health care reform efforts is forcing an expansion of the services provided by PC individuals and teams. Emerging models of care are being implemented, and previously unidentified fields of study such as care coordination and transitional care are growing into full independent programs of their own. Outcome measures have been determined and results are being tracked. Although PC has been considered a generalist practice, there is still a role for the specialty practice of the CNS in each of the three spheres. The potential impact of the CNS role in PC is limitless.

■ DISCUSSION QUESTIONS

- Research indicates that many patients have experienced an adverse event associated with the transition from the inpatient setting to home. Have you ever encountered this scenario in your practice or in your personal life? What was the nature of the adverse event? What might have been done to decrease the chances of the occurrence of this event?
- Many health care practice settings include team-based care. Have you worked within a team? Who were the members and what were their disciplines? What was the purpose of the team? Did you achieve all your goals? What made the team function well together and what caused challenges?
- Care coordination has been a nursing responsibility for a long time. How do you perform care coordination in your current role? Do you incorporate functions to improve care across transitions? Have you ever called a health care professional in another setting to discuss the care of a patient that you were handing off to them?

■ ANALYSIS AND SYNTHESIS EXERCISES

- Think about where the patients in your care setting go for their PC needs. Reach out to that care team and find out if they are using a team-based model and whether they consider their practice a PCMH. Who are the members of their care team and what are their functions? Compare the description of their practice with national criteria and make your own determination on whether they are following the PCMH model.
- Discuss the role of the PC provider with one or more patients. Are they familiar with the possibility of an NP in that position? What are their thoughts about the use of APRNs as independent providers? Provide the patient(s) with evidence supporting NP practice.

- ED visits are considered a utilization outcome for many care coordination projects. Contact an ED employee and discuss why patients with nonurgent concerns choose to visit the ED rather than their PC office. Design a project that could decrease ED utilization for nonurgent patient visits.

REFERENCES

American Academy of Family Physicians (AAFP). (2012, September 18). *Primary care for the 21st century.* Retrieved September 12, 2013, from http://www.aafp.org/dam/AAFP/documents/about_us/initiatives/AAFP-PCMHWhitePaper.pdf?cmpid=npp12_ad_com_na_van_1

American Association of Nurse Practitioners (AANP). (2013). *Nurse practitioners in primary care.* Retrieved September 1, 2013, from http://www.aanp.org/images/documents/publications/primarycare.pdf

American Association of Nurse Practitioners (AANP). (n.d.). *Clinical outcomes: The yardstick of educational effectiveness.* Retrieved September 2, 2013, from http://www.aanp.org/images/documents/publications/clinicaloutcomesyardstick.pdf

American Nurses Association (ANA). (2012, June). *The value of nursing care coordination: A white paper of the American Nurses Association.* Retrieved September 6, 2013, from http://www.nursingworld.org/carecoordinationwhitepaper

APRN Consensus Work Group & the National Council of State Boards of Nursing APRN Advisory Committee. (2008). *Consensus model for APRN regulation: Licensure, accreditation, certification & education.* Retrieved October 1, 2013, from https://www.ncsbn.org/7_23_08_Consensue_APRN_Final.pdf

Association of American Medical Colleges (AAMC). (n.d.). *Physician shortages to worsen without increases in residency training.* Retrieved September 2, 2013, from https://www.aamc.org/download/286592/data

Bodenheimer, T., & Grumbach, K. (2007). *Improving primary care: Strategies and tools for a better practice.* New York, NY: McGraw-Hill.

Centers for Medicare and Medicaid Services (CMS). (n.d.). *Comprehensive primary care initiative.* Retrieved September 6, 2013, from http://innovation.cms.gov/initiatives/comprehensive-primary-care-initiative

Coleman, E. (n.d.). *National Quality Forum: Specifications for the three-item care transition measure – CTM3.* Retrieved September 1, 2013, from http://www.caretransitions.org/documents/CTM3Specs0807.pdf

Coleman, E. A., & Boult, C. E. (2003). Improving the quality of transitional care for persons with complex care needs. *Journal of the American Geriatrics Society, 51,* 556–557. Retrieved September 6, 2013, from http://www.caretransitions.org/documents/Improving%20the%20quality%20-%20JAGS.pdf

Coleman, E. A., Smith, J. D., Raha, D., & Min, S. J. (2005). Posthospital medication discrepancies. *Archives of Internal Medicine, 165,* 1842–1847.

Donelan, K., DesRoches, C. M., Dittus, R. S., & Buerhaus, P. (2013). Perspectives of physicians and nurse practitioners on primary care practice. *New England Journal of Medicine, 368*, 1898–1906.

Forster, A. J., Murff, H. J., Peterson, J. F., Gandhi, T. K., & Bates, D. W. (2003). The incidence and severity of adverse events affecting patient after discharge from the hospital. *Annals of Internal Medicine, 138*, 161–167.

Green, L. V., Savin, S., & Lu, Y. (2013). Primary care physician shortages could be eliminated through use of teams, nonphysicians, and electronic communication. *Health Affairs, 32*, 11–19.

Hastings, S. N., Schmader, K. E., Sloane, R. J., Weinberger, M., Goldberg, K. C., & Oddone, E. Z. (2007). Adverse health outcomes after discharge from the emergency department: Incidence and risk factors in a veteran population. *Journal of General Internal Medicine, 22*, 1527–1531.

Institute for Healthcare Improvement (IHI). (2013a). *IHI triple aim initiative.* Retrieved October 1, 2013, from http://www.ihi.org/offerings/Initiatives/TripleAim/Pages/default.aspx

Institute for Healthcare Improvement (IHI). (2013b). *IHI triple aim measures.* Retrieved from http://www.ihi.org/offerings/Initiatives/TripleAim/Pages/MeasuresResults.aspx

Institute of Medicine (IOM). (1996). *Primary care: America's health in the 21st century.* Washington, DC: National Academies Press.

Institute of Medicine (IOM). (2010). *The future of nursing: Leading change, advancing health.* Washington, DC: National Academies Press. Retrieved September 6, 2013, from http://books.nap.edu/openbook.php?record_id=12956&page=R1

Institute of Medicine (IOM). (2012). *Primary care and public health: Exploring integration to improve population health.* Washington, DC: National Academies Press.

The Joint Commission (TJC). (2013). *Primary care medical home.* Retrieved September 1, 2013, from http://www.jointcommission.org/accreditation/pchi.aspx

Klein, S. (2011). The Veterans Health Administration: Implementing patient-centered medical homes in the nation's largest integrated delivery system. *The Commonwealth Fund, 16*, pub. 1537.

Lachman, V. D. (2012). Ethical challenges in the era of health care reform. *MedSurg Nursing, 21*, 248–245.

Longworth, D. L. (2011). Accountable care organizations, the patient-centered medical home, and health care reform: What does it all mean? *Cleveland Clinic Journal of Medicine, 78*, 571–582.

Muller, A., McCauley, K., Harrington, P., Jablonski, J., & Strauss, R. (2011). Evidence-based practice implementation strategy: The central role of the clinical nurse specialist. *Nursing Administration Quarterly, 35*, 140–151.

Mundinger, M. O., Kane, R. L., Lenz, E. R., Totten, A. M., Tsai, W.-Y., Cleary, P. D., & Shelanski, M. L. (2000). Primary care outcomes in patients treated by nurse practitioners or physicians. *JAMA, 283*, 59–68.

National Association of Clinical Nurse Specialists (NACNS). (2004). *Statement on clinical nurse specialist practice and education* (2nd ed.). Harrisburg, PA: Author.

National Association of Clinical Nurse Specialists (NACNS). (2010, June). *Clinical nurse specialists – practitioners contributing to primary care: A briefing paper.* Retrieved September 6, 2013, from http://www.nacns.org/docs/PrimaryCareBriefing.pdf

National Association of Clinical Nurse Specialists (NACNS). (2013, September). *Achieving specialty competency for clinical nurse specialists.* Retrieved September 6, 2013, from http://www.nacns.org/docs/NACNS-SpecialtyPaper.pdf

National Center for Medical Home Implementation. (n.d.). *Medical home recognition & accreditation programs.* Retrieved September 1, 2013, from http://www.medicalhomeinfo.org/national/recognition_programs.aspx

National Committee for Quality Assurance (NCQA). (2013). *Start to finish: Patient-centered medical home (PCMH) recognition.* Retrieved September 1, 2013, from http://www.ncqa.org/Programs/Recognition/PatientCenteredMedicalHomePCMH.aspx

National Governors Association (NGA). (2012). *The role of nurse practitioners in meeting increasing demand for primary care.* Retrieved September 6, 2013, from http://www.nga.org/files/live/sites/NGA/files/pdf/1212NursePractitionersPaper.pdf

National Quality Forum (NQF). (2006). *NQF-endorsed definition and framework for measuring care coordination.* Retrieved September 2, 2013, from http://janus.pscinc.com/dualeligibles/Workgroups/CC/112911/NQF%20CareCoordination%20definition%20and%20framework.pdf

National Quality Forum (NQF). (2010). *Preferred practices and performance measures for measuring and reporting care coordination.* Retrieved September 2, 2013, from http://www.qualityforum.org/Publications/2010/10/Preferred_Practices_and_Performance_Measures_for_Measuring_and_Reporting_Care_Coordination.aspx

National Transitions of Care Coalition (NTOCC). (2008). *Transitions of care measures.* Retrieved September 6, 2013, from http://www.ntocc.org/Portals/0/PDF/Resources/TransitionsOfCare_Measures.pdf

Naylor, M. D. (2012). Advancing high value transitional care: The central role of nursing and its leadership. *Nursing Administration Quarterly, 36*, 115–126.

Newhouse, R. P., Stanik-Hutt, J., White, K. M., Johantgen, M., Bass, E. B., Zangaro, G., & Weiner, J. P. (2011). Advanced practice nurse outcomes 1990–2008: A systematic review. *Nursing Economics, 29*, 230–250.

Nielsen, M., Langner, B., Zema, C., Hacker, T., & Grundy, P. (2012). *Benefits of implementing the primary care patient-centered medical home: A review of cost & quality results, 2012.* Retrieved September 12, 2013, from http://www.pcpcc.org/sites/default/files/media/benefits_of_implementing_the_primary_aare_pcmh.pdf

Patient-Centered Primary Care Collaborative (PCPCC). (2013). *Defining the medical home.* Retrieved September 12, 2013, from http://www.pcpcc.org/about/medical-home

Peikes, D., Zutshi, A., Genevro, J., Smith, K., Parchman, M., & Meyers, D. (2012, February). *Early evidence on the patient-centered medical home.* Retrieved September 6, 2013, from http://pcmh.ahrq.gov/ portal/server.pt/community/pcmh_home/1483/pcmh_ evidence_evaluation_v2

Poghosyan, L., Lucero, R., Rauch, L., & Berkowitz, B. (2012). Nurse practitioners workforce: A substantial supply of primary care providers. *Nursing Economics, 30,* 268–294.

Sargen, M., Hooker, R. S., & Cooper, R. A. (2011). Gaps in the supply of physicians advance practice nurse and physician assistants. *Journal of the American College of Surgeons, 212,* 991–999.

Shinseki, E. K. (2009, April 22). *Veterans Health Administration national leadership board strategic planning summit.* Retrieved September 5, 2013, from http://www.va.gov/opa/speeches/2009/09_ 0422.asp

Tringali, C. A., Murphy, T. H., & Osevala, M. L. (2008). Clinical nurse specialist practice in a care coordination model. *Clinical Nurse Specialist, 22,* 231–239.

Growing a Clinical Nurse Specialist Practice in a Rehabilitation Setting

Kathleen L. Dunn

Rehabilitation nurses assist individuals with disabilities or chronic disease toward maximal health through health restoration, maintenance, and promotion (Association of Rehabilitation Nurses, 2008; Mauk, 2012). The Association of Rehabilitation Nurses (2008) notes that "rehabilitation nursing is a philosophy of care, not a work setting or a phase of treatment" (p. 7). An advanced practice rehabilitation nurse

> conducts comprehensive assessment and demonstrates a high level of autonomy and expert skill in diagnosis and treatment in the management of complex responses of individuals, families, groups and communities to health problems stemming from altered functional ability and altered lifestyle. (Association of Rehabilitation Nurses, 1996, p. 4)

The advanced practice nurse may also "direct care or manage systems of care for complex patient/family/community populations" (Association of Rehabilitation Nurses, 1996, p. 6). This chapter discusses the clinical nurse specialist (CNS) role and practice as demonstrated through the opening of a new acute and rehabilitation spinal cord injury (SCI) unit.

PROBLEM

As an experienced SCI rehabilitation CNS, I was recruited for the CNS position at a new SCI and disease (SCI/D) unit in a Veterans' Affairs (VA) medical center. My first responsibilities were to develop essential clinical programs and support opening the unit, a situation with both challenges and opportunities. A major challenge was my lack of experience working within the VA health care system. I also would be working with a nursing staff that had little or no experience in rehabilitation or SCI/D nursing, including registered nurses (RNs) and licensed vocational nurses (LVNs). The hospital did not employ nurses' aides. Opportunities included the ability to help design a program and unit from the beginning, to expand my CNS practice, and to develop new staff in this specialty area. I would be establishing practice standards and norms, training new staff, and helping create a unit culture—all in addition to ordering specialty equipment and supplies to meet the needs of this patient population.

GOALS

The overall goal was to have the inpatient unit and home care program open within 3 months. To meet this goal, the following initiatives had to be completed:

1. Develop the new CNS position, including procedures for clinical consultation with nurses on other units caring for SCI patients
2. Develop interprofessional policies and procedures, including admission criteria, scope of service, and procedures for admission, care coordination, and discharge
3. Develop nursing policies and procedures specific to the program and unit, including standard procedures for everything from bowel, bladder, and skin management to management of complex medical emergencies such as autonomic dysreflexia
4. Orient, educate, and train the entire interprofessional team
5. Select and order equipment and supplies
6. Develop a seamless system of care between the SCI/D clinic, inpatient unit, home care program, and our external and internal stakeholders

IMPLEMENTATION/MOVING FORWARD

I had just 3 months from starting the CNS position in a new, largely empty building to admitting the first patient. There was a long "to do" list. As a CNS new to the VA, I had to focus on developing working relationships that would be essential to the opening of the new unit. In addition to developing relationships with the new nurse manager and unit physician, this position would require frequent collaboration with other medical center CNSs and nurse managers, with staff in other areas of the hospital, and with the SCI/D center therapy, counseling, and administrative staff. I would also need to learn how to work with a physician's assistant (PA) on the inpatient unit (a new experience for me) and to develop relationships with discharge planners and case managers at local trauma centers, as well as Department of Defense medical facilities in our region.

The acting nurse manager had been a professional colleague and friend for many years. Having her as my supervisor initially necessitated a change in our relationship; however, she was also experienced in the VA system and was invaluable to me in helping me learn both the formal and informal methods of getting the job done and the patients' needs met. She was a nurse practitioner (NP) with an extensive background of working with CNSs, and she was very comfortable with the CNS role. At the time there were four CNSs at this medical center, all unit based. They were my major source of support and also a resource for learning how the informal chain of command worked—how things "really get done around here." I began participating in nursing service committees and task forces and collaborated on hospital-based special projects. I also spent a lot of time getting to know the SCI physician and PA. The acting nurse manager and I often discussed role boundaries and expectations for the nursing staff and the medical staff (including the PA). Initially, the PA wanted sign-off approval of nursing policies and procedures. We disagreed. Redefining and setting boundaries and clarifying roles continued through the first year.

Working with a nursing staff who had little or no experience in rehabilitation or SCI nursing was a challenge. Most staff had previous experience in medical-surgical or long-term care nursing only. Rehabilitation nursing requires a paradigm shift in perspective of the nurse–patient relationship and the roles of a nurse in teaching, coaching, and guiding versus direct caregiver. Staff education had to emphasize cognitive/affective competencies as well as psychomotor competencies. Disability awareness training had to be integrated with learning skills such as body mechanics for transfers, and bowel care. I was not able to participate in all the new nursing staff interviews. This meant that I did not meet most of the nursing staff until they began orientation, which made needs assessment much more difficult.

Emphasis was placed on key issues required for patient and staff safety, but quality of care also had to be addressed. Many of the orientation classes would be provided in an interprofessional group, so they had to meet the needs of a varied staff. I worked extensively with the nurse manager, who had obtained information about similar orientation programs at other VA SCI centers and who also helped me identify guest faculty from both our facility and other VA SCI centers. Some of these presentations were scheduled prior to my hire; however, I became responsible for coordinating the presentations and bridging the gaps in content.

I had developed educational materials over the years, and while it was helpful to have a large collection of audiovisual materials; additional educational programs and materials had to be created. The medical center's media center helped with this and videotaped staff orientation presentations. I also ordered additional teaching materials, including videotapes, models, books, and journals, as well as equipment such as projectors and videotape players.

During orientation, key people from other hospital departments were invited, including other CNSs, staff from Prosthetics and Central Supply, and leadership from departments such as social work and psychology. The combined team orientation lasted a week, with an additional week for nursing staff only. Class formats included didactic presentations, skills labs, and disability "experiences," with ample opportunities for discussion and questions. The nursing classes consisted of specific nursing skills, such as intermittent catheterization, application of external condom catheters, and transfers skills, as well as classes on rehabilitation nursing theory, primary nursing, care planning, and working in an interprofessional team.

The unit was custom designed for SCI care, with large bathrooms that were fully wheelchair accessible; however, some important and necessary features were not included. A medication room was missing, hand-washing facilities were not available at the nurses' station, and the space allocated for bowel care and showers was an outdated holdover from old VA SCI unit designs. In addition, there were no plans for office space on the unit and no plans for a staff lounge and/or classroom. Working together, the acting nurse manager and I were able to have space reallocated and minor modifications made for all these needs. The shower/bowel care area was redesignated (though not remodeled) for equipment storage because the accessible bathrooms in each patient room were adequate. Our success was, in part, related to the manager's extensive experience in the VA system and her ability to work within her established networks/relationships. This experience underscored the need to put relationship building on the top of my priority list.

Rehabilitation care involves a lot of different specialized equipment and supplies; opening a new unit required evaluating and selecting these items. Some equipment was already in place, including beds, bedside stands, med carts, chart racks, and commode chairs. Upon further investigation, however, some of this was not appropriate for rehabilitation patients. The over-toilet shower/commode chairs, for example, did not fit the unit toilets. I found suitable replacements and was able to negotiate a trade-in of 15 previously purchased chairs for chairs that would fit over the toilets.

Other specialized patient equipment needs included hands-free nurse call bells, positioning and transfer equipment, and bathing assistance equipment. Specialized supplies had to be evaluated and ordered, such as external condom catheters, straight and indwelling catheters, urinary drainage bags, and wound care supplies. Vendors were contacted for samples, and I worked closely with the nurse manager of Central Supply to ensure that sufficient supplies would be on hand prior to the opening of the unit.

I was responsible for developing many of the clinical policies and procedures. Some of this work could be based on previous experience, others were developed from the literature, and some others were based on policies at other VA and private sector SCI centers. Collaboration with the SCI physician and other hospital departments was critical, and many meetings were needed to work out details. For example, a standard procedure and an accompanying nurse competency for managing episodes of autonomic dysreflexia (an emergency in SCI patients) was necessary to be able to respond appropriately and quickly to this emergency situation. Arriving at consensus on the protocol involved consideration of nursing scope of practice, level of practice competency, internal VA regulations, and state nurse practice guidelines, along with evidence-based best practices as described in the literature.

As CNS, I was designated to determine criteria for nurse competence. I developed both learning modules and competency assessment methods, including written tests, return demonstrations, and clinical case study simulations and methods for documenting and maintaining competency records.

Clinical policies and procedures were also needed for treatments and procedures such as intermittent catheterization programs, bowel care programs, and a self-medication program. These were developed collaboratively with appropriate disciplines and in compliance with both Veterans Health Administration (VHA) and the hospital's existing policies.

I would also be responsible for preadmission screening for those patients referred to the center for both acute care and rehabilitation following a new SCI. I designed screening forms, developed materials to give to referral sources about our program for both their information and patients and families, and arranged to make site visits to the referring facilities (if within the county) to assess the patient, provide information, and coordinate a smooth transfer. I worked closely with the SCI chief so that we were in agreement on criteria for admission, assessment parameters, and appropriate medical stability for these patients. This involved making many phone calls to facilities referring patients out of the area and screening by phone when needed. I visited the local Navy hospital to establish a contact there with the appropriate case managers and social workers and to become familiar with their units and facility.

IMPLEMENTATION

The unit had to be ready for our first admission on Friday of the week the educational programs were completed. Organizing supplies and setting up patient rooms was a priority. As is typical for CNSs who focus on "making it happen," I found myself helping an LVN install patient televisions on Thursday afternoon. A good CNS has many diverse skills. Being mechanically inclined and having the ability to work with hand tools is a definite asset!

The first few patients admitted to the new SCI unit were medically stable and needed hospitalization only for tests and procedures. As the unit CNS, I worked side by side with the nursing staff, helping them develop competence and confidence. When the first emergency admission occurred at the end of the first week, I stayed on the unit for 14 hours to assist with management of the patient's pyelonephritis and autonomic dysreflexia. Over the next few weeks I averaged 10- to 12-hour days so that staff were adequately supported both in routine care delivery and with problem solving. I also consulted and made some home visits with our new SCI home care nurse, and I consulted with the new SCI NP in the outpatient clinic to help them problem-solve and develop increased expertise in SCI nursing. These were long and tiring days, but it was necessary in order for the unit to be successful.

EVALUATION AND OUTCOMES

We initially opened with eight inpatient beds, and by the end of 3 months increased this to 15. By the end of 9 months, we had 18 inpatient beds open and had hired and oriented two more groups of staff, including nurses, therapists, a physician, and another PA. Some staff found that SCI and rehabilitation nursing was not for them and left quickly. A few had unsatisfactory performance and were terminated. Several found that SCI and rehabilitation nursing was their calling and remained for many years.

Overall, staff believed they were well prepared to provide patient care, and they also noted how important it was to them to have ready access to CNS support when confronted with actual patient care situations that were unfamiliar or unanticipated.

The new nurse manager and I worked closely with other SCI center leadership staff to develop a unit culture and spirit of camaraderie. This spirit extended to unit-based social events such as potluck lunches and beach parties. We even obtained donated polo shirts with the unit logo for all the staff.

The first year was tough, with turnover of both medical and therapy leadership staff and some nursing staff. Feedback from patients was helpful both to identify areas where we were meeting or exceeding the expectations of our clients and to identify areas for improvement. Care delivery was modified based on our assessment of what was and was not working,

with frequent staff and patient input. We found that we needed frequent contacts with the medical staff and other leadership, so a SCI leadership committee was established to review progress toward unit goals and to work together on process improvement projects.

Materials developed for the initial orientation proved invaluable for use in subsequent orientations. I continued to use some of the videotaped lectures for a number of years until the content became dated, meanwhile developing more easily updated materials consistent with evidence-based practice (EBP).

I started screening new injury referrals as soon as we opened. I coordinated services with the discharge coordinator or social worker at the referring facility, with eligibility and the transfer coordinator at our hospital, and with external case managers for different insurances or the Department of Defense. The SCI physician accepted or declined these admissions based on my data collection and recommendations. While having a CNS perform screenings and assessments is not unique in the world of rehabilitation nursing, it is quite unusual within VA SCI centers. The ability of the CNS to both assess the patient and coordinate complex systems to achieve a smooth transition to our unit has been invaluable to the success of our program.

MY CNS PRACTICE TODAY

In the years that have passed since first opening the unit, my CNS role has evolved. Currently, I am also the case manager for new injury rehabilitation SCI patients (averaging one to four patients at a time on our 28-bed unit). I continue to coordinate revision of and development of evidence-based nursing policies and procedures and the SCI personal care attendant training program. I also implement SCI new nurse orientation and in-services, and chair the SCI interprofessional patient/staff education committee. I review and approve all requests for specialty mattresses and beds for all system outpatients, and chair the hospital pressure ulcer task force. I provide direct care to patients, with a special interest in sexuality education and counseling. I coordinate and lead the SCI unit interprofessional weekly wound care rounds, and I also coordinate activities to meet Commission for Accreditation of Rehabilitation Facilities standards.

Since opening the unit 25 years ago, I have worked with six different SCI nurse managers, six different supervisors, and four different SCI chief physicians. None of the original staff nurses are currently working on the unit. I have had to learn to be flexible in working with other leadership staff with vastly different leadership styles and approaches to patient care. Being able to adjust to changes in leadership and personnel, with differences in philosophy and approach, while maintaining focus and commitment to rehabilitation nursing principles has remained a keystone of my practice.

My participation in national nursing and interprofessional organizations has resulted in invitations to present and publish nationally and internationally. I coordinate a panel of other SCI advanced practice nurses who answer health-related questions on a website for people with SCI (sci.rutgers.edu). I have represented both the Association of Rehabilitation Nurses and the American Association of SCI Nurses on the Steering Committee for the Consortium for Spinal Cord Medicine (which develops and publishes clinical practice guidelines). I served on a national task force for implementation of safe patient handling and movement programs within the VA health care system and served as a National Association of Clinical Nurse Specialists (NACNS) representative to the American Nurses Credentialing Center (ANCC) Core CNS certification exam Content Expert Panel. In 2008 I was the first nurse inducted into the Spinal Cord Hall of Fame, and received the Association of Rehabilitation Nurses Advanced Practice award. I was honored with the Secretary of Veterans Affairs Nursing Excellence (Expanded Role) award in 2012. With a new SCI unit building in the early planning stages, I am able to bring my years of experience and expertise to the table for a radically different and improved facility sometime in the future.

Opening a new unit and watching it grow and mature was one of the major accomplishments of my career. The CNS, as the clinical expert in specialty-focused advanced nursing practice, is ideally prepared to coordinate physical facility design, develop care delivery systems and processes, evaluate outcomes, and make continued corrections to adjust and adapt to new technology, science, and clinical evidence. My first and last passion is being a CNS in SCI rehabilitation nursing. Finding your passion, working in a stimulating environment with a network of peers, and making a difference for patient outcomes is the ultimate success in a nursing career.

REFERENCES

Association of Rehabilitation Nurses. (1996). *Scope and standards of advanced clinical practice in rehabilitation nursing.* Glenview, IL: Author.

Association of Rehabilitation Nurses. (2008). *Standards and scope of rehabilitation nursing.* Glenview, IL: Author.

Mauk, K. L. (2012). *Rehabilitation nursing: A contemporary approach to practice.* Burlington, MA: Jones & Bartlett Learning.

Exploring Clinical Nurse Specialist Practice in the Emergency Department

Garrett K. Chan

OVERVIEW OF EMERGENCY NURSING AND EMERGENCY DEPARTMENT PATIENT POPULATIONS

Clinical nurse specialists (CNSs) in the emergency department (ED) are master generalists. CNSs in emergency care must be educated in many aspects of human physiology, growth, and development across the life span and have expertise in several physiological, pathophysiological, psychological, social, and public health systems. Inherent in emergency clinical practice is a sense of uncertainty and unpredictability, as patients arrive to the ED unannounced and with chief complaints rather than with diagnoses common in other practices in health care. Clinicians need to be prepared to care for anyone with any disease or injury process who presents to the ED. Emergency nurses are trained to assess whether the patient has a life-threatening condition, to assist in making a diagnosis, and to initiate diagnostic and resuscitative interventions in an effort to stabilize the patient's condition (Arslanian-Engoren, 2009). Differential diagnosis is a cornerstone of emergency nursing practice. Understanding many pathophysiological, psychological, social, and public health issues and creating a differential diagnosis list are core activities of emergency nursing because the exact diagnosis of a patient is unknown.

Emergency nurses work in close collaboration with other disciplines such as medicine with every patient encounter. Respiratory therapy and social services are disciplines that are consulted on a daily basis. In the ED, the team approach to every patient is embedded in the care delivery system. All disciplines work together to achieve the same goal: to diagnose the patient's underlying illness and initiate treatment to stabilize the patient's condition. Family-centered care and patient education are also core activities of emergency nursing. Throughout the history of emergency nursing, there is much overlap between the medicine and nursing disciplines (Snyder, Keeling, & Razionale, 2006). For example, emergency nurses are educated and trained to diagnose myocardial ischemia by looking at electrocardiograms and understanding laboratory values. Alternatively, emergency physicians are involved with discharge planning and education of patients.

The patient census can fluctuate wildly throughout the course of a day. In addition, the ED has been described as a place of transition (Chan, 2004). Patients do not usually stay in the ED for the duration of their hospital stay (Sun et al., 2013). Rather, they are either discharged to home or admitted to an inpatient unit or to another hospital for specialty care. The focus of ED care is to stabilize the patient's condition and begin treatment with a referral to another service or to the patient's primary care provider for further follow-up.

An important aspect of emergency CNSs' work is to have direct clinical contact with patients who present with complex issues or who are severely ill or injured (Proehl, 2003). These clinical encounters provide opportunities for the emergency CNS to demonstrate, perform, implement, or role model clinical skills of advanced health and social assessment, nursing and medical differential diagnoses, and psychomotor skills. Additional unique issues that have influenced emergency practice include overcrowding and lack of experienced nurses and physicians (Institute of Medicine [IOM], 2006). In addition, the encounters provide an opportunity to assess the knowledge and behavior of clinicians and teach or debrief depending on the situation. Supporting the spheres of influence of nursing and organizations depends on the assessment of clinical practice within the department. Domains of advanced practice nursing in emergency care settings include critical care, urgent care, primary care, behavioral medicine, public health, and social medicine (Chan & Garbez, 2006).

Lewandowski and Adamle (2009) identified three substantive areas of CNS practice: (a) to manage the care of complex and vulnerable populations; (b) to educate and support interprofessional staff, and (c) to facilitate change and innovation within health care systems. These substantive areas of practice clearly differentiate CNS practice from other advanced practice registered nursing roles. To further build upon the National Association of Clinical Nurse Specialists (NACNS) CNS core competencies (NACNS, 2010) and Lewandowski and Adamle's substantive areas of practice, the Emergency Nurses Association (ENA) conducted a competency validation study to create specialty-specific competencies (ENA, 2011). As many CNS programs are moving toward the National Council of State Boards of Nursing (NCSBN) Consensus Model Regulatory Language (National Council of State Boards of Nursing, 2012), there is some concern that specialist educational content can be lost when focusing solely on adult/gerontology or family/across the life span population foci content. Therefore, the ENA CNS specialty competencies can help guide the didactic and clinical content in any population-focused CNS educational program to preserve the specialty-specific education and training.

Problem Identification

Providing safe patient care is paramount within hospitals today. Many factors are responsible for the threats to safe patient care. There is a growing concern about the number of experienced nurses who are aging and getting ready for retirement and an increasing number of novice nurses, as well as high turnover rates of nurses in the workforce (Glynn & Silva,

2013). Additional factors that may lead to less safe patient care include lack of mentoring and coaching as well as an increased physician workload leading to a decreasing amount of time for collaboration (Glynn & Silva, 2013). Novice nurses report the need for increased assistance from experienced nurses to help them socialize into the role of the professional nurse, for recognition and support, and to support their clinical decision making (Phillips, Kenny, Esterman, & Smith, 2013). Common themes surrounding novice nurses' near-miss or adverse events include an increased need for clinically focused critical thinking, seeking assistance from experienced nurses, knowledge of unit and workflow patterns, first-time experiences in situations, time constraints, handoffs, influence of peer pressure and social norms, losing the big picture, and novice nurses helping other novice nurses (Ebright, Urden, Patterson, & Chalko, 2004). There is an increased workload for staff nurses, which leaves little time for mentoring, coaching, and supervision of more novice nurses (Institute of Medicine Committee on the Work Environment for Nurses & Patient Safety Board on Health Services, 2004). Physician inexperience, organizational factors and pressures that inhibit interprofessional practice, and communication breakdown are other factors that threaten safe patient care. To ensure that process improvement (PI) projects are successful, there is a tendency to put pressure on the CNS to implement other parts of the role, by evaluating practices and outcomes and performing audits that take them away from direct patient care. These factors contribute to the need to have CNSs at the bedside providing direct patient care as well as coaching to staff.

With the proliferation of regulatory agency standards and quality initiatives such as the National Quality Forum and the Institute for Healthcare Improvement (IHI), hospitals struggle to meet all of these mandates for improving care in the hospital setting. CNSs are educated and well positioned within hospitals to lead the efforts through committee work to comply with these mandates. However, with the increased amount of committee and quality improvement work the CNS engages in, CNSs spend less time in the central activity of all advanced practice nurses—direct clinical practice.

CNS direct clinical practice can be the answer to addressing the issues surrounding patient safety and mentoring less experienced nurses to provide better care. In addition, direct clinical practice can provide the CNS with opportunities to identify staff learning needs and system or process breakdowns. The following exemplar illustrates these concepts and domains of emergency advanced practice nursing and highlights the three spheres of influence of CNS practice.

Exemplar

Practice Innovation. In my daily practice as the ED CNS, I would round in the department at least twice a day—once in the morning before turning on my computer and beginning to check my e-mails and once in the early afternoon. Often, I would round at 6:30 a.m. to talk with the night shift to ask if there were any unusual incidents or concerns during that time. However, on this particular day, I happened to round in the ED at 8 a.m.

The ED was quiet, as there were only three patients. I walked by one of the ED resuscitation rooms and glanced inside. I saw one ventilated patient and three nurses around the patient's bed. As I continued to walk toward the charge nurse desk, I decided to turn around and see what was going on in that room because I thought it was unusual that three very experienced nurses were standing around one patient.

I walked into the room, greeted the nurses, and asked them what was going on with the patient. The primary nurse gave me report. Ms. H was a 14-year-old female who was flown to our hospital from a rural hospital after ingesting a whole bottle of isoniazid in a suicide attempt. Ms. H was paralyzed, sedated, and being mechanically ventilated in the ED awaiting a pediatric intensive care unit (PICU) bed.

Still wondering why there were three nurses at the patient's bedside, I took this opportunity to assess the situation by performing a health and physical assessment and doing some bedside teaching, explaining what I was looking for in each step of the health and physical assessment and paying close attention to the expected normal and potentially abnormal findings in a patient who overdoses on isoniazid. As we were completing the physical exam and reviewing the charting on this patient, the cardiac monitor alarm sounded. The patient's heart rate suddenly went from 80 beats per minute to 180 beats per minute, and the blood pressure was 200/105 mmHg. The primary nurse informed me that this was the third time this had happened to the patient.

I quickly ran through my differential diagnosis list for probable causes of sudden-onset tachycardia:

1. Seizure secondary to metabolic acidosis
2. Atrial fibrillation/flutter
3. Narrow-complex tachycardias (i.e., multifocal atrial tachycardia, paroxysmal supraventricular tachycardia, atrioventricular [AV] nodal reentrant tachycardia, ectopic atrial tachycardia, junctional tachycardia)
4. Unstable or stable wide-complex tachycardias (i.e., unknown type, AV reentrant tachycardia, torsades de pointes, or ventricular tachycardia—monomorphic or polymorphic)
5. Thyrotoxicosis
6. Pheochromocytoma
7. Hypoglycemia
8. Hypovolemia/hemorrhage
9. Fever
10. Fear/anxiety
11. Other illicit drug ingestion (e.g., cocaine package rupture, which often occurs to "body packers" or "mules" who traffic packages of cocaine by ingesting them)

As the CNS in a Level-2 trauma center ED in California, I had to be familiar with the patient demographics and public health issues in my community. For example, in the San Francisco Bay Area, multidrug-resistant tuberculosis is on the rise and becoming an epidemic in our communities. Therefore, it was important that I stay informed of the Public Health Department's recommendations for surveillance and treatment of tuberculosis. From my CNS education about advanced pathophysiology, pharmacology, and physical assessment, I recognized that this patient was in metabolic acidosis from the isoniazid overdose.

Symptoms of isoniazid overdose include nausea, vomiting, altered mental status, slurred speech, hallucinations, blurred vision, seizures, and coma. I arrived at the diagnosis that this patient was having a seizure secondary to metabolic acidosis. However, because the patient was being paralyzed and sedated, the patient was not exhibiting the tonic/clonic activity typical of this type of seizure.

I had the nurse draw an arterial blood gas and contact pharmacy to mix more of the antidote, vitamin B6, as well as a sodium bicarbonate drip. We had the ED physician come in to collaborate with us on our findings. The ED physician agreed with my plan of care.

The arterial blood gas results came back as pH = 6.9, PaCO2 = 17 mmHg; PaO2 = 180 mmHg; HCO3 = 6 mmHg; Anion Gap = 30, indicating severe metabolic acidosis with an anion gap. The patient received more vitamin B6 and lorazepam for her seizures, and she was placed on a sodium bicarbonate drip to correct her severe metabolic acidosis. I made a referral to social services to support the family during this time of crisis. Psychiatry was consulted to follow Ms. H during her hospital stay. Ms. H was then transferred to the PICU and made a full recovery. She was discharged to the care of a local psychiatrist in her home town.

The CNS in the ED is called upon to effect changes in the three spheres of influence of patient/client, nursing, and organizations using direct clinical practice skills, education, consultation, research, and change-agent skills. To affect patient care and outcomes, the CNS in EDs must be present in the department. Maintaining a presence in the ED allows the CNS to be visible and to establish or maintain credibility as an expert clinician among the staff. In addition, to affect patient care and outcomes, the CNS in EDs must be present in the department to understand the skill level of clinicians, to evaluate current practices of staff, to provide immediate coaching and teaching, to observe the processes of care, to identify opportunities for improvement, and to elicit current issues from the staff. If aspects of clinical care are not well understood, then planned interventions to address issues or to change processes potentially will not succeed because the CNS does not intimately understand the issues or processes. Additionally, if the staff do not perceive the CNS as being credible, then attempts at PI will be seen as extraneous, superfluous, or inappropriate. The goal of this practice innovation is to provide leadership, education, coaching, and mentoring to staff in an effort to ensure that quality care is being delivered and to create a culture of excellent care. This goal can be attained through four interventions: direct patient care, bedside teaching, coaching and mentoring of clinicians, and providing evidence-based resources.

To incorporate these four interventions into CNS practice, CNSs in emergency care settings can integrate many activities into their daily routine. First, CNSs can conduct daily rounds in the department across all shifts (i.e., day shift, evening shift, night shift). I would commonly round in the department twice a day—once at 6:30 a.m. at the change of shift to check in with the night staff to determine if there were any issues that occurred during their shift, and once at around 3 p.m. Rounding at 6:30 a.m. allowed me to be present when the day shift nurses arrived so they knew I was always available if they needed my assistance. During this time, I would take the opportunity to informally remind the staff nurses of any PI projects the ED was working on and provide rationale for the PI project. Often, staff nurses would either question or have questions regarding the PI project. Rounding with the staff provided the opportunity for the nurses to understand the goals or be educated about the necessity of the PI project. The afternoon rounds provided me with an opportunity to observe and assess nursing practice and care or administrative processes, to assist the department if busy, to assist staff in troubleshooting or managing breakdowns, and to be available to answer questions or provide resources.

Second, my pager was included in all group paging to alert me of any trauma or major medical (i.e., patients *in extremis* or in full arrest) alert. When available, I would attend these resuscitations to provide coaching to novice nurses or to experienced nurses in unusual situations, to assist the health care team in incorporating new technology or medications, to assess potential learning needs of the staff, to ensure that evidence-based interventions were being included in the care, to acknowledge and reinforce examples of excellent caring interventions, and to debrief and problem-solve with staff regarding any issues of concern or breakdown. Participating in care of the highest acuity patients afforded me the opportunity to be visible in the department and maintain credibility with staff, to practice my skills of advanced health and physical assessment, to use psychomotor skills in highly stressful situations, and to work as a team player in the ED.

Third, I scheduled myself regularly as a staff nurse to fill 4- or 8-hour shifts across all shifts. These scheduled shifts allowed me to assess and monitor the flow of patients in the ED, to care for patients and maintain clinical competency with patients across all acuity levels and body systems (e.g., obstetric complaints, ear/nose/throat complaints), to be available to staff for any questions they might have, and to establish credibility with staff in that I could care for all patients who came to the ED. In terms of filling a sick call shift, I avoided being seen as someone who had nothing else to do but to fill in for someone who called in sick or covering lunches or breaks. In extreme circumstances, I would relieve nurses so that they could take a much-needed break or would agree to work to fill an empty slot in the schedule.

Lastly, I realized that I could not be present in the department 24 hours a day, 7 days a week. Therefore, in order maintain a presence, I developed or participated in the development of educational materials, policies, procedures, and resource guides that were evidence based. For example, I developed a vasoactive medication binder that listed all the intravenous vasopressor and antiarrhythmic medications and included indications, contraindications, standard concentrations, drip rate charts, adverse side effects, and pediatric through geriatric considerations. Another resource guide was the appropriate assessment and documentation of the neurologic exam in patients with altered level of consciousness due to pathology or medications. At the bottom of each resource I created, I wrote my name and pager number in the event that anyone had a question or concern about the resource.

Empirical indicators to evaluate experience and expertise have been difficult to define (Institute of Medicine Committee on the Work Environment for Nurses & Patient Safety Board on Health Services, 2004). Proxy measures of ED quality care include patient flow indicators such as waiting room time, average length of stay, and the number of patients who left without being seen. Clinical performance indicators such as time to 12-lead electrocardiogram, time to antibiotic administration in community-acquired pneumonia, and medication error rates are captured for national quality/PI initiatives. Patient satisfaction has also been identified as a proxy measure of quality care. However, when including questions about nursing care in patient satisfaction surveys, such as "care and concern shown by nurses" and "courtesy shown to your family and friends," which are asked of the lay public, an incompetent nurse may show a great deal of concern and care for a patient and family yet not be competent in the technical or social skills required to expertly take care of a patient or family. While these indicators are important in determining whether there are process issues that can be corrected, they do not measure the "near misses" or capture the true expertise of nurses caring for patients in the ED.

Adherence to benchmark standards, facilitating practice change, creation of clinical resources, implementation of clinical standards, and educational needs assessment potentially averted forces that could have created a sentinel event when I was in the department providing direct clinical care. Additionally, living the clinical practice of a staff and advanced practice nurse, I advocate for or implement processes that support successful changes in practice that are feasible for staff nurses in the ED. Administrators look to the CNS as an expert clinician/practitioner to speak to practice changes that provide safe patient care.

CONCLUSION

Direct patient care is a hidden or often deleted part of CNS practice in the face of other organizational demands such as The Joint Commission preparation, Magnet Hospital preparation, committee work, and project management. Yet, direct patient care is an invaluable and core aspect of CNS practice. Since I incorporated these interventions into my practice, I realized that staff were very accepting of changes and improvements I would attempt to institute. One nurse said to me that she would incorporate a process change because she knew that I understood the challenges and issues that staff nurses deal with in their daily practice. Without that sense of understanding of the issues of staff nurses, changes to care processes might fail. Competency in the patient/client sphere of influence can take the form of direct care clinician or consulting roles and can maintain the competency of the CNS, identify core issues for the ED, educate nurses to improve nursing and other disciplines' care

practices, provide evidence-based rationale for care practices where appropriate, and improve the quality of care for patients. Additionally, emergency CNSs need to stay informed and promote individual state scopes of practice, participate in national discourses that advance the role of the CNS, and utilize specialty-specific competencies to guide education and practice.

REFERENCES

Arslanian-Engoren, C. (2009). Explicating nurses' cardiac triage decisions. *Journal of Cardiovascular Nursing, 24*(1), 50–57. doi:10.1097/01 JCN.0000317474.50424.4f

Chan, G. K. (2004). End-of-life models and emergency department care. *Academic Emergency Medicine, 11*(1), 79–86.

Chan, G. K., & Garbez, R. O. (2006). Education of advanced practice nurses for emergency care settings: Emphasizing shared competencies and domains. *Advanced Emergency Nursing Journal, 28*(3), 216–225.

Ebright, P. R., Urden, L., Patterson, E., & Chalko, B. (2004). Themes surrounding novice nurse near-miss and adverse-event situations. *Journal of Nursing Administration, 34*(11), 531–538.

Emergency Nurses Association (ENA). (2011). Competencies for clinical nurse specialists in emergency care. Retrieved from http://www.ena .org/practice-research/Practice/Quality/Documents/ CNSCompetencies.pdf

Glynn, P., & Silva, S. (2013). Meeting the needs of new graduates in the emergency department: A qualitative study evaluating a new graduate internship program. *Journal of Emergency Nursing, 39*(2), 173–178. doi:10.1016/j.jen.2011.10.007

Institute of Medicine (IOM). (2006). *Hospital-based emergency care: At the breaking point.* Washington, DC: National Academies Press.

Institute of Medicine Committee on the Work Environment for Nurses and Patient Safety Board on Health Services. (2004). *Keeping patients safe: Transforming the work environment of nurses.* Washington, DC: National Academies Press.

Lewandowski, W., & Adamle, K. (2009). Substantive areas of clinical nurse specialist practice: A comprehensive review of the literature. *Clinical Nurse Specialist, 23*(2), 73–90; quiz 91–72. doi:10.1097/ NUR.0b013e31819971d0

National Association of Clinical Nurse Specialists (NACNS). (2010). *Clinical nurse specialist core competencies.* Retrieved from www.nacns.org/docs/ CNSCoreCompetenciesBroch.pdf

National Council of State Boards of Nursing. (2012). *NCSBN consensus model for APRN regulation.* Retrieved from https://www.ncsbn.org/aprn.htm

Phillips, C., Kenny, A., Esterman, A., & Smith, C. (2013). A secondary data analysis examining the needs of graduate nurses in their transition to a new role. *Nurse Education in Practice.* Advance online publication. doi:10.1016/j.nepr.2013.07.007

Proehl, J. A. (2003). The role of the clinical nurse specialist in the emergency department. In V. A. Keough (Ed.), *Advanced practice nursing: Current practice issues in emergency care* (2nd ed.). Des Plaines, IL: Emergency Nurses Association.

Snyder, A., Keeling, A., & Razionale, C. (2006). From "first aid rooms" to advanced practice nursing: A glimpse into the history of emergency nursing.

Advanced Emergency Nursing Journal, 28(3), 198–209.

Sun, B. C., Hsia, R. Y., Weiss, R. E., Zingmond, D., Liang, L. J., Han, W., ... Asch, S. M. (2013). Effect of emergency department crowding on outcomes of admitted patients. *Annals of Emergency Medicine, 61*(6), 605–611 e606. doi:10.1016/j.annemergmed.2012.10.026

Establishing a Private Practice for Diabetes Self-Management

Patricia S. Moore

POPULATION SERVED

Diabetes mellitus is defined as a group of metabolic diseases characterized by hyperglycemia (American Diabetes Association [ADA], 2013a). The etiology of diabetes mellitus (diabetes) is multifactorial and includes defects in insulin secretion and/or insulin action. The underlying mechanisms of diabetes are the result of genetic and environmental influences such as autoimmune process and insulin resistance. Diabetes is classified by the mechanism that influences the onset of the disease. The classification categories include prediabetes, impaired fasting glucose and impaired glucose tolerance, type 1 diabetes, type 2 diabetes, gestational diabetes, and other types of diabetes that result from concurrent diseases, drugs, or chemicals (ADA, 2013a). Diabetes affects children and adults of all ages and ethnicity, with an estimated prevalence rate in the United States of 8.3%, or 25.8 million people (U.S. Department of Health and Human Services Centers for Disease Control and Prevention [CDC], 2011). The predominant form of diabetes is type 2, accounting for 90% to 95% of diagnosed cases. Due to the chronic nature of the disease, multiple complications such as retinopathy, nephropathy, neuropathy, and cardiovascular disease commonly occur in people with diabetes (ADA, 2013a).

Providing health care for the person with diabetes is a complex process that involves a team approach from a variety of disciplines such as nursing, medicine,

dietary, and social work. A plan of care is formulated as an individualized therapeutic alliance among the person with diabetes, his or her family, and the health care team. The person with diabetes and his or her family are encouraged to assume an active role in the management of diabetes by implementing self-management strategies (ADA, 2013b). The role of the diabetes clinical nurse specialist (CNS) is to promote the health of people with diabetes through the diagnosis and treatment of illnesses associated with disease.

In my CNS practice, participation in the care and management of the person with diabetes included the pharmacologic and nonpharmacologic management of the disease as well as the complications that result from the disease. As a member of the health care team, I focused on the delivery of care within the three spheres of influence as described in the National Association of Clinical Nurse Specialists' (NACNS, 2004) *Statement on Clinical Nurse Specialist Practice and Education*, specifically patient/client, nurses/nursing practice, and organization/system.

CNS PRACTICE PROBLEM

The patient population that I have served in my role as a diabetes CNS has primarily been adults with impaired fasting and glucose tolerance, type 1, type 2, and gestational diabetes. My initial CNS practice was based in a university, tertiary health care system as a member of a multidisciplinary team that provided care to preconceptual and pregnant women with diabetes. After approximately 7 years, however, an opportunity to develop a diabetes center in a regional hospital system closer to my home became available.

During the development stages of the diabetes center, a number of visits were arranged to observe a variety of diabetes centers, including hospital-based centers as well as a CNS-owned and operated independent diabetes center. Additionally, a community needs survey was conducted with potential customers of the diabetes center, which included physicians, hospital nursing staff, and clients with diabetes and their families. The survey outcomes demonstrated an interest by the respondents to expand the diabetes services outside the traditional setting and into a community setting. The hospital acknowledged the interest and initially sought office space in a free-standing retail location. However, a final decision was made to locate the diabetes center within the main hospital building.

Although the hospital location was convenient, it did not serve the needs of all clients. Over the ensuing 2.5 years, it became evident that a significant percentage of potential clients would not attend a hospital-based diabetes program for a variety of reasons, including the expense of the hospital diabetes program; appointment times were not available during the evening and weekend hours; the primary care physician would not refer to a hospital program; the fear of a hospital setting; and inconvenient parking. In addition, my availability to provide individualized CNS care to clients and family members was gradually diminished as my responsibilities were redefined and a greater amount of time was devoted to completion of administrative and committee duties. As a result, I reached the conclusion that establishing a CNS entrepreneurial private practice in a community-based setting would allow me the opportunity to better serve the needs of my clientele.

CNS PRACTICE INNOVATION

My goal was to set up a CNS diabetes private practice in a community-based setting to implement a diabetes self-care management program for clients. Prior to setting up the private practice, it was important for me to understand the legal and financial aspects of establishing a nursing entrepreneurial business. A literature search was conducted to gather information about establishing a private practice in nursing. The search was expanded to include articles on the development and management of medical and nutrition practices in a community setting. Meetings were arranged with a variety of business advisors, including the director of

a business development center, a lawyer with expertise in business development, and an accountant with small business experience. The discussions with each of the experts centered on (a) the type of business entities that could be legally established for a nursing practice, (b) liability issues, and (c) tax advantages/disadvantages. Each advisor provided pamphlets, books, and Internet site resources for review.

A variety of legal structures were available for the establishment of a private practice, including sole proprietorship, partnership, limited liability company, and S corporation (S corp). The business advisors explained the benefits and liabilities of each structure and how they are regulated by the state and federal agencies. Upon their advice, the practice was established as an S corp, with the designation as a Professional Corporation. Once the formal name for the corporation was chosen, the legal advisor submitted the application to the state to designate a new corporation. The application included the name of the corporation, the owner, and the primary purpose of the corporation. Upon receiving approval from the state, an application for liability insurance as a self-employed CNS was submitted to the malpractice insurance company.

ESTABLISHING THE NEW OFFICE

Although very few CNSs were in private practice at that time, I was fortunate to meet a mental health CNS in my community who had already established her private practice. After indicating my interest in sharing office space, she agreed to relocate her office to a larger space that would accommodate my practice. Before we looked at available office space, we developed a conceptual model for the office. The model included the amount of square footage that would be required for two office spaces, a waiting room for clients and families, and storage space.

A variety of office locations were available in the community; however, the selection of the final location was based on the conceptual model and other important factors. These factors included accessibility of the office to persons with disabilities, a centralized location within the community setting, availability of a bus route near the office location, business signage, familiarity of the location to referral sources and potential clients, monthly cost of rent and utilities, and leasing terms. A final location was selected that most closely matched these requirements.

Once a location had been selected, a meeting was arranged with the leasing agent to discuss more specific details that applied to the office rental. These included: office building rules and regulations, rent deposit and monthly charges, average utility costs and hook-up deposits, availability of telephone and cable service, liability issues, and business insurance requirements. A tentative lease was presented for review. The terms were negotiated and adapted to our needs; specifically, the lease allowed us to rent on a year-to-year basis with first option to renew or decline in subsequent years. The percent increase in rent for the second year was established and added to the lease. Once the lease had been signed, the deposit and first month's rent paid, and the business insurance policy purchased, we were allowed access to the office space.

The diabetes office was arranged to enhance the delivery of care to clients and family members. A conference table was added to enhance discussion and education. Education materials were obtained from a variety of diabetes sources, including printed and video materials from the diabetes professional organizations. Additionally, educational materials were developed to support self-management diabetes strategies such as sick-day rules, glucose monitoring schedules, and nutritional support tools. Office supplies were purchased, including a desk, computer, telephone/fax machine, portable TV/VCR, educational videos, and a filing cabinet with a lock to store patient records.

Office hours were established to meet the needs of clients and families. Daytime, evening, and weekend hours were offered. Appointment times were set to allow for flexibility in scheduling. Two-hour sessions were allowed for new clients, which included a 90-minute client and family interaction and 30 minutes for documentation. Return visits were set for 30- to 60-minute client sessions with 15 to 30 minutes between visits for documentation. Clients were provided with return appointment cards that included the office telephone and pager numbers as well as an after-hours number. Clients were scheduled for return visits based on their self-management needs. The return intervals varied from 1 to 4 weeks with the number of sessions determined by the client's progress and ability to master the self-management skills.

MARKETING

In order to establish a collaborative model with physicians, all clients were required to have a physician referral. Therefore, the initial marketing was targeted to the medical community. Appointments were arranged with key physicians to discuss the new diabetes practice. These physicians, who were familiar with my services, had routinely referred clients to me for ongoing diabetes management and self-management education. Pamphlets were developed for distribution

to the physicians and office staff, which described the goals of the practice, types of clients appropriate for referral, referral methods, location, hours, charges, and contact information. Each practice was provided with referral forms that were designed as a checklist to indicate the type of services requested, such as diabetes self-management, nutritional counseling, insulin initiation, and self-monitoring of blood glucose. Referral forms were either faxed to the office or given to the client and brought to the initial meeting. These pamphlets and referral forms were also mailed to all primary care and specialty practice physicians. Additional marketing efforts were targeted at nurses in the acute care setting, a home care agency, and to the staff of a community free health clinic.

Prior to scheduling the first client, potential customers received an open house invitation to tour the new office location. Invitations were sent to all potential customers, as outlined previously, as well as business advisors and faculty from the CNS program. Signage listing the name of the new business was placed in strategic locations inside and outside on building marquees. Advertisements announcing the new practice were placed in the community newspaper each week for approximately 3 months, then monthly for another 3 months. Business cards were designed and printed and distributed to all potential customers.

CLIENT VISIT

The initial visit was usually 90 minutes in duration. During this visit, the client's health history was reviewed. The client was interviewed about the duration of diabetes, complications, comorbid diseases and conditions, current pharmacologic regimen, literacy level, and family history. An assessment was conducted with each client to include (a) knowledge of diabetes; (b) concurrent and potential illness; and (c) culture, age-related factors, and lifestyle behaviors that influenced self-management strategies. Additionally, the client was interviewed about his or her diet plan, exercise routine, and nonpharmacologic treatment strategies. Self-monitored blood glucose and laboratory results were reviewed when available. A physical exam was conducted that included vital signs and neurologic and vascular exams of the lower extremities. Treatment, education, and self-management goals were discussed, and behavioral goals were mutually established with the client and family. Follow-up visits, ranging from 15 to 60 minutes in duration, included a review of the outcomes of self-management strategies, a physical exam, and a review of treatment and education goals.

A variety of nurse-sensitive outcomes were used to measure the outcomes of the self-management sessions, including knowledge, diabetes management, blood glucose control, diet, disease process, health behaviors, health resources, illness care, medication, preconception, pregnancy, treatment regimen, neurological status, nutritional status, risk control regarding cardiovascular health, sensory function and proprioception, sexual function and symptom control, peripheral tissue perfusion, vital signs status, and weight control (Moorhead, Johnson, Mass, & Swanson, 2012).

A chart was established for each new patient. The chart contained the following documents: treatment consent form, physician's referral form, laboratory findings, medication sheet, personal and family history, initial visit history and physical summary, and follow-up visit encounter forms. The initial visit summary was dictated and the notes typed up at the end of the day. Eventually, as more clients were referred to the office, a medical transcriptionist was hired to transcribe dictations. All transcribed notes were reviewed and edited for accuracy. Copies of all notes were faxed to the referring physicians. All charts were maintained and kept in a locked filing cabinet.

OBTAINING PROVIDER NUMBERS, DETERMINING CHARGES, AND ESTABLISHING BILLING METHODS

In setting up the practice, a decision was made that it would be advantageous to clients to bill insurance companies for the CNS services. As a result of the previous hospital experience, it was estimated that 30% of the potential clients for the new diabetes office would have insurance coverage through a company insurance plan, 40% would be covered under Medicare, 20% would be covered by Medicaid (state coverage for the indigent), and 10% would be private pay. An application was completed to obtain provider numbers for Medicare and Medicaid early in the process of setting up the office. A meeting was scheduled with a local third-party insurance agency to provide an overview of my services and to apply as a provider. Additionally, an application was submitted to a large national insurance company that provided coverage in my region.

Charges for the self-management sessions were determined by a variety of methods. The current copy of the physician fee schedule was downloaded from the Internet, charges and reimbursement rates were discussed with my CNS mental health partner, and a voluntary survey was conducted with local providers. A flat-rate charge was established for new clients. Charges for returning clients were based on time, with increments of 15, 30, 45, and 60 minutes. Clients were advised of the charges in advance of the self-management session, and a handout of billing procedures was made available. A 20% copayment was collected at the time of each visit.

A detailed review of the American Medical Association (AMA, 2013) *Current Procedural Terminology Coding Manual* was used to determine the evaluation and management codes appropriate for the CNS services. In order to facilitate billing, a superbill was developed that listed the specific code and associated charge. This superbill was used as a reference when billing the insurance company or client.

The Centers for Medicare and Medicaid Services (CMS, 2013) professional paper claim form (CMS-1500) was completed for each self-management session. Initially, the billing forms were completed by hand and mailed to Medicare, Medicaid, and the appropriate insurance company. As the practice became busier, a billing software program that could function on a desktop computer was purchased from a medical supply company. Eventually, a billing company was hired to manage the billing process, including completion of the 1500 form, submission to insurance companies, resubmission of bills as necessary, posting of payments, and billing of clients for outstanding balances. The billing company also directly billed private-pay clients as well. The billing company handled notices to clients whose bills were in arrears and submitted bills to a collection agency as necessary. This process allowed me to concentrate on the provision of services and provided a degree of separation of the services from the payment issues.

CNS CORE COMPETENCIES RELATED TO PRACTICE INNOVATION

In my role as a diabetes CNS, I designed and implemented an innovative practice solution that provided diabetes self-management services to people with diabetes and their families in a community-based setting. I utilized nurse-sensitive outcomes to evaluate program and client outcomes. As a change agent, I advanced the practice of nursing among other nurses. Hospital staff nurses, home care nurses, and other advanced practice nurses, such as nurse practitioners and nurse midwives, contacted me with questions and routinely referred clients to my office. Additionally, I advanced the practice of nursing within a network of providers. Physicians from a variety of specialties, including obstetrics, family practice, and internal medicine, routinely referred clients to my office for advanced practice nursing intervention. I interacted frequently with podiatrists, ophthalmologists, optometrists, and wound specialists to discuss issues and provide referrals.

PRACTICE INNOVATION OUTCOMES

The CNS diabetes practice was a successful endeavor in many ways. The number of client referrals increased over the years. Initially, client referrals were received from the five key physicians who were familiar with my services from the hospital. Eventually, providers from a variety of specialties referred clients to the practice, including obstetrics, family practice, internal medicine, orthopedics, surgery, and podiatry. Additionally, endocrinologists from surrounding communities began to refer clients. Nursing referrals were accepted when the primary care provider agreed to the referral. These referrals were initiated by nurses in the acute care setting, home care, public health, and nurse practitioner providers. The best source for referrals originated from the clients themselves by word of mouth. Clients routinely referred family, friends, and coworkers to the practice. The primary care physicians were usually agreeable to the word-of-mouth referrals; however, in the rare case when a referral was denied, the client was instructed to contact the regional hospital diabetes center.

Maximum reimbursement for charges was successfully obtained from Medicare and Medicaid, as well as the majority of insurance companies and clients. One large national insurance company that initially declined my request to become a provider eventually recruited me as a preferred provider. Over the years, the practice generated enough money to cover the operating expenses and my salary.

Although the CNS practice was very successful, I discontinued the practice after 8 years due to personal reasons. However, the business and marketing skills that were developed from the practice were invaluable for establishing my future entrepreneurial endeavor, a nurse-owned and operated wellness company.

REFERENCES

American Diabetes Association (ADA). (2013a). Diagnosis and classification of diabetes mellitus. *Diabetes Care, 36*, S67–S74.

American Diabetes Association (ADA). (2013b). Standards of medical care in diabetes-2013. *Diabetes Care, 36*, S11–S66.

American Medical Association (AMA). (2013). *Current procedural terminology: CPT professional 2014* (2014 ed.). Chicago, IL: Author.

Centers for Medicare and Medicaid Services (CMS). (2013). *Medicare billing: Form CMS-1500.* Retrieved September 8, 2013, from http://www.cms.gov/Medicare/CMS-Forms/CMS-Forms/Downloads/CMS1500805.pdf

Moorhead, S., Johnson, M., Mass, M. L., & Swanson, E. (2012). *Nursing outcomes classification: Measurement of health outcomes* (5th ed.). St. Louis, MO: Elsevier Mosby Sanders.

National Association of Clinical Nurse Specialists (NACNS). (2004). *Statement on clinical nurse specialist practice and education* (2nd ed.). Harrisburg, PA: Author.

U.S. Department of Health and Human Services, Centers for Disease Control and Prevention (CDC). (2011). *National diabetes fact sheet, 2011.* Retrieved from http://www.cdc.gov/diabetes/pubs/pdf/ndfs_2011.pdf

Rapid Response Exemplar: Maturation and Refinement of a Rapid Response Program

Tracey Loudon and Victoria Church

At its foundation, the work of the clinical nurse specialist (CNS) supports nurses, patients, and organizations so that all may achieve excellent results. Change theory and implementation science are key components for the CNS in both education and practice. Mastering these processes supports successful program implementation and improved outcomes. Additionally, understanding the culture of an organization, including historical perspective and the compelling need for change, has the potential to increase the success of a new program or established program.

PRACTICE OVERVIEW

The Portland Veterans Affairs Medical Center (PVAMC) is a Magnet-designated facility that is academically affiliated with the Oregon Health and Sciences University (OHSU). Of the 140 medical-surgical (MS) beds, 80 have telemetry monitoring capabilities. An additional 20 beds are designated for inpatient psychiatry. There are 8 operating suites and 24 intensive care beds. The emergency department (ED) is a Level-2 center, which is defined as a trauma center that in collaboration with a Level-1 center provides 24-hour comprehensive care of all essential specialties. The ED is a 19-bed unit that experienced 28,496 visits, and the hospital had 9,814 inpatient discharges in 2011.

Admissions are exclusively adult and predominantly geriatric male patients, with an increasing trend for female and younger veterans entering into the Veterans Affairs (VA) health care system. The surgical ward population includes general, vascular, orthopedic, neurological, urological, bariatric, thoracic, and/or cardiac surgery patients. Surgical programs also include liver and kidney transplant. The medical ward population includes patients with acute and chronic cardiac, pulmonary, neurological, renal, and metabolic diseases. PVAMC also has an active cardiac and vascular interventional program. Our veteran population is afflicted with multiple comorbidities including coronary artery disease (CAD), congestive heart failure (CHF), chronic obstructive pulmonary disease (COPD), diabetes, hypertension, metabolic syndrome, a complex subgroup with alcohol and substance abuse, and homelessness. These coexisting disease states in a geriatric population mean that high acuity and complex patients present on our five MS wards. The patient population also carries with it the additional risk of cognitive challenges, especially in light of the presence of posttraumatic stress disorder (PTSD) in many of the veterans.

As CNSs, our core goal is to improve patient outcomes. Our role is made up of several integral components. These include (a) assessing multiple levels of systems; (b) identifying problems at the staff, patient, and system levels; (c) developing and implementing corrective action plans; and (d) evaluating outcomes. We are also available for clinical consultation by all team members and lead educational sessions for staff on a variety of topics related to our patient population and programs. Direct patient care may be performed during our consultative process or during the mentorship of staff in acquiring specific skills. At PVAMC, there is an active CNS workgroup that consists of 11 members who represent multiple specialties such as MS, perioperative, diabetes, transplant, wound ostomy, infectious disease, and critical care. The group of 11 CNSs meets regularly at CNS subcommittee meetings. Additionally, the CNSs hold membership within the advanced practice registered nurse (APRN) committee that consists of CNSs, nurse practitioners (NPs), and certified registered nurse anesthetists (CRNAs). The APRN meetings include members who are locally, regionally, and nationally affiliated and collaborate on programs nationwide. The local CNS group has facilitated the integration of evidence into practice utilizing multiple strategies that include the development and implementation of evidence-based fact sheets within our facility.

Professional memberships in the American Association of Critical Care Nurses (AACN), Sigma Theta Tau, and the Society of Medical Surgical Nurses facilitate the ability of the CNSs to maintain current knowledge of local and national resources. In addition, one of the authors is on the board of the local AACN chapter. Subscriptions to online services with organizations such as the Institute for Healthcare Improvement (IHI), the National Database for Nursing Quality Indicators (NDNQI), the National Center for Patient Safety, and the National Guideline Clearing House assist with staying up-to-date on research and practice standards.

One of the authors of this chapter, Ms. Church, has been a CNS for 27 years. She came to PVAMC in 2003 as a MS CNS. In 2011, she transitioned from being a full-time MS CNS to a part-time MS CNS, dedicating approximately 20% of her time to practice. The rest of her time became focused around the role of associate director within our Northwest Innovation Center (NWIC). During Ms. Church's transition in 2010, the other author, Ms. Loudon, completed her CNS practicum at the VA and was hired as the CNS for the critical care unit.

PROBLEM IDENTIFICATION

In 2000, the Institute of Medicine (IOM) published *To Err is Human: Building a Safer Health System*, the landmark report that revealed the health care system to be fraught with error. This publication (Kohn, Corrigan, & Donaldson, 2000) noted that approximately 100,000 hospital deaths per year were not related to the patients' admitting diagnoses. The report pinpointed four categories of error: (a) diagnostic, (b) treatment, (c) prevention, and (d) other (further identified as communication failures, equipment failures, and other systems failures). Driven by the IOM report, the IHI (2004) developed its *100,000 Lives Campaign*, which focused on saving lives in hospitals. In addition, the IOM report served as a catalyst for change in patient advocate groups, insurers, and regulating bodies like The Joint Commission (TJC). The call for improved safety in our health care system began to spread nationwide. In 2009, TJC introduced National Patient Safety Goal (NPSG) 16, "improve the identification and response to clinical deterioration in hospital-ward patients" (Jones, DeVita, & Bellomo, 2011). The IOM and IHI were instrumental in increasing awareness of gaps in health care, which contributed to both the national and international surges in momentum to develop rapid response systems as a patient safety strategy (Schmid, Hoffman, Happ, Wolf, & DeVita, 2007).

"Failure to rescue" is a term first introduced by Silber in 1992 (Schmid et al., 2007). The term is used to identify key contributors of poor outcomes similar in nature: (a) inadequate monitoring, (b) failure to recognize deterioration, (c) failure to plan or act, and (d) failure in communication. This relatively new concept began to gain more attention as agencies like Medicare disclosed that nearly 17% of all patient safety incidents were related to system failures that could be attributed to one of the elements of the "failure to rescue" scenario (Schmid et al., 2007). Schmid et al. (2007) define *failure to rescue* as the "inability to save a patient's life after the development of a complication in the hospital that was not present on admission" (Schmid et al., 2007, p. 188). Such failures exist, in part, due to the deeply enculturated hierarchies found in our health care system. The hesitation of a nurse to question the authority of a physician, a nurse having been conditioned not to call, or a call made by a nurse having been ignored—these examples demonstrate a system with flaws. Other instances of failure to rescue could be attributed to communication errors. Nursing staff may not be able to convey the urgency of the situation in order to effectively articulate the changes they see in the patient's condition. All of these examples could be attributed to cultural barriers such as a lack of confidence on the part of the nurse in his or her own assessments, or a nurse feeling intimidated by certain physicians that he or she must contact (Winters et al., 2013).

It is not uncommon for a nurse to feel intimidated solely due to differences in communication style.

Historically, nurses are storytellers and include many details of the patient's hospitalization that may not always seem pertinent to the situation. Physicians typically prefer concise, organized information and a clear reason for the discussion. Nurses are not always prepared when they call the physician. Instead, the nurse should be able to present all the details necessary to make decisions over the phone, or off site. The nurse should also feel confident and prepared to make recommendations regarding the patient's needs. In 2006, TJC added NPSG No. 2, the call to "Implement a standardized approach to 'hand-off' communications, which included an opportunity to ask and respond to questions" (TJC, 2006). The compelling need for this new NPSG is a sobering revelation. Sixty percent of all sentinel events are related to communication failures (Halm, 2013). Many organizations have chosen to adapt the Situation, Background, Assessment, and Recommendation (SBAR) tool to fulfill this requirement and are using it extensively in handoff communication situations. The SBAR tool promotes organized, concise transfer of information and includes a recommendation from the nurse for follow-up or further action, allowing him or her to function to the highest level of his or her licensure.

Because of failures in systems to meet the needs of patients experiencing worsening conditions and the previously identified system flaws, the IHI began to develop a means to quickly provide critical care resources at the bedside. Their effort gave rise to rapid response teams (RRT). Once activated, the role of the RRT is to assess and treat patients on nursing wards who are experiencing changes that might be indicative of a worsening condition. These response teams' composition is varied, but typically consists of critical care personnel including physicians, nurses, and respiratory therapists. In 2000, the Conwy and Denbighshire National Health Service (NHS) Trust in Wales developed and adopted a novel assessment strategy called Modified Early Warning Score (MEWS). It is a scoring system that utilizes physiologic signs (vital sign parameters and level of consciousness), assigns a score based on the degree of deviation from normal parameters, and then sums the scores. The higher the score, the greater the deviation from normal, and theoretically, the greater the level of concern. Along with the score, the system included an action algorithm that contained recommended interventions for each level of concern/alarm. The aim is to assist in identifying patients at risk for cardiac arrest so that the RRT may intervene preemptively (Moon, Cosgrove, Lea, Fairs, & Cressey, 2011). Moon and colleagues (2011) reported that patients with higher MEWS scores had an increased risk of death. Therefore, early identification is critical in the prevention of increased morbidity and mortality.

In 2010, Chan and colleagues (Chan, Jain, Nallnotku, Berg, & Sasson, 2010) performed a systematic review and meta-analysis of RRT-related literature in the field. They looked at 18 studies, and, out of 1.3 million admissions, found that RRT was associated with a reduced rate in cardiopulmonary arrests (approximately 34%) outside of the intensive care unit (ICU). Despite this result, Chan and colleagues could not show a statistically significant mortality benefit (Chan et al., 2010). In a more recent systematic review, however, Winters and colleagues found moderately strong evidence to support that Rapid Response Systems (RRS)/RRT are effective in decreasing cardiopulmonary arrest rates and mortality (Winters et al., 2013). It has taken at least 15 years for RRS/RRT to demonstrate a mortality benefit, which suggests that there is more work to do on these types of responses.

INITIAL PROBLEM IDENTIFICATION AND INTERVENTIONS

In 2003, Ms. Church reviewed 6 months of data that revealed a baseline incidence of six to eight failure to rescue (FTR) cases a month from a total of 90 MS beds. In terms of body systems involved in the FTR, respiratory decompensation was the leading cause, followed in turn by cardiac and neurological decompensation. According to chart reviews with a focus on the causative factors of the FTR incidences, failure to rapidly detect patient decompensation was attributed to 40% of the cases, and failure to obtain resources for the decompensating patient was attributed to the remaining 60%. It became very clear during the review and participation in FTR cases that the bedside nurse on the MS unit was pivotal in identifying early signs of decompensation. In addition, the second and third most pivotal links impacting FTR were early access to clinical resources and early intervention. Ms. Church developed an intervention model with the goal of improved patient outcomes evidenced by a decrease in cardiac and respiratory arrest as well as a decrease in the incidence of FTR.

Participation in intervention development and implementation included bedside staff, the charge nurses and nursing managers of each MS unit, and the charge nurses and nursing management of the ICU. During a 6-month period in 2004, PVAMC implemented five initial interventions in order to: (a) expand the scope of assessment, and improve the assessment skills and documentation of these activities on the wards; (b) improve communication between the wards and ICU; (c) establish 24/7 clinical resources for ward RNs; (d) establish educational programs that incorporated high-fidelity simulation

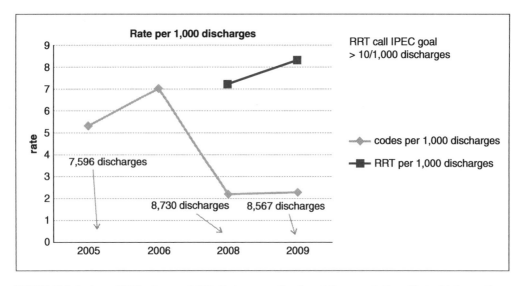

FIGURE 42.1 Code and RRT rates per 1,000 discharges reflective of the cumulative effect of interventions. RRT, rapid response teams.

(HFS) modalities related to FTR, resource utilization, communication, and cardinal sign identification; and (e) change the source of ICU bed availability from the nonclinical bed control personnel.

Documentation strategies in expanding the scope of assessment included the introduction of a cardinal sign note that established an ability to review all charts independent of code event documentation. Improving communications in the wards and having readily available clinical resources were key strategies in the intervention. One of the lasting results of these strategies was the establishment of a system whereby the medical and surgical charge nurses would contact the ICU charge nurse directly about any patient experiencing cardinal signs of change. If the patient could not be stabilized on the ward, the information related to bed availability would then be communicated directly with the ward team. Previously, the process was to have the ward team contact a nonclinical individual in bed control to ascertain ICU bed availability. The ICU charge was also available to come to the bedside for a coassessment as well as to bring respiratory therapy to the bedside. A formal RRT was not part of the initial intervention due to resistance at the provider level. An educational program targeted to the MS RN that included HFS modalities related to FTR, resource utilization, communication (SBAR), and cardinal sign identification was driven by chart reviews of FTR occurrences. Part of this intervention was to develop reference sheets for the key cardinal signs and resources available to the MS wards. The HFS scenarios were mandatory for all ward RNs and certified nursing assistants (CNAs).

Within 3 months of implementation, the incidence of FTR had declined from the baseline of six to eight per month to only one per month. Consistently, the remaining FTR incidents involved patients identified as exhibiting cardinal signs, but who, due to lack of ICU bed availability, could not be transferred. The incidence of FTR continued to remain at one per month for the next 6 months. During this time PVAMC addressed other factors of ICU throughput, shift report, and transfer (handoff) report. Of note, the incidence of code team responses in the MS wards decreased by 80% while survival from codes improved from 68% to 95% (Figure 42.1).

This level of success brought about a positive change in responsiveness for provider participation in the rapid response program. A formal RRT team was established, with members consisting of ICU charge nurse, respiratory therapist, and the senior ICU resident. In 2007, the Veterans Health Administration (VHA) selected our facility as a national best-practice example for initiation of a successful rapid response program. As part of this work, an online systemwide multimedia education for VA nurses was developed.

GOALS FOR PRACTICE INNOVATION

In 2011, Ms. Loudon came to the VA as a novice CNS in critical care. After completing orientation, she was asked to take over the lead role in the rapid response program. At that time, she was told by nursing leadership that the incidence of FTR, code responses, and RRTs was on the rise. Nursing leadership requested an evaluation of the causative factors and aksed her to determine if the evaluation revealed an opportunity to improve the program. If the assessment determined that there was room to improve veteran outcomes, Ms. Loudon was to develop and implement an appropriate intervention plan.

INNOVATION SPECIFICS: APPLICATION OF MEWS

The first step was to review the historical aspects of the program, including the qualitative and quantitative data. The history revealed that Ms. Church had transitioned from the rapid response program facilitator role in 2010, and thus, the rapid response program had been without a facilitator for 1 year. Additionally, the facilitator role had included holding 18 HFS sessions with MS staff every quarter. These sessions had been discontinued when Ms. Church was unable to continue to coordinate their implementation due to job duties that had shifted. Even though the CNS attempts to develop solutions that are independently sustainable, system stability is not always achievable. A level of facilitation, mentorship, and oversight is required to maintain outcomes. In order to determine if this was the main contributing factor, Ms. Loudon first had to establish credibility in the MS wards that would allow completion of a comprehensive evaluation. She also had to establish credibility with response team members outside of the critical care unit. Thus, a request was made to become a member of the code committee and review the data for code and RRT responses as well as cardinal sign note documentation. Second, Ms. Loudon began participating in HFS with the MS staff to evaluate the training and clinical capabilities of the nursing staff.

In the spring of 2011, the IHI held an information-sharing expedition called *Modified Early Warning Systems, the Next Level of Rapid Response*. I made a request for our facility to participate in this program and invited staff and clinical leadership to participate. The IHI expedition team introduced participants to MEWS. MEWS is a scoring system that utilizes physiologic signs (vital sign parameters, level of consciousness), and may include additional parameters such as urine output, oxygen saturation, or increasing oxygen needs. Each vital signs (VS) parameter and physiologic finding is assigned points ranging from zero to three, depending on the degree of deviation from normal parameters. The points are then summed. Depending on the MEWS score, concern or alarm is categorized in ranges from green (considered normal) to red (considered red alert or high concern). As identified earlier in this chapter, a high MEWS score signals an increase in deviation from normal. Along with the score, the system includes an action algorithm, which contains recommended interventions for each level of concern/alarm.

The authors guided participants through an organizational assessment. One MS unit had agreed to participate in the project. The IHI expedition team/rapid cycle improvement team requested that nursing staff check VS on one nursing unit, make an assessment, and compare them to the established MEWS criteria from participating hospitals. The local rapid cycle improvement team was encouraged to take the tool and modify it to fit the facility structure and practice. Most of the parameters fit the PVAMC population with the exclusion of the respiratory rate (RR). With the exception of the RR, the nursing staff assessed the VS of 20 veterans on one nursing unit and found them to be normal for all of our subjects. The tool as-is had an RR of 16 to 20 as normal, which is the commonly accepted normal range for RR. Any number above 20 was considered to be abnormal and would be assigned an appropriate point value. The PVAMC assessment revealed that most of the veterans were breathing at 22 respirations per minute. The team wanted to make a more accurate prediction of decline, so the tool was modified to incorporate the context presented by the PVAMC patient population (see Figure 42.2). Consequently, the RR range was increased to exclude points for an RR of 22 and consider 22 to be within the defined limits of normal. A literature review of the MEWS tool revealed multiple authors stating that the RR is one of the most sensitive indicators for predicting decline, and is, therefore, a critical component in the effectiveness of any intervention. Unfortunately, the RR is also the least accurately assessed VS parameter and the least often recorded. Knowing that the RR is the most valuable parameter, we knew that we had to educate the nursing staff, including the nurses' aides and RNs. It was imperative to increase staff awareness of the need for careful monitoring and recording of the RR to get the best information for detecting deterioration in our veterans.

The team made a few other adjustments to the tool as well. Specifically, the team chose to use increased oxygen need rather than oxygen saturation. If a patient whose previous oxygen requirement was 2 L per nasal cannula now required 3 L, or if a patient had previously been on room air and now required 2 L, the veteran score would be increased by one point. This meant that the patient's oxygen needs had changed (were increasing).

In addition to VS parameters and oxygenation, the tool contains a level of consciousness assessment. When the team presented the MEWS to the Code Committee in early planning stages, one of the providers was concerned that nursing would wait to call until the veteran presented a high score. The provider wanted to be notified with any change in neurological status, so we added the comment "For any change in neurological status, notify provider" in red at the bottom of both sides of our tool. The team emphasized to the nursing and medical group that the MEWS is a tool, not a substitute for nursing assessment.

PVAMC MEWS

Modified Early Warning System Tool & Action Algorithm **MEWS Criteria**								
Score		3	2	1	0	1	2	3
HR			≤ 40	41–50	51–100	101–110	111–129	≥ 130
Systolic BP		< 70	71–90	91–100	101–180	181–200	201–220	> 220
RR			< 8	8–11	12–24	25–29		≥ 30
Oxygen		For increasing oxygen requirement add one			+1			
Temp	F	< 93.1	< 93.2–95		95.1–99.5	99.6–101.3	> 101.4–104	104.1
	C	< 34	34–35		35.1–37.5	37.6–38.5	38.6–40	> 40.1
CNS/LOC **Any neuro change requires notification of provider**		Unresponsive	Responds to pain only	Response to voice	Alert		Confused or agitated	

Attention: Any significant change from baseline or any single parameter with a score of 3, notify provider

Action Algorithm

MEWS	Inpatient –Action	
0–2	Green	Re-score using routine vitals. Observe Q2–4 hours
3	Yellow	VS and reassessment in 2 hours. Calculate MEWS Inform Charge RN Place on telemetry? (obtain order)
4	Orange	VS and reassessment in 1 hour. Inform Charge RN Notify MD Consult CCU Charge nurse
5–6	Red	VS and reassessment minimum every 30 minutes with MEWS score Notify Charge RN Notify MD **Call RRT.** Possible ICU consult

Attention: Any significant change from baseline or any single parameter with a score of 3, notify provider

FIGURE 42.2 PVAMC MEWS tool.

MEWS, modified early warning score; PVAMC, Portland Veterans Affairs Medical Center.

Introducing an additional assessment tool such as the MEWS into an established nursing culture required leadership support. It had to make sense and have value to the frontline staff affected by the change. The MEWS has strong face validity. It sounded good in concept to experienced clinical managers, our director, and other CNSs. Fortunately, the frontline nursing staff could see the benefit of having another tool in their tool kit to enhance patient care and wanted to evaluate the tool in practice. Thus, the tool was piloted on one nursing unit with one staff nurse and was assessed using the Plan, Do, Study, Act (PDSA) principles for process improvement. The team chose an enthusiastic nurse with less than 2 years of clinical experience to pilot the tool. We asked her to calculate the MEWS score for each of her patients. We wanted to know if the tool was easy to use and how long it took to calculate a score for each of her patients. She used the tool with her patient assignment, found it easy to use, and thought that it might help her identify and report changes in her patients. The next steps were to have several nurses try out the tool, then expand to an entire floor.

Of note, we originally planned to trial the MEWS on one nursing unit prior to moving to the other wards. As with most organizations, at times our nurses must float to different nursing units. This allowed us the opportunity to introduce the tool to a nurse float from a different unit. She took the idea to her manager, who then contacted us and asked if their unit could use the tool as well. The other unit's nurses were enthusiastic about the possibility of incorporating the tool into their workflow. The team consulted as a group and decided that we could extend to this second unit. The project then spread virally as additional nursing units became aware of the initiative. They wanted to have the tool available for their patients and nurses as well.

MEWS includes an action algorithm of recommended interventions depending on the MEWS score. We chose to identify four condition ranges: (a) Green, (b) Yellow Alert, (c) Orange Alert, and (d) Red Alert. Green Condition (normal) ranges between 0 and 2. The recommendation is to rescore using routine VS every 8 hours, or as ordered and indicated. Then the nurse is to observe every 2 to 4 hours thereafter. Yellow Alert Condition (caution) is a score of 3. The recommendation is that VS should be repeated in 2 hours, a MEWS recalculation should be performed, the charge nurse should be notified, and the patient should be considered for telemetry. Orange Alert is a score of 4. The nurse should reassess in 1 hour with an MEWS score, the charge nurse and physician should be notified, and the ward is encouraged to notify the ICU charge nurse. Early notification and awareness provide the ICU charge nurse an opportunity to review bed availability and make plans for an admission. Red Alert is a score of 5 or 6. Patients with this score need to be reassessed at a minimum of every 30 minutes. The recommendation is to recalculate MEWS and to notify the charge nurse, physician, and ICU charge. Additionally, this is the level at which the team recommended calling an RRT. Not all patients with a high MEWS score end up coding. However, all patients who code have a high MEWS score. The tool is more sensitive than specific in terms of its ability to identify deterioration.

There is currently no delta (or change from baseline) for the VS in the tool and this is a noted limitation. As an example, if the patient had a systolic blood pressure of 160, and it is now 119/50 (greater than a 40-point drop), this significant change would be part of a positive screen for possible sepsis but is not addressed in the MEWS as it currently exists. In an attempt to show a baseline change, we added an alert at the bottom of each side of the card that reads, *Attention: Any significant change from baseline or any single parameter with a score of three, notify provider.* The team also updated the Cardinal Sign Note template, which the ward staff completes for any patient who exhibits cardinal signs or has an escalating MEWS score.

EVALUATION AND OUTCOMES

Our aim in implementing the MEWS tool was to decrease codes and improve recognition of deterioration on our inpatient nursing units. As reported in the literature, the tool also supports an increased rate of VS assessment and documentation in the electronic record.

What the team did not know when the project began was that there would be several unanticipated additional benefits attributed to use of the tool. The nurses reported feeling empowered when they made condition update phone calls to our physician colleagues. The tool provided them with objective data to report. Moreover, the tool helped them to articulate changes with increasing confidence. Additional unanticipated benefits included an easier, facilitated transfer to a higher level of care when a patient's needs exceeded the level of nursing care available on a MS unit. When a patient has a score of greater than five, the nurse, per the action algorithm, must complete VS and a MEWS every 30 minutes. With an assignment of three to four additional patients, this requirement is not sustainable for long periods, therefore necessitating the transfer to the ICU bed.

We do not have a step-down unit at our hospital. The tool has helped our nurses to articulate with objective data that the patient may need a higher level of care. Our team supports the use of the MEWS to provide the patient with the nursing hours required by his or her condition or level of acuity. If the patient has higher nursing needs, the patient may require a "higher dose" of nursing.

Rapid Response Event Evaluation

Unit managers and frontline nursing staff value feedback and follow-up after an RRT event. Chart audits are completed on each RRT event and placed in a database for internal tracking. The manager of the ward where the call occurred is sent an e-mail with an event summary, any need for follow-up, or if there were issues with the call that needed further addressing. Rapid response calls are discussed quarterly in the RRT subcommittee meeting, and monthly in the Code Committee meeting. When learning needs are recognized, or if education is requested by a team or group of nurses, a HFS learning session has been developed. This feedback loop allows for continual process improvement and reinforcement of skills that allow for sustained improvement in veteran care.

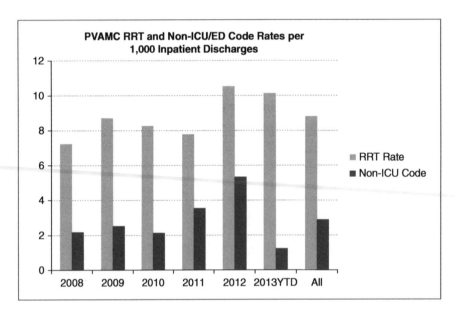

FIGURE 42.3 Non-ICU code and RRT rates.

ED, emergency department; ICU, intensive care unit; RRT, rapid response teams.

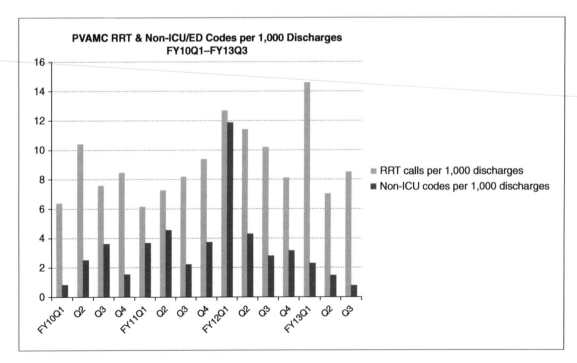

FIGURE 42.4 Non-ICU and RRT codes per 1,000 discharges per quarter 2010 to 2013.

ED, emergency department; ICU, intensive care unit; RRT, rapid response teams.

Outcomes: Rapid Response and Code Events 2011 to 2013

In the spring of 2011, PVAMC was introduced to the MEWS system, which was used to update our rapid response program. We adapted the tool to meet our needs. We piloted the tool with one nurse, on one patient, in one day. The nurse liked the tool and found it easy to use. Moreover, our hospitalists like the idea that the tool both helps to guide reassessment through use of an action algorithm and to support improved documentation of VS. Our innovation spread virally. Seventy-five percent of our nurses found the tool to be either helpful or extremely helpful. We incorporated the MEWS into our simulation education and cardinal signs of change in-services. Over the course of the implementation phase, we have seen desirable outcomes. Our RRT events have increased, and our non-ICU/ED/noninpatient care areas code rates have decreased (Figures 42.3 and 42.4). It is difficult to say that these changes are related to the MEWS, as we have additional interventions that may have contributed to our outcomes. Perhaps the MEWS has helped support nurses to objectively communicate their "gut" feelings, or to support their assessment with greater confidence. In any case, we are pleased with our trends and expect to continue to see our code event rate decrease.

RRT Summary

Our rapid response program continues to evolve and mature. Key to this successful program implementation at PVAMC is strong leadership support, a compelling need for change, and frontline staff who are able to see the value of the change. New interventions and more sophisticated systems are certain to be available in the future. Device integration and automated notification of positive sepsis screens and MEWS are already integrated into some electronic systems. Technology will eventually improve screening and will alert providers when thresholds either have been met or have been exceeded. Care and outcomes will continue to improve. Providing nurses and staff with the tools, education, and simulated experiences that they need to be successful is the one of the most satisfying parts of the work of the CNS.

REFERENCES

Chan, P., Jain, R., Nallnotku, B., Berg, R., & Sasson, C. (2010). Rapid response teams: A systematic review and analysis. *Archives of Internal Medicine, 170*(1), 18–26.

Conwy & Denbighshire National Health Service (NHS) Trust (2000). *Modified early warning score: Reducing harm from deterioration.* Retrieved October 27, 2013, from http://www.patientsafetyfirst.nhs.uk/Content .aspx?path=/interventions/Deterioration

Halm, M. (2013). Nursing handoffs: Ensuring safe passage for patients. *American Journal of Critical Care Nursing, 22*(2), 158–162.

Institute for Healthcare Improvement (IHI). (2004). *100K lives campaign.* Retrieved October 27, 2013, from http://www.ihi.org/offerings/Initiatives/PastStra tegicInitiatives/5MillionLivesCampaign/Documents/ Overview%20of%20the%20100K%20Campaign.pdf

The Joint Commission (TJC). (2006). *Patient safety goal #2.* Retrieved October 27, 2013, from http:// www.ed-qual.com/Emergency_Medicine_News/ED_ News_2006_JCAHO_Patient_Safety_Goals.htm

Jones, D., DeVita, M., & Bellomo, R. (2011). Rapid-response teams. *New England Journal of Medicine, 365*(2), 139–146.

Kohn, L., Corrigan, J., & Donaldson, M. (Eds.). (2000). *To err is human: Building a safer health system.* Washington, DC: National Academy Press.

Moon, A., Cosgrove, J. F., Lea, D., Fairs, A., & Cressey, D. M. (2011). An eight year audit before and after the introduction of modified early warning score (MEWS) charts, of patients admitted to a tertiary referral intensive care unit after CPR. *Resuscitation, 82,* 150–154.

Schmid, A., Hoffman, L., Happ, M. B., Wolf, G., & DeVita M. (2007). Failure to rescue: A literature review. *Journal of Nursing Administration, 37*(4), 188–198.

Winters, B., Weaver, S., Pfoh, E., Yang, T., Cuong Pham, J., & Dy, S. (2013). Rapid-response systems as a patient safety strategy: A systematic review. *Annals of Internal Medicine, 158*(5 pt. 2), 417–442.

Specialty Practice Organizations in Nursing

Michelle L. Treon and Diana Jones

ACADEMY OF MEDICAL-SURGICAL NURSES
East Holly Avenue, Box 56
Pitman, NJ 08071–0056
Phone: 866–877-2676
E-mail: AMSN@ajj.com
Website: http://www.amsn.org/
Specialty: Medical-surgical
Basic Certification: Certified Medical-Surgical
Registered Nurse (CMSRN)
Advanced Certification: None
Certifying Organization: Medical-Surgical Nursing
Certification Board

ACADEMY OF NEONATAL NURSING
1425 N. McDowell Blvd, Suite 105
Petaluma, CA 94954
Phone: 707–795-2168
E-mail: None
Website: http://www.academyonline.org
Specialty: Neonatal
Basic Certification: None
Advanced Certification: None
Certifying Organization: N/A

AIR AND SURFACE TRANSPORT NURSES
ASSOCIATION
7995 East Prentice Avenue, Suite 100
Greenwood Village, CO 80111
Phone: 800–897-NFNA (6362)
E-mail: astna@gwami.com
Website: http://www.astna.org

Specialty: Emergency
Basic Certification: Certified Emergency Nurse
(CEN); Certified Flight Registered Nurse (CFRN);
Certified Transport Registered Nurse (CTRN);
Certified Pediatric Emergency Nurse (CPEN)
Advanced Certification: None
Certifying Organization: Board of Certification for
Emergency Nursing (BCEN); Pediatric Nursing
Certification Board (PNCB)

AMERICAN ACADEMY OF AMBULATORY
CARE NURSING
East Holly Avenue, Box 56
Pittman, NJ 08071–0056
Phone: 800–262-6877
E-mail: aaacn@ajj.com
Website: http://www.aaacn.org
Specialty: Ambulatory
Basic Certification: Ambulatory Care Nursing
Certification (RN-BC)
Telehealth Nursing Certification—retired, but available for renewal for currently certified candidates.
Advanced Certification: None
Certifying Organization: American Nurses
Credentialing Center (ANCC)

AMERICAN ACADEMY OF NURSING
1000 Vermont Avenue NW, Suite 910
Washington, DC 20005
Phone: 202–777-1170
E-mail: info@aannet.org

Website: http://www.aannet.org
Specialty: Health Policy & Nursing Practice
Basic Certification: None
Advanced Certification: None
Certifying Organization: N/A

AMERICAN ASSEMBLY FOR MEN IN NURSING, THE

P.O. Box 130220
Birmingham, AL 35213
Phone: 205–956-0146
E-mail: aamn@aamn.org
Website: http://www.aamn.org
Specialty: General
Basic Certification: None
Advanced Certification: None
Certifying Organization: N/A

AMERICAN ASSOCIATION OF CRITICAL-CARE NURSES

101 Columbia
Aliso Viejo, CA 92656–4109
Phone: 800–899-AACN (2226)
E-mail: info@aacn.org
Website: http://www.aacn.org
Specialty: Critical care
Basic Certification: Critical Care Registered Nurse (CCRN: adult, neonatal, pediatric); Tele-ICU Acute/Critical Care Nursing, Adult (CCRN-E); Progressive Care Certified Nurse (PCCN); Nurse Manager and Leader (CNML); Cardiac Medicine Certification, Adult (CMC); Cardiac Surgery Certification, Adult (CSC)
Advanced Certification: Acute Care Nurse Practitioner, Adult-Gerontology (ACNPC-AG); Clinical Nurse Specialist, Wellness through Acute Care (ACCNS: Adult-Gerontology, Pediatric, Neonatal); Acute Care Nurse Practitioner, Adult (ACNPC); Acute Care Clinical Nurse Specialist (CCNS: Adult, Pediatric, Neonatal)
Certifying Organization: AACN Certification Corporation

AMERICAN ASSOCIATION OF DIABETES EDUCATORS

200 W. Madison Street, Suite 800
Chicago, IL 60606
Phone: 800–338-3633
E-mail: membership@aadenet.org
Website: http://www.diabeteseducator.org/
Specialty: Diabetes
Basic Certification: Certified Diabetes Educator (CDE)
Certifying Organization: National Certification Board for Diabetes Educators (NCDBE)

Advanced Certification: Board Certified in Advanced Diabetes Management (BC-ADM)
Certifying Organization: Via AADE partnership with Castle World

AMERICAN ASSOCIATION OF LEGAL NURSE CONSULTANTS

330 N. Wabash Avenue
Chicago, IL 60611
Phone: 877–402-2562
E-mail: info@aalnc.org
Website: http://www.aalnc.org
Specialty: Legal
Basic Certification: Legal Nurse Consultant Certified (LNCC)
Advanced Certification: None
Certifying Organization: American Nurses Credentialing Cerner (ANCC)

AMERICAN ASSOCIATION OF MANAGED CARE NURSES

4435 Waterfront Drive, Suite 101
Glen Allen, VA 23060
Phone: 804–527-1905
E-mail: via website
Website: http://www.aamcn.org
Specialty: Managed care
Basic Certification: Certification in Managed Care Nursing (CMCN)
Advanced Certification: None
Certifying Organization: American Board of Managed Care Nursing (ABMCN)

AMERICAN ASSOCIATION OF NEUROSCIENCE NURSES

8735 W. Higgins Road, Suite 300
Chicago, IL 60631
Phone: 888–557-2266 (U.S. only)
Phone: 847–375-4733
E-mail: info@aann.org
Website: http://www.aann.org
Specialty: Neuroscience
Basic Certification: Certified Neuroscience Registered Nurse (CNRN); Stroke Certified Registered Nurse (SCRN)
Advanced Certification: None
Certifying Organization: American Board of Neuroscience Nursing (ABNN)

AMeRICAN ASSOCIATION OF NURSE ATTORNEYS, THE

3416 Primm Lane
Birmingham, AL 35216
Phone: 877–538-2262
E-mail: TAANA@primemanagement.net

Website: http://www.taana.org
Specialty: Legal
Basic Certification: None
Advanced Certification: None
Certifying Organization: N/A

AMERICAN ASSOCIATION OF OCCUPATIONAL HEALTH NURSES

7794 Grow Drive
Pensacola, FL 32514
Phone: 800–241-8014
E-mail: AAOHN@dancyamc.com
Website: http://www.aaohn.org
Specialty: Occupational health
Basic Certification: Certified Occupational Health Nurse (COHN); Certified Occupational Health Nurse-Specialist (COHN-S)
Advanced Certification: None
Certifying Organization: The American Board of Occupational Health Nurses (ABOHN)

AMERICAN ASSOCIATION OF SPINAL CORD INJURY NURSES

c/o Paralyzed Veterans of America
801 Eighteenth Street, NW
Washington, DC 20006–3517
Phone: 800–424-8200
E-mail: info@pva.org
Website: http://www.pva.org/
Specialty: Neuro
Basic Certification: None
Advanced Certification: None
Certifying Organization: N/A

AMERICAN HOLISTIC NURSES ASSOCIATION

100 SE 9th Street, Suite 3A
Topeka, KS 66612–1213
Phone: 800–278-2462
E-mail: info@ahna.org
Website: http://www.ahna.org
Specialty: Holism
Basic Certification: Holistic Nurse-Certified (HN-C); Holistic Baccalaureate Nurse, Board Certified (HNB-BC)
Advanced Certification: Advanced Holistic Nurse, Board Certified (AHN-C); Advanced Practice Holistic Nurse, Board Certified (APRN, APHN-BC)
Certifying Organization: American Holistic Nurses' Certification Corporation

AMERICAN NEPHROLOGY NURSES' ASSOCIATION

East Holly Avenue, Box 56
Pittman, NJ 08071–0056
Phone: 856–256-2320
E-mail: anna@ajj.com
Website: http://www.annanurse.org
Specialty: Renal
Basic Certification: Certified Nephrology Nurse (CNN); Certified Dialysis Nurse (CDN); Certified Clinical Hemodialysis Technician (CCHT); Certified Clinical Hemodialysis Technician-Advanced (CCHT-A)
Advanced Certification: Certified Nephrology Nurse-Nurse Practitioner (CNN-NP); Certified Nephrology Nurse (baccalaureate or master's in nursing; CNN)
Certifying Organization: Nephrology Nursing Certification Commission (NNCC)

AMERICAN NURSES ASSOCIATION AMERICAN NURSES CREDENTIALING

Center 8515 Georgia Avenue, Suite 400
Silver Spring, MD 20910–3492
Phone: 1–800-284-CERT (2378)
E-mail: Various, see website directory: http://www. nursecredentialing.org/FunctionalCategory/ ContactUs
Website: http://www.nursecredentialing.org/
Specialty: Credentialing
Basic Certification: Ambulatory Care Nursing (RN-BC); Cardiac Rehabilitation Nursing (RN-BC) *Retired;* Cardiac-Vascular Nursing (RN-BC); Certified Vascular Nurse (RN-BC) *Retired;* College Health Nursing (RN-BC) *Retired;* Community Health Nursing (RN-BC) *Retired;* Faith Community Nursing *New-Available starting 2014;* Forensic Nursing-Advanced (AFN-BC); General Nursing Practice (RN-BC) *Retired;* Gerontological Nursing (RN-BC); High-Risk Perinatal Nursing (RN-BC) *Retired;* Home Health Nursing (RN-BC) *Retired;* Informatics Nursing (RN-BC); Medical-Surgical Nursing (RN-BC); Nurse Executive (NE-BC; awarded as RN-BC); Nurse, Executive, Advanced (NEA-BC); Nursing Case Management (RN-BC); Nursing Professional Development (RN-BC); Pain Management Nursing (RN-BC); Pediatric Nursing (RN-BC); Perinatal Nursing (RN-BC) *Retired;* Psychiatric-Mental Health Nursing (RN-BC); Public Health Nursing-Advanced (APHN-BC); School Nursing (RN-BC) *Retired;* Guided Care Nursing (certificate holder only); Fundamentals of Magnet (certificate holder only)
Advanced Certification Specifically for the CNS: Adult Health CNS (ACNS-BC); Adult-Gerontology CNS (AGCNS-BC) *New-Available starting April 2014;* Adult Psychiatric-Mental Health CNS (PMHCNS-BC); Child/Adolescent Psychiatric-Mental Health CNS (PMHCNS-BC); CNS Core (CNS-BC) *Retired;*

Gerontological CNS (GCNS-BC); Home Health CNS (HHCNS-BC) *Retired;* Pediatric CNS (PCNS-BC); Public/Community Health CNS (PHCNS-BC) *Retired*

Certifying Organization: American Nurses Credentialing Center (ANCC)

AMERICAN NURSING INFORMATICS ASSOCIATION

200 E. Holly Avenue
Sewell, NJ 08080
Phone: 866–552-6404
E-mail: ania@ajj.com
Website: http://www.ania.org
Specialty: Informatics
Basic Certification: Informatics Nursing (RN-BC)
Advanced Certification: None
Certifying Organization: American Nurses Credentialing Center (ANCC)

AMERICAN ORGANIZATION OF NURSE EXECUTIVES

155 N. Wacker Drive, Suite 400
Chicago, IL 60606
Phone: 312–422-2800
E-mail: aone@aha.org
Website: http://www.aone.org
Specialty: Administration
Basic Certification: Certified in Executive Nursing Practice (CENP); Certified Nurse Manager and Leader (CNML)
Advanced Certification: None
Certifying Organization: AONE Credentialing Center in partnership with American Association of Critical Care Nurses (AACN)

AMERICAN PSYCHIATRIC NURSES ASSOCIATION

3141 Fairview Park Drive, Suite 625
Falls Church, VA 22042
Phone: 855–863-APNA (2762)
E-mail: Various, see http://www.apna.org/i4a/pages/index.cfm?pageid=3291
Website: http://www.apna.org
Specialty: Mental health
Basic Certification: See ANCC section for information
Advanced Certification: See ANCC section for information
Certifying Organization: Via American Nurses Credentialing Center (ANCC)

AMERICAN SOCIETY FOR PAIN MANAGEMENT NURSING

P.O. Box 15473
Lenexa, KS 66285–5473

or
18000 W. 105th Street
Olathe, KS 66061–7543
Phone: 888–34A-SPMN (342–7766)
E-mail: aspmn@goamp.com
Website: http://www.aspmn.org
Specialty: Pain management
Basic Certification: Pain Management Nursing (RN-BC)
Advanced Certification: None
Certifying Organization: Via American Nurses Credentialing Center (ANCC)

AMERICAN SOCIETY OF PERIANESTHESIA NURSES

90 Frontage Road
Cherry Hill, NJ 08034–1424
Phone: 877–737-9696
E-mail: aspan@aspan.org
Website: http://www.aspan.org
Specialty: Anesthesia
Basic Certification: Certified Post-Anesthesia Nurse (CPAN); Certified Ambulatory Perianesthesia Nurse (CAPA)
Advanced Certification: None
Certifying Organization: The Accreditation Board for Specialty Nursing Certification

ASSOCIATION FOR NURSING PROFESSIONAL DEVELOPMENT (ANPD)

330 N. Wabash Avenue, Suite 2000
Chicago, IL 60611
Phone: 800–489-1995
E-mail: info@anpd.org
Website: www.anpd.org
Specialty: Staff development
Basic Certification: See ANCC
Advanced Certification: See ANCC
Certifying Organization: American Nurses Credentialing Center (ANCC)

ASSOCIATION FOR PROFESSIONALS IN INFECTION CONTROL AND EPIDEMIOLOGY

1275 K Street, NW, Suite 1000
Washington, DC 20005–4006
Phone: 202–789-1890
Phone: 800–650-9570
E-mail: info@apic.org
Website: http://www.apic.org
Specialty: Infection control
Basic Certification: Certified in Infection Prevention and Control (CIC)
Advanced Certification: None

Certifying Organization: Certification Board for Infection Control and Epidemiology (CBIC)

ASSOCIATION FOR RADIOLOGIC AND IMAGING NURSING

7794 Grow Drive
Pensacola, FL 32514
Phone: 866–486-2762
E-mail: ARIN@dancyamc.com
Website: http://www.arinursing.org
Specialty: Radiology
Basic Certification: Certified Radiology Nurse (CRN)
Advanced Certification: None
Certifying Organization: Radiologic Nursing Certification Board (RNCB)

ASSOCIATION FOR VASCULAR ACCESS (AVA)

5526 West 13400 South, Suite 229
Herriman, UT 84096
Phone: 877–924-AVAI (2821)
E-mail: AVA@avainfo.org
Website: http://www.avainfo.org
Specialty: Vascular
Basic Certification: VA-BC
Advanced Certification: None
Certifying Organization: Vascular Access Certification Corporation (VACC)

ASSOCIATION OF NURSES IN AIDS CARE (ANAC)

3538 Ridgewood Road
Akron, OH 44333–3122
Phone: 800–260-6780
E-mail: anac@anacnet.org
Website: http://www.anacnet.org
Specialty: Medical-surgical
Basic Certification: AIDS Certified Registered Nurse (ACRN)
Advanced Certification: Advanced AIDS Certified Registered Nurse (AACRN)
Certifying Organization: HIV/AIDS Nursing Certification Board (HANCB)

ASSOCIATION OF PEDIATRIC HEMATOLOGY/ ONCOLOGY NURSES (APHON)

4700 W. Lake Avenue
Glenview, IL 60025–1485
Phone: 847–375-4724
E-mail: info@aphon.org
Website: http://www.aphon.org
Specialty: Hematology/Oncology
Basic Certification: Certified Pediatric Hematology/ Oncology Nurse (CPHON)
Advanced Certification: None

Certifying Organization: Oncology Nursing Certification Corporation (ONCC)

ASSOCIATION OF PERIOPERATIVE REGISTERED NURSES (AORN)

2170 South Parker Road, Suite 400
Denver, CO 80231
Phone: 800–755-2676
E-mail: custsvc@aorn.org
Website: http://www.aorn.org and http://www.cc-institute.org
Specialty: Perioperative
Basic Certification: Certification in Perioperative Nursing (CNOR); Certified Registered Nurse First Assistant (CRNFA)
Advanced Certification: Clinical Nurse Specialist Perioperative Certification (CNS-CP)
Certifying Organization: Competency & Credentialing Institute (CCI)

ASSOCIATION OF REHABILITATION NURSES (ARN)

8735 W. Higgins Road, Suite 300
Chicago, IL 60631–2738
Phone: 800–229-7530
E-mail: info@rehabnurse.org
Website: http://www.rehabnurse.org
Specialty: Rehabilitation
Basic Certification: Certified Rehabilitation Registered Nurse (CRRN)
Advanced Certification: Certified Rehabilitation Registered Nurse-Advanced (CRRN-A)
Certifying Organization: Rehabilitation Nursing Certification Board (RNCB)

ASSOCIATION OF WOMEN'S HEALTH, OBSTETRIC AND NEONATAL NURSES (AWHONN)

2000 L Street, NW, Suite 740
Washington, DC 20036
Phone: 800–673-8499
E-mail: customerservice@awhonn.org
Website: http://www.awhonn.org
Specialty: Women's health
Basic Certification: None
Advanced Certification: None
Certifying Organization: N/A

CASE MANAGEMENT SOCIETY OF AMERICA (CMSA)

6301 Ranch Drive
Little Rock, AR 72223
Phone: 501–225-2229
E-mail: cmsa@cmsa.org
Website: http://cmsa.org
Specialty: Case management

Basic Certification: Accredited Case Manager (ACM); Certified Case Manager (CCM); Certified Disability Management Specialist (CDMS); Case Management Administrator Certification (CMAC); Care Manager Certified (CMC); Certified Managed Care Nurse (CMCN); Certified Nurse Case Manager (RN-C); Certified Orthotist (CO); Certified Occupational Health Nurse (COHN); Certified Prosthetist (CP); Certified Prosthetist-Orthotist (CPO); Certified Professional in Disability Management (CPDM); Certified Professional in Healthcare Quality (CPHQ); Certified Professional in Utilization Management (CPUM); Certified Professional in Utilization Review (CPUR); Certified Rehabilitation Counselor (CRC); Certified Rehabilitation Registered Nurse (CRRN); Certified Social Work Case Manager (CSWCM); Health Care Quality and Management (HCQM); Registered Nurse Case Manager (RN-BC)

Advanced Certification: Continuity of Care Certification-Advanced (A-CCC); Certified Advanced Social Work Case Manager (CASWCM); Certified Rehabilitation Registered Nurse-Advanced (CRRN-A)

Certifying Organization: Specific to particular certification; see http://cmsa.org/Individual/Education/AccreditationCertification/tabid/209/Default.aspx

DERMATOLOGY NURSES ASSOCIATION (DNA)

15000 Commerce Parkway, Suite C
Mt. Laurel, NJ 08054
Phone: 800–454-4362
E-mail: DNA@dnanurse.org
Website: http://www.dnanurse.org
Specialty: Dermatology
BaSic Certification: Dermatology Nurse Certified (DNC)
Advanced Certification: Dermatology Certified Nurse Practitioner (DCNP)
Certifying Organization: American Board of Nursing Specialties (ABNS)

DEVELOPMENTAL DISABILITIES NURSES ASSOCIATION (DDNA)

P.O. Box 536489
Orlando, FL 32853–6489
Phone: 800–888-6733
E-mail: None
Website: http://www.ddna.org
Specialty: Developmental disabilities
Basic Certification: Registered Nurse Certification in Developmental Disability Nursing (CDDN); Developmental Disabilities Certified (DDC)
Advanced Certification: None

Certifying Organization: DDNA Certification Committee

EMERGENCY NURSES ASSOCIATION (ENA)

915 Lee Street
Des Plaines, IL 60016–6569
Phone: 847–460-4123
E-mail: education@ena.org
Website: http://www.ena.org
Specialty: Emergency
Basic Certification: Certified Emergency Nurse (CEN); Certified Flight Registered Nurse (CFRN); Certified Pediatric Emergency Nurse (CPEN); Certified Transport Registered Nurse (CTRN)
Advanced Certification: None
Certifying Organization: American Board of Nursing Specialties (ABNS)

ENDOCRINE NURSES SOCIETY (ENS)

P.O. Box 211068
Milwaukee, WI 53211
Phone: 414–421-3679
E-mail: endo.nurses@sbcglobal.net
Website: http://www.endo-nurses.org
Specialty: Endocrine
Basic Certification: None
Advanced Certification: None
Certifying Organization: N/A

HOSPICE AND PALLIATIVE NURSES ASSOCIATION (HPNA)

One Penn Center West, Suite 229
Pittsburgh, PA 15276–0100
Phone: 412–787-9301
E-mail: hpna@hpna.org
Website: http://www.hpna.org
Specialty: Palliative care
Basic Certification: Certified Hospice and Palliative Nurse (CHPN); Certified Hospice and Palliative Licensed Nurse (CHPLN); Certified Hospice and Palliative Pediatric Nurse (CHPPN); Certified Hospice and Palliative Care Administrator (CHPCA)
Advanced Certification: Advanced Certified Hospice and Palliative Nurse (ACHPN)
Certifying Organization: National Board for Certification of Hospice and Palliative Nurses (NBCHPN)

INFUSION NURSES SOCIETY

315 Norwood Park South
Norwood, MA 02062
Phone: 781–440-9408
E-mail: ins@ins1.org

Website: http://www.ins1.org
Specialty: General
Basic Certification: Certified Registered Nurse
  Infusion (CRNI)
Advanced Certification: None
Certifying Organization: Infusion Nurses
  Certification Corporation (INCC)

NATIONAL ASSOCIATION OF ORTHOPEDIC NURSES (NAON)

330 N. Wabash Avenue, Suite 2000
Chicago, IL 60611
Phone: 800–289-NAON (6266)
E-mail: naon@orthonurse.org
Website: http://www.orthonurse.org
Specialty: Orthopedics
Basic Certification: Orthopedic Nurse Certified
  (ONC)
Advanced Certification: Orthopedic Clinical Nurse
  Specialist-Certified (OCNS-C); Orthopedic Nurse
  Practitioner-Certified (ONP-C)
Certifying Organization: Orthopedic Nurses
  Certification Board (ONCB)

NATIONAL GERONTOLOGICAL NURSING ASSOCIATION (NGNA)

3493 Lansdowne Drive, Suite 2
Lexington, KY 40517
Phone: 800–723-0560
E-mail: info@ngna.org
Website: http://www.ngna.org
Specialty: Gerontology
Basic Certification: See ANCC
Advanced Certification: See ANCC
Certifying Organization: American Nurses
  Credentialing Center (ANCC)

NATIONAL LEAGUE FOR NURSING (NLN)

61 Broadway, 33rd Floor
New York, NY 10006
Phone: 212–812-0300
E-mail: generalinfo@nln.org
Website: http://www.nln.org
Specialty: General
Basic Certification: None
Advanced Certification: Certified Nurse Educator
  (CNE)
Certifying Organization: NLN's Certification
  Governance Committee
**Formerly National Nursing Staff Development
  Organization (NNSDO) is Association for
  Nursing Professional Development (ANPD); see
  ANPD listing**

ONCOLOGY NURSING SOCIETY (ONS)

125 Enterprise Drive
Pittsburgh, PA 15275
Phone: 866–257-4ONS (4667)
E-mail: customer.service@ons.org
Website: http://www.ons.org
Specialty: Oncology
Basic Certification: Oncology Certified Nurse
  (OCN); Certified Pediatric Hematology Oncology
  Nurse (CPHON); Certified Breast Care Nurse
  (CBCN)
Advanced Certification: Advanced Oncology
  Certified Nurse Practitioner (AOCNP); Advanced
  Oncology Certified Clinical Nurse Specialist
  (AOCNS)
Certifying Organization: Oncology Nursing
  Certification Organization (ONCC)

SOCIETY OF OTORHINOLARYNGOLOGY AND HEAD-NECK NURSES (SOHN)

207 Downing Street
New Smyrna Beach, FL 32168
Phone: 386–428-1695
E-mail: info@sohnnurse.com
Website: http://www.sohnnurse.com
Specialty: Ear, nose, throat
Basic Certification: Certification in
  Otorhinolaryngology and Head-Neck Nursing
  (CORLN)
Advanced Certification: None
Certifying Organization: National Certifying Board
  of Otorhinolaryngology and Head-Neck Nurses
  (NCBOHN)

SOCIETY OF PEDIATRIC NURSES (SPN)

7044 S. 13th Street
Oak Creek, WI 53154
Phone: 414–908-4950
E-mail: s.lorenz@pedsnurses.org
Website: http://www.pedsnurses.org
Specialty: Pediatrics
Basic Certification: See ANCC
Advanced Certification: See ANCC
Certifying Organization: American Nurses
  Credentialing Center (ANCC)

SOCIETY OF UROLOGIC NURSES AND ASSOCIATES (SUNA)

East Holly Avenue, Box 56
Pitman, NJ 08071–0056
Phone: 888–827-7862
E-mail: suna@ajj.com
Website: http://www.suna.org
Specialty: Genitourinary

Basic Certification: Certified Urologic Registered Nurse (CURN); Certified Urologic Associate (CUA)

Advanced Certification: Certified Urologic Nurse Practitioner (CUNP); Certified Urologic Clinical Nurse Specialist (CUCNS); Certified Urologic Physician's Assistant (CUPA)

Certifying Organization: Certification Board for Urologic Nurses and Associates (CBUNA)

SOCIETY FOR VASCULAR NURSING (SVN)

100 Cummings Center Suite, 124 A
Beverly, MA 01915
Phone: 888–536-4SVN (4786)
E-mail: none
Website: http://www.svnnet.org
Specialty: Vascular
Basic Certification: See ANCC
Advanced Certification: See ANCC
Certifying Organization: American Nurses Credentialing Center (ANCC)

WOUND, OSTOMY AND CONTINENCE NURSES SOCIETY (WOCN)

15000 Commerce Parkway, Suite C
Mt. Laurel, NJ 08054
Phone: 888–224-WOCN (9626)
E-mail: info@wocncb.org
Website: http://www.wocn.org and
http://www.wocncb.org/ (Certification Board)
Specialty: General

Basic Certification: Certified Wound, Ostomy and Continence Nurse (CWOCN); Certified Wound Ostomy Nurse (CWON); Certified Wound Care Nurse (CWCN); Certified Continence Care Nurse (CCCN); Certified Ostomy Care Nurse (COCN); Certified Foot Care Nurse (CFCN)

Advanced Certification: Advanced Practice Wound, Ostomy, and Continence Nurse (CWOCN-AP); Advanced Practice Certified Wound Ostomy Nurse (CWON-AP); Advanced Practice Certified Wound Care Nurse (CWCN-AP); Advanced Practice Certified Continence Care Nurse (CCCN-AP); Advanced Practice Certified Ostomy Care Nurse (COCN-AP)

Certifying Organization: Wound, Ostomy, and Continence Nursing Certification Board (WOCNCB)

Index